Foundations of Pediatric Audiology

Fred H. Bess

Judith S. Gravel

Foundations of Pediatric Audiology

Identification and Assessment

Fred H. Bess
Judith S. Gravel

PLURAL
PUBLISHING
INC.

5521 Ruffin Road
San Diego, CA 92123

e-mail: info@pluralpublishing.com
Web site: http://www.pluralpublishing.com

49 Bath Street
Abingdon, Oxfordshire OX14 1EA
United Kingdom

Typeset in 10/12 Times New Roman by SoCal Graphics
Printed in the United States of America by McNaughton and Gunn

ISBN-13: 978-1-59756-108-2
ISBN-10: 1-59756-108-8

Library of Congress Cataloging-in-Publication Data

Foundations of pediatric audiology / [edited by] Fred H. Bess, Judith
    S. Gravel.
        p. ; cm.
    Includes bibliographical references and index.
    ISBN-13: 978-1-59756-108-2 (softcover)
    ISBN-10: 1-59756-108-8 (softcover)
    1. Hearing disorders in children.   2. Deaf children.   I. Bess, Fred
H.   II. Gravel, Judith.
    [DNLM: 1. Hearing Loss—Collected Works.   2. Child.   3. Evoked
Potentials, Auditory, Brain Stem—physiology—Collected Works.
4. Hearing Tests—methods—Collected Works. 5. Infant.   WV 271
F771 2006]
    RF291.5.C45F682 2006
    618.92'09789—dc22
                                                2006023288

CONTENTS

Speech Audiometry

SECTION III. ELECTROPHYSIOLOGIC/PHYSIOLOGIC METHODOLOGY

Aural Acoustic Immittance

Auditory Evoked Potential

Evoked Otoacoustic Emissions

PREFACE

The papers included in this compilation of readings entitled *Foundations of Pediatric Audiology* were selected because, in our view, they represent the basis for the practice of pediatric audiology. Many hours of discussion and deliberation were required to select the articles included in the Table of Contents. The original pool of articles was at least twice the number ultimately used. Space limitations necessitated that we restrict the number of articles included in each section. Based on our collective experiences with teaching pediatric audiology, we deemed these final selections critical to a student's understanding of the fundamental principles of our field. In our opinion, these studies represent the foundation of research and opinion that subserves the clinical screening and evaluation procedures utilized daily in the practice of pediatric audiology.

Several criterion guided our selection of articles for this volume. We considered only papers that appeared in refereed journals. In addition to the inclusion of many classic papers, readers will note that several more recent articles appear in the book. This information, which builds on the foundation of our profession, has been brought about mostly by rapid changes in technology and changes in the demographics of young children with hearing impairment. Pediatric audiology practice is a dynamic process that must constantly be modified as new evidence emerges.

A second criterion was that the selected articles specifically address infants and children. Hence, we did not include many seminal papers within particular categories. Presumably, these basics are required reading in introductory-level and advanced courses in audiology. For example, in the section on evoked otoacoustic emissions (EOAEs), we did not include Kemp's 1978 classic description of cochlear emissions (D.T. Kemp, 1978, *JASA* 64:1386-1391). Rather, we selected articles for the section that examined the specific description and measurement of EOAEs in infants and children, as well as their application in clinical practice. Finally, we acknowledge that this compilation of studies also reflects our individual biases following more than fifty combined years of experience in pediatric audiology teaching and practice.

This book of readings has been divided into five sections that broadly address the identification and assessment of children with hearing loss. Following each section we have listed additional readings for those who desire to explore any topic in greater depth. We intentionally have omitted the areas of aural habilitation and educational audiology, including papers addressing traditional amplification, assistive device technology (such as FM personal and classroom systems), and cochlear implants. Once again, this decision was based on space limitations.

Section I contains studies that examine the development of audition in infants—an area frequently overlooked in pediatric audiology training. Much of the relevant work often appears in journals outside our discipline, primarily those that focus on research in the area of developmental psychology. An appreciation of these fundamental aspects of auditory behavior is basic to our understanding of normal auditory development in infants and to our understanding of the profound impact that an auditory impairment in early life may have on the young child.

Section II begins with the classic paper of Jerger and Hayes on the importance of the test-battery approach to pediatric audiologic practice. As we incorporate new test techniques and technology into clinical practice (as in Sections II and III) the importance of the cross-check principle cannot be overemphasized. Section II then presents the background literature for our current practice of behavioral audiologic assessment and speech audiometry. Although our field has benefited immeasurably from new techniques in auditory electrophysiology, behavioral audiometry continues to occupy an integral role in pediatric practice. Operant audiometry has become the practice standard for the audiologic assessment of the infant and young child. Through this behavioral procedure, we may assess and monitor hearing sensitivity reliably in the young child, making appropriate referrals for medical intervention and pursuing further auditory remediation when necessary. Results obtained through speech audiometry afford us valuable insight into the functional consequences of hearing loss in the young child. Subsequently, this knowledge also serves as the foundation for the formulation of habilitative strategies.

Section III presents studies in aural acoustic immittance, auditory evoked potentials, and evoked otoacoustic emissions. Heretofore, the auditory evaluation of difficult-to-test populations has presented enormous challenges for the pediatric audiologist. Now acoustic immittance assessment for evaluating middle ear function and acoustic reflex function is considered part of the routine audiometric test battery. The Auditory Brainstem Response (ABR) has afforded clinicians a valid and reliable test method for assessing auditory system integrity in the youngest of babies as well as in the most compromised of children. The rapid development of the auditory steady-state response (ASSR) procedure suggests new techniques will continue to improve efficiency and frequency-specificity of electrophysiologic assessment procedures. Although clearly a valuable tool, the clinical utility of evoked otoacoustic emissions assessment has yet to be fully delineated. All of these measures have contributed so substantially to the practice of pediatric audiology that it is difficult to remember clinical work without them.

Section IV presents literature that provides background in newborn hearing screening protocols, the development of current auditory screening techniques, and a summary of the multisite clinical trial that examined performance characteristics of various screening tests, in a report from one of the larger statewide programs currently undertaking universal newborn screening. The latter half of the screening section presents a series of exchanges published in the literature, wherein the efficacy of universal newborn hearing screening (UNHS) is debated. We have included these diverse opinions regarding the issue of universal newborn hearing screening because we believe that students should be well informed on this topic. It is important that they read the full extent of opinion surrounding this significant and controversial public health issue. Undoubtedly, UNHS and the follow-up of infants with early identified hearing loss will present ever increasing challenges for our field for years to come.

Finally, Section V presents a series of papers on the effects of hearing loss in special populations of children, those often overlooked due to the minimal nature of their auditory impairments. Specifically, the section addresses children with unilateral sensorineural hearing loss, recurrent otitis media, and minimal sensorineural hearing impairment.

After an overview of each section, we have included references and additional readings. Readers are encouraged to review these materials which will build further on the foundation of knowledge compiled in this volume.

Clearly, there has been an explosion of knowledge and technology in all areas of pediatric audiology. The student interested in this discipline must appreciate the breadth of our research history as well as the current advancements in our field. Our rich and varied literature subserves the fundamentals of the profession. Research is the foundation for evidence-based, clinical decision-making in day-to-day pediatric audiology practice.

We thank Mary Sue Fino-Szumski and Georgia M. Walker for all of their efforts in the development of this book. In addition, we thank Shelia Lewis whose work brought this book to publication.

Fred H. Bess and Judith S. Gravel

I. Development of Auditory Function

Section I presents selected articles in developmental psychoacoustics, a literature that is often overlooked in the training of pediatric audiologists. Perhaps this is because developmental psychoacoustics and pediatric audiology are often considered very different fields: One involves basic research in normal auditory development, the other, direct clinical service to infants and children with hearing disabilities. Moreover, developmental psychologists study audition in stringently selected cohorts of, for example, typically developing babies, whereas pediatric audiologists assess hearing in the individual infant (Carney, 1992).

Knowledge of normal auditory abilities should serve as a framework for the comprehensive and developmentally appropriate audiologic assessment of young infants as well as in the strategic planning of their aural habilitation. Very young infants with normal hearing demonstrate an impressive auditory repertoire that includes binaural processing, frequency and temporal resolution, and speech sound discrimination. Study of the ontogeny of normal audition provides the pediatric audiologist with a greater appreciation of the potentially profound impact that congenital and acquired hearing impairments may have on child development. Furthermore, many of the behavioral paradigms used by developmental psychoacousticians in their laboratories have been adapted for use in the pediatric audiologic test armamentarium. Researchers will continue to develop and refine their techniques in order to improve their reliability, efficiency, and effectiveness as tools for the study of the development of audition in infants and young children. Thus, clinicians should also appreciate this literature as a source of behavioral procedures that may be modified for practical application in the clinical setting.

The studies included in Section I deal specifically with the development of audition in infants. The Additional Readings listed at the conclusion of this section provide references to other excellent developmental psychoacoustic studies of neonates, infants, and children for the interested reader. In the series of articles chosen for this section, we begin with a study by Nozza and Wilson who examined threshold sensitivity at 1000 and 4000 Hz in quiet and noise in infants 6- and 12-months-of-age and in adults. As expected, infants of both ages had absolute thresholds that were poorer than adult listeners. Masked threshold data, however, suggested that frequency selectivity of infants was proportional to adults. Threshold sensitivity data in quiet suggested that differences in infants' responses between the 1000 Hz and 4000 Hz signals varied in a manner different from that observed in adult listeners. Nozza and Wilson discuss age effects and the potential impact of developmental factors on estimates of auditory function. Next, Olsho and colleagues examined hearing sensitivity in 3-, 6-, and 12-month-old infants. Using a behavioral observer-based psychophysical procedure (OBP), these researchers obtained pure-tone thresholds from babies at 250 through 8000 Hz. Olsho and colleagues concluded that thresholds of 6- and 12-month-old infants are about 10 to 15 dB less sensitive than those of adults; 3-month-old infants' thresholds are poorer than those of adults by 15 to 30 dB. Olsho and coworkers provide a discussion of the sensory and nonsensory factors that affect threshold acquisition

Muir, Clifton, and Clarkson studied the development of spatial hearing by examining auditory localization abilities in infants from birth to 7 months of age. They found that newborns turned their heads toward the source of a sound, but that 1- and 2-month-old infants did not orient toward sounds. By 3 months of age, orienting toward sounds was again demonstrated. According to these authors, this pattern represents a developmental change in sound localization, from reflexive (subcortical) activity to a more mature, purposeful (cortical) auditory-motor response. Later, we shall see that the development of mature visual searching for the source of a sound is requisite behavior for conditioned audiometry techniques (see Section II—Behavioral Methodology; Audiometric Assessment).

Schneider, Morrongiello, and Trehub further examined the important question of whether frequency resolution changes with development. By studying the size of the critical band (auditory filter width) in infants, children, and adults, Schneider and coworkers concluded that critical bandwidths do not change with age. Although absolute unmasked and masked thresholds of their youngest subjects were higher than those of the older children and adults, the width of the auditory filter did not appear to change substantially with development.

Next, Werner and associates studied auditory temporal acuity in three groups of infants, one year of age and younger (3- and 6-month-old babies), using a gap-detection paradigm. They found that temporal resolution (gap detection) was poorer in babies than in adults but that both groups resolved temporal cues similarly as a function of frequency. Werner and colleagues concluded that although absolute abilities differ, similar mechanisms appear to be governing temporal resolution throughout the course of development. The classic study of Eilers, Wilson, and Moore used a technique known as visually reinforced infant speech discrimination (VRISD), a variant of the operant head-turn procedure.Though methodologic issues were raised by Nozza (1987), the Eilers paper demonstrated that speech discrimination could be reliably examined in infants.

Finally, Kuhl and colleagues studied the phonetic perception of infants at 6 months of age. Babies from the United States and Sweden were tested using variants of native and non-native vowel prototypes. Babies from both countries demonstrated better discrimination of vowel prototype variants derived from their native language versus those variants of the foreign language. Thus, these authors demonstrated that linguistic experiences before the age of 6 months have already begun to shape the infant's auditory perceptual set.

As the most qualified professional to examine hearing in the young child, the pediatric audiologist should have a thorough appreciation of the relationship between the maturation of auditory function and normal child development. Moreover, incorporating the principles and techniques used by developmental psychologists for the objective behavioral study of infant audition can strengthen the behavioral test battery clinicians use daily for the assessment of hearing in young children. Clearly, the rich literature in developmental psychoacoustics is important to the foundation of knowledge that supports the practice of pediatric audiology today.

REFERENCES

Carney, A.E. 1992. Bridging the gap between developmental psychoacoustics and pediatric audiology. In L.A. Werner and E.W. Rubel (Eds.), *Developmental psychoacoustics* (pp. 333-349). Washington, D.C.: American Psychological Association.

Nozza, R.J. 1987. Infant speech-sound discrimination testing: Effects of stimulus intensity and procedural model on measures of performance. *Journal of the Acoustical Society of America* 81:1928-1939.

Additional Readings

Allen, P., Wightman, F., Kistler, D., and Dolan, T. 1989. Frequency resolution in children. *Journal of Speech and Hearing Research* 32:317-322.

Ashmead, D.H., Davis, D.L., Whalen, T., and Odom, R.D. 1991. Sound localization and sensitivity to interaural time differences in human infants. *Child Development* 62:1211-1226.

Clifton, R., Morrongiello, B., and Dowd, J. 1984. A developmental look at an auditory illusion: The precedence effect. *Developmental Psychobiology* 17:519-536.

Field, J., Muir, D., Pilon, R., Sinclair, M., and Dodwell, P. 1980. Infants' orientation to lateral sounds from birth to three months. *Child Development* 51:295-298.

Morrongiello, B.A., Fenwick, K.D., and Chance, G. 1990. Sound localization acuity in very young infants: An observer-based testing procedure. *Developmental Psychology* 26:75-84.

Muir, D., and Field, J. 1979. Newborn infants orient to sounds. *Child Development* 50:431-436.

Olsho, L.W., Koch, E.G., Halpin, C.F., and Carter, E. 1987. An observer-based psychoacoustic procedure for use with young infants. *Developmental Psychology* 23:627-640.

Werner, L.A. 1992. Interpreting developmental psychoacoustics. In L.A. Werner and E.W. Rubel (Eds.), *Developmental psychoacoustics* (pp. 47-88). Washington, D.C.: American Psychological Association.

Werner, L.A., and Gillenwater, J.M. 1990. Pure-tone sensitivity of 2- to 5-week old infants. *Infant Behavior and Development* 13:355-375.

Wightman, F., Allen, P., Dolan, T., Kistler, D., and Jamieson, D. 1989. Temporal resolution in children. *Child Development* 60:611-624.

Masked and Unmasked Pure-Tone Thresholds of Infants and Adults: Development of Auditory Frequency Selectivity and Sensitivity

Robert J. Nozza* and Wesley R. Wilson

University of Washington, Seattle

Detection thresholds for pure tones (1000 Hz and 4000 Hz) in noise and in quiet were estimated for infants at 6 months and 12 months of age and for adults. A visually reinforced head-turn procedure under control of a PDP - 11/03 minicomputer was used. An adaptive protocol with a 5-dB step size was employed for the threshold estimates. Infant thresholds were poorer than adult thresholds in each condition. In noise, infant-adult differences were 8 dB (6-month-old infants) and 6 dB (12-month-old infants) at each frequency. In quiet, infant-adult differences were 14 dB (6-month-old infants) and 12 dB (12-month-old infants) at 1000 Hz but were only 7 dB (6-month-old infants) and 5 dB (12-month- old infants) at 4000 Hz. The masking data suggest that infants are at only a slight disadvantage in detecting a target in a background of noise and are consistent with a frequency selectivity mechanism that is proportional to that of adults. The detection-in-quiet data, with greater correspondence among the groups at 4000 Hz than at 1000 Hz, support the notion that hearing sensitivity varies with frequency in a different way in infants than in adults. Data on task performance reveal significant age effects, and the possibility that such effects have biased the observed differences in the estimates of sensory function among the groups is considered.

Recent studies of infant auditory detection have added greatly to our understanding of both auditory development and the behavioral methods used in its assessment. Detection-in-quiet data from various studies are equivocal, however, on whether infant hearing thresholds vary with frequency in a way different from adult hearing thresholds and whether infant hearing thresholds change between 6 and 12 months of age (Schneider, Trehub, & Bull, 1980; Sinnott, Pisoni, & Aslin, 1983; Trehub, Schneider, & Endman, 1980; Wilson & Moore, 1978; Wilson, Moore, & Thompson, 1976). Detection-in-noise data suggest that infants are less able to detect a signal in noise than are adults (Bull, Schneider, & Trehub, 1981; Trehub, Bull, & Schneider, 1981).

In each of those studies, a behavioral procedure that includes a head-turn response followed by visual reinforcement was used. While to some extent the behavioral techniques are similar among the various studies, substantial differences in the stimuli, the response, the threshold-estimating procedure, and the subject-screening criteria leave open the question of procedural differences which may account for the discrepancies in the data.

HEAD-TURN RESPONSE AND AUDITORY DETECTION

The head turn is a specific and easily observable behavior of infants. Infants as young as 5fi months can be conditioned to make a head turn in response to an auditory stimulus when attractive visual stimuli are provided as reinforcement (Moore, Thompson, & Thompson, 1975; Moore, Wilson, & Thompson, 1977). The visually reinforced head-turn response is robust and can be maintained for many trials over repeated sessions.

The head-turn response has been used in two ways in assessing auditory function. It was originally developed as a conditioned orientation reflex (COR) response and, as such, requires that signals be presented from one of two loudspeakers located to either side of the infant (Suzuki & Ogiba, 1961). A head turn toward the speaker from which the sound comes is considered a correct response and is rewarded by activation of a visual stimulus located in the direction of the speaker. A head turn toward the opposite speaker, or no identifiable head turn, is considered incorrect and no reinforcement is provided. It is a turn-right or turn-left response that is contingent on localizing the signal.

Subsequent to the development of the COR procedure, a unilateral head-turn procedure emerged (Moore et al., 1975, 1977). It requires that the infant make a head turn to only one side for visual reinforcement independent of the locus of the stimulus. This procedure is similar to a go/no-go discrimination procedure. Wilson et al. (1976), Wilson and Moore (1978), Goldman (1979), and Sinnott et al. (1983) have used the unilateral head-turn task with an adaptive (staircase) procedure (Dixon & Mood, 1948) for estimating thresholds of infants between 6 and 12 months old using frequency-specific stimuli (warbled tones and

Reprinted by permission of authors and American Speech-Language-Hearing Association. Copyright 1984. *Journal of Speech and Hearing Research,* 27, pp. 613-622.

*Current affiliation: Department of Otolaryngology, Division of Audiology, Children's Hospital of Pittsburgh.

pure tones). Wilson and Moore (1978) have also introduced the use of earphones into this infant assessment protocol.

Trehub et al. (1980) used a different modification of the COR (localization) head-turn procedure to study infant auditory sensitivity. They have removed the condition of *no response* as a possible alternative by making the trial intervals unlimited in duration and forcing a choice, right or left, to be made. This is then a two-alternative, forced-choice (2AFC) procedure. Trehub et al. (1980) used this procedure in conjunction with a method of constant stimuli and octave bands of noise to develop group psychometric functions for infants at ages 6, 12, 18, and 24 months.

RECENT DATA ON INFANT HEARING THRESHOLDS

Differences in hearing thresholds between infants and adults, as determined by behavioral procedures, are much smaller than previously believed, according to recent studies (Goldman, 1979; Schneider et al., 1980; Sinnott et al., 1983; Trehub et al., 1980; Wilson & Moore, 1978; Wilson et al., 1976). Considering the potential effects on the data of poor infant attention abilities and lack of motivation, the findings suggest that the head-turn procedure has largely overcome problems related to behavioral assessment of hearing in infants. However, there are unanswered questions regarding the degree to which infant and adult thresholds are similar. Infant-adult differences range from 5 to 30 dB across studies for stimuli in the 200- to 4000-Hz range. Also, there are equivocal data regarding the differences between infant and adult thresholds as a function of frequency, as well as regarding threshold changes during the first year of life (Sinnott et al., 1983; Trehub et al., 1980; Wilson & Moore, 1978). Trehub et al. (1980) reported larger differences in the low frequencies than in the high frequencies between infants and adults and found significant differences between 6-month-old and 12-month-old infants. Wilson and Moore (1978) and Wilson et al. (1976) found no significant differences either in shape of the threshold curves with age or in threshold among the two infant groups. Their protocol, however, used a 10-dB step size developed primarily for clinical use and was not designed to find subtle differences in the shape of the hearing threshold curve between groups.

A question that arises when comparing data from the two (2AFC and go/no-go) procedures (Aslin, Pisoni, & Jusczyk, 1983) relates to the localization head-turn task which may confound the development of sensitivity with the development of localization. Since localization is a function of a different process for signals of high frequency than for signals of low frequency, differences in rate of development of those processes may bias responses for some signals relative to others.

A problem that exists in all behavioral research relates to the differences between infants and adults in attention, memory, motivation, and cognition. While a task can be made similar for groups in spite of large differences in developmental stage, some differences in behavior may never be eliminated. Trehub et al. (1980) have argued that their localization procedure minimizes concerns over response biases because it is a 2AFC procedure. Added to that is their finding that infant and adult behavioral thresholds are almost the same at very high test frequencies-—10000 and 19000 Hz (Schneider et al., 1980). If there were a response bias on the part of the infants in the threshold-test procedure, they argued, then the infants could not produce thresholds at levels similar to the adult threshold levels at any frequency. Implicit in their argument is the assumption that infants have identical sensory capability to adults at those test frequencies and that equal behavioral thresholds in the 2AFC procedure should be interpreted to mean equal sensory capability. This logic ignores the possibility that infant sensory capability is better than that of adults in the high frequencies and that the similarity in behaviorally obtained thresholds still results from a procedural or response bias. There is no evidence that infants are behaving in a similar way to adults in all aspects of the behavioral task. Similarity of the behavioral thresholds of the two groups at one or two test frequencies does not establish that the two groups have similar sensory capability and similar, criterion-free, unbiased response strategies.

Another potential for bias in the existing infant threshold data comes from the failure to use adequate screening criteria for subject selection. Studies that have produced behavioral threshold data on infants have not been aggressive at ruling out the possibility that mild middle-ear pathology influences the data. In adults, high negative pressure and/or middle-ear effusion can cause some shift in hearing threshold. Because the incidence of middle-ear pathology is greatest among infants during the first year of life and its effects on hearing in that group is unknown, it is important that researchers in the area of auditory development take care to screen out subjects with questionable middle-ear status.

MASKING AND FREQUENCY SELECTIVITY

While detection of a signal in quiet is important, there is also a need to understand detection of a signal in noise. The effect that a noise has on detectability of a signal is critical to our understanding of how the auditory system analyzes auditory input. Since the auditory system behaves as a filter (cf. Evans, 1974), the extent to which a noise influences our ability to detect a signal is a function of the characteristics of the filter. The variation of masked thresholds with frequency reflects the changes in auditory filter bandwidth as a function of frequency.

In adults, masked threshold (using broadband maskers) increases with increasing signal frequency in a manner proportional to estimates of frequency difference limen (DL) and direct estimates of auditory-filter bandwidth (e.g., the critical band). There are no data regarding the frequency selectivity of the developing human auditory system that have been acquired with a strict behavioral protocol excepting the work of Olsho, Schoon, Sakai, Turpin, and Sperduto (1982) on frequency DL. The masking data that do exist (Bull et al., 1981; Trehub et al., 1981) reveal substantial differences between infants and adults. These data were collected without the intention of estimating frequency selectivity and do not allow interpretation for that purpose. Differences of 16-25 dB between infant and adult masked thresholds (Bull et al., 1981) suggest that infants are operating at a disadvantage in our noisy world and may suggest poor frequency selectivity.

Critical ratio. Fletcher (1940) attempted to estimate auditory filter bandwidth indirectly based on detection-in-noise data. Under the assumption that the energy in that portion of the masker (noise) allowed to pass through the auditory filter is equivalent to the energy in the signal at masked threshold (S), the estimate of bandwidth is equal to the ratio S/N_0 (N_0 = spectrum level of noise masker) (Hawkins & Stevens, 1950; Reed & Bilger, 1973). This indirect estimate of filter bandwidth is known as the critical ratio (Zwicker, Flottorp, & Stevens, 1957). Critical ratios are proportional to direct estimates of critical bandwidth but do not correspond exactly.

PURPOSE

This research was designed to use the unidirectional head-turn response procedure with a rigid psychophysical protocol to estimate detection thresholds in infants and adults in quiet and in noise. The detection-in-noise data were collected to allow for interpretation as critical ratios so that some information on frequency selectivity could be obtained. Finally, data on subject task performance were analyzed to determine if suggested developmental trends could be attributed to developmental differences in ability to respond in the test situation rather than in ability to hear.

METHODS

SUBJECTS

Subjects were divided into three groups: infants, 6.5 months (mean age = 196.5 days); infants, 12.5 months (mean age = 378 days); and adults, 18-22 years old. Of the 110 subjects who participated altogether, 60 subjects, 20 in

each age group, completed the study. Subjects were paid for participating.

Infants. Infant subjects were drawn randomly from a subject pool maintained by infant-perception research laboratories at the University of Washington. Subjects were screened initially through a telephone interview with a parent. Infants with a history of neonatal health problems, recent ear disease (within the last 30 days), recent cold (within the last 2 weeks), family history of hearing impairment, or high-risk birth (e.g., prematurity, low birth weight, etc.) were not included. Infants were given a tympanometric evaluation on each visit and any with middle-ear pressure in excess of negative 100 mm H_2O in the test ear were screened out. Tympanometry followed data collection on each visit because some infants react negatively to the procedure, making it more difficult to complete the behavioral test procedure.

Adults. The adult subjects were also screened for recent ear disease, history of hearing impairment, noise exposure history (recent or chronic), and tympanometric configuration using the same criteria as for infants. None had experience as a subject in auditory research.

INSTRUMENTATION

Stimuli. The sinusoidal test signals (1000 and 4000 Hz) were generated by a Wavetek Model 182 function generator, passed through a digital attenuator (Charybdis) and introduced to the auxiliary input of the left channel of a Maico MA-24 two-channel audiometer. Subjects listened monaurally (left ear) over a TDH-49 earphone with Telephonics Model 51 earphone cushion (Michael & Bienvenue, 1980). The active earphone/cushion and an inactive or "dummy" earphone and cushion were mounted in a small metal headband sized for children, with sponge cushioning added where contact with the top of the infant's head is made. For detection-in-noise testing, a white-noise masker, produced by a noise generator in the right channel of the MA-24 audiometer, was present at the earphone throughout the session.

The stimulus was 500 ms in duration and was presented five times in a 4-s trial interval (500 ms on/300 ms off). The audio switch, digital attenuator, and experimental logic were controlled by a PDP 11/03 laboratory computer.

Calibration. Spectral analyses of the test signals and the white-noise masker were performed upon the acoustic output of the TDH-49 as input to a Bruel and Kjaer 2203 sound-level meter with artificial ear and 6-cc coupler. A 1-in. (.25-mm) pressure microphone (Type 4132) was used. The output of the sound-level meter was fed electronically to a Hewlett-Packard Spectrum Analyzer (3582A). The noise was analyzed in the steady state and had a uniform intensity per cycle (+ or −2 dB) from 20 to 6000 Hz. The intensity of the noise was 63.5 dB SPL and the noise spectrum level was 26 dB SPL in the area centered around each test signal—1000 and 4000 Hz.

Energy at the second harmonic of the test signals was more than 48 dB down when analysis was done on the gated signal at each frequency. The rise time of the audio switch was 40 ms and the fall time was 10 ms. Intensity levels of the pure-tone signals and the white-noise masker were checked each data-collection day. A frequency counter allowed constant monitoring of the signal frequency, which never varied more than 2 Hz from the nominal test frequency, during testing.

Test environment. Testing was done in a single-wall sound-treated room (Tracoustics) situated inside a second large single-wall sound-treated room (IAC) which serves as the control room. Noise levels inside the test room are-within the limits specified for earphone testing (ANSI S3.1-1977) at the test frequencies.

The test room has been described in detail elsewhere (Moore & Wilson, 1978). The room is equipped with a loudspeaker, a smoked-black plexiglass column housing two stacked mechanical toys, a small round table, and two chairs (see Figure 1 for details).

Reinforcers. Four different mechanical toys were used as visual reinforcers. Two were used during each session, one above the other in the plexiglass enclosure. A probability generator in the base of the enclosure randomly lighted and activated either the top or the bottom toy when signaled by the computer. There was no systematic variation in the particular toy used or in their relative position in the plexiglass column from session to session.

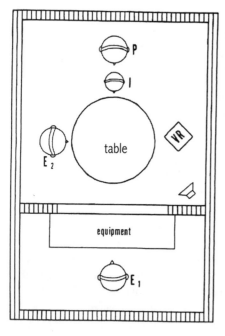

E₁	Experimenter 1
E₂	Experimenter 2
P	Parent
I	Infant
VR	Visual Reinforcer

E_1 Experimenter 1
E_2 Experimenter 2
P   Parent
I   Infant
VR Visual Reinforcer

PROCEDURES

Experimenters. Experimenter 1 (E_1) was the same for each subject in the study. Experimenter 2 (E_2) was one of two trained graduate-student assistants. Each E_2 had at least 20 hr of experience with the infant head-turn procedure prior to the beginning of this research.

Infant subjects. The procedure required the infant to detect an auditory stimulus and make an operant head-turn response for reinforcement by a visual stimulus (Moore et al., 1975). In the present study the infant was seated on the parent's lap in the sound-treated test room. The parent listened to music through headphones throughout the test sessions. E_2 was in communication with E_1 throughout each session through a talkback system. During the test sessions the infant was visually attracted toward midline with toys by E_2. An experimental trial was initiated from the control room by E_1 when the infant was in a quiet, ready state with eyes at midline.

To initiate the trial, E_1 pressed a key on the computer terminal and the computer selected the trial type (control trial, $p = .33$; or a stimulus trial, $p = .67$) on a quasirandom basis. Trial-type selection was restricted so that no trial type was chosen more than four times consecutively. Removal of trial-type selection from experimenter control reduced the potential for examiner bias in determining infant readiness. E_2 was alerted to the start of a trial by an audio signal sent through her headset. The trial signal remained on throughout the trial. E_2, unaware of the trial type, observed the infant during the trial interval and pressed a response button on a handswitch if a criterion head turn (45° rotation toward the reinforcement column) occurred. The button was interfaced with the computer such that a response during a stimulus interval automatically activated the toy reinforcer for 3 s. Such a response was recorded as a *hit*. If during a stimulus interval no response occurred, the trial was scored as a *miss*. On control trials, responses by E_2 were scored as *false alarms* and failures to respond were scored as *correct rejections*. Reinforcement was provided for *hits* on a 100% schedule.

Adult subjects. The procedure used with adult subjects was almost identical to that used with the infants. Rather than requiring a head-turn response, adults were given the response button and instructed to press it whenever they heard the test stimulus. Correct responses caused activation of the visual reinforcement apparatus. The toys were removed so only the lights went on when adults scored *hits*. This form of feedback was given the adults to make their tests as similar to those of the infants as possible. Control trials were included at the same rate and under the same conditions for adults as for infants.

TEST PROTOCOL

Training only was done during the first session. Following successful completion of training, each infant was assigned randomly to one of two groups—Group I for detection-in-noise (critical ratio) measures and Group II for detection-in-quiet (sensitivity) measures. Each subject was required to provide a threshold estimate at both frequencies (1000 and 4000 Hz). Test frequency order was counterbalanced to eliminate order effects with each frequency being tested on a separate visit. The test sessions averaged approximately 15 min. For any infant who failed to complete a session or failed to meet criteria for stimulus control on a session (see below), that test condition was repeated after the three originally scheduled visits. A second failure on any test condition caused exclusion of that subject. Infants were scheduled until 10 at each age had completed the required test at each frequency.

Adults were assigned to groups and test conditions in the same way as were the infants. No training was provided to the adults. Each was given instructions to listen for the signal and press the response button as soon as the signal was heard. Each also was told that a correct detection of the signal would cause the light in the reinforcer to turn on and that the feedback thus provided might be useful in making judgments regarding the task. Instructions were deliberately vague so that adult subjects would use their own criteria for responding. In that way the procedure would be as similar as possible for both infant and adult subjects.

Threshold estimate. Detection thresholds were estimated using an adaptive (staircase) procedure (Dixon & Mood, 1948; Levitt, 1971). The intensity of the initial stimulus presentation was at a level presumed to be above threshold for all subjects for the test condition. For detection-in-noise estimates, the starting signal intensity was 80 dB SPL and the white-noise masker was continuously present at the earphone at 63.5 dB SPL. For detection-in-quiet estimates the starting intensity was 50 dB SPL. Following each correct response to a signal (i.e., a *hit*), the intensity on the next stimulus trial was reduced 10 dB. A 10-dB step size was used only during the first descending run of the session. When a stimulus trial occurred without a response (first *miss*), the step size changed to 5 dB and the intensity for the next stimulus trial was increased. Each *hit* caused a 5-dB reduction in stimulus intensity and each *miss* caused a 5-dB increase. No intensity changes were made based on responses to control trials. Figure 2 provides an illustration of changes of intensity associated with a threshold determination for one subject.

Stimulus trials were presented until nine turnaround points (changes from *failure to respond* to *response*, or vice versa) were established. Threshold was defined as the mean of the intensity levels of the final eight turnaround points. Thresholds estimated in this way are approximations of the 50% point on the psychometric function (Dixon & Mood, 1948).

Stimulus control. Two measures of stimulus control, false-alarm rate and staircase symmetry, were employed to minimize the possibility that data obtained within a given session were unreliable.

1. *False-alarm rate.* False alarms—responses during control trials—at a rate greater than 25% during threshold estimation resulted in exclusion of the data.

2. *Staircase symmetry.* Adaptive procedures produce unbiased estimates when the subject is alert, motivated, and generally attentive to the task. Lapses in attention during a session produce a staircase, or response record, that is biased and usually appears asymmetrical. Since asymmetry in a staircase may indicate a biased estimate of a threshold value (Levitt, 1971), there must be a means of assessing consistency throughout the course of a session. This is critical with infant subjects, as Moore et al. (1975, 1977) and Trehub et al. (1980) have shown that infants respond less than 100% even when signals are well above threshold. Based on pilot data, it was determined that with a 5-dB step size most infants show a 10-15-dB variability in turnaround values determined by runs in a given direction (i.e., ascending or descending runs). Threshold sessions in which variability in turnaround values exceeded 15 dB resulted in exclusion of the data.

RESULTS

To provide the 40 infant subjects (20 at each age) necessary for data analysis, 88 infants—46 at 6 months, 42 at 12 months—were seen. Twenty-two adults were seen to provide the 20 adults necessary, with one failing to meet the tympanometry criterion and one failing to meet a stimulus-control criterion. Table 1 summarizes the reasons for exclusion of infant subjects.

DETECTION THRESHOLDS

Detection-in-noise (Group I). Mean detection-in-noise thresholds for 1000-Hz and 4000-Hz pure tones in white noise with a 26-dB spectrum level were, for 6-month-old infants, 50 dB ($SD = 4.4$) and 55 dB ($SD = 3.6$) SPL, respectively; for 12-month-old infants, 48 dB ($SD = 2.2$) and 53 dB ($SD = 1.9$) SPL, respectively; and for adults, 42 dB ($SD = 2.5$) and 47 dB ($SD = 1.2$) SPL, respectively. Figure 3 plots these detection-in-noise thresholds by group and frequency (left ordinate). The derived critical ratios, based on the masked thresholds, are also found in Figure 3 (right ordinate). The adult data from this study agree very well with previous research (Hawkins & Stevens, 1950; Reed & Bilger, 1973).

The data were evaluated with a two-way analysis of variance with repeated measures (Winer, 1971). The two main effects, age and frequency, are significant ($p < .01$). There is no Age ˘ Frequency interaction. A multiple comparison of means across age, done with a Newman-Keuls analysis (Winer, 1971), reveals a significant difference between the thresholds of the 6-month-old infants and adults ($p < .01$) and a significant difference between the 12-month-old infants and adults ($p < .01$). The difference between the two infant groups is not statistically significant.

Detection-in-quiet (Group II). Mean thresholds for each age group are shown in Figure 4. Thresholds in quiet for 1000-Hz and 4000-Hz pure tones were, for 6-month-olds, 20 dB ($SD = 6.0$) and 16 dB ($SD = 3.6$) SPL, respectively; for 12-month-olds, 18 dB ($SD = 3.7$) and 14 dB ($SD = 6.1$) SPL, respectively; and for adults, 6 dB ($SD = 4.8$) and 9 dB ($SD = 2.9$) SPL, respectively. The adult data from this research agree well with previous research (Watson, Franks, & Hood, 1972).

The data were evaluated with a two-way analysis of variance with repeated measures (Winer, 1971). The age main effect is significant ($p < .01$), but the frequency main effect is not. There is a significant interaction between age and frequency ($p < .05$). A multiple comparison of means across age done with a Newman-Keuls analysis (Winer, 1971) reveals a significant difference between each of the infant groups and the adult group ($p < .01$). The difference between the two infant groups is not significant.

PERFORMANCE MEASURES

Number of trials to meet training criterion. The mean number of trials to reach criterion was tabulated for all subjects who completed training. In addition to the 10 selected subjects in each group, subjects who were eventually excluded from the study for a variety of other reasons (Table 1) are included in this analysis. Altogether, 73 subjects (43 at 6 months, 30 at 12 months) completed training, with the mean number of trials to meet training being 22 for the 6-month-olds and 14 for the 12-month-olds. The difference between the means is significant (t test, $p < .01$).

Trials per session. The mean number of trials to complete a session for 6-month-olds was 28.5; for 12-month-olds, 24.9; and for adults, 23.0. A three-way analysis of variance with repeated measures was done on the number of trials to complete each session for all subjects. Masking condition, age, and the number of trials for each of the two tests for each subject are the factors. The only main effect to reach significance is age ($p < .01$). Since age is the only significant factor, the trials per session were collapsed across masking condition and frequency. There are no significant interactions. A multiple comparison on the ordered means for trials per session was done. The dif-

ference between the 6-month-old infants and the adults is significant ($p < .01$), the difference between the two infant groups is significant ($p < .05$), and the difference between the 12-month-old infants and the adults is not significant.

False-alarm rate. The mean false-alarm rate for 6-month olds was 11.5%; for 12-month olds, 7.7%; and for adults, 2.6%. A three-way analysis of variance with repeated measures was done with false-alarm rate as the dependent variable. Again, the only significant main effect ($p < .01$) is age. The false-alarm rate was collapsed for masking condition and test frequency and multiple comparisons were made on the mean data by age. The difference between the 6-month-olds and the adults is significant ($p < .01$), the difference between the 6- and 12-month-olds is not significant, and the difference between the 12-month-olds and the adults is significant ($p < .05$). There are no interactions between masking condition, test frequency, and/or age in this analysis.

Staircase symmetry. The final measure of performance in the procedure is the assignment of a value for the variability, or symmetry, in the staircase (tracking record) for each session. In this study, 15 dB was the maximum allowable difference between turnaround points determined on runs in a given direction. The mean for the staircase symmetry data for 6-month-olds was 8.9; for the 12-month-olds, 6.6; and for adults, 3.1. The main effect of age is significant ($p < .01$), as is the three-way interaction between condition, age, and test frequency. Since age is the only main effect, multiple comparisons were made with masking condition and test frequency collapsed. The difference between 6-month-olds and adults is significant ($p < .01$), the difference between the 6- and 12-month-olds is not significant, and the difference between the 12-month-olds and adults is significant ($p < .05$). All two-way interactions are not significant. Another way of viewing staircase variability is to measure the standard deviation of the turnaround points in each session. An ex post facto computation reveals similar age differences with standard deviations of 5.63 for 6-month-olds, 4.67 for 12-month-olds, and 3.70 for adults.

TYMPANOMETRIC SCREENING

The largest subset of data not included in the primary analyses comes from those subjects failing the tympanometric screening. The data from those failing tympanometric screening in the masking group is undifferentiated from those passing tympanometric screening. The data of interest come from the group tested in quiet. In the 6-month group, 11 subjects who failed the screening provided at least one behavioral threshold which met all other performance criteria. In the 12-month group, 4 subjects provided a valid threshold test but failed the tympanometric screening. Only one adult was excluded for failing the tympanometric screening.

Table 2 displays the data relating to the effects of middle-ear status on infant hearing thresholds. Three groups are represented, and in order to understand the significance of the table it is important that the subjects included in each group be explicitly described.

Excluded group. This consists of all data provided by infants who failed the tympanometric screening but passed all other performance criteria. That is, they provided a valid threshold according to the experimental protocol but had excessive negative pressure in the middle ear.

Screened group. The screened group includes all valid threshold tests provided by infants who passed the tympanometric screening. This includes not only those represented in the primary analysis of this research, but also those data from infants who could provide only a single valid frequency. (In order to be included in the primary analysis, subjects had to provide data at each threshold. Some infants provided data at one frequency and not the other, so they could not be included in the primary analysis. They are included in this analysis because the infants failing the tympanometric screening, in almost every case, provided only a single threshold.)

Unscreened group. The unscreened group is simply the total sample of valid threshold data without regard for tympanometry. That is, it includes the combined data from the excluded and the screened groups.

Because the data from these groups are a by-product of the study, it should be noted that the sample sizes are small and unequal. The mean thresholds and variability measures from the excluded group are an indication of the effects that high negative middle-ear pressure and/or reduced compliance of the tympanic membrane have on infant hearing. The data from the unscreened group represent findings that would have been considered "normal," had active middle-ear screening been omitted.

DISCUSSION

In terms of sensitivity, the 2-dB difference in favor of the 12-month-old infants relative to the 6-month-olds for each experimental condition is not significant and is not evidence that auditory function changes during the second half of the first year of life. The data for the two infant groups, therefore, are treated as a single group, except where specifically noted, in the following discussion.

Infant detection thresholds are different from adult thresholds. In quiet, threshold estimates of infants are not only less sensitive than those of adults, but they also have a different relationship as a function of frequency. The plot of the relationship of hearing threshold to frequency represents the sensitivity curve. In this study, only two points on that curve have been estimated and the slope of the line between those points differs for the two groups (Figure 4). The greater similarity at 4000 Hz than at 1000 Hz between infants and adults is consistent with the findings of Trehub et al. (1980). Several possible explanations for such a difference must be considered before conclusions on auditory development are drawn.

At the outset, it should be noted that although the slope of the adult sensitivity curve is consistent with existing data (Watson et al., 1972), the difference between thresholds at 1000 Hz and 4000 Hz within each group in this study is not statistically significant. The remainder of the discussion, therefore, treats the different threshold-by-frequency relationship between infants and adults as an apparent trend which still needs further study.

In early behavioral auditory research with infants, differences in responses to stimuli of different frequencies could not be assigned definitely to sensory capability because of the nature of the response that was used. Data that depend on reflexive behavioral activity, such as that used in behavioral observation audiometry (BOA), are clouded by questions of bias in the infant's willingness to respond. The fact that infant minimum-response levels are different for one stimulus as compared to another may not relate directly to the detection thresholds for the stimuli. That is, the qualitative aspects of the stimulus rather than the detectability of the stimulus may be responsible for eliciting reflexive responses from infants in such a procedure. The incorporation of a specific operant response and reinforcement contingencies into behavioral assessment of the auditory function of infants has reduced questions regarding the stimulus-frequency bias because the response is associated with the reinforcer, not the stimulus. Under the visually reinforced head-turn procedure, there is no evidence that willingness to respond is influenced by stimulus features. Therefore, the greater sensitivity to the 4000-Hz pure tone than to the 1000-Hz pure tone in the infant data is probably not due to some response bias that favors 4000-Hz signals.

There are physiologic differences between infants and adults which may contribute to the threshold-curve difference. Infant ear canals are smaller and shorter than those of adults. It is likely that the resonant peak of the infant ear canal is higher than that of the adult and may account for at least some of the difference in slope of sensitivity in these data. Middle-ear impedance differences also favor higher frequencies in infants (Hecox, 1975).

Moore and Wilson (1978) found differences in earphone response level as compared to soundfield response level for 500-Hz signals in infants. They questioned whether poor cushion-to-pinna coupling caused acoustic leakage. Such leakage would cause greater loss of acoustic energy in the low frequencies than in the high frequencies, thus reducing signal energy at the tympanic membrane. In a subsequent study, however, Hesketh (1983) has measured ear canal sound pressure levels in infants and adults for pure tones (500 and 1000 Hz) under earphones, and found no significant differences. Also, there are soundfield data which reveal a greater difference between adult and infant thresholds in the low frequencies (Sinnott et al., 1983; Trehub et al., 1980).

The head-turn procedure may contribute to the relatively poorer low-frequency thresholds in infants. Infants are not quite as good as adults in waiting quietly between trial intervals in a threshold-test session. Adults often will sit still and even hold their breath in anticipation of a stimulus trial, thus optimizing the environment for detection of a low-level signal. Infants are often moving, reaching, and/or vocalizing between trials. Masking effects are likely on at least some occasions and may be sufficient to influence the group data. Physiologic-masking effects are greater in the low than in the high frequencies when testing adults under earphones (Anderson & Whittle, 1971; Rudmose, 1982; Shaw, 1974). In testing infants, the level of activity and vocalization may result in greater physiologic-masking across a broader frequency spectrum, which would be consistent with greater differences in threshold between infants and adults at 1000 Hz versus 4000 Hz.

Finally, the concept of auditory development must not be thought of as ending at some point in childhood. Developmental change is a continuous process. Perhaps the differences between the infant and adult sensitivity curves are influenced as much by adult desensitization in the high frequencies over time as by changes in infancy. It is known that high-frequency hearing reveals the effects of our noisy environment before low-frequency hearing does. Bredberg (1967) found evidence of cochlear lesions in "normal" young-adult ears. Therefore, it seems reasonable that these effects may already be present in young-adult subjects such as those in this experiment.

MIDDLE-EAR STATUS

An issue that is critical to conclusions regarding auditory development and the differences in auditory function between infants and adults is the status of the middle ear of each subject. Infants are more likely than adults to have an abnormal middle-ear condition, and an abnormal middle-ear condition often causes elevated hearing thresholds. In none of the studies focusing on developmental sensitivity has there been an active attempt to assess middle-ear status of the subjects. This alone weakens any conclusions that might be drawn regarding normal developmental change during infancy and between infancy and adulthood.

In this research, a high proportion of infants who passed subjective screening criteria, such as recent medical history and parental report, presented with high negative middle-ear pressure. Thresholds of subjects screened out by tympanometry reveal the effects of middle-ear abnormality on individual ears and on group data. These findings are consistent with data from studies of the effects of middle-ear abnormality in other populations (Brooks, 1979).

The data that resulted from the tympanometric screening of subjects are important from both the clinical and the normative-research perspectives. On the clinical side, it is important that we learn what the effects of middle-ear abnormality are on developing human auditory systems. Mean thresholds for all infants in the excluded group were 12 dB (1000 Hz) and 13 dB (4000 Hz) higher than those of the screened group and had greater variability.

In terms of research in normal auditory development, two things are apparent. First, the threshold values of a group of randomly selected, unscreened infants is poorer than those of a group screened for abnormal middle-ear status using simple tympanometric criteria. Data on normal sensitivity in infants may be adversely affected when active steps are not taken to rule out middle-ear condition. The unscreened group in this research was screened by birth history and parental report of recent ear disease. Studies in which the screening consists of such methods, or a judgment as to whether the infant has a cold on the test day (Trehub et al., 1980), risk inclusion of infants with middle-ear abnormalities. Second, there may be a greater effect on group data in 6-month-olds than in 12-month-olds, as evidenced by the higher rate of failure on the tympanometry criterion in the younger group in this study. Studies in which unscreened data are used to represent developmental changes in auditory function may have exaggerated differences between groups or may suggest differences where none exist. This is important to consider when attempting to chart the normal developmental process.

MASKING AND CRITICAL RATIOS

Masked thresholds of infants show the same variation with frequency as do those of adults. The 6-8-dB difference (7-dB for all infants combined) between the infants and adults at each test frequency is somewhat less than the differences found in the only other masking study (Bull et al., 1981) which used a relatively frequency-specific (octave band of noise) stimulus. It is difficult to explain this discrepancy except in terms of the different methodological approaches and different stimuli. It is encouraging to note the small degree of difference between infants and adults in detecting pure tones in a background of noise. It would appear that infants are not as disadvantaged when listening in poor conditions as was suggested by the Trehub et al. (1981) and Bull et al. (1981) data. It is also reassuring to see that the masked thresholds have the same relationship with frequency for the infants as for the adults. This suggests a common frequency-selective mechanism in each group.

When the infant masked thresholds from this study are interpreted as critical ratios, very large estimates of auditory filter bandwidth result. The dependence of the critical ratio on the threshold value permits shortcomings in the detection paradigm to bias the estimate of frequency selectivity. That is, a nonsensory variable that causes the infant to provide a detection threshold biased upward by only a few decibels, such as lapses of attention during the tracking procedure or selection of a high stimulus level as criterion for response, would cause a substantial inflation of the critical ratio.

TASK VARIABLES

There is evidence in the data on task-related variables to support the notion that the subject groups behaved differently in the procedure used in this experiment. Measures of stimulus control, such as false-alarm rate and variability in the tracking procedure, have significant age effects. Although the data on sensory function were gathered with a procedure that is nearly the same for each group, they in fact arise from subject populations which differ in ways that are important in the stimulus-response paradigm. It is not possible to assign a value to the effect of the task-related differences on sensory data. However, it is reasonable to assume that, based on these data, at least some of the age-related differences in the detection thresholds come not from sensory capability differences but from other factors related to the task.

The ability of infants to perform reliably in a sophisticated behavioral procedure is no longer in doubt. There is now every reason to pursue issues of auditory development with vigor. Such efforts include, of course, the continued study of infant behavior as it relates to the stimulus-response paradigm used in auditory discrimination and perception tasks. The differences in task performance among the groups is important to consider. Norms must be developed for each group because of differing ability to operate under stimulus control as a function of age. Although the response may be the same for 6- and 12-month-olds, the reliability of performance may be different. Our methods have improved substantially in recent years, but there are still limitations regarding the head-turn procedure, and there remains a need for reliable behavioral techniques for infants below 6 months old.

The success and sensitivity of the head-turn procedure is strong evidence for its careful use in the clinical setting as well. From a clinical perspective, the small observed differences between 6- and 12-month behavioral thresholds are insignificant, as long as variability remains the same for each group. The correspondence between tympanometric data and hearing threshold in infants is very similar to the correspondence seen in older children and adults. While negative middle-ear pressure is not always accompanied by thresholds outside a normal range, the potential for elevated thresholds is great and the effects are measurable in group data. This is most important in studies of normal development and in the search for the definition of consequences of middle-ear pathology in the young.

ACKNOWLEDGMENTS

This work was supported in part by a grant from the Deafness Research Foundation. The authors gratefully acknowledge the help of the late K.H. Lee, Electronics Engineer, in development and maintenance of the experimental equipment used in this study. We also wish to thank Linda Hesketh for her assistance in data collection and preparation of the manuscript and Stephanie Cannon for her assistance in data collection.

REFERENCES

Anderson, C.M.B., & Whittle, L.S. (1971). Physiological noise and the missing 6 dB. *Acustica*, 24, 261-272.

American National Standards Institute. (1977). *American National Standard criteria for permissible ambient noise during audiometric testing* (S3.1-1977). New York: ANSI.

Aslin, R.N., Pisoni, D.B., & Jusczyk, P. W. (1983). Auditory development and speech perception in infancy. In M.M. Haith & J.J. Campos (Eds.), *Handbook of child psychology, Vol II: Infancy and developmental psychobiology* (4th ed., pp. 573-687). New York: Wiley & Sons.

Bredberg, G. (1967). The human cochlea during development and ageing. *Journal of Laryngology and Otology*, 81, 739-758.

Brooks, D.N. (1979). Otitis media and child development. Design factors in the identification and assessment of hearing loss. *Annals of Otology, Rhinology, and Laryngology*, 88 (Suppl. 60), 29-47.

Bull, D., Schneider, B.A., & Trehub, S.E. (1981). The masking of octave-band noise by broad-spectrum noise: A comparison of infant and adult thresholds. *Perception & Psychophysics*, 30, 101-106.

Dixon, W.J., & Mood, A.M. (1948). A method for obtaining and analyzing sensitivity data. *Journal of the American Statistical Association*, 43, 109-126.

Evans, E.F. (1974). Auditory frequency selectivity and the cochlear nerve. In E. Zwicker & E. Terhardt (Eds.), *Facts and models in hearing: Proceedings of the Symposium on Psychophysical Models and Physiological Facts in Hearing* (pp. 118-129). Berlin: Springer.

Fletcher, H. (1940). Auditory patterns. *Reviews of Modern Physics*, 12, 47-65.

Goldman, T.M. (1979). *Response of infants to warble-tone signals presented in soundfield using visual reinforcement audiometry.* Unpublished thesis, University of Cincinnati.

Hawkins, J.E., & Stevens, S.S. (1950). The masking of pure tones and of speech by white noise. *Journal of the Acoustical Society of America*, 22, 6-13.

Hecox, K. (1975). Electrophysiological correlates of human auditory development. In L.B. Cohen & P. Salapatek (Eds.), *Infant perception: From sensation to cognition* (Vol 2, pp. 151-191). New York: Academic Press.

Hesketh, L.J. (1983). *Pure-tone thresholds and ear-canal pressure levels in infants, young children, and adults.* Unpublished thesis, University of Washington, Seattle.

Levitt, H. (1971). Transformed up-down methods in psychoacoustics. *Journal of the Acoustical Society of America*, 49, 467-477.

Michael, P.L., & Bienvenue, G.R. (1980). A comparison of acoustical performance between a new one-piece earphone cushion and the conventional two-piece MX-41/AR cushion. *Journal of the Acoustical Society of America*, 67, 693-698.

Moore, J.M., Thompson, G., & Thompson, M. (1975). Auditory localization of infants as a function of reinforcement conditions. *Journal of Speech and Hearing Disorders*, 40, 29-34.

Moore, J.M., & Wilson, W.R. (1978). Visual reinforcement audiometry (VRA) with infants. In S.E. Gerber & G.T. Mencher (Eds.), *Early diagnosis of hearing loss* (pp. 177-214), New York: Grune & Stratton.

Moore, J.M., Wilson, W.R., & Thompson, G. (1977). Visual reinforcement of head-turn responses in infants under 12-months of age. *Journal of Speech and Hearing Disorders*, 42, 328-334.

Olsho, L.W., Schoon, C., Sakai, R., Turpin, R., & Sperduto, V. (1982). Preliminary data on frequency discrimination in infancy. *Journal of the Acoustical Society of America*, 71, 509-511.

Reed, C.M., & Bilger, R.C. (1973). A comparative study of S/N_0 and E/N_0. *Journal of the Acoustical Society of America*, 53, 1039-1044.

Rudmose, W. (1982). The case of the missing 6 dB. *Journal of the Acoustical Society of America*, 71, 650-659.

Schneider, A.A., Trehub, S.E., & Bull, D. (1980). High-frequency sensitivity in infants. *Science*, 207, 1003-1004.

Shaw, E.A.G. (1974). The external ear. In W.D. Keidel & W.D. Neff (Eds.), *Handbook of sensory physiology* (Vol. 1, pp. 455-490). New York: Springer-Verlag.

Sinnott, J.M., Pisoni, D.B., & Aslin, R.N. (1983). A comparison of pure tone auditory thresholds in human infants and adults. *Infant Behavior and Development*, 6, 3-17.

Suzuki, T., & Ogiba, Y. (1961). Conditioned orientation reflex audiometry. *Archives of Otolaryngology*, 74, 192-198.

Trehub, S.E., Bull, D., & Schneider, B.A. (1981). Infants' detection of speech in noise. *Journal of Speech and Hearing Research*, 24, 202-206.

Trehub, S.E., Schneider, B.A., & Endman, M. (1980). Developmental changes in infants' sensitivity to octave-band noises. *Journal of Experimental Child Psychology*, 29, 282-293.

Watson, C.S., Franks, J.R., & Hood, D.C. (1972). Detection of tones in the absence of external masking noise. I. Effects of signal intensity and signal frequency. *Journal of the Acoustical Society of America*, 52, 633-643.

Wilson, W.R., & Moore, J.M. (1978). *Pure-tone earphone thresholds of infants utilizing visual reinforcement audiometry (VRA).* Paper presented at the Annual Convention of the American Speech and Hearing Association, San Francisco.

Wilson, W.R., Moore, J.M., & Thompson, G. (1976). *Sound-field auditory thresholds of infants utilizing visual reinforcement audiometry (VRA).* Paper presented at the Annual Convention of the American Speech and Hearing Association, Houston.

Winer, B.J. (1971). *Statistical principles in experimental design.* New York: McGraw-Hill.

Zwicker, E., Flottorp, G., & Stevens, S.S. (1957). Critical band width in loudness summation. *Journal of the Acoustical Society of America*, 29, 548-557.

Received April 4, 1984
Accepted September 10, 1984

Requests for reprints should be sent to Robert Nozza, Children's Hospital of Pittsburgh, Division of Audiology, 125 De Soto Street, Pittsburgh, PA 15213.

Pure-Tone Sensitivity of Human Infants[a]

Lynne Werner Olsho

Department of Otolaryngology, RL-30, University of Washington, Seattle, Washington 98195

Elizabeth G. Koch

University of Virginia, Charlottesville, Virginia 22903

Elizabeth A. Carter

Virginia Commonwealth University, Richmond, Virginia 23284

Christopher F. Halpin and Nancy B. Spetner

University of Virginia, Charlottesville, Virginia 22903

(Received 7 October 1987; accepted for publication 29 June 1988)

Pure-tone thresholds at frequencies ranging from 250 to 8000 Hz were estimated for 3-, 6-, and 12-month-old infants and for adults, using the Observer-based Psychoacoustic Procedure (OPP). Sounds were presented monaurally using an earphone. Psychometric functions of infants were similar to those of adults, although 3-month-olds had shallower functions at higher frequencies. The thresholds of 6- and 12-month-old infants were 10-15 dB higher than those of the adults, with the difference being greater at lower frequencies. This result is in general agreement with results from other laboratories. The thresholds of 3-month-olds were 15-30 dB higher than those of adults. The greatest difference between 3-month-olds and adults was at 8000 Hz. This threshold difference is smaller than that reported in earlier behavioral studies; higher thresholds at high frequencies have been previously reported for newborn and 3-month-old infants. The relative contributions of sensory and nonsensory variables to these age differences are discussed.

PACS numbers: 43.66. Cb [NFV]

INTRODUCTION

One of the most fundamental characterizations of hearing is the shape of the audibility curve, the function relating absolute sensitivity to acoustic frequency. It follows that any description of auditory development should address age-related changes in the shape of this curve. Several studies have described this curve for human infants older than 6 months of age. The shape of the audibility curve has not been established for younger infants.

For infants older than 6 months, the absolute value of the reported infant threshold varies considerably across studies. The average thresholds reported are summarized in Table I. All but one of these studies (Hoversten and Moncur, 1969) used some variation of Visual Reinforcement Audiometry (VRA) (Moore *et al.*, 1975; Moore and Wilson, 1978), an operant discrimination paradigm, to obtain thresholds. However, studies differ in the stimulus employed, the mode of stimulus presentation (earphone versus loudspeaker), psychophysical paradigm (two-alternative, forced-choice versus go/no-go), and def-

inition of threshold. Some of these differences are also noted in Table I. While these factors undoubtedly contribute to the variability between studies, there is no obvious relationship between methodological variables and the thresholds obtained.

Despite the between-study variability in absolute value of the threshold, several of these studies suggest that, by 6 months of age, thresholds are somewhat close to those of adults at higher frequencies (Trehub *et al.*, 1980; Schneider *et al.*, 1980; Sinnott *et al.*, 1983; Nozza and Wilson, 1984). To make this trend more evident, in Fig. 1, infant thresholds are plotted in decibels *re:* thresholds of adults in the same study. The results of Hoversten and Moncur (1969), the only study not using a conditioning procedure, clearly stand out from the others. At the same time, the range of thresholds expressed *re:* adults is generally smaller than the range of thresholds expressed in dB SPL. The agreement among some of the studies in the shape of the curve for older infants can also be seen.

There are reasons to believe that the audibility curve of younger infants will differ in shape from that of older infants and adults. First, since the shape of the audibility curve in adults is largely determined by the characteristics of the external and middle ears, and since at least some of these characteristics have been shown to change postna-

[a]A preliminary report of these data was made at the Fall 1986 Meeting of the Acoustical Society of America in Anaheim, CA [*J. Acoust. Soc. Am.* Suppl. 1 80, S123 (1986)].

Table 1. Summary of studies of infant absolute sensitivity, 6 to 24 months postnatal age. (VRA = visual reinforcement audiometry, infant reinforced for headturn by presentation of mechanical toy; 2AFC = two-alternative, forced-choice.)

Study	Stimuli	N	Age (mos.)	Procedure	Mean threshold: dB SPL (dB re: adults) (standard deviation) Frequency (Hz)							
					250	500	1000	2000	4000	8000	10000	19000
Hoversten and Moncur (1969)	30-s tones, sound field	22	8	Behavioral observation two observers, ascending method of limits		45 (33) a			50 (58) a			
Trehub et al. (1980)	Continuous octave-band noise, sound field	89[c]	6	VRA 2AFC	38[d] b a	33[c] (24) a	25 (22) a	28 b a	23 (19) a		18 (8) a	
		74[c]	12		27[d] b a	25[c] (16) a	19 (16) a	16 b a	17 (13) a		10 (0) a	
		76[c]	18		31[d] b a	24[c] (15) a	18 (15) a	20 b a	14 (10) a		19 (9) a	
Schneider et al. (1980)	Continuous octave-band noise, sound field		6	VRA 2AFC							24 (6) a	41 (8) a
			12,18								22 (4) a	38 (5) a
			24								19 a a	31 b a
Moore and Wilson (1978)	2-s, 5% warbled tones Earphone	9	6-7	VRA, go/no-go		38 b	25 b		23 b			
		10	12-13			31 b	27 b		25 b			
	Sound field	9	6-7			18 b	18 b		16 b			
		10	12-13			21 b	16 b		14 b			
Berg and Smith (1983)	250-ms tones Earphone	12	6	VRA, go/no-go		23 (11) (5.8)		20 (10) (4.8)		29 (15) (4.1)		

Table I. (Continued.) Summary of studies of infant absolute sensitivity, 6 to 24 months postnatal age. (VRA = visual reinforcement audiometry, infant reinforced for headturn by presentation of mechanical toy; 2AFC = two-alternative, forced-choice.)

Study	Stimuli	N	Age (mos.)	Procedure	Mean threshold: dB SPL (dB re: adults) (standard deviation) Frequency (Hz)							
					250	500	1000	2000	4000	8000	10000	19000
Berg and Smith (1983) continued		6	10			27 (15) (5.6)		17 (7) (4.3)		23 (9) (5.3)		
	Sound field	12	10			20 (7) (3.9)		18 (12) (5.4)		21 (11) (5.0)		
		12	14			19 (6) (4.4)		20 (14) (5.6)		21 (11) (5.8)		
		6	18			19 (6) (6.8)		18 (12) (7.1)		21 (11) (4.5)		
Sinnott, Pisoni, and Aslin (1983)	1-s tones, sound field	11–16/ frequency	7–11	VRA, go/no-go	38 (22) (8.53)	30 (21) (11.8)	31 (23) (10.2)	36 (24) (9.0)	34 (27) (12.3)			
	0.5-s tones, sound field	2–7/ frequency				34 (23) (4.98)	35 (26) (7.51)	37 (23) (10.6)	31 (23) (7.79)	25 (18) (9.97)		
Nozza and Wilson (1984)	500-ms tones, earphone	screened[f] 11, 1K 12, 4K	6	VRA, go/no-go			21 (14) (5.72)		16 (7) (4.20)			
		unscreened[f] 17					23 (16) (7.30)		20 (11) (10.00)			
		12 screened[f]					18 (11) (3.62)		14 (5) (6.10)			
		17 unscreened[f]					22 (15) (9.40)		15 (6) (6.75)			

[a] No variability estimate available; thresholds calculated from group psychometric functions.
[b] No adults tested.
[c] Each subject contributed (one) trial at each of four levels at each of five frequencies.
[d] Actual frequency 200 Hz.
[e] Actual frequency 400 Hz.
[f] Tympanometric screening, criterion for inclusion when screened = pressure peak greater than −100 mm H_2O.

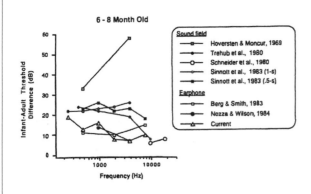

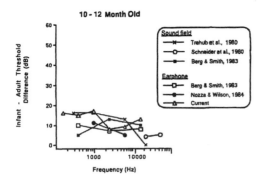

Figure 1. Average infant-adult threshold difference as a function of frequency for several studies and two infant age groups. Studies are included if the infants tested were older than 6 months of age, and if adult subjects were tested as part of the study. Within a study, only frequencies where both infants and adults were tested are included.

tally in humans (McLellan and Webb, 1957; Saunders *et al.*, 1983), one might expect to see postnatal changes in sensitivity on that basis alone. Second, in other mammals, behavioral and physiological thresholds tend to mature first at low to middle frequencies (reviewed by Rubel, 1978). By one estimate (Javel *et al.*, 1986), the auditory system of a 3-month-old human infant would be similar in maturity to the auditory system of a 6-week-old cat. There are no behavioral data for cats between 1 month of age and adulthood, so it is difficult to estimate when kitten thresholds reach adult levels. However, Ehret and Romand (1981) compared detection thresholds of 1-month-old kittens to adult cats and found a difference in sensitivity on the order of 50 dB above 10000 Hz, but only 40 dB at 1000 Hz and 30 dB at 500 Hz. Thus, over the age range in cats (6-9 weeks) that supposedly corresponds to the period between 3 and 6 months in humans, changes in high-frequency sensitivity are occurring. Third, the results of the few studies of young infants' responsiveness to sound (Hutt *et al.*, 1968; Weir, 1976; Eisele *et al.*, 1975; Hoversten and Moncur, 1969) suggest that, prior to 3 months, infants are relatively insensitive to high-frequency sounds.

Only Hoversten and Moncur (1969) have reported thresholds for 3-month-olds: 55 dB SPL at 500 Hz (43 dB

re: average threshold of young adults tested in the same study) and 65 dB SPL at 4000 Hz (73 dB *re*: adult threshold). However, for 8-month-olds tested in the same study, thresholds also increased between 500 and 4000 Hz (see Table I and Fig. 1). Because this is the opposite of what is most often reported for 6- to 18-month-olds, Hoversten and Moncur's data do not provide strong evidence for insensitivity to high frequencies at 3 months. Thus neither general sensitivity nor the shape of the audibility curve has been established for infants younger than 6 months of age.

The purpose of the current article is to examine changes in the shape of the audibility curve of human infants between 3 and 12 months of age. Thresholds were estimated over a broader frequency range than in Hoversten and Moncur's (1969) study of 3-month-olds and employed a conditioning procedure. Unlike earlier studies, the same procedure (Olsho *et al.*, 1987b) was used to obtain thresholds for infants at all ages tested.

I. Method

A. Subjects

The data described were collected as part of four separate studies: (1) a preliminary study of absolute thresholds and frequency discrimination (Olsho, 1984); (2) a longitudinal study of frequency discrimination (Olsho *et al.*, 1987b); (3) a cross-sectional study of frequency discrimination (Olsho *et al.*, 1987b); and (4) a cross-sectional study of absolute thresholds at certain frequencies undertaken for the purposes of the present article. The numbers of exclusions from each of the first three studies are given in the respective articles. In the fourth group, five other babies were tested who did not provide thresholds, either because the false alarm rate was too high or because the psychometric function was flat. Data from four other infants were lost due to equipment failures. The total number of infants included from each study at each age and frequency is shown in Table II.

Subjects in the preliminary and frequency discrimination studies were selected and recruited as described by Olsho (1984) and Olsho *et al.* (1987b), respectively. In all groups, each infant was tested within 2 weeks of the required age. In addition, all infant subjects met the following criteria for inclusion, as reported by their parents: (1) full-term birth, with no complications of delivery or perinatal course; (2) normal postnatal developmental course; (3) never diagnosed as having hearing loss; (4) free of colds; (5) no occurrence of middle ear infection within 3 weeks prior to testing, and no more than two prior occurrences of ear infections; and (6) no family history of congenital hearing loss.

Table II. Breakdown of subjects by age, frequency, design, and study.

Frequency (Hz)	Design CS[a]	L[b]	Study '84[c]	87[d]	Current[e]	Total
3 mos.						
250	10	0	6	0	4	10
500	5	10	0	15	0	15
1000	17	11	6	22	0	28
2000	17	0	0	0	17	17
4000	5	10	5	10	0	15
8000	10	0	0	0	10	10
6 mos.						
250	10	0	6	0	4	10
500	5	10	0	15	0	15
1000	8	9	6	11	0	17
2000	10	0	0	0	10	10
4000	6	10	6	16	0	22
8000	10	0	0	0	10	10
12 mos.						
250	10	0	6	0	4	10
500	3	7	0	10	0	10
1000	3	7	0	10	0	10
2000	11	0	0	0	11	11
4000	4	7	0	11	0	11
8000	11	0	0	0	11	11

[a]CS = cross sectional. Infant participated at one age only.

[b]L = longitudinal. Infant participated at two or more ages.

[c] '84 = Olsho (1984). Infants were also tested in frequencydiscrimination.

[d] '87 = Olsho *et al.* (1987b). Infants were also tested in frequency discrimination.

[e] "Current" refers to infants tested at a single age for the purposes of this study.

Six adults were included, aged 18 to 26. Each adult listened at each frequency from 250 to 8000 Hz. None had other experience listening in psychoacoustic experiments. None reported hearing problems, and thresholds were similar to those obtained in our laboratory in other studies using a similar procedure with adults.

B. Stimuli and Apparatus

The stimuli were pure tones generated using a Wavetek (model 171) oscillator. Tone bursts ranging in frequency from 250 to 8000 Hz, 500-ms in duration with 500 ms between bursts, were used. The rise and fall times of each burst were 10 ms. Stimuli were presented in trains of 10 bursts/trial. The tones were switched by a Coulbourn (S84-04) rise-fall gate and attenuated by Coulbourn programmable (S85-08) and manual (S85-02) attenuators. These devices were controlled by an Apple II Plus microcomputer using locally developed software. The computer also controlled stimulus and trial timing and recorded observer judgments.

Two different types of earphones were used to deliver sounds to the right ear. The subjects in the preliminary group listened over TDH-49 headphones in MX-41/AR cushions, which were held in place by two elastic bands with velcro closures (after Moore and Wilson, 1978). The remaining subjects (including the adults) were tested using a Toshiba RM-3 or Sony MDR-E242 "Walkman™"-style earphone held in the infant's ear with micropore tape. The response characteristics of these earphones are described by Olsho *et al.* (1987a, b). Briefly, the response is relatively flat (within 4 dB), from 250 to 4000 Hz, rolling off by about 8 dB at 8000 Hz. For all of the frequencies in this study, the amplitude of the second harmonic was at least 45 dB below that of the fundamental. Both earphones were calibrated using a 6-cmΔ coupler (Bruel & Kjaer 4152) with a 1-in. microphone (type 4144) and a Bruel & Kjaer (2215) sound level meter, using octave-band filters, linear scale. The Walkman™-style phones just fit in the center opening of the MX-41/AR cushion; the MX-41/AR cushion was used to hold the small earphone in place during calibrations. No differences in the infant thresholds obtained with these two types of earphones were noted. However, the number of infants (18 total) listening with the TDH-49 earphone was rather small. Ambient noise levels (octave band) in the test room were measured using a 6-cmΔ coupler (Bruel & Kjaer 4152) with a 1-in. microphone (type 4144) and a Bruel & Kjaer (2215) sound level meter, using octave-band filters, linear scale, with the earphone in place on the coupler at the baby's approximate location in the test booth. The levels were 17 dB SPL at 250 Hz, 11 dB SPL at 500 Hz, 10 dB SPL at 1000 Hz, 13.5 dB SPL at 2000 Hz, 15.5 dB SPL at 4000 Hz, and 15 dB SPL at 8000 Hz.

Testing was conducted inside a single-walled, sound attenuating room (IAC). The infant sat on a parent's lap in the room, facing a window into the control booth and a video camera. There was a table in front of the parent and infant. An assistant sat at the table to the infant's left. The "visual reinforcer," a mechanical toy enclosed with lights in a smoked Plexiglas box, was positioned to the infant's right. The mechanical toy could not be seen until the lights inside the box were turned on under computer control.

C. Procedure

Infants were tested using the Observer-based Psychoacoustic Procedure (OPP). Full details of the procedure are described by Olsho *et al.* (1987a); additional information is given in Olsho *et al.* (1987b).

With the infant seated on the parent's lap, the earphone was placed on the infant's right ear. The parent and an assistant who sat in the test room wore headsets to prevent them from hearing the sounds presented to the infant. The assistant manipulated toys on the table to direct the infant's gaze at midline, but tried not to get the infant so involved with the toys on the table that the infant ignored the auditory stimuli. Neither adult knew when a trial was in progress.

The observer watched the infant through the window and on the video monitor. When the infant was quiet and attending to the toys on the table, the observer began a trial. A flashing LED indicated to the observer that a trial was in progress. A train of tone bursts was presented to the infant on a given trial with a probability of 0.65. The observer did not know whether a stimulus was being presented during the trial. The observer watched the infant during the trial and made a judgment as to whether or not a sound had been presented. The observer received feedback at the conclusion of each trial.

A test run typically lasted 20 min. The session consisted of two phases, training and testing. During training, the stimulus intensity was between 60 and 70 dB, depending on the frequency. If the observer judged that a sound had occurred on a signal trial, the visual reinforcer was activated as soon as the observer made the judgment and continued for 4 s after the end of the stimulus presentation. If the observer missed a signal trial, the reinforcer was activated for 4 s at the conclusion of the stimulus train. If the observer judged that a sound had occurred on a no-signal trial, an error (false alarm) was scored. If the observer judged that no stimulus had occurred on a no-signal trial, this was scored as a correct rejection, but in no case was the reinforcer activated following a no-signal trial. Thus the observer was trained to use the infant's behavior in anticipation of the onset of the visual reinforcer as the basis of the judgment. The infant was reinforced for responding in such a way that the observer could make correct judgments, since the visual reinforcer was activated sooner and for a longer duration when the infant made an observable anticipatory response on a signal trial. Typical behaviors used were head turns; changes in facial expression, especially eye widening; increases or decreases in activity; or breaks in eye contact with the toys being manipulated on the table. Head turns were more frequently observed in 6- and 12-month-olds than in 3-month-olds, but other behaviors were used for some infants in each age group. Once the observer had reached a criterion of four of the last five signal trials correct and four of the last five no-signal trials correct, the training phase ended.

During testing, the visual reinforcer was activated only when the observer judged that a sound had been presented when a signal trial had actually occurred. Stimulus intensity was varied during testing to estimate threshold, following PEST rules (Taylor and Creelman, 1967). The PEST rules essentially generate a binary search, attempting on each reversal to halve the distance between the current level and level of the last reversal. The only exception that we made to these rules was that stimulus intensity stayed at a given level for at least four trials before a decision to change the level was considered. Thus, if the observer was correct on three or four trials at a given level, the level went down on the next trial by an amount specified by the PEST rules. If the observer was correct on fewer than three trials, the level went up on the next trial. This aspect of the procedure makes it more conservative and more resistant to brief lapses of attention on the part of the infant or the observer, since a few missed trials due to inattentiveness would lead to one or two increases in level rather than several increases. The observer was required to maintain a false alarm rate below 0.25 during testing. Testing was continued until either 50 signal trials had been completed, or the observer's false alarm rate exceeded 0.25, or the infant's state precluded further testing. An example of an infant test protocol is shown in Fig. 2.

Thresholds were estimated as the 70.7% "yes" point on the best-fitting psychometric function for each infant, using probit analysis (Finney, 1970) and maximum likelihood criterion (Hall, 1968, 1981). The threshold from a run was used only if (1) at least 30 signal trials had been obtained; (2) the false alarm rate for the run was 0.25 or below; and (3) the slope of the best-fitting psychometric function was greater than zero. For about 25% of the sessions, thresholds were not obtained. Except for the infants noted as exclusions above, thresholds were subsequently obtained at a later visit. The entire procedure (training and testing) was repeated on all visits. Comparison of thresholds obtained in first versus subsequent visits revealed no consistent differences.

Adult thresholds were obtained using the same general procedure except that the adults were instructed to

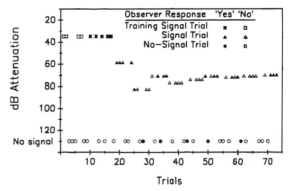

Figure 2. Example of infant adaptive trial-by-trial protocol. The subject was a 6-month-old tested at 500 Hz. Testing began on trial 18.

raise their hands when they heard a train of tone bursts. An observer in the control room recorded a "yes" response when-ever the adult did so. The reinforcer was activated as feedback, with the same contingencies as described for the infants. Order of testing at the six frequencies was randomized for each subject.

II. RESULTS

A. PSYCHOMETRIC FUNCTIONS

We examined age-group average psychometric functions at each frequency (Fig. 3). The purpose of this

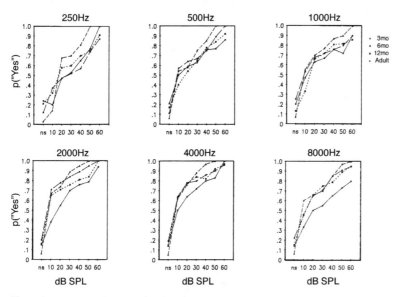

Figure 3. Average psychometric functions for 3-, 6-, and 12-month-old infants and for adults at six frequencies. Each point represented combines all trials within a 10-dB range around the level indicated.

analysis was to characterize performance in this procedure; note that thresholds were calculated from individual best-fitting functions, not from the age-group averages. The age-group average functions were obtained by calculating the percent of "yes" responses on all signal trials within a 10-dB range of the given stimulus intensity for all subjects at each frequency and age. The functions exhibit three trends:

(1) Infants' functions, particularly those of 3-month-olds, tend to be somewhat shallower than adults' functions. Where there are differences among infant age groups, namely, at higher frequencies, the 6- and 12-month-olds tend to have similar slopes, which are steeper than those of the 3-month-olds.

(2) Infant functions often do not reach 100% "yes" within the range of intensities employed. In most cases, the slope of the infant age-average psychometric function in the region of 50-60 dB is still relatively steep, implying

that the function might reach 100% at still higher intensities. However, it is possible that the infant psychometric functions actually asymptote at a performance level less than 100% "yes."

(3) In most conditions, adult performance is quite similar to infant performance at low stimulus intensities. As the intensity of the stimulus is increased, however, adult performance increases at a faster rate than does infant performance. The meaning of this difference is not clear.

We also examined the average slope of the individual best-fitting psychometric functions for each age and frequency bearing in mind that the slope estimates were based on no more than 50 trials. Psychometric function slopes increased progressively with age: The mean slope and standard error for 3-month-olds was 0.07 ± 0.14 z units/dB, for 6-month-olds, 0.13 ± 0.17 z units/dB, for 12-month-olds, 0.30 ± 0.02 z units/dB, and for adults 0.38 ± 0.01 z units/dB. There did not appear to be any consistent pattern of change with frequency for any of the age groups.

We feel that the psychometric function slopes of infants are, in fact, somewhat shallower than those of older individuals because this pattern emerges in both the age-average group functions and in the individual best-fitting functions. Whether the age difference in slope is frequency specific is not clear at this point. However, in general, the infant psychometric functions are qualitatively similar to those of adults.

B. THRESHOLDS

Average thresholds, estimated from the best-fitting psychometric function for each subject, for each age and frequency, are shown in Fig. 4. For frequencies above 250 Hz, there was a decrease in average thresholds between 3 and 6 months, which was more pronounced at higher frequencies. Between 12 months and adulthood, there was a further decrease in threshold, but the change was greater at lower frequencies. The average thresholds of 6- and 12-month-olds were essentially identical at all frequencies.

Comparison of each age group to the adults revealed that the difference between the 6-month-olds and the adults was smaller at higher frequencies, in agreement with other studies of this age group (Trehub *et al.*, 1980; Sinnott *et al.*, 1983). However, this result did not hold for

3-month-olds: The largest difference between 3-month-olds and adults occurred at 8000 Hz.

We tested the significance of these trends using analysis of variance, separately comparing each group of infants to the adults. Because each adult was tested at all frequencies while each infant was tested at only one frequency, the error terms for testing effects involving frequency were calculated separately for the two age groups and then pooled (Winer, 1971, pp. 371-378). For the 3-month-old versus adult comparison, all the effects in the age ˘ frequency analysis were significant: age $[F(1,119) = 459.03, p < 0.0001]$, frequency $[F(5,119) = 48.73, p < 0.0001]$, and age ˘ frequency $[F(5,119) = 2.81, p < 0.05]$. Pairwise comparisons between 3-month-old and adult means indicated significant differences at each frequency, $p < 0.01$ for all comparisons. However, the significant interaction supports the claim that the 3-month-olds' audibility curve does not parallel that of the adults.

For the 6-month-olds, the age $[F(1,109) = 52.62, p < 0.0001]$ and frequency $[F(5,109) = 29.36, p < 0.0001]$ effects were significant. However, the age ˘ frequency interaction was not significant $[F(5,109) = 1.07, p > 0.25]$. As Fig. 4 shows, this failure to find a significant interaction between age and frequency in this comparison may well have been due to the great variability between infants in some conditions. In fact, pairwise comparisons did show that the 6-month-olds differed from the adults at 250, 1000, and 2000 Hz ($p < 0.02$ in each case), but not at 500, 4000, or 8000 Hz ($p > 0.2$ in each case).

The effects of this variability are apparent when the 12-month-old versus adult comparisons are considered. Not only were the age $[F(1,88) = 207.04, p < 0.0001]$ and frequency $[F(5,88) = 99.96, p < 0.0001]$ effects significant, but the interaction was significant as well $[F(5,88) = 2.65, p < 0.05]$. Given that the average thresholds have not changed between 6 and 12 months, this difference must result from the decrease in variability between 6 and 12 months. Pairwise comparisons between the 12-month-olds and adults at each frequency revealed that all differences were significant ($p < 0.05$ in all cases). However, as the significant interaction implies, the age difference was smaller at higher frequencies.

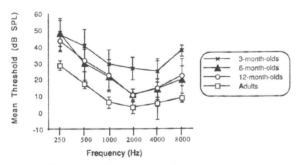

Figure 4. Mean thresholds (± 1 s.d.) as a function of frequency for 3-, 6-, and 12-month-old infants and for adults.

To summarize, the average thresholds of 3-month-olds are higher than those of adults, by 15-20 dB between 250 and 4000 Hz, and by about 30 dB at 8000 Hz. By 6 months, sensitivity at high frequencies improves; at 250 Hz, thresholds are still elevated by about 15 dB, but, at 8000 Hz, the difference between infants and adults is less than 10 dB. Thus the period between 3 and 6 months is marked by a 20-dB improvement in sensitivity at 8000 Hz. Between 3 and 6 months, the amount of threshold improvement increases regularly with increasing frequency across the frequency range. Essentially no change occurs between 3 and 12 months at 250 Hz. The only notable change between 6 and 12 months is a decrease in variability. The low-frequency age difference is resolved between 12 months and adulthood. Studies of absolute thresholds among older children suggest that low-frequency thresholds may not reach adult levels until school age or later (e.g., Schneider *et al.*, 1986; Elliott and Katz, 1980).

III. DISCUSSION

Two major conclusions can be drawn from these results. First, pure-tone thresholds improve between 3 months and adulthood. Second, the timing of this improvement is frequency dependent: Between 3 and 6 months, the improvement is greater at higher frequencies; improvement at low frequencies does not occur until some time after 12 months.

In general, the results for 6- and 12-month-olds are in good agreement with those of previous studies. This is evident in Fig. 1, where the results of this study are plotted in decibels *re*: adult thresholds, along with the results of the earlier studies. The infant-adult differences observed here are of the same magnitude as those previously reported in conditioning studies using earphones and show a similar tendency to decrease at higher frequencies.

A decrease in variability was also noted here between 6 and 12 months of age, especially at 4000 and 8000 Hz. Nozza and Wilson (1984) also reported a decrease in variability at 4000 Hz between 6 and 12 months, but only for infants who were not screened by tympanometry on the test date (see Table I). Thus at least some of the variability in performance we see, particularly at high frequencies at 6 months, may stem from variation in middle ear function.

This study represents the first report of absolute thresholds for 3-month-olds over a broad frequency range. The current results differ from those of Hoversten and Moncur (1969) in two respects. First, the thresholds reported here are much lower. Three-month-olds achieved thresholds of 15-30 dB relative to those of adults here; Hoversten and Moncur (1969) report infant-adult differences of 40-70 dB. The use of visual reinforcement in

OPP undoubtedly accounts for some of this difference. Similar threshold improvements are seen among older infants when reinforcement procedures are compared to nonreinforced behavioral observations (Moore *et al.*, 1975). Second, the difference between 3-month-olds and adults is not particularly pronounced at 4000 Hz: Three-month-olds' thresholds at 500 Hz average about 23 dB higher than those of adults, while at 4000 Hz they average about 19 dB higher. Hoversten and Moncur (1969) report a 43-dB infant-adult difference at 500 Hz and a 73-dB difference at 4000 Hz. The reason for the discrepancy between the studies is not clear, but it should be noted that Hoversten and Moncur also reported a pronounced threshold elevation at 4000 Hz for 8-month-olds and that no other laboratory has reported such a result for older infants.

The greatest difference between 3-month-olds and adults in the current study (almost 30 dB) occurred at 8000 Hz. It could be argued on that basis that human infants are similar to other mammals in demonstrating an early insensitivity to high-frequency sound. However, a simple "low frequencies first" rule does not describe the pattern reported here very well. Despite the early insensitivity at 8000 Hz, by 6 months behavioral thresholds at higher frequencies approach those of adults. Thus it is difficult to describe any general developmental sequence for mammalian auditory behavior. Such a description awaits a better understanding of the sources of infant-adult differences in behavioral thresholds, as well as a more detailed account of the development of auditory behavior in other mammals.

To what extent can the age differences described be attributed to sensory immaturity? Immaturity of the response system and/or of the connections between the sensory and response systems may influence the thresholds we obtain (see discussion by Olsho, 1986). Moreover, adult pure-tone thresholds are influenced by learning and by other variables not inherent in the auditory system. These variables appear to have a greater effect at low frequencies (Watson *et al.*, 1972; Zwislocki *et al.*, 1958). One might also argue that the demands of the detection task in the OPP and VRA experiments are actually greater for the infants than for the adults, since the infant's attention is divided between the assistant's table-top toys and the auditory stimulus. It is not clear whether the effect of divided attention would be frequency dependent. Thus there are variables such as learning and attention that would be expected to affect adult performance. In the case of learning, at least, the effect may be frequency specific.

It would not be difficult to believe that these variables would have an exaggerated effect on the performance of an individual with limited processing resources,

and could contribute to the differences between infants and adults in detection thresholds. Along the same lines, Olsho *et al.* (1988) found that adults show a greater effect of practice in discrimination of low frequencies, and that this effect could account for part of the difference between infants and adults in frequency discrimination.

We would argue on several grounds that there is little difference between 6-month-olds and adults in absolute sensitivity. First, the size of the average difference in thresholds is not large, and some 6- and 12-month-olds have thresholds that fall within the adult range at each frequency. Second, the psychometric functions of infants at these ages are quite similar to those of adults tested under similar conditions, suggesting that the function reflects a similar underlying process at each age. Third, 6- to 12-month-old infants differ most from adults in the frequency range where practice appears to have the greatest effect on adult thresholds (Watson *et al.*, 1972; Zwislocki *et al.*, 1958). Thus age differences at low frequencies are likely to reflect poorer infant performance under apparently more difficult listening conditions.

Such arguments, however, do not account for the differences between 3-month-olds and older listeners. First, the age difference is considerably larger in this case, and we rarely see 3-month-olds with thresholds in the adult range. Second, although individual psychometric function slopes are quite variable, the age-group average psychometric function of 3-month-olds also appears to grow shallower, relative to older listeners, at higher frequencies. This suggests, at least to us, an insensitive system. While nonauditory factors, such as lapses of attention, might also produce a flatter psychometric function, these factors would also be expected to produce a function with a lowered upper asymptote. It is difficult to draw any strong conclusions about an upper asymptote from these data, since it is not clear that asymptotic performance was reached at any frequency except 4000 Hz. However, there is no evidence of a correlation between function slope and upper asymptote among the 3-month-olds, as would be predicted if lapses of attention were responsible for the observed differences. Thus, although incomplete, the psychometric function data are consistent with a sensitivity difference between 3-month-olds and older listeners. Third, even if practice or learning account for the low-frequency threshold difference, such factors cannot explain why the difference between 3-month-olds and adults is greatest at 8000 Hz.

If the differences between 3-month-olds and adults reflect immaturity of the auditory system at 3 months, it is still not clear where the immaturity lies. An obvious potential contributor to the threshold differences between infants and adults is the resonance of the external ear. Unfortunately, the results of the only study to examine infant concha-ear canal resonance directly (Kruger and Ruben, 1987) are at variance with predictions based on ear canal length and compliance (McLellan and Webb, 1957; Saunders *et al.*, 1983). At this point, then, it is difficult to assess possible external ear effects. In addition, threshold differences at 250 or 500 Hz obviously require another explanation. Middle ear effects (Relkin, 1986), including undetected middle ear effusions, must be considered along with immaturity of the cochlea and auditory nervous system (Rubel *et al.*, 1984), in addition to the nonauditory factors discussed above.

ACKNOWLEDGMENTS

This research was supported by NIH grant NS 24525 to L.W. Olsho. The authors thank Trent Davis, Jay Gillenwater, Pat Feeney, Cam Marean, and JoAnn Chavira-Bash for assistance in data collection, graphics, and manuscript preparation, and Richmond Memorial Hospital, Martha Jefferson Hospital, and the University of Virginia Hospital for help with subject recruitment. We also thank Ed Burns for critical reading of the manuscript.

REFERENCES

Berg, K.M., and Smith, M.C. (1983). "Behavioral thresholds for tones during infancy," *J. Exp. Child Psychol.* 35, 409-425.

Ehret, G., and Romand, R. (1981). "Postnatal development of absolute thresholds in kittens," *J. Comp. Physiol. Psychol.* 95, 304-311.

Eisele, W.A., Berry, R.C., and Shriner, T.H. (1975). "Infant sucking response patterns a conjugate function of change in the sound pressure level auditory stimuli," *J. Speech Hear. Res.* 18, 296-307.

Elliott, L.L., and Katz, D.R. (1980). "Children's pure-tone detection," *J. Acoust. Soc. Am.* 67, 343-344.

Finney, D.J. (1970). *Probit Analysis* (Cambridge U.P., Cambridge, England).

Hall, J.L. (1968). "Maximum likelihood sequential procedure for estimation of psychometric functions," *J. Acoust. Soc. Am.* 44, 370.

Hall, J.L. (1981). "Hybrid adaptive procedure for estimation of psychometric functions," *J. Acoust. Soc. Am.* 69, 1763-1769.

Hoversten, G.H., and Moncur, J.P. (1969). "Stimuli and intensity factors in testing infants," *J. Speech Hear. Res.* 12, 677-686.

Hutt, S.J., Hutt, C., Lenard, H.G., von Bernuth, H., and Muntjewerff, W.J. (1968). "Auditory responsivity in the human neonate," *Nature* 218, 888-890.

Javel, E., Walsh, E.J., and McGee, J.D. (1986). "Development of auditory evoked potentials," in *Advances in Neural and Behavioral Development*, edited by R.N. Aslin (Ablex, Norwood, NJ), Vol. 2.

Kruger, B., and Ruben, R.J. (1987). "The acoustic properties of the infant ear: A preliminary report," *Acta Oto-Laryngol.* 103, 578-585.

McLellan, M.S., and Webb, C.H. (1957). "Ear studies in the newborn infant." *J. Pediatr.* 51, 672-677.

Moore, J.M., Thompson, G., and Thompson, M. (1975). "Auditory localization of infants as a function of reinforcement conditions," *J. Speech Hear. Disord.* 40, 29-34.

Moore, J.M., and Wilson, W. (1978). "Visual Reinforcement Audiometry (VRA) with infants," in *Early Diagnosis of Hearing Loss*, edited by S.E. Gerber and G.T. Mencher (Grune & Stratton, New York).

Nozza, R.J., and Wilson, W.R. (1984). "Masked and unmasked pure-tone thresholds of infants and adults: Development of auditory frequency selectivity and sensitivity," *J. Speech Hear. Res.* 27, 613-622.

Olsho, L.W. (1986). "Early development of human frequency resolution," in *The Biology of Change in Otolaryngology*, edited by R.J. Ruben, T.R. Van De Water, and E.W. Rubel (Elsevier, Amsterdam).

Olsho, L.W. (1984). "Preliminary results of an observer-based method for infant auditory testing," Paper presented at the International Conference for Infant Studies, New York.

Olsho, L.W., Koch, E.G., and Carter, E.A. (1988). "Nonsensory factors in infant frequency discrimination," *Infant Behav. Dev.* 11, 205-222.

Olsho, L.W., Koch, E.G., Halpin, C.F., and Carter, E.A. (1987a). "An observer-based psychoacoustic procedure for use with young infants," *Dev. Psychol.* 23, 627-640.

Olsho, L.W., Koch, E.G., and Halpin, C.F. (1987b). "Level and age effects in infant frequency discrimination," *J. Acoust. Soc. Am.* 82, 454-464.

Relkin, E. (1986). "Functional development of the middle ear," *ASHA Rep.* 28, 61 (A).

Rubel, E.W. (1978). "Ontogeny of structure and function in the vertebrate auditory system," in *Handbook of Sensory Physiology: Vol. 9. Development of Sensory Systems*, edited by M. Jacobson (Springer, New York).

Rubel, E.W., Born, D.E., Deitch, J.S., and Durham, D. (1984). "Recent advances toward understanding auditory system development," in *Hearing Science*, edited by C.I. Berlin (College-Hill, New York).

Saunders, J.C., Kaltenbach, J.A., and Relkin, E.A. (1983). "The structural and functional development of the outer and middle ear," in *Development of the Auditory and Vestibular Systems*, edited by R. Romand and R. Marty (Academic, New York).

Schneider, B.A., Trehub, S.E., and Bull, D. (1980). "High- frequency sensitivity in infants," *Science* 207, 1003-1004.

Schneider, B.A., Trehub, S.E., Morrongiello, B.A., and Thorpe, L.A. (1986). "Auditory sensitivity in preschool children," *J. Acoust. Soc. Am.* 79, 447-452.

Sinnott, J.M., Pisoni, D.B., and Aslin, R.M. (1983). "A comparison of pure tone auditory thresholds in human infants and adults," *Infant Behav. Dev.* 6, 3-17.

Taylor, M.M., and Creelman, C.D. (1967). "PEST: Efficient estimates on probability functions," *J. Acoust. Soc. Am.* 41, 782-787.

Trehub, S.E., Schneider, B.A., and Endman, M. (1980). "Developmental changes in infants' sensitivity to octave-band noises," *J. Exp. Child Psychol.* 29, 283-293.

Watson, C.S., Franks, J.R., and Hood, D.C. (1972). "Detection of tones in the absence of external masking noise. I. Effects of signal intensity and signal frequency," *J. Acoust. Soc. Am.* 52, 633-643.

Weir, C. (1976). "Auditory frequency sensitivity in the neonate: A signal detection analysis," *J. Exp. Child Psychol.* 21, 219-225.

Winer, B.J. (1971). *Statistical Principles in Experimental Design*, (McGraw-Hill, New York).

Zwislocki, J., Maire, F., Feldman, A.S., and Rubin, H. (1958). "On the effect of practice and motivation on the threshold of audibility," *J. Acoust. Soc. Am.* 30, 254-262.

The Development of a Human Auditory Localization Response: A U-Shaped Function[*]

Darwin W. Muir
Queen's University

Rachel K. Clifton and Marsha G. Clarkson
University of Massachusetts

Abstract   *Research during the past 10 years on the neonatal head-turn response to off-centred rattle sounds is reviewed, and various procedural and stimulus conditions that influence the probability of eliciting a correct response are identified. Also, the existence of a U-shaped developmental function is confirmed in a cross-sectional study of 104 infants between 3 days and 7 months of age. Neonates responded reliably, but slowly; the response decreased in frequency and magnitude between 1- 3 months of age and increased again by 4- 5 months of age. Speculation that this U-shaped function reflects a maturational shift in locus of control from subcortical to cortical structures was supported by the infants' responses to the precedence effect (PE), which is thought to be cortically mediated. The PE was produced by playing the rattle sound through two loudspeakers with the output of one delayed by 5 ms, relative to the other; adults perceive only one sound at the leading loudspeaker. As predicted, neonates failed to respond to the PE, and the onset of correct PE responses corresponded closely to the upswing in the U-shaped function for SS responses. Other explanations for the temporary decline in orientation responses to sound are also discussed.*

Résumé   *Nous avons passé en revue les recherches depuis 10 ans sur le mouvement de la tête en réponse à des sons de hochet décentrés et nous avons identifié des procédures variées et des conditions de stimulus qui influencent la probabilité de déclencher une réponse correcte. Nous avons aussi confirmé l'existence d'une fonction développementale en forme de U dans une étude cross-section impliquant 104 enfants âgés de 3 jours à 7 mois. Les nouveaux-nés répondaient s û rement mais lentement; la réponse diminuait en fréquence et en magnitude entre 1 et 3 mois et augmentait encore à partir de 5 mois. L'idée que cette fonction en forme de U reflète un déplacement du lieu de contrôle, lors du processus de maturation, des structures sous-corticales aux structures corticales, était appuyée par les réponses des enfants à l'effet de précédence (PE) dont le contrôle serait cortical. Le PE était produit par le son du hochet dans deux haut-parleurs dont l'émission de l'un était différée de 5 ms relativement à l'autre; les adultes perçoivent seulement le premier son émis et non le second. Tel que prévu, les nouveaux-nés ne répondaient pas au PE et l'arrivée des réponses PE correctes correspondait de près avec la branche ascendante de la fonction en forme de U pour les réponses SS. D'autres explications pour le déclin temporaire des réponses d'orientation au son sont aussi discutées.*

Investigators who studied children's hearing at the turn of the century observed that neonates might startle to loud sounds, but that directional responses, such as head turning toward a sound source, did not occur until infants were around 3-4 months of age (see Chrisman, 1892). Piaget (1952), in his classic longitudinal studies, reported that, although his newborns crudely located visual targets, they also failed to turn toward sounds until they were several months old. He suggested that infants developed a multimodal representation of space only after actively exploring the relationship between the visual image of objects and their auditory and tactile properties through reciprocal assimilation. This gradual integration model of perceptual development was in line with normative studies in the clinical literature on large infant populations who were observed to begin turning reliably toward a

sound's source displaced along the horizontal plane between 3-5 months of age and later on to sounds displaced along the vertical median plane (see Table 1).

These normative results contrast with a widely cited paper by Wertheimer (1961) who reported that a newborn reliably flicked his eyes toward a brief, clicking sound when it was presented beside one or the other ear. Subsequent, carefully-controlled studies by Turkewitz and others confirmed that neonates turn their eyes toward off-centred sounds of moderate intensities on the majority of trials and away from loud sounds (e.g., Butterworth &

[*]This research was supported by grants from Natural Sciences and Engineering Research Council (A0044) awarded to P.C. Dodwell and D.W. Muir, the National Institute of Health (NS-23771) to R. Clifton and M. Clarkson, and a National Institute of Mental Health Research Scientist Award (MH-00332) to R. Clifton. We wish to thank Fran Sherriff, Helen Killen, and Beth Pater for collecting the data, the parents and their infants who participated in the study, and Renée Desjardins for her indispensable help in preparing this manuscript. Address reprint requests to D. Muir, Department of Psychology, Queen's University, Kingston, Ontario, Canada K7L 3N6.

Table 1. Age (in months) at Which Infants First Localized Sounds Along the Horizontal and Vertical Median Plane (Adapted from Muir, 1985).

Authors	Localization Responses	
	Horizontal	Vertical
Gesell & Amatruda (1947)	4-5	—
Bayley (1969)	4-5	—
Uzgiris & Hunt (1975)	3-5	—
Chun, Pawsat, & Forster (1960)	5-6	7-8
Watrous, McConnell, Sitton, & Fleet (1975)[a]	3-5 (14%)	0%
	6-8 (49%)	8%
	9-12 (29%)	32%
Northern & Downs (1978)	4-7	9-13

[a]Watrous et al. (1975) give the percentages of responses elicited at different ages.

Castillo, 1976; Turkewitz, 1977). These and other observations led Bower (1978) to propose the intriguing notion that newborns possess a primitive unity of the senses at birth. He suggested that infants represent various amodal properties of stimuli (e.g., intensity, rhythm) within a common perceptual space but cannot differentiate between modalities (e.g., sights from sounds), an ability which emerges with age. Bower (1977) offered exciting evidence that young infants are innately sensitive to the natural correlation between sights and sounds. He reported that a congenitally blind 4-month-old spontaneously used the acoustic signals from an ultrasonic echo-location device to reach out and touch various silent objects and people. Finally, Wishart, Bower, and Dunkeld (1978) reported that 4- to 5-month-olds reached for an invisible sounding object presented in the dark as often as they did when it was presented silently in the light. This retrieval of invisible sounds ceased by 7 months of age and reappeared again at 11 months.

We were influenced by Bower's ideas and puzzled by the discrepancy between the normative head-turning to sound literature in Table 1 and the neonatal eye-movement literature. Also, early informal reports by Hammond (1970) and Wolff (1959), a study by Mills and Melhuish (1974), and the normative data presented by Brazelton (1973) for his popular Neonatal Behavioral Assessment Scale all indicated that human newborns would orient toward off-centred rattle sounds and voices.

REVIEW OF NEONATAL ORIENTATION TOWARD OFF-CENTRED RATTLE SOUNDS (1979 TO 1989)

In all of the studies reviewed in Table 2, neonates were tested under controlled laboratory conditions using an adaptation of Brazelton's (1973) procedure. Briefly, experimenters held 2- to 3-day-olds in a semi-supine position so that their head movements were unrestrained and they faced the ceiling either between two loudspeakers or, in a few studies, with a fake silent rattle (control stimulus) next to one ear and a live rattle next to the other ear. The rattle sound was produced by rhythmically shaking a small, plastic, container partially filled with popcorn kernels at a rate of about 2 shakes per s. The major improvements in Brazelton's procedure common to all studies in Table 2 include: presenting the sound for 20 s or until a response occurred, balancing the visual/tactile stimulation (e.g., loudspeaker next to each ear), and using blind test procedures (i.e., both the person holding the infant and the one scoring videorecordings of the infant's behavior were deaf to stimulus location). Interobserver agreement across studies for scoring the direction and latency of both the first and largest head rotation (usually the same) ranged between 86-100%. The first 6 studies in Table 2 were conducted in D. Muir's laboratory at Queen's University and the others in R. Clifton's laboratory at the University of Massachusetts, Amherst.

In Table 2, variables that may influence neonatal performance are listed as follows: nature of the sound source and its position, sound intensity, proportion of lateral versus silent/midline control trials, and criterion for scoring the occurrence of a head turn. The summary of results includes the percentage of correct responses on trials when a head turn occurred, the percentage of no-turn trials, and the latency to complete the maximum head turn and the degree of rotation. This latency measure includes time to initiate a turn (usually 5-7 s) plus time to complete the movement (3-4 s). Although some details vary between studies, several generalizations can be made. Under conditions where neonates turned reliably toward off-centred sounds, they averaged 89% correct across studies. For conditions where the normal rattle sound was presented 90° from their midline, newborns averaged 9.5 s to complete their major head turn of 56°. Various conditions which appear to modulate the probability of a rattle sound eliciting head turning are considered next.

PROCEDURAL EFFECTS

Under certain conditions neonates fail to respond on a number of trials (see Table 2). It is striking that the number of no-turn trials averaged across studies for conditions where the number of correct head turns was reliably above chance was 4% in Muir's laboratory compared with 49% in Clifton's. In some cases, but not all, Clifton's group used a slightly stricter response criterion than Muir's; however, it is unlikely such a small difference (5-10°) would make such a large impact, especially given the large head turns typically reported by both groups.

Several other procedural variations are likely candidates, such as differences in the presence of competing

Table 2. Review of Neonatal Headturning Responses to Off-Centred Rattle Sounds

Study	Procedural Variables					Results for Maximum Head Turn			
	Rattle Stimulus	± Position from Midline	Intensity dB (SPL)	Probability of Lateral vs. Control Trials	Head Turn Criterion	Correct % of Turns	No Turn	M Latency to Complete Major Turn	Head Turn
Muir & Field (1979)	live	90°	80	1.00	>5°	87*	0%		
	recorded	90°	80	0.73a	>5°	81*	9	8.0 s	45-68°
Muir & Clifton (1985)	live	60°	72	1.00	>30°	100*	0		
Forbes (1979)	recorded	90°	76	0.67a	>0°	100*	10	8.4 s	68°
		45°				61	0		53°
Field et al. (1980)	live	90°	80	0.73a	>5°	84*	5	5 s	>67°
Fisher-Fay (1981)	recorded	90°	68/80	0.33	>0°	78*	0	9 s	45°
Kellman (1984)	recorded	90°	86	0.50a	>30°	23	0	—	78°
Clifton et al. (1981)	recorded	90°	80	0.33b	>10°	95*	41	11.1 s	—
	precedence (7 ms)					38	89		
Morrongiello et al.	recorded	90°	80	0.25b	>15°	100*	54	—	—
	precedence (5,20,50 ms)					85	95		
Morrongiello & Clifton 1984	recorded	90°	76-82	1.00	>15°	93*	39	10.3 s	—
	>1.8 kHz					100*	41		
	1-3 kHz					95*	47		
	<1.6 kHz					72	70		
Clarkson et al. (1982)	recorded	90°	80	0.75a	>10°	91*	55		—
				0.50a		81*	64		
				0.25a		76	83		
Clarkson et al. (1985) Exp. 1, Fig. 1	recorded continuous	90°	64-70	0.80b	10-15°	82*	46	12.3 s	35-40°
	discontinuous					87*	41		
Exp. 2, Fig. 2	duration 1 s			1.00	>20°	85*	63	11.5 s	
	duration 5-20 s					73*	49		
Clarkson & Clifton (in press)	recorded duration: .5-.014 s	90°	65-75	—		44	75	9.8 s	35-40°
	rate: ≤1.5/s					36	58		
	rate: 2/s					66*	30	—	

Note: a silent control, b midline or PE control, *p < .05

visual stimuli. As noted by Muir and Clifton (1985), when infants were centred at the beginning of each trial, Clifton's infants directly faced a black circular visual target produced by the lens of a videocamera 0.5 m away against a moderately lit white ceiling. In Muir's laboratory, the videocamera was 1.5 m away and was difficult or impossible to see because testing was carried out either under very dim illumination or in complete darkness. Thus, Clifton's neonates may not have turned toward the sound's source on some trials because they were attending to the visual target. Evidence supporting this speculation comes from three auditory-visual conflict studies (see Muir & Clifton for details) in which neonates were presented, in the dark, with a visual target 30° to one side of midline when the rattle sound was presented 60°-90° from midline on the opposite side. Under these conflict conditions, newborns turned toward the sound source on only 55% of the trials.

Another factor contributing to the probability of eliciting a neonatal head turn toward off-centred sounds is the proportion of control trials in the experimental design. For the most part, in Muir's laboratory, the probability of lateral versus control trials was greater than .71, whereas in several studies from Clifton's laboratory this probability ranged from .25 to .33. When Clarkson, Morrongiello, and Clifton (1982) manipulated the control- trial density, they found that once the probability of lateral trials dropped below .50 the incidence of responding was so low (17%) that directional responses could not be differentiated from chance levels. Although this factor is important, other factors must be operating to control the neonate's orientation response to off-centred sounds because of several counter instances (see Table 2).

A third factor that may reduce the probability of responding is habituation. The number of lateral sound trials in a session ranged between 8-10 in Muir's laboratory and between 8-16 in Clifton's laboratory. Although Clifton's more lengthy procedure may have contributed to the large number of trials on which no response was recorded, she did not obtain a significant degree of habituation in her studies (Muir & Clifton, 1985). However, using an almost identical procedure, Zelazo, Brody, and Chaika (1984) have demonstrated a reliable decline in head turning toward a 78 dB rattle sound. After an unspecified number of warm-up trials, they allowed each infant to reach a habituation criterion consisting of no turn or turning away from the sound source on 3 of 4 consecutive trials. Their infants reached this criterion in an average of 14 trials and responded again when a novel rattle sound was subsequently introduced. Interestingly, although they did not give details concerning incorrect responses in their first study, Weiss, Zelazo, and Swain (1988) report that neonates reliably turned away when the

same sound was repeated again during post-habituation no- change control trials.

Finally, neonates may turn their heads away from a sound's location if the sound is too loud. As shown in Table 2 (Column 4) the maximum sound level in the majority of studies was approximately 80 dB SPL (range = 64-82 dB). When Kellman (1984) used an 86 dB, recorded rattle sound, her newborns turned away from the source on 73% of the trials, significantly more often than on silent control trials. Her results are not surprising given the reports of contralateral eye movements elicited by intense sounds, reviewed above.

STIMULUS EFFECTS

Various manipulations of stimulus characteristics have been motivated by efforts to determine the nature of neonatal head orientation responses. These manipulations were chosen based on an initial conceptualization of the neonate's response as a subcortically-mediated reflex directed by large disparities in binaural cues. In the absence of a true sense of spatial localization, the newborn might successfully orient toward a sound by either turning until input at the ears was balanced or, even more simply, tracking the sound by turning toward the side with the more intense and/or earlier arriving sound. Other stimulus manipulations have been directed at testing configurations shown in animal research to be cortically mediated. Neonatal head turning should be disrupted under such conditions.

One might expect that if neonates were seeking to balance the input to their two ears, they would point their heads at different sound locations along the horizontal plane. However, their response is very imprecise. As shown in Table 2, the average degree of head rotation toward a sound positioned 90° from midline varies across studies from 40° to 68°. Although responses to sounds at other locations have not been studied extensively, in one experiment, neonates' directional responses for stimuli located only 45° from midline were not reliably different from those on centre or silent control trials (Forbes, 1979 in Muir, 1982). Apparently, to elicit optimal responding from neonates, the sound source should be located more than 60° from midline (see Table 2).

Studies on stimulus duration revealed that our implicit assumption that neonates require a continuous, long lasting sound was wrong. The long latency of the newborn's response (see Table 2) originally suggested that a full 20 s of stimulation might be needed to elicit and maintain a head orientation response. We speculated that newborns might track the location of sound sources by monitoring the continuous changes in interaural cues that accompany head movements. To determine whether continuous sounds were necessary, Clarkson, Clifton, and Morrongiello (1985, Exp. 1) repeatedly presented brief rattle sounds (14, 100, & 500 ms) in trains lasting 20 s. The proportion of correct responses was equally high for the stimulus trains (87%) and a continuous control stimulus (82%). Apparently, continuous sound is not necessary to elicit neonatal responding, but the total stimulus duration of 20 s did not preclude the infants' use of a tracking mechanism. We speculated that if newborns track the location of sound sources, then only signals lasting as long as the typical response latency should elicit reliable responding. Clarkson et al. (Exp. 2) tested this possibility by presenting newborns with rattle stimuli varying in duration between 1 s and 20 s (see Table 2). While the number of no-response trials increased from about 50% to 63% as the length of the segments decreased from 20 s to 1 s, the proportion of correct responses remained high (85%). Thus, Clarkson and Clifton (in press) concluded that rapidly repeating brief sounds are as effective as continuous ones and that continuous sounds ending before any response begins will engage the neonatal head-turning response.

If, as we speculated, infants are using binaural cues to direct their head turn, then a spectral composition that eliminates or distorts these cues might influence the accuracy of neonatal responses. Both the interaural time (ITD) and intensity (IID) cues used by adults to localize sounds along the horizontal plane (Mills, 1972) are coded at low levels in the auditory pathway, in the medulla's superior olivary complex and midbrain's inferior colliculus (see Erulkar, 1972; Masterton & Imig, 1984). Because these structures appear to be functional at birth (see Hecox, 1975), either cue or both may mediate the neonatal head-turn response. Although no studies have directly manipulated these cues in newborns, Morrongiello and Clifton (1984) noted that different cues predominate when adults localize sounds containing frequencies above and below 1600 Hz, IID and ITD, respectively. Morrongiello and Clifton filtered the standard rattle stimulus which normally has a broadband spectrum between 50- 8000 Hz. They reported that neonates reliably turned toward the stimuli containing mid- and high-frequencies but made significantly fewer correct responses to the low frequency (< 1600 Hz) stimulus (see Table 2). No turn trials increased and per cent correct dropped for the low frequency stimulus. Kelly (1987) reported a similar trend of earlier orienting to high frequencies (16 kHz) compared to low (2 kHz) in young rats. He cautioned that differences in orientation could be due to either higher thresholds for low frequency sound or more difficulty in using the localization cues available in those frequencies. Pure tone sensitivity appears to follow a complex developmental course during human infancy (Olsho, Koch, Carter, Halpin, &

Spetner, 1988), so resolving these issues may be difficult.

The results of a study by Muir and Harris (see Muir, 1985) suggest that neonates can locate a sound source when normal localization cues are distorted. They tested two babies born with unilateral atresia and microtia; their right external ear canal was blocked by an unresolved meatal plug and the pinna was missing. This condition results in a constant interaural intensity difference, but may not have interfered with the ITD cue to the same extent, given intact inner structures. One might have expected these neonates to turn toward the louder side in the direction of their normal ear if the IID cue predominated or to perform at chance levels if they could not locate the sound. Instead, in repeated test sessions, both infants turned toward the recorded rattle sound reliably irrespective of its direction. They averaged between 72-83% correct when tested at term (40 weeks gestational age). Although the stimulus input cannot be specified for these infants, their performance indicates that gross distortion of normal input does not produce chance responding.

Two stimulus manipulations have been used to study the level of processing involved in the newborn's head orientation responses: very brief signals and precedence effect signals. Evidence from human adults and animals suggests that the localization of brief sounds may be mediated by the auditory cortex (Kavanagh & Kelly, 1988; Sanchez-Longo & Forster, 1958). For example, decorticate mammals do not effectively localize single, brief stimuli (Kavanagh & Kelly, 1987) or slowly-repeated ones (Riss, 1959), while the same animals responded reliably to rapidly-repeating signals. Given the relative immaturity of the newborn's auditory system, particularly cortical regions (Yakovlev & Lecours, 1967), we speculated that they might be impaired in the localization of brief sounds. To test this possibility, Clarkson and Clifton (in press) presented newborns with single rattle sounds (14 & 500 ms). Neither brief stimulus elicited reliable responding, whereas these same signals elicited reliable responding when they were rapidly repeated (Clarkson et al., 1985, Exp. 1). To determine whether newborns would also respond to slowly-repeated brief signals, Clarkson and Clifton (in press) repeated 14 ms rattle segments at three rates (2/s, 1.5/s, & 1/s) for 10 s. Only the most rapidly-repeating stimulus elicited reliable correct responding (66%). Thus, newborns showed a selective impairment in orienting to brief sounds, possibly reflecting a relative immaturity in cortical regions of the central nervous system.

The second stimulus manipulation that may separate cortical and subcortical levels of processing sound involves a phenomenon known as the precedence effect (PE). The PE is produced by feeding the same sound through two loudspeakers with one output leading the other by a few ms. Under such delay conditions, an adult's perception is of one sound image emanating from the leading loudspeaker, that is, no sound at the lagging loudspeaker. The PE has been described as part of an echo suppression mechanism to separate the perception of a sound's true location from echoes in a reverberatory environment (e.g., Green, 1976). The PE can be demonstrated in a variety of species other than humans and appears to require the operation of an intact auditory cortex. For example, Whitfield, Cranford, Ravizza, and Diamond (1972) reported that cats with cortical lesions were able to localize single source (SS) sounds but were impaired in their localization of PE sounds. Clifton and colleagues (Clifton, Morrongiello, Kulig, & Dowd, 1981; Morrongiello, Clifton, & Kulig, 1982) found that newborns would orient reliably toward the active loudspeaker on SS trials, but failed to turn their head reliably toward either loudspeaker on PE trials (see Table 2). Clifton et al. (1981) speculated that the response to SS stimuli was based on binaural cues processed at the brain stem level, whereas localization of PE stimuli would be shown later in development, reflecting maturation in the central auditory system.

DEVELOPMENTAL COURSE OF ORIENTATION RESPONSES TOWARD OFF-CENTRED RATTLE SOUNDS

One must conclude from the above review that, immediately following birth, human infants will readily turn toward off-centred sounds if they are tested under certain procedural and stimulus conditions. This conclusion contrasts with the one derived from the early normative studies reviewed above (Table 1), which document the onset of reliable localization responses to be around 3-4 months of age. Several longitudinal studies were dedicated to resolving this issue. Muir, Abraham, Forbes, and Harris (1979) tested four infants bi-weekly from birth through 4 months of age. Three turned reliably toward rattle sounds presented 90° off-centre at birth (87-100% correct), while one performed at chance. They averaged 56% correct between 1-3 months of age, and all four turned reliably again (80-100% correct) at 4 months of age. Using the same procedure, Field, Muir, Pilon, Sinclair, and Dodwell (1980) tested 11 infants once each month from birth to 3 months of age. Their infants turned toward the rattle sound on approximately 80% of the trials at birth, 1 and 3 months of age, but responded correctly less than 60% of the time at 2 months of age. Finally, Muir (1985) reported that 45 preterm infants, born at least 6 weeks prior to their expected delivery date, responded correctly

on 76% of the trials at term, 40% at 3 months and 91% at 6 months of age, post term.

Although several explanations have been offered to account for this U-shaped developmental function, including habituation and visual competition (see Muir, 1982, 1985; Muir et al., 1979), only a cortical maturation hypothesis (e.g., Muir & Clifton, 1985) has received much experimental attention. As discussed earlier, the newborn's auditory head-turning response may be viewed as a subcortically- mediated reflex. The temporary decrease in responding after the first month of life may reflect a shift to cortical control which at first inhibits and then modulates the subcortical centres mediating such reflexes (Drillien & Drummond, 1977; McGraw, 1943). Two sets of results support the idea that our infants may have experienced a transition from reflexive head turning toward a sound's general direction to perceiving the sound at a specific locus in auditory space. First, the preterm results described above support an explanation based on maturation, rather than experience. Although these infants had more than 1fi months of auditory experience prior to their term tests, the U-shaped developmental function followed their maturational rather than their chronological age. Second, Clifton, Morrongiello, and Dowd (1984) extended the comparison of SS and PE stimuli to two older age groups, 2- and 6-month-olds. They presented an 8-s computer generated train of clicks, rather than a rattle sound, and obtained poor responses from 2- month- olds to both the PE and SS stimuli but highly accurate performance to both stimuli from 6-month-olds. They tentatively related both the reappearance of frequent head turning toward the SS stimuli and the emergence of PE responses by older infants to maturation of the auditory cortex.

PRECEDENCE EFFECT AND SINGLE SOURCE RESPONSES BETWEEN BIRTH AND 7 MONTHS OF AGE

In the present study[1], we attempted to confirm the existence of the U-shaped function using the tape-recorded version of the rattle sound employed in our previous neonatal studies. We tested a large number of subjects throughout the transition period established by earlier work. Finally, we wished to compare the developmental functions for both SS and PE stimuli to evaluate the following predictions derived from the cortical maturation hypothesis: (1) Neonates were expected to orient reliably toward off-centred SS, but not PE, stimuli; (2) at interme-

---

[1]Portions of this data were presented by Clifton, Muir, Clarkson, Ashmead, and Sherriff in a poster entitled "Development of auditory localization in infants" at the meeting of the Society for Research in Child Development, Toronto, April, 1985.

Table 3. Percentage of Trials on Which Headturns Were Either Toward or Away From the Sound or No Turn Occurred for Each Age Group and Stimulus Type.

				Single Source				Precedence Effect			
Groups											
	N										
Age (M, range[a])	M + F	M	F	T	A	NT	TA + T	T	A	NT	TA + T
Birth (3 days)	14	9	5	75	21	4	78	50	46	4	52
1 mo. (35 ± 4)	10	4	6	52	20	28	72	45	32	23	58
2 mo. (61 ± 8)	10	4	6	55	28	18	68	38	32	30	54
3 mo. (95 ± 9)	10	5	5	78	20	2	75	65	30	5	68
4 mo. (128 ± 7)	20	11	9	92	8	0	92	76	24	0	76
5 mo. (158 ± 7)	20	11	9	99	1	0	99	90	8	2	91
6 mo. (185 ± 8)	10	4	6	98	2	0	98	92	5	3	95
7 mo. (214 ± 5)	10	4	6	100	0	0	100	95	5	0	95

Note: The percentage of toward (T), away (A), and no turn (NT) columns are based on the total number of trials, whereas the ratio (T/A + T) columns are based on trials when a turn occurred.
[a]Range is expressed in days.

diate ages the response to SS stimuli should diminish; and (3) at older ages the developmental functions for both SS and PE stimuli should coincide.

METHOD

Subjects: The subjects were 104 infants who represented 1 of 8 monthly (±8 days) age groups between birth and 7 months of age. Details of age and sex are given for each age group in Table 3. Newborns (all 3-day-olds) were recruited in the local hospital and tested as described above for studies in Table 2 (detailed in Muir & Field, 1979). Older infants were identified from birth announcements in the local newspaper, recruited by telephoning their parents, and tested after obtaining informed parental consent.

Procedure: The stimulus was a stereophonic tape recording of a rhythmically-shaken rattle which could be delivered through an amplifier to one or two loudspeakers. When infants were in the proper position facing forward, one loudspeaker was 90° left and the other 90° right of centre, at a distance of about 1.3 m along an extension of the interaural axis between their two ears. The tape recording had the same sound sequence on both channels, but one channel's signal led the other by 5 ms. On PE trials both channels were operating, while on SS trials, the same tape recording was played with the sound on one channel turned off and the volume increased to match the intensity of the PE stimulus (65 dB SPL over a background noise of 48 dB). Switches controlled which loudspeaker was leading on PE and active on SS trials. Visual distractions were minimized by testing neonates in dim illumination (described in Muir & Clifton, 1985) and older infants in a sound treated room with the walls and recording equipment draped in black and illuminated

indirectly by a shielded, 25-Watt lamp placed behind the infant.

During testing, newborns, 1-, and 2-month-olds were held in a semisupine position by a nurse (newborns) or their mothers (1- to 2-month-olds) while the older babies were seated on their mothers' laps. When they were in a quiet alert state, each infant received two blocks of four stimulus trials with SS and PE trials presented once on each side per block in random order. Their heads were centred between the loudspeakers at the beginning of a trial by the experimenter who flashed a small red light mounted directly below an infra-red sensitive camera which recorded a frontal view. Each stimulus lasted 20 s or until the infant turned to face the sound source. Later, observers naive to stimulus location scored the latency (time between stimulus onset and completion of the head turn), magnitude (scored in 15° segments on either side of midline), and direction of major (> 30°) head turns from edited videorecords. Interrater agreement was > 88% on all measures.

RESULTS

The average number of trials on which infants turned toward the SS and PE stimuli and the respective standard errors are plotted for each age group in Figure 1. As predicted, a U-shaped developmental function was obtained with the SS stimulus, but not with the PE stimulus. An ANOVA (Age ˇ Sex ˇ Stimulus) performed on the angular transformation (cf. Kirk, 1982, p. 83) of this percentage data confirmed our impression. As predicted, performance varied with age, $F(7, 88) = 18.56, p < .001$, and stimulus, $F(1, 88) = 32.62, p < .001$. The three-way interaction was also significant, $F(7, 88) = 3.01, p < .006$. To correct the alpha levels for multiple tests, we always

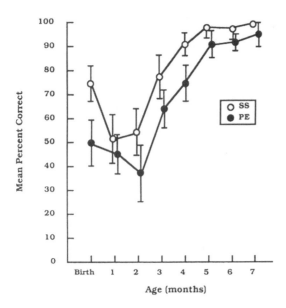

Figure 1. Average percent of total trials on which infants turned toward the single source (SS) and precedence effect (PE) stimuli plotted as a function of age. Standard errors are indicated by the vertical bar for each point.

employed conservative simple effects analyses to follow up any age effects. The analyses contrasting SS and PE performance at each age revealed that the superior SS localization response occurred only at birth, $F(1, 88) = 23.33$, $p < .001$, and at 4 months of age, $F(1, 88) = 9.73$, $p < .003$. Indeed, at both ages when infants displayed a difference, 89% of them turned more often toward the SS than the PE stimulus.

Further tests of the simple interaction (Sex ˜ Stimulus) at each age revealed significant effects at birth, 1, and 4 months; however, the results for the two youngest ages are not discussed due to small ns and the 1-month-old's performance being at chance levels. The interaction at 4 months of age may be important: Females performed well on both PE (84%) and SS (89%) stimuli, whereas males performed poorly on PE (67%) relative to SS (94%) stimuli. This finding must be considered tentative because a subsequent analysis restricted to the transition ages of 3-, 4-, and 5-month-olds revealed only a trend for the age by stimulus by sex interaction, $F(2, 44) = 2.87$, $p = .068$. Given this caveat, the observation that males do not differ from females in their response to SS stimuli but lagged behind in their response to the more complex PE stimuli is provocative. That the precedence effect differentiates between the sexes fits with our interpretation of it as a "higher level" localization task. It is noteworthy that the onset of three relatively complex visual abilities, stereopsis, fusion (rivalry), and vernier acuity, also appears earlier in females than males in this same age range (see Gwiazda, Bauer, & Held, this volume).

The decrease in correct responding during the transition period could be due to an overall drop in head turning behavior or to increased contralateral turns. To present a complete picture, the results for percentages of turns toward, away, and no turns are given for SS and PE trials in Table 3. Clearly, the incidence of no-turn trials increased in the 1- and 2-month-olds compared with both newborns and the older infants. The ratio of toward to away turns also decreased during this period of decline. An Age ˜ Sex ˜ Stimulus ˜ Direction (toward vs. away) ANOVA on the angular transformation of the percentage data confirmed this impression. Performance varied as a function of age, $F(7, 88) = 7.89$, $p < .001$, and overall more turns were directed toward than away from both stimuli, $F(1, 88) = 355.19$, $p < .001$. Also, both the direction by age, $F(7, 88) = 15.56$, $p < .001$, and direction by stimulus, $F(1, 88) = 30.09$, $p < .001$, interactions were significant, reflecting the presence of the U-shaped function. In the fourth column for each stimulus condition, we present the percentage of turns toward the stimuli based on the number of trials on which a turn occurred (as in the studies summarized in Table 2). Follow-up analyses of the interaction with age indicated that there were more turns toward the stimulus at all ages (i.e., all ps $< .01$) except at 1 and 2 months when the number of toward and away turns did not differ. A follow-up analysis of the direction by stimulus interaction indicated significantly more turns toward than away for both SS and PE stimuli, but the effect was much larger for the former (see Table 3). One striking feature in Table 3 is that the percentage correct for PE is almost identical to those for SS between 3 and 5 months of age, except that they lag behind the SS by 1 month.

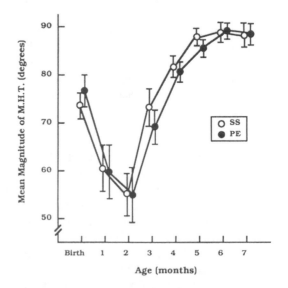

Figure 2. The average magnitude of turns toward single source (SS) and precedence effect (PE) stimuli plotted as a function of age. Standard errors are indicated by vertical bars for each point.

A second aspect of the infants' responses to off-centred sounds that changed with age was the extent of the response. The average magnitudes of the infants' head turns toward the SS and PE stimuli are plotted as a function of age in Figure 2. An ANOVA (Age ˘ Sex ˘ Stimulus) performed on this data revealed only one main effect of age, $F(7, 88) = 21.62$, $p < .001$. Age differences in the degree of head rotation appear to parallel the U-shaped age function for per cent correct with the SS stimulus. Infants rotated their heads about 75° toward the stimuli at birth, to a lesser extent between 1-2 months of age (55°-60°), to a greater extent between 3-4 months of age (70°-82°), and almost 90° (the actual stimulus location) by 5-6 months of age. A significant 3-way interaction was also obtained with this measure, $F(7, 88) = 3.57$, $p < .01$, but, in this case, the simple interactions (Sex ˘ Stimulus) were significant only at the younger ages.

The third characteristic of the infants' head-turning response which changed with age was its speed. This is illustrated in Figure 3 where the latency to complete a head turn toward each stimulus is plotted as a function of age. The ANOVA (Age ˘ Sex ˘ Stimulus) performed on this data revealed only a significant effect of age, $F(7, 88) = 27.12$, $p < .001$. The relatively slow head turn (averaging 7-12 s) typically exhibited by infants between birth and 2-3 months of age shifted to a brisk (1.5-2.5 s) accurate response by 5 months of age.

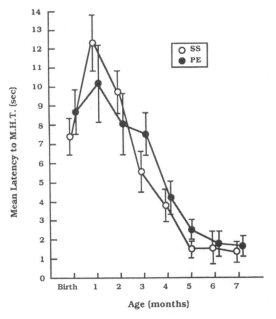

Figure 3. Average latency to complete a head turn toward single source (SS) and precedence effect (PE) stimuli plotted as a function of age. Standard errors are indicated by vertical bars for each point.

DISCUSSION

The present results resolve the conflict between the late appearance of accurate auditory localization responses by older infants assessed in normative studies (Table 1) and the reliable orientation responses repeatedly observed in neonatal studies (Table 2). In all major respects our cross-sectional data match those obtained in prior neonatal and longitudinal studies to a remarkable extent. Muir and Field (1979) recorded correct responses on 81% of the trials while the present group were correct on 78%. Both percentage correct scores and turn magnitude of the correct responses declined between 1-3 months of age and improved dramatically by 4 months of age. Finally, between 1 and 5 months the latency shortened by about 2 s per month to an asymptote of about 1.5 s. Interestingly, the largest gain in latency was between 2 and 4 months, accompanying the shift to reliable responding after the transition period. Although the precise timing may vary among infants, the latency, frequency, and per cent correct of the head-turning response improved together when infants reached the ascending arm of the U-shaped developmental function. We should stress that it is not impossible to obtain reliable responding to SS sound at 2 months of age. Several investigators who used a female voice stimulus managed to elicit significantly more responses toward than away from the sound in 2-month-olds (Clifton et al., 1984; Field, DiFranco, Dodwell, & Muir, 1979). However, the present data demonstrate that responses become more difficult to elicit at 1-2 months than either before or after this age when a standard stimulus is used between birth and 7 months.

The qualitative changes in the response support the speculation that the reappearance of SS responses and the initial appearance of responses to the precedence effect herald the onset of cortical function. In this regard, the present data replicate and extend Clifton's work on the precedence effect (Clifton et al., 1981, 1984), in that we have documented that infants who reliably orient toward SS stimuli at birth fail to do so when presented with PE stimuli. For both stimuli, responding during the transition period was equally poor and improved between 3-5 months of age. Although performance was virtually identical for both stimuli at 6 months of age, the age tested by Clifton et al. (1984), we did discover a small but reliable difference at 4 months of age when responding to PE stimuli was lower than to SS stimuli. Four months appears to be a transition age for onset of the precedence effect. Some infants are responding equivalently to both stimuli, whereas others show a lag in response to PE stimuli. The interaction of stimulus type with sex may be relevant here. Nine out of 20 infants responded equivalently and b of these were females; 9 out of 20 responded more to SS than PE stimuli and b of these were males. What we do not know from these data is whether the nine infants with equivalent responding at 4 months had experienced a relative lag in PE earlier in their development. We expected the responses to SS and PE either to coincide closely or to show a lag favoring SS stimuli in older infants because PE stimuli are more complex. As Clifton et al. pointed out,

> to obtain the precedence effect, the ears must receive four inputs, two from the leading and two from the lagging sound, whereas single- source stimuli have only two inputs. Thus, the precedence effect involves perceptually more complex stimuli and presents the brain with a task of input suppression (1984, p. 521).

The cortical maturation hypothesis does not contradict and may complement a cognitive explanation of the U-shaped developmental function. There is a notable correspondence between the onset age for both the decline and recovery of reliable head turning toward sounds and the first 3 substages of Piaget's (1952) sensorimotor period. Oversimplifying his theory, reflexive responses in each sensory modality operate independently between birth and 1 month of age, coordination between sensory-motor schemes begins to develop between 1-3 months of age, and intentional responding directed at external events first appears around 4-5 months of age (see Cowan, 1978; Warren, 1984). During the second stage (our transition period), although infants can assert their independence from the constraints of simple reflexive behavior, they still may not have the ability to coordinate the various motor schemes needed to engage in interactions with certain external events. Thus, they may appear to be disorganized. Another behavior that follows a similar developmental course is arm-hand movements directed toward visual objects. According to von Hofsten (1984) prereaching in the neonatal period is followed by a decline prior to the onset of intentional reaching at 4 to 5 months of age. As the infants emerge from the transition period with a perceptual system in which objects are located at specific positions in space, they begin to display direct interactions with external objects. This may explain why a variety of new behaviors appear around 4 months of age.

The age of onset of reaching for both visible and invisible sounding objects appears to coincide with the recovery of reliable orientation toward off-centred sounds. As mentioned previously, Wishart et al. (1978) were first to observe that 4- to 5-month-olds would reach equally often for an invisible sounding object presented in the dark and visible objects presented in the light. Recently, in a cross-sectional study, Stack, Muir, Sherriff, and Roman

(in press) also observed that infants started to reach on a majority of trials for invisible sounds presented in the dark beginning at 4 months of age. Infants' responses to the sounds in the dark were not as accurate as those to visual targets, and explicit pairing of auditory and visual stimuli appeared to be necessary to elicit frequent reaches toward the invisible sounds at this age. Perris and Clifton (1988) found that 7-month- olds who were exposed to sounding objects in the light would reach accurately for this sounding object in the dark presented at different locations on either side of midline. Infants clearly appreciate that sounds can signal an object's location in space by 4-5 months of age, and further research using the reaching measure in conjunction with the head- turning response should enable us to investigate their developing ability to locate invisible sounds in depth (see Perris & Clifton) as well as at elevations off the horizontal plane.

To conclude, during the past 10 years we have identified the proper stimulus conditions to elicit a highly reliable, slow head-turn response toward off-centred sounds from neonates. Perhaps the most surprising result was that continuous sound is not needed to drive the head turn which led Clarkson et al. (1985) to speculate that the response is a "triggered motor pattern" rather than an attempt to balance binaural disparity cues. We have also established that the slow but accurate neonatal response decreases in frequency and magnitude between 1-3 months of age. By 4-5 months of age infants again orient toward sounds, now with a shorter latency, larger magnitude, and greater accuracy than neonates. We have speculated that this U-shaped developmental function reflects a maturational shift in locus of control from subcortical to cortical structures. One line of evidence supporting this interpretation is the work on the precedence effect, which is thought to be cortically mediated. As predicted, neonates fail to respond to the precedence effect, and a correspondence exists between the upswing in the U-shaped function and the onset of appropriate precedence effect responding, although there is an initial superiority of SS stimuli. At about the same age, reaching to both visual and auditory targets appears, which implies that infants are coordinating motor schemes across modalities and may be perceiving objects in a 3-dimensional auditory- visual space. Perhaps the absence of an integrated perceptual space is reflected in the frustrated attempts to obtain orienting toward sounds during the dip in the U-shaped function. Certainly it provided part of the motivation for the development of testing procedures not dependent on the head-turn response to determine the young infant's auditory frequency and intensity thresholds (see Olsho, Koch, Halpin, & Carter, 1987). Finally, these findings imply that training blind infants to use ultrasonic spatial sensors at an early age will be frustrated as well (see review by Humphrey, Muir, Dodwell, & Humphrey, 1988).

REFERENCES

Bayley, N. (1969). *Bayley scales of infant development.* New York: Psychological Corporation.

Bower, T.G.R. (1977). Blind babies see with their ears. *New Scientist,* 73, 255-257.

Bower, T.G.R. (1978). Perceptual development: Object and space. In E.C. Carterette & M.P. Friedman (Eds.), *Handbook of perception* (Vol. 8). New York: Academic Press.

Brazelton, T.B. (1973). *Neonatal Behavioral Assessment Scale.* London: Spastics International Medical Publications.

Butterworth, G., & Castillo, M. (1976). Coordination of auditory and visual space in newborn human infants. *Perception,* 5, 155-160.

Chrisman, O. (1892). The hearing of children. *Pedagogical Seminary,* 2, 397-404.

Chun, R.W.M., Pawsat, R., & Forster, F.M. (1960). Sound localization in infancy. *Journal of Nervous & Mental Disorders,* 130, 472-476.

Clarkson, M.G., & Clifton, R.K. (in press). Acoustic determinants of newborn orienting. In M.J. Weiss & P.R. Zelazo (Eds.), *Newborn attention.* Norwood, NJ: Ablex.

Clarkson, M.G., Clifton, R.K., & Morrongiello, B.A. (1985). The effects of sound duration on newborns' head orientation. *Journal of Experimental Child Psychology,* 39, 20-36.

Clarkson, M.G., Morrongiello, B.A., & Clifton, R.K. (1982). Stimulus-presentation probability influences newborns' head orientation to sound. *Perceptual & Motor Skills,* 55, 1239-1246.

Clifton, R.K., Morrongiello, B.A., & Dowd, J.M. (1984). A developmental look at an auditory illusion: The precedence effect. *Developmental Psychobiology,* 17, 519-536.

Clifton, R.K., Morrongiello, B.A., Kulig, J.W., & Dowd, J.M. (1981). Newborns' orientation toward sound: Possible implications for cortical development. *Child Development,* 52, 833-838.

Cowan, P.A. (1978). *Piaget with feeling.* Toronto: Holt, Rinehart, & Winston.

Drillien, C.M., & Drummond, M.B. (1977). (Eds.). *Neurodevelopmental problems in early childhood: Assessment and management.* London: Blackwell.

Erulkar, S. (1972). Comparative aspects of spatial localization of sound. *Physiological Review,* 52, 237-337.

Field, J., DiFranco, D., Dodwell, P., & Muir, D. (1979). Auditory-visual coordination in 2fi- month-old infants. *Infant Behavior and Development,* 2, 113-122.

Field, J., Muir, D., Pilon, R., Sinclair, M., & Dodwell, P. (1980). Infants' orientation to lateral sounds from birth to three months. *Child Development,* 51, 295-298.

Fisher-Fay, A. (1981). *The effect of a visual stimulus on auditory localization in the newborn infant.* Unpublished honors thesis, Queen's University, Kingston, Ontario.

Forbes, B. (1979). *Auditory localization in newborns.* Unpublished honors thesis, Queen's University, Kingston, Ontario.

Gesell, A.L., & Amatruda, C.S. (1947). *Developmental diagnosis: Normal and abnormal child development, clinical methods and pediatric applications* (2nd ed). New York: Hoeber.

Green, D. (1976). *An introduction to hearing.* Hillsdale, NJ: Lawrence Erlbaum.

Gwiazda, J., Bauer, J., & Held, R. (1989). From visual acuity to hyperacuity: A ten-year update. *Canadian Journal of Psychology,* 43, 109-120.

Hammond, J. (1970). Hearing and response in the newborn. *Developmental Medical Child Neurology,* 12, 3-5.

Hecox, K. (1975). Electro-physiological correlates of human auditory development. In L.B. Cohen & P. Salapatek (Eds.), *Infant perception: From sensation to cognition* (Vol. 2, pp. 151-191). New York: Academic Press.

Hofsten, C. von. (1984). Developmental changes in the organization of prereaching movements. *Developmental Psychology,* 20, 378-388.

Humphrey, G.K., Muir, D.W., Dodwell, P.C., & Humphrey, D.E. (1988). The perception of structure in vectorpatterns by 4-month-old infants. *Canadian Journal of Psychology,* 42, 35-43.

Kavanagh, G.L., & Kelly, J.B. (1987). Contribution of auditory cortex to sound localization by the ferret. *Journal of Neurophysiology,* 57, 1746-1766.

Kellman, D. (1984). *The effect of intensity on the habituation of the head turn and startle response.* Unpublished honors thesis, Queen's University, Kingston, Ontario.

Kelly, J.B. (1987). The development of sound localization and auditory processing in mammals. In R.N. Aslin (Ed.), *Advances in neural and behavioral development* (Vol. 2, pp. 205-234). Norwood, NJ: Ablex.

Kirk, R.E. (1982). *Experimental design: Procedures for the behavioral sciences* (2nd ed.). Belmont, CA: Wadsworth.

Masterton, R.B., & Imig, T.J. (1984). Neural mechanisms for sound localization. *Annual Review of Physiology,* 46, 275-287.

McGraw, M.B. (1943). *The neuromuscular maturation of the human infant.* New York: Columbia University Press.

Mills, A.W. (1972). In J.V. Tobias (Ed.), *Foundations of modern auditory theory* (Vol. 2, pp. 301-345). New York: Academic Press.

Mills, M., & Melhuish, E. (1974). Recognition of mother's voice in early infants. *Nature,* 252, 123-124.

Morrongiello, B.A., & Clifton, R.K. (1984). Effects of sound frequency on behavioral and cardiac orienting in newborn and five-month-old infants. *Journal of Experimental Child Psychology,* 38, 429-446.

Morrongiello, B.A., Clifton, R.K., & Kulig, J.W. (1982). Newborn cardiac and behavioral orienting responses to sound under varying precedence- effect conditions. *Infant Behavior & Development,* 5, 249-259.

Muir, D.W. (1982). The development of human auditory localization in infancy. In R.W. Gatehouse (Ed.), *Localization of
sound: Theory and applications* (pp. 220-243). Groton, CT:
Amphora Press.

Muir, D.W. (1985). The development of infants' auditory spatial
sensitivity. In S.E. Trehub & B. Schneider (Eds.), *Auditory
development in infancy* (pp. 51-83). New York: Plenum
Press.

Muir, D., Abraham, W., Forbes, B., & Harris, L. (1979). The
ontogenesis of an auditory localization response from birth
to four months of age. *Canadian Journal of Psychology, 33,*
320-333.

Muir, D.W., & Clifton, R. (1985). Infants' orientation to the
localization of sound sources. In G. Gottlieb & N.
Krasnegor (Eds.), *The measurement of audition and vision
during the first year of life: A methodological overview* (pp.
171-194). Norwood, NJ: Ablex.

Muir, D., & Field, J. (1979). Newborn infants orient to sounds.
Child Development, 50, 431-436.

Northern, J.L., & Downs, M.P. (1978). *Hearing in children.*
Baltimore, MD: Waverly Press.

Olsho, L.W., Koch, E.G., Carter, E.A., Halpin, C.F., & Spetner,
N.B. (1988). Pure-tone sensitivity of human infants.
Journal of the Acoustical Society of America, 84,
1316-1324.

Olsho, L.W., Koch, E.G., Halpin, C.F., & Carter, E.A. (1987). An
observer-based psychoacoustic procedure for use with
young infants. *Developmental Psychology, 23,* 627-640.

Perris, E.E., & Clifton, R.K. (1988). Reaching in the dark toward
sound as a measure of auditory localization in 7-month-old
infants. *Infant Behavior & Development*, 11, 477-495.

Piaget, J. (1952). *The origins of intelligence in children.* New
York: International Universities Press.

Riss, W. (1959). Effect of bilateral temporal cortical ablation on
discrimination of sound direction. *Journal of
Neurophysiology*, 22, 374-384.

Sanchez-Longo, L.P., & Forster, F.M. (1958). Clinical significance of impairment of sound localization. *Neurology,* 8,
119-125.

Stack, D.M., Muir, D.W., Sherriff, F., & Roman, J. (in press).
Development of infant reaching in the dark to luminous
objects and invisible sounds. *Perception.*

Turkewitz, G. (1977). The development of lateral differentiation
in the human infant. *Annals of the New York Academy of
Science, 299,* 309-318.

Uzgiris, I.C., & Hunt, J.McV. (1975). *Assessment in infancy.*
Chicago: University of Illinois Press.

Warren, D.H. (1984). *Blindness and early childhood* (2nd Ed.)
New York: American Foundation for the Blind.

Watrous, B.S., McConnell, F., Sitton, A.B., & Fleet, W.F. (1975).
Auditory responses of infants. *Journal of Speech and
Hearing Disorders,* 40, 357- 366.

Weiss, M.J., Zelazo, P.R., & Swain, I.U. (1988). Newborn
response to auditory stimulus discrepancy. *Child
Development,* 59, 1530-1541.

Wertheimer, M. (1961). Psychomotor coordination of auditory
and visual space at birth. *Science,* 134, 1692.

Wishart, J.G., Bower, T.G.R., & Dunkeld, J. (1978). Reaching in
the dark. *Perception,* 7, 507-512.

Whitfield, I., Cranford, J., Ravizza, R., & Diamond, I. (1972).
Effects of unilateral ablation of auditory cortex in cat on
complex sound localization. *Journal of Neurophysiology,*
35, 718-731.

Wolff, P. (1959). Observations on newborn infants. *Psychoso-
matic Medicine,* 21, 110-118.

Yakovlev, P.I., & Lecours, A. (1967). The myelogenetic cycles of
regional maturation of the brain. In A. Minkowski (Ed.),
Regional development of the brain in early life.
Philadelphia: F.A. Davis & Company.

Zelazo, P.R., Brody, L.R., & Chaika, H. (1984). Neonatal habituation and dishabituation of head turning to rattle sounds.
Infant Behavior and Development, 7, 311-321.

Size of Critical Band in Infants, Children, and Adults

Bruce A. Schneider, Barbara A. Morrongiello, and Sandra E. Trehub

University of Toronto, Mississauga, Ontario, Canada

Masked thresholds at two signal frequencies (0.8 and 4 kHz) were obtained from listeners aged 6.5 months, 2 years, 5 years, and 20.5 years in the presence of constant spectrum level, narrow-band maskers of differing bandwidths. Consistent with the classical results of Fletcher (1940), masked threshold for all age groups increased with bandwidth up to a critical width, beyond which further increases in bandwidth were ineffective in increasing threshold. These critical widths (estimates of critical band size) did not change substantially with age (critical widths for infants were no more than 50% larger than those of adults) despite substantial changes in masked thresholds with age. Thus, contrary to previous claims, changes in auditory filter width cannot account for developmental changes in masked or absolute thresholds.

The concept of a critical band or auditory filter has been invoked in virtually every auditory phenomenon (e.g., Moore, 1982; Scharf, 1970) and has been the concern of numerous studies in auditory psychophysics and auditory psychophysiology. Indeed, the perception of many auditory events seems to depend on whether the energy in the stimulus is contained within a limited frequency region (i.e., a critical band) or is spread across two or more such regions. Consider, for example, the classic experiment by Fletcher (1940), in which listeners were required to detect the presence of a pure tone centered in narrow-band noises of different bandwidths, with the spectrum level (dB per cycle) of each noise band held constant. (Because the spectrum level was held constant, the total power in the masker was proportional to the bandwidth of the masker.) Fletcher found that pure-tone thresholds increased with bandwidth (total power) up to a certain point, beyond which no further increases in threshold were observed, in spite of enormous changes in masker bandwidth and power. This basic result has been confirmed a number of times (e.g., Greenwood, 1961; Schafer, Gales, Shewmaker, & Thompson, 1950; Swets, Green, & Tanner, 1962), indicating that only the energy in a narrow frequency region centered on a pure tone is effective in masking that pure tone. As Scharf (1970) has documented, the dependency of masked thresholds on critical bandwidth is but one of many instances in which auditory phenomena function differently within and across critical bands.

Because of the importance of the critical band concept, any theory of auditory development would be incomplete without some understanding of how the critical band or auditory filter changes with age. For example, there are substantial adult-infant differences in masked thresholds (Bull, Schneider, & Trehub, 1981; Nozza & Wilson, 1984; Trehub, Bull, & Schneider, 1981), and these differences decline exponentially over the first decade of life (Schneider, Trehub, Morrongiello, & Thorpe, 1989). Changes in the size of the critical band could easily account for these developmental trends (Schneider & Trehub, 1985). Figure 1 (upper panel) illustrates how this might occur. The solid horizontal line represents the spectrum level (N_0) of a band-limited Gaussian noise (i.e., flat power spectrum), the vertical arrow represents the power in a 0.8-kHz pure tone, and the dashed vertical lines indicate the upper and lower boundaries of the critical band centered at 0.8 kHz. In line with the notion of an auditory filter or critical band, we assume that energy falling outside the critical band cannot affect quantities calculated from energy within the band. Therefore, only the portion of the masker that falls within the critical band is effective in masking the pure tone at its center. Suppose that threshold is reached when the ratio of signal power to noise power in the critical band exceeds some criterion value, that is, when

$$I_s/I_{ncb} = C, \qquad (1)$$

where I_s is the power in the pure tone, I_{ncb} is the noise power within the critical band, and C is the threshold constant. Because the spectrum of a Gaussian noise is flat, it is clear that $I_{ncb} = N_0 \cdot CB$, where CB is the width of the critical band. Now suppose that the criterion signal-to-noise ratio, C, remains unchanged throughout development but that the size of the critical band decreases with age. Because the noise power in the critical band is proportional to bandwidth, then as critical bandwidth shrinks

Copyright © 1990 by the American Psychological Association. Reprinted with permission. *Journal of Experimental Psychology: Human Perception and Performance*, 16 (3), pp. 642-652.

This research was supported by grants from the Medical Research Council of Canada and from the University of Toronto. We thank K.J. Kim, Marilyn Barras, Donna Laxdal, and Elizabeth Olszewska for assistance in data collection.

Barbara A. Morrongiello is currently affiliated with the Department of Psychology, University of Western Ontario, London, Ontario, Canada N6A 3K7.

Correspondence concerning this article should be addressed to Bruce A. Schneider, Department of Psychology, Erindale Campus, University of Toronto, Mississauga, Ontario, Canada L5L 1C6.

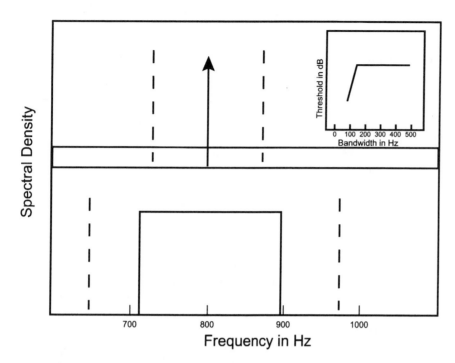

Figure 1. Schematic representation of critical bandwidth for 800-Hz pure tone (upper panel) and for 800-Hz, a-octave band of noise (lower panel). (Insert in the upper panel illustrates how threshold should change as a function of bandwidth, according to critical band model.)

Irwin, Stillman, and Schade (1986) measured the width of the auditory filter in two 6-year-olds, two 10-year-olds, and two adults by having them detect a pure tone centered in a spectral notch in a band of noise. The signal power necessary for detection was determined as a function of notch width. There were no significant differences in auditory filter widths between 10-year-olds and adults, but the auditory filter widths of 6-year-olds were about 30% larger than those of the two older groups, a difference that is much too small to account for the differences in masked thresholds between these age groups.

In the present experiment, we attempted to determine the size of the critical band with the classic paradigm used by Fletcher, modified, as required, for the limitations of young participants. In the classic measurement procedure, pure-tone thresholds are determined in a background of band-limited Gaussian noise. The bandwidth of the masker, but not its spectrum level, is increased systematically to observe how the bandwidth of the noise affects the threshold of the pure tone. For a constant-spectrum rectangular band of noise, the total power in the masker is proportional to the bandwidth. We would expect, therefore, that the threshold for the signal would continue to increase with increasing bandwidth, until the bandwidth matched or exceeded the critical band. Beyond that point, further increases in bandwidth should not affect tone threshold. The insert in the upper panel of Figure 1 shows how the threshold for a 0.8-kHz pure tone should vary as a function of the bandwidth of a constant spectrum level masker.

In our adaptation of this technique for infant participants, we used a two-alternative, forced-choice procedure (Bull et al., 1981; Schneider et al., 1989; Trehub et al., 1981) that we have used previously to determine masked thresholds in infants, children, and adults. We used a-octave bands of noise instead of pure tones to permit direct comparisons with these earlier studies and to reduce amplitude variation in the signal measured at different locations in the sound field (Dillon & Walker, 1982) while still retaining adequate frequency specificity. The infant or child sits in one corner of the test chamber

with age, the signal power required for threshold decreases proportionally. A number of studies (Bull et al., 1981; Nozza & Wilson, 1984; Schneider et al., 1989; Trehub et al., 1981) have shown that the masked threshold of infants is 8-15 dB higher than that of adults. If changes in masked threshold are to be accounted for by changes in critical band size, then the size of the critical band in infants should be 6 to 30 times as large as it is in adults.

Despite the importance of the concept of an auditory filter to a theory of auditory development, we know of only two attempts to measure its size in nonadult populations. Olsho (1985) used a visually reinforced head-turning technique to determine psychophysical tuning curves for infants. The listener's task in this procedure is to detect a low-level probe of fixed frequency and intensity when it is presented simultaneously with a masker tone of the same or different frequency (Chistovich, 1957; Small, 1959; Zwicker, 1974). The level of the masking tone is adjusted to determine the masker intensity at which the listener can no longer detect the probe tone. As the frequency separation between masker and probe increases, so does the masker intensity required to suppress the perception of the probe tone. The width of the resulting tuning curve is considered to be a behavioral measure of auditory filter width. Olsho (1985) found no substantial differences in the widths of the tuning curves for infants and adults, but infants were more susceptible to masking effects.

with a masking noise presented over loudspeakers to the left and right. During a trial, the test signal, a a-octave band of noise, is presented over one of the two loudspeakers, the signal remaining on until the infant or young child turns 45° to the right or left. Older children press one of two buttons to indicate the location of the sound. For all listeners, correct responses are reinforced visually with a toy located near the loudspeaker; incorrect responses result in a short intertrial delay. In the present experiment, four values of signal intensity were used at each of the eight bandwidths of a constant-spectrum masking noise to determine how threshold for the signal changes as a function of the bandwidth of the masking noise.

In line with the adult research, we expected that thresholds for the a-octave band signal would increase with masker bandwidth until the width of the masker reached a critical value, after which further increases in bandwidth would be ineffective in raising threshold. The theoretical value of the bandwidth at which this transition takes place should not be the same as that found for the masking of pure tones by narrow-band noises. We have illustrated the reasons for this in Figure 1 (lower panel), where we represent the signal as a rectangular, a-octave band centered on 0.8 kHz. The critical band for a 0.8-kHz pure tone is indicated by the dashed vertical lines in the upper panel. Note that some portion of the energy in the signal falls outside the critical band for a 0.8-kHz tone. Clearly, energy in a masker that falls outside the critical band centered on 0.8 kHz will be effective in masking this signal because a portion of the energy in the signal itself falls outside this bandwidth. If, on the other hand, we consider critical bands centered on the lower ($f1$) and upper ($f2$) cutoff frequencies for the a-octave band (indicated by the dashed vertical lines in the lower panel of Figure 1), then energy in the masker at frequencies to the left of the leftmost dashed line and to the right of the rightmost dashed line should be ineffective in masking the a-octave band. The lower cutoff frequency is given by $f1 - 0.5*\mathrm{CB}(f1)$ and the upper cutoff frequency by $f2 + 0.5*\mathrm{CB}(f2)$. By using tables of critical bandwidth as a function of frequency (Scharf, 1970), the effective upper and lower cutoff frequencies are calculated to be 647 and 973 Hz, respectively, for a a-octave band of noise centered at 0.8 kHz, for an effective critical bandwidth of 326 Hz. Similarly, the effective critical bandwidth for a 4-kHz, a-octave band of noise is calculated to be 1.62 kHz. Therefore, the threshold for a 0.8-kHz, a-octave band noise should no longer increase with masker bandwidth once the bandwidth exceeds 326 Hz. A similar pattern should hold for a 4-kHz, a-octave band signal, but with the transition from a rising to a constant threshold level occurring near 1.62 kHz. These theoretical calculations,

which represent an upper limit on expected critical band size, were used to evaluate the effectiveness of our procedure in measuring critical bands in adults and the relative sizes of critical bands in infants and children.[1]

METHOD

SUBJECTS

Infant and child participants were recruited primarily from letters sent to local families. Adult participants were university students who responded to posted notices. There were 733 participants; 270 were 6.5 months old (±1 month), 245 were 2 years old (±1 month), 109 were 5 years old (±3 months), and 109 were approximately 20.5 years old (17-25 years). All infants and children were healthy, born at term, had no history of ear infections, and were free of colds at the time of testing. Of the infants and children who were tested, 234 were excluded from the final sample because of failure to meet a training criterion (75 and 27 from the 6.5-month and 2-year group, respectively), 111 because of side biases (56 and 55 from the 6.5-month and 2-year group, respectively; and 21 because of fussing during the session (all from the 2-year group).

APPARATUS

The apparatus was identical to that used in Schneider et al. (1989). The a-octave signals were produced by filtering the output of a white noise generator (General Radio, model 1381) with a Bruel and Kjaer bandpass filter (model 1617). Third-octave bands were chosen as signals to provide good frequency specificity while still minimizing amplitude variation at different positions in the sound field (Dillon & Walker, 1982) and to keep testing conditions as close as possible to those in Schneider et al. (1989). The rate of decrease in energy on either side of the band was greater than 60 dB/octave. During signal presentation, the a-octave band was added to the background noise over one of the speakers.

The narrow-band background noise was produced by filtering an independent white noise generator (General Radio, model 1381) with a programmable Wavetek (System 716) bandpass filter. The rate of decrease in energy on either side of the band was 115 dB/octave. We set

---

[1]In calculating these theoretical bandwidths, we used Scharf's (1970) estimates of critical bandwidth and assumed that subjects were attending to critical bands centered on the cutoff frequencies of the noise signal. More effective listening strategies (see Discussion) or the use of smaller estimates of critical band size (see Green, 1988) would result in a smaller estimate of the theoretical bandwidth for these a-octave-noise signals. Thus these values of 326 Hz at 0.8 kHz and 1.62 kHz at 4 kHz should be considered upper boundaries on the effective size of the critical band.

the filter to a wideband (0.1 to 20 kHz) and used an equalizer (Altec-Lansing 729) to compensate for the acoustic properties of the sound-attenuating chamber so as to provide a background noise in the sound field with a relatively flat spectrum. Calibrations of this background noise showed that the sound pressure levels obtained at a-octave intervals for both left and right speakers were within 1.5 dB of the expected levels for white noise (see Figure 1 in Schneider et al., 1989). During a session, the upper and lower cutoff frequencies of the Wavetek filter were set to present the desired narrow-band noise (see Table 1). The spectrum level of the masking noise was set to 0 dB for the 6.5-month-olds and to 10 dB for the 2- and 5-year-olds and for adults. Electronic switches (rise/fall times = 40 ms) were used to turn the signals and maskers on and off.

The loudspeakers were placed in an Industrial Acoustics sound-attenuating chamber (double-wall, measuring 3 ˇ 2.8 ˇ 1.8 m) 1.8 m from the center of the listener's chair, which occupied one corner of the room. A chair for the experimenter was located in the corner opposite the listener's chair. Each loudspeaker was at a 45° angle to the listener's left and right. Below each loudspeaker was a four-chamber, smoked Plexiglas box with four different mechanical toys that served to reinforce correct responses. Adjacent to each loudspeaker was a portable color television set (Sony Trinitron, model KV-1911), which was also used for reinforcement during the second session for the 5-year-old children. The viewing screen was blacked out during the periods of nonreinforcement.

CALIBRATION

Sound pressure levels were calibrated with a Bruel and Kjaer impulse precision sound-level meter (model 2204) without the listener present but at the approximate location of the listener's head. Readings on the linear scale were taken with a 0.5-inch (1.3-cm) microphone directed at the loudspeaker producing the signal. Sound pressure measurements were taken within a 1-square-foot (approximately 0.1 m≈) area centered on the approximate location of a subject's ear for signals and maskers. Signal/masker ratios (in dB) were determined at the center of this 1-square-foot (0.1 m≈) area and at eight other points along the perimeter. The standard deviation of these signal/ masker ratios for both 0.8- and 4-kHz signals was ≤1 dB for all but the broadband masker, in which the standard deviation was about 1.6 dB. Thus, head movements in the younger subjects were unlikely to have exerted a significant effect on the results.

The signal levels used were determined on the basis of pilot testing and were the same for all bandwidths tested. They were 30, 38, 46, and 54 dB for both the 0.8- and 4-kHz signals for nonadult participants. Signal levels for adults were 16 dB lower than those for children at 0.8 kHz, and 12 dB lower than those for children at 4 kHz.

Table 1 shows both the nominal bandwidths used and their equivalent rectangular widths. Because the rate of attenuation on either side of the nominal cutoff frequencies was not infinite, the actual power in the band was greater than $N_0 (f2 - f1)$, where N_0 is the average power in a one-cycle wideband of noise and $f1$ and $f2$ are the nominal lower and upper cutoff frequencies of the band. Therefore, equivalent rectangular bandwidths were calculated. The equivalent rectangular bandwidth is the width of a hypothetical rectangular band of noise with the same gain at its center frequency as the actual band of noise, and whose total power is the same as the power in the noise band actually presented to the listeners. The equivalent rectangular bandwidths for the 0.8 and 4 kHz a-octave bands were 185 and 926 Hz, respectively.

Table 1. Nominal Bandwidths (NB) and Equivalent Rectangular Bandwidths (ERB) in Hz for Maskers Centered at 0.8 and 4 kHz.

0.8 kHz		4 kHz	
NB	ERB	NB	ERB
0	84	0	421
100	185	400	823
200	285	800	1224
300	385	1200	1625
400	486	1600	2027
600	686	2000	2428
800	887	2400	2829
9800	10370	9800	10370

Note. Upper and lower cutoff frequencies for all but the largest nominal bandwidth were symmetrically located above and below the signal frequency. The largest band at both frequencies had nominal cutoffs of 0.2 and 10 kHz.

PROCEDURE

During the test session, the 5-year-old children and the adults were seated in a test chair equipped with a push button on each arm. They were instructed to indicate their judgment of the location of the signal by pressing the button on the corresponding side; these responses were recorded automatically. For the 6.5-month-old infants and 2-year-old children, the parent sat in the test chair with the child on his or her lap, facing the experimenter. The required response was a head turn of 45° or greater, which the experimenter recorded by means of a hand-held push button. During the test session, the parent (if present) and the experimenter wore headphones with continuous broadband noise to prevent them from detecting the locus of the test signal.

A within-subjects design was used with four levels of signal intensity crossed with eight bandwidths of noise to yield 32 Signal Intensity ˜ Bandwidth combinations. We tested each of these 32 combinations for a single signal frequency within a single session. Whenever possible, we tested each subject in two sessions with signal frequency changed between sessions. Of the 6.5-month-olds, 70 completed both sessions, 37 completed only one session at 0.8 kHz, and 32 completed only one session at 4 kHz. Data were included for all subjects tested at a particular frequency. Of the 2-year-olds, 59 completed both sessions, 41 completed only one session at 0.8 kHz, and 42 completed only one session at 4 kHz. Of the 5-year-olds, 103 completed both sessions, 3 completed only one session at 0.8 kHz, and 3 completed only one session at 4 kHz. Of the adults, 102 completed both sessions and 7 completed only one session at 0.8 kHz. The center frequency of the signal (0.8 or 4 kHz) was changed across sessions.

Because there were only 32 trials per session, each listener experienced each level of Bandwidth ˜ Intensity combination only once in each session. A trial began with the simultaneous presentation of the narrow-band masker over the left and right loudspeakers. The experimenter presented a signal over one of the loudspeakers by pressing a button only when the masker was on and the child was looking directly ahead. Thus, the delay between masker onset and signal onset was variable and was determined by the subject's head orientation. The signal and masker remained on until the listener responded, either by a head-turn of at least 45°, in the case of younger children, or by a button press, in the case of older children and adults. Responses terminated the masker and signal, with correct responses resulting in reinforcement (the presentation of an animated toy) and incorrect responses producing a 4-s time-out before the beginning of the next trial.

To ensure that all of the infants and children tested could perform the task of identifying the location of the signal, we used a training criterion with sound intensity well above threshold. Initially, the signal (either a 0.8 or 4-kHz a-octave band noise) was presented at an intensity of 65 dB in the presence of a narrow-band masker (750 to 850 Hz for the 0.8-kHz signal and 3.8 to 4.2 kHz for the 4-kHz signal). The same narrow-band masker was used throughout training. During the training period, we alternated the location of the signal on successive trials between left and right loudspeakers until the child made four successive correct responses. We have found this alternation procedure to reduce side biases resulting from random selection of the sound location during the early training trials. (In no instance has this procedure generated a continuing strategy of response alternation in infants.) We then reduced the intensity by 10 dB and continued the alternation until the listener again made four successive correct responses. When this criterion was reached, the actual test series began. The training criterion for adults required only two successive correct responses at each training intensity.

The test phase, which consisted of 32 trials, immediately followed the training phase. Each trial consisted of a single instance of one of the masker bandwidths combined with one of the signal intensities. To preclude the occurrence of several successive instances of the lowest intensity, the stimuli were randomized as follows. Eight random permutations of the four intensity levels were generated (for each listener) so that all four intensity levels were represented in a block of four trials. The narrow-band masker associated with each of these intensity levels was randomly assigned (again for each subject), with the constraint that each masker appeared only once combined with a given intensity level. Assignment of signal to loudspeaker location was randomized with the constraints that an equal number of signals appeared on the left and right loudspeakers and that no more than three successive trials had signal presentation from the same side.

Listeners who showed an extreme side bias were eliminated from the final sample. The criterion for exclusion involved 11 or more errors during a session, with 75% or more of these errors occurring on a single side. All participants eliminated on the basis of side bias were from the 6.5-month and 2-year-old groups.

Note that, in this procedure, the bandwidth of the masker changed from trial to trial, requiring that the masker be turned on and off for each trial. In our previous masking studies (Bull et al., 1981; Schneider et al., 1989), the masker was on continuously during the entire session. Changing the masker was disruptive for the youngest participants, as indicated by their high failure rates in the training phase. For example, 27% of the 6.5-month-olds failed to meet our standard training criterion as compared with 19% of the 6.5-month-olds in the Schneider et al. (1989) experiment. Furthermore, 28% of the infants who met the training criterion in this study were subsequently eliminated because of side biases in the test phase as compared with 10% in the Schneider et al. (1989) experiment, again indicating that the younger listeners were experiencing some difficulty with the procedure. Nevertheless, 51% of the 6.5-month-olds and 58% of the 2-year-olds successfully completed the requisite test sessions.

RESULTS

In Figure 2, the percentage of correct responses is plotted as a function of the intensity of the 0.8-kHz signal for each of the eight bandwidths of the masker for the 6.5-month-olds and adults. (The bandwidths of the maskers are specified in terms of the equivalent rectangular bandwidths.) For both infants and adults, the psychometric functions were displaced to the right as bandwidth increased until it exceeded about 400 Hz, whereupon further increases in bandwidth produced no further shifts in

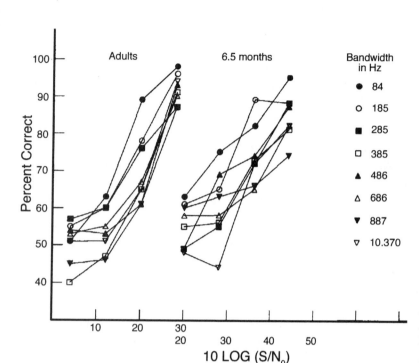

Figure 2. Percentage of correct responses as a function of intensity of 0.8-kHz signal for each of eight effective rectangular bandwidths for 6.5-month-olds and adults.

the psychometric functions. A similar pattern held at the other ages, as well as for all ages tested with the 4-kHz signal.

The psychometric functions were used to determine thresholds for both signal frequencies at each masker bandwidth for the four age groups. Threshold was defined as the intensity corresponding to 68% correct. We chose this value because at some of the larger bandwidths used with the 4-kHz signal, performance never reached 75% correct at the highest intensity values tested. Use of a 68% criterion permitted the threshold value to be determined by linear interpolation between the two intensities on either side of this point in all but two cases (5-year-olds: 4-kHz signal, masker bandwidth 10.4 kHz; adults: 4-kHz signal, masker bandwidth 2.8 kHz). Because the psychometric functions approached but did not reach 68% for these two cases, thresholds were defined as the highest stimulus intensity presented.

Figure 3 (lower right panel) shows how threshold changes as a function of masker bandwidth for adults tested with the 0.8-kHz signal. Figure 4 (lower right panel) plots the equivalent function for the 4-kHz signal. In each figure, the ordinate is the threshold signal-to-noise ratio (total signal power/N_0) expressed in dB. For the 0.8-kHz signal, a horizontal straight line was fit to threshold values for masker bandwidths larger than 326 Hz, the predicted upper limit for the critical band in this experiment. For bandwidths less than that value, a second straight line was fit to the data, with the constraint that the line must intersect the horizontal portion of the function at 326 Hz. A

similar procedure with a transition bandwidth of 1.62 kHz was used to fit a function to the data in Figure 4. The adult data in Figures 3 and 4 correspond quite closely to the expected pattern.

The data for the three younger age groups are also plotted along with the data from adults in Figures 3 and 4 for the 0.8- and 4-kHz signals, respectively. In both cases, horizontal lines were fit to the threshold values when maskers exceeded the predicted upper limit for the critical band. Straight lines intersecting these horizontal lines at the calculated critical bandwidth were fit to the threshold values for maskers less than the calculated critical widths. Although the data were more variable at the younger ages, these theoretical functions provide a good description of the manner in which thresholds change as a function of bandwidth. For maskers of less than critical width, thresholds increased with bandwidth at all ages and at both signal frequencies, with the exception of 6.5-month-olds at 4 kHz. For the 6.5-month-olds at 4 kHz, thresholds for subcritical bandwidths, although less than those for supracritical widths, did not increase systematically with bandwidth. Thresholds for supracritical widths were roughly constant for all ages at both signal frequencies.

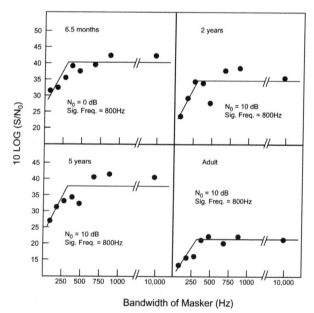

Figure 3. Thresholds at four different ages for 0.8-kHz signal as a function of effective rectangular banwidth of the masker.

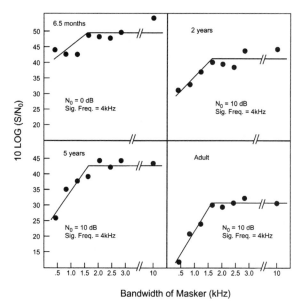

Figure 4. Thresholds at four different ages for 4-kHz signal as a function of effective rectangular banwidth of the masker.

DISCUSSION

SIZE OF THE CRITICAL BAND FOR a-OCTAVE BAND SIGNALS

Figures 3 and 4 show that signal threshold rises with masker bandwidth until the masker bandwidth exceeds the predicted upper limit for the critical band, after which no further increases in threshold are evident. The absence of further masking after the upper limit is exceeded confirms that energy in the masker that is spectrally remote from the signal is ineffective in masking the signal. It should be noted, however, that for subcritical masker bandwidths, threshold increases much more rapidly with bandwidth than one would expect if detection of the signal were based on a critical band centered on the signal[2] However, if subjects listen in critical bands above or below the center frequency of the signal, quite rapid increases in threshold with masker bandwidth are possible. To see why this would be the case, consider what happens when the bandwidth of the masker is less than the bandwidth of the signal. Figure 5 shows the spectral density functions for a rectangular masker (bandwidth = 84 Hz) and for a a-octave 0.8-kHz signal (bandwidth =

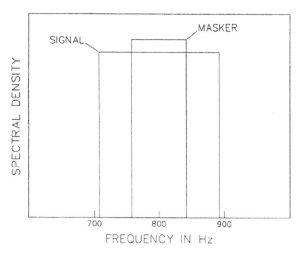

Figure 5. Spectral density functions for rectangular masker (bandwidth = 84 Hz) and for rectangular a-octave 0.8-kHz signal (band width = 185 Hz).

185 Hz). Note that a considerable portion of the energy in the signal falls outside of the masker bandwidth. Imagine a rectangular critical band whose upper frequency is set to the lower edge of the masker. Such a critical band would not be affected by the energy in the masker because all of the energy in the masker is at frequencies above the range of this critical band. Therefore, as long as the energy in the signal falling within this critical band exceeded that required for absolute threshold, detection would occur. Figure 6 (upper panel) plots the signal-to-noise ratio required for detection within this critical band as a function of the bandwidth of the masker for widths up to 185 Hz.[3] Above 185 Hz, it is assumed that the signal-to-noise ratio required for detection is constant, an assumption consistent with a critical band whose width is less than that of a-octave signal. Note that below a masker bandwidth of 185 Hz (the width of the signal), the function rises steeply with bandwidth, much more steeply than the actual data points plotted in this figure.

....

[2]Assume a masker whose bandwidth was identical to the critical band. If we reduce the masker bandwidth by half, we reduce the power in the critical band by 3 dB, which, in turn, should lower the threshold for the signal by 3 dB. If the effective bandwidth is 326 Hz in Figure 3, then signal threshold for a masker bandwidth of 163 Hz should be reduced by 3 dB. Similarly, signal threshold for a masker whose width is 81.5 Hz should be 6 dB lower than for a broadband masker. In Figure 3, however, the threshold for an 81.5-Hz band is considerably more than 6 dB lower than that for a broadband noise.

[3]At 0.8 kHz, the ideal a-octave filter is a rectangular band of energy whose width is 185 Hz (713-898 Hz). Assume an 84-Hz rectangular masker centered at 0.8 kHz. Assume, further, a critical band whose upper boundary occurs at 758 Hz. None of the energy in the masker falls within this critical band, but $(758 - 713)/185 = 9/37$ of the energy in the a-octave signal falls within this band. Let y dB SPL be the threshold value for a pure tone centered in this band. It follows that the sound pressure for a a-octave band of noise (centered at 0.8 kHz) would have to be $y + 10*\log(37/9)$ dB to ensure that the energy from the signal falling into this critical band reached threshold. (We assume here that a narrow-band noise exactly filling the critical band would be at threshold when its power equals the power in a pure tone at threshold.) In general, the intensity required for threshold for the a-octave band noise would be $y + 10* \log(185/800 - MBW/2 - 713)$, where y is the threshold for a pure tone centered in a critical band whose upper boundary is $800 - MBW/2$ Hz, where MBW is the bandwidth of the masker. Note that this model represents the ideal situation for ideal (i.e., rectangular) signals and noise. Pure-tone thresholds in the sound field were taken from Robinson and Whittle (1964).

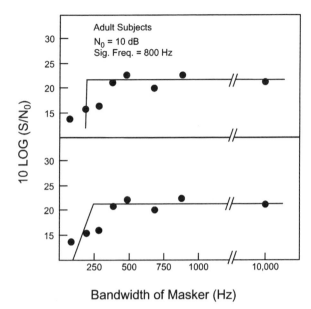

Figure 6. *Upper panel.* Predicted threshold for a-octave 0.8-kHz signal in a model that assumes the subject listens at a critical band situated just below the lower bandwidth of the masker (see text). (Predicted threshold assumes rectangular bandwidths for both maskers and signals.) *Lower panel.* Predicted threshold for a-octave 0.8-kHz signal in a model that assumes the subject listens at a critical band sufficiently remote from the masker that any residual energy from the masker falling in that critical band is ineffective at masking a signal centered in that band (see text). (Actual spectral density functions for the signals and maskers were used in calculating this model. Data points are adult thresholds from this condition.)

Figure 6 shows that off-frequency listening should produce a sharp rise in threshold as the bandwidth of the masker approaches the bandwidth of the a-octave signal. One reason why the predicted rise in threshold is much steeper than the actual rise (see Figures 3 & 4) is due to the fact that our masker and signal bands are not really rectangular. Figure 7 plots the actual spectral density functions for the 0.8 kHz, a-octave band signal and for two bandwidths of masker (nominal bandwidths of 0 and

100 Hz). Note that if the upper edge of the critical band is placed on the nominal lower cutoff frequency in the masker, some of the energy in the masker will fall into that critical band. Therefore the energy in the signal falling within this critical band will be partially masked by the energy in the masker that also falls within this band. The upper edge of the critical band, however, can be progressively lowered until the amount of energy in the critical band due to the masker is decreased to the point at which it is no longer an effective masker. In plotting the predicted function in the lower panel of Figure 6, we located the critical band so that the energy falling within it from the masker is just below threshold for effective masking.[4] We then adjusted the intensity of the a-octave signal so that the amount of energy from the signal falling within that critical band was just at absolute threshold. The signal intensity (in terms of signal-to-noise ratio) that would produce a threshold response in this critical band is shown in the lower panel of Figure 6 along with the actual data points for that experiment. A comparison of upper and lower panels shows that the nonrectangular nature of the actual bandwidths will affect the rate at which the threshold for the signal increases with bandwidth. Moreover, the actual rate of increase with bandwidth will be affected by random noise in the system and may not be as steep as the theoretical calculations in Figure 6 would indicate.

Figure 6 shows that off-frequency listening will produce rapid increases in masked threshold until the bandwidth of the masker exceeds the bandwidth of the signal.[5] If the size of the critical band is less than the bandwidth of the signal, then no further masking should occur once

---

[4] It is generally assumed that energy in a critical band is no longer effective in masking a pure tone at its center when the total energy from the masker falling into that critical band is less than or equal to the energy of a threshold pure tone at the center of the band. In deriving the predicted function in the lower panel of Figure 6, for each masker bandwidth, we searched for the critical band such that the energy falling in that critical band from the masker just equaled the threshold energy for a pure tone in the center of that band. A linear interpolation applied to the data of Robinson and Whittle (1964) was used to determine the threshold value for a pure tone at the center of the band. A linear interpolation of the data from Scharf (1970) was used to determine the bandwidth of the critical band in that frequency region. The spectral density functions of Figure 7 were used to determine the amount of energy falling into that critical band from both the signal and the masker. The predicted threshold for the a-octave signal was taken to be $y + 10*\log(x/z)$, where y is the estimated threshold value for the pure tone at the center of the critical band, x is the total energy in the a-octave signal, and z is the energy in the a-octave signal between f_l and f_u, where f_l and f_u are the lower and upper boundaries of the critical band. This predicted function is shown in the lower panel of Figure 6. The predicted function for the 4-kHz a-octave signal provided a better fit to the 4-kHz data than did the predicted function for the 0.8-kHz data.

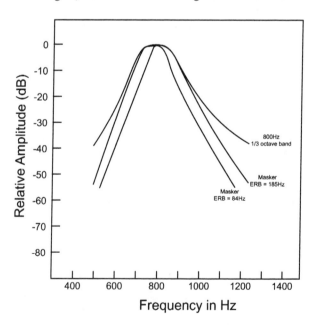

Figure 7. Spectral density for a-octave, 0.8-kHz signal and for two maskers with nominal bandwidths of 0 and 100 Hz.

the bandwidth of the masker exceeds the bandwidth of the signal. The obtained functions for adults indicate, however, that the effective size of the critical band is larger than the bandwidth of the a-octave signal but does not exceed the upper boundary suggested by the arguments presented in the introduction. Therefore, energy within half a critical bandwidth of the upper and lower cutoff frequencies of a-octave signals appears to be effective in masking those signals; energy falling outside of this region is ineffective.

DEVELOPMENTAL CHANGES IN CRITICAL BAND SIZE

In Figures 3 and 4, the same values for the effective critical band were used to derive the straight-line functions fit to the data. An examination of Figures 3 and 4 reveals that the fit of the functions to the data is not as good for infants and children as it is for adults. At 4 kHz, the intersecting straight-line functions account for 49%, 82%, 90%, and 98% of the variance in thresholds for the 6.5-month-old, 2-year-old, 5-year-old, and adult participants, respectively. At 0.8 kHz, the same pattern holds in that the function accounts for a greater proportion of the variance in the adult data (73%, 59%, 59%, and 77% of the variance for 6.5-month-old, 2-year-old, 5-year-old, and adult participants, respectively). The better fit for adults might arise because their performance is less variable than that of infants and children or because the effective critical band is larger in children than in adults.

We evaluated the latter possibility in two ways. First, by visual inspection of Figures 3 and 4, we attempted to pinpoint the exact bandwidth at which there is no further increase in thresholds for the younger listeners. An examination of Figure 3 shows no clear evidence of further increases in threshold as bandwidth increases beyond 500 Hz. This impression was confirmed by determining the best-fitting two-part functions to the data in Figure 3. The two-part function consisted of a linear ramp that ended at the effective critical bandwidth and a horizontal section that continued beyond that bandwidth. The value of the effective critical bandwidth was varied systematically until a value was found for which the sum of squared deviations of the data points from the function was at a minimum. The largest best-fitting effective critical band was 485 Hz for 5-year-olds. Thus, a least-squares analysis supports the visual impression that thresholds are independent of bandwidth for masker bandwidths greater

than 500 Hz. If we assume that 500 Hz is an upper boundary on the effective critical band for the younger age groups, then the effective critical band for the younger ages is no more than 54% larger than the effective critical band of adults.

Visual inspection of Figure 4 indicates that there are no further increases in threshold beyond 2 kHz at any age. The transition points for the best-fitting functions for all but the 6.5-month-olds are less than 2 kHz. (The best-fitting function for the 6.5-month-olds has a maximum of 2.4 kHz, which can be attributed to the fact that the thresholds for the first three bandwidths do not increase with bandwidth.) Thus, results at this frequency indicate that, for children 2 years and older, the size of the effective critical band is, at most, 50% larger than it is for adults.

Perhaps developmental changes in the size of the critical band depend, in part, on certain features of our measurement procedure, which requires judgments of localization as opposed to detection. It is possible, in principle, for detection and localization thresholds to differ and for the extent of such differences to depend on the age of the listener and the frequency of the signal. Trehub and Schneider (1987) demonstrated, however, that in a quiet background, listeners 1, 3, 5, and 20 years of age localized, in a two-loudspeaker localization task, all stimuli that they could detect in a single-loudspeaker detection task. Moreover, there were no interactions between frequency (0.4 and 10 kHz) and type of task (detection or localization). Schneider et al. (1989) have reported similar findings for the localization of octave-band signals in broadband noise. Thus the available data suggest that, for band-limited noise, detection and localization thresholds are comparable, and are independent of stimulus frequency.

Because the signals in the present experiment occurred in the context of identical broadband maskers presented over loudspeakers on each side of the listener, it is possible that there was some degree of binaural unmasking. Two factors suggest, however, that the contribution of unmasking to the observed developmental changes would be negligible. First, very little unmasking occurs when the spectrum level of the masker is as low as in the present experiment (see Durlach & Colburn, 1978, p. 437). Second, Nozza (1987) and Schneider, Bull, & Trehub (1988) have shown that binaural unmasking occurs in infants, but to a lesser extent than in adults. Thus, even with some unmasking, the adult-infant difference attributable to this factor would be of little consequence.

The present results are consistent with the findings of Olsho (1985) and Irwin et al. (1986) in indicating that the width of the critical band changes very little from infancy to adulthood. If this is true, then how do we account for the higher masked thresholds in children compared with adults? Even if we assume that the in-

---

[5]Given off-frequency listening, we would not expect our measure of the critical band to be smaller than the width of the a-octave signal. Thus, even though other investigators (see Green, 1988, for a summary) have arrived at critical bands less than half those suggested by Scharf (1970) in situations that are similar to ours, our data cannot address this issue.

fant's critical band is 50% larger than that of the adult, this increase in the critical band size should result in a mere 1.75-dB increase in threshold. In the present experiment, however, as in others (Bull et al., 1981; Irwin et al., 1986; Nozza & Wilson, 1984; Olsho, 1985; Schneider et al., 1989; Trehub et al., 1981), the child-adult difference in masked thresholds is on the order of 8-15 dB. Clearly, changes in critical band size can account for no more than 1-2 dB of this difference.

Schneider et al. (1989) argue that the most likely source of these developmental changes is a nonlinear change in the representation of intensity, given that the size of the critical band does not change substantially with age. Their argument is based on the following observations. First, linear changes at any stage in the auditory processing chain cannot account for changes in masked threshold. For example, consider a simple change in the mechanical efficiency with which signals are delivered to the basilar membrane. If the efficiency, say, of the outer and middle ear improves by 10 dB from childhood to adulthood, this improvement would not change the signal-to-noise ratio in a masking experiment because the improved efficiency would enhance both signal and noise by the same amount. Because masked thresholds have been shown to depend only on the signal-to-noise ratio for moderate to high levels of the masker, one can conclude that linear changes in sensitivity could not affect masked threshold because such changes leave the signal-to-noise ratio unchanged.

Child-adult differences could also be due to differential motivation and attention. However, differential attention should affect not only the threshold but also the slopes of the psychometric functions. But Schneider et al. (1989) found no differences in the slopes of the psychometric functions between children over 1 year of age and adults. This finding, in conjunction with the fact that highly motivated older children could not match adult performance, suggests that attention and motivation cannot account for much of this adult-child difference.

If linear changes in sensitivity, motivational and attentional factors, and changes in critical band size do not account for the observed differences in masked threshold, then the source of the differences must lie in nonlinear changes in signal processing. Because the peripheral auditory system is essentially linear, the locus of these nonlinear changes is likely to be found in more central processes. It would be of considerable interest to explore the nature of these changes and their relation to maturational changes in the nervous system.

REFERENCES

Bull, D., Schneider, B.A., & Trehub, S.E. (1981). The masking of octave-band noise by broad-spectrum noise: A comparison of infant and adult thresholds. *Perception & Psychophysics, 30,* 101-106.

Chistovich, L. (1957). Frequency characteristics of the masking effect. *Biofizika, 2,* 714-725.

Dillon, H., & Walker, G. (1982). Comparison of stimuli used in sound field audiometric testing. *Journal of the Acoustical Society of America, 71,* 161- 172.

Durlach, N.I., & Colburn, H.S. (1978). Binaural phenomena. In E.C. Carterette & M.P. Friedman (Eds.), *Handbook of perception: Vol. IV. Hearing* (pp. 365-466). Orlando, FL: Academic Press.

Fletcher, H. (1940). Auditory patterns. *Review of Modern Physics, 12,* 47-65.

Green, D.M. (1988). Audition: Psychophysics and perception. In R.C. Atkinson, R.J. Hernstein, G. Lindzey, & R.D. Luce (Eds.), *Stevens' handbook of experimental psychology: Vol. 1* (2nd ed., pp. 327-376). New York: Wiley.

Greenwood, D.D. (1961). Auditory masking and the critical band. *Journal of the Acoustical Society of America, 33,* 484-502.

Irwin, R.J., Stillman, J.A., & Schade, A. (1986). The width of the auditory filter in children. *Journal of Experimental Child Psychology, 41,* 429-442.

Moore, B.C.J. (1982). *An introduction to the psychology of hearing* (2nd ed.). Orlando, FL: Academic Press.

Nozza, R.J. (1987). The binaural masking level difference in infants and adults: Developmental changes in binaural hearing. *Infant Behavior and Development, 10,* 105-110.

Nozza, R.J., & Wilson, W.R. (1984). Masked and unmasked pure-tone thresholds of infants and adults: Development of auditory frequency selectivity and sensitivity. *Journal of Speech and Hearing Research, 27,* 613-622.

Olsho, L.W. (1985). Infant auditory perception: Tonal masking. *Infant Behavior and Development, 8,* 371-384.

Robinson, D.W., & Whittle, L.S. (1964). The loudness of octave bands of noise. *Acustica, 14,* 24-25.

Schafer, T.H., Gales, R.S., Shewmaker, C.S., & Thompson, P.O. (1950). The frequency selectivity of the ear as determined by masking experiments. *Journal of the Acoustical Society of America, 22,* 490-496.

Scharf, B. (1970). Critical bands. In J.V. Tobias (Ed.), *Foundations of modern auditory theory* (Vol. 1, pp. 157-202). Orlando, FL: Academic Press.

Schneider, B., Bull, E., & Trehub, S.E. (1988). Binaural unmasking in infants. *Journal of the Acoustical Society of America, 83,* 1124-1132.

Schneider, B.A., & Trehub, S.E. (1985). Behavioral assessment of basic auditory abilities. In S.E. Trehub & B.A. Schneider (Eds.), *Auditory development in infancy* (pp. 104-114). New York: Plenum Press.

Schneider, B.A., Trehub, S.E., Morrongiello, B.A., & Thorpe, L.A. (1989). Developmental changes in masked thresholds. *Journal of the Acoustical Society of America, 86,* 1733-1742.

Small, A. (1959). Pure-tone masking. *Journal of the Acoustical Society of America, 31,* 1619-1625.

Swets, J.A., Green, D.M., & Tanner, W.P. (1962). On the width of critical bands. *Journal of the Acoustical Society of America, 34,* 108-113.

Trehub, S.E., Bull, D., & Schneider, B.A. (1981). Infants' detection of speech in noise. *Journal of Speech and Hearing Research,* 24, 202-206.

Trehub, S.E., & Schneider, B.A. (1987). Problems and promises of developmental psychophysics: Throw out the bath water but keep the baby. In M. Teghtsoonian & R. Teghtsoonian (Eds.), *Fechner Day 87* (pp. 43-47). Northampton, MA: International Society for Psychophysics.

Zwicker, E. (1974). On a psychophysical equivalent of tuning curves. In E. Zwicker and E. Terhardt (Eds.), *Facts and models in hearing* (pp. 132-141). Berlin, Federal Republic of Germany: Springer.

Received October 4, 1988
Revision received June 16, 1989
Accepted July 19, 1989

Infant Auditory Temporal Acuity: Gap Detection

Lynne A. Werner and G. Cameron Marean
University of Washington

Christopher F. Halpin
University of Virginia

Nancy Benson Spetner and Jay M. Gillenwater
University of Washington

Werner, Lynne A.; Marean, G. Cameron; Halpin, Christopher F.; Spetner, Nancy Benson; and Gillenwater, Jay M. Infant Auditory Temporal Acuity: Gap Detection. Child Development, 1992, 63, 260-272. The development of auditory temporal acuity during infancy was examined in 3-, 6-, and 12-month-old infants and in adults using the gap detection paradigm. Listeners detected a series of gaps, or silent intervals, of variable duration in a broadband noise. In order to vary the acoustic frequencies available to the listener, a high-pass noise was used to mask frequencies above specified cutoffs. High-pass maskers with cutoffs of 500, 2,000, and 8,000 Hz were used. The minimum detectable gap was determined using the Observer-based Psychoacoustic Procedure. The thresholds of 3- and 6-month-olds were considerably poorer than those of the adults, although the effect of masker condition was about the same for these 3 groups. The thresholds of 12-month-olds were significantly worse than the adults when the stimulus was unmasked or when the masker cutoff frequency was 2,000 or 8,000 Hz. When the masker cutoff frequency was 500 Hz, 12-month-olds fell into 2 groups: some had gap thresholds that were about the same as 3- and 6-month-olds, while some had gap thresholds that approached those of adults. In a second experiment, a larger group of 12-month-olds were tested with a 500-Hz masker cutoff. Average performance of 12-month-olds was about the same as that of 3- and 6-month-olds in Experiment 1. Some infants attained thresholds close to those of adults. Thus, gap detection thresholds are quite poor in infants, although the similarity of the effect of frequency on performance in infants and adults suggests that the mechanisms governing temporal resolution in infants operate qualitatively like those in adults.

Temporal cues have frequently been shown to be critical to both human and nonhuman communication (e.g., Gottlieb, 1985; Pisoni, 1977). Moreover, a relation between temporal acuity and the ability to understand speech has been demonstrated among human listeners (e.g., Dreschler & Plomp, 1980). The few studies examining the development of temporal acuity suggest that immaturity of this capacity may even persist into childhood. Davis and McCroskey (1980) determined the duration of a silent interval between two tone bursts required for children to report hearing two sounds rather than one sound. The threshold duration decreased progressively between 3 and 11 years. A similar age effect was observed for all tone frequencies and intensities. Irwin, Ball, Kay, Stillman, and Rosser (1985) measured gap detection threshold, or the minimally detectable silent interval in a continuous sound, for children and adults. They found that 6-year-olds had higher gap detection thresholds than older children or adults. This effect was more pronounced at lower intensities and when a low-frequency noise band was the stimulus. In contrast, Wightman, Allen, Dolan, Kistler, and Jamieson (1989) found that 6-year-olds were adultlike in gap detection at both 400 and 2,000 Hz. These investigators reported that 3-year-olds were poorer than adults in gap detection at both frequencies; however, they were also able to simulate the thresholds of these children by assuming that the children were inattentive on a high proportion of trials. Thus, whether temporal resolution is mature among preschool and school age children is not clear.

Morrongiello and Trehub (1987) have published the only developmental study of temporal resolution that included infant subjects. They found that adults responded to a smaller change in the duration of a repeated noise burst than did 5.5-year-old children, who in turn respond-

Preliminary report of these data was made at the Midwinter Meeting of the Association for Research in Otolaryngology, Clearwater Beach, FL, February 1986. Requests for reprints should be addressed to L.A. Werner, CDMRC, WJ-10, Box 47, University of Washington, Seattle, WA 98195. This research was supported by NIH grant DC00396 to L.A. Werner. C. Halpin's current address is: Massachusetts Eye and Ear Infirmary, Audiology Dept., 243 Charles St., Boston, MA 02114. N. Spetner's current address is: AT&T Bell Laboratories, Rm. 2D-602A, Crawfords Corner Road, Holmdel, NJ 07733-1988.

ed to smaller changes in duration than did 6-month-old infants. While these age differences may result from differences in temporal acuity, one cannot dismiss the possibility that they result from immaturity of performance factors (e.g., attention) not directly related to the auditory system.

The purpose of the current study was to assess temporal acuity among human infants. A gap detection technique, similar to that employed in earlier studies (e.g., Fitzgibbons & Wightman, 1982; Irwin et al., 1985; Irwin, Hinchcliffe, & Kemp, 1981) was used. Because several studies of infants in our own as well as other laboratories suggest that the rate of auditory development depends on sound frequency (e.g., Olsho, 1984; Olsho, Koch, Carter, Halpin, & Spetner, 1988; Olsho, Koch, & Halpin, 1987; Schneider, Trehub, & Bull, 1980; Sinnott, Pisoni, & Aslin, 1983; Trehub, Schneider, & Endman, 1980), the effect of frequency on the development of temporal processing was of particular interest.

The manipulation of stimulus frequency in the gap detection paradigm is not a trivial problem. A pure tone is the most frequency specific sound that might be used. The most straightforward way to introduce a gap of known duration into a sound is to abruptly switch the sound off and on again. However, this abrupt switching creates spectral "splatter" (i.e., the spectrum of the stimulus will contain energy at a range of frequencies around that of the original pure tone). While use of a narrow band of noise rather than a pure tone alleviates this problem to some extent, it does not eliminate it. Furthermore, the waveform of a noise band has pronounced variations in amplitude that may be confused with a gap. The frequency and extent of such amplitude variations are related to the bandwidth of the stimulus and, hence, usually to the stimulus frequency. Thus, one explanation for the pronounced age difference in gap detection of low frequency noise bands observed by Irwin et al. (1985) is that younger children were more easily confused by these "dips" in the waveform than were older listeners.

In the current study, an interrupted broadband noise was the stimulus in all conditions. The duration of the interruption, or gap, was varied to determine gap detection threshold. Frequency was manipulated by varying the low-frequency cutoff of a continuous high-pass masking noise presented simultaneously with the interrupted stimulus. A broadband noise contains energy over the entire range of audible frequencies. When gaps are introduced in a broadband noise, the listener can use information in any frequency region to detect the gaps. A high-pass noise contains only frequencies above its low-frequency cutoff. With such a noise presented at a sufficiently high intensity, the portion of the broadband stimulus above the cutoff of the masker would be inaudible. Only those frequencies

below the cutoff would be available for detecting gaps in the broadband stimulus. While this stimulus configuration avoids the problems inherent in the use of noise bands, it confounds frequency with bandwidth. In other words, as the cutoff frequency of the masker is increased, the bandwidth of the stimulus that can be used to detect gaps also increases. Shailer and Moore (1983, 1985) have shown, however, that in the range of bandwidths used here, the effects of bandwidth are minimal compared to the effects of stimulus frequency for adult listeners.

EXPERIMENT 1

Method

Subjects. The infant subjects were 17 3-month-olds, 19 6-month-olds, and 14 12-month-olds. These subjects provided 86 acceptable data sets. An additional 84 sessions were attempted but excluded for the following reasons: training criterion not met (21); insufficient data (7); false alarm rate too high (51); psychometric function slope not greater than zero (5). About half of the excluded sessions were from the infants who eventually contributed thresholds to the final data set. The rest were from seven 3-month-olds, nine 6-month-olds, and eight 12-month-olds who never provided usable data, typically because they did not return for testing after the first or second session. All subjects met the following criteria for inclusion: (1) fullterm gestation and normal pre-, peri-, and postnatal developmental course; (2) no history of hearing dysfunction and no family history of congenital hearing loss; (3) no occurrence of middle ear infections within 2 weeks of testing and no more than 2 prior occurrences of middle ear problems. All infants completed testing within 2 weeks of the age given.

Eleven 20-30-year-olds were the adult subjects. All were undergraduate or graduate students. All reported normal hearing and no history of hearing dysfunction. None of the adult subjects had prior experience listening in psychophysical or other auditory experiments. Adults were tested in two sessions; one of the adult subjects completed only one session.

Data with respect to subject race, gender, and socioeconomic status were not systematically collected.

Stimuli and apparatus. Two independent noise generators (Coulbourn S81-02) were used to produce the stimulus and masker. The stimulus noise was presented at a spectrum level[1] of 30 dB SPL. Gaps were created in the noise by gating the stimulus off and on with a rise/fall time less than 1 ms. Gap duration could be varied between 0 and 125 ms in 1-ms steps. A series of 10 gaps, each gap followed by 500 ms of noise, constituted a "signal" trial. Using this rather long "intergap interval" ensured that subjects could not use changes in the overall loudness of the stimulus to detect gaps. Although this procedure meant that trial duration changed as gap duration changed, once gap duration reached near threshold values, the resulting change in duration would be negligible.

The masker noise was high-pass filtered with cutoffs of 500, 2,000, or 8,000 Hz (i.e., frequencies above the cutoff were passed by the filter, while frequencies below the cutoff were not). These frequencies would be expected to result in different levels of performance in adults, and they represent frequencies where infants perform differentially relative to adults in other tasks (e.g., Olsho, 1984; Olsho, Koch, & Halpin, 1987; Olsho et al., 1988; Schneider et al., 1980; Sinnott et al., 1983; Trehub et al., 1980). Two Krohn-Hite 3343 filters in series were used to achieve a nominal filter slope of 96 dB/oct.≈ The masker level, 35 dB pressure spectrum level, was chosen so that when the unfiltered masker noise was presented simultaneously with the interrupted stimulus, no gaps were detected by a panel of adult pilot subjects. The same spectrum level of the masker was then maintained in all conditions. The stimulus, and, in masked conditions, the masker were turned on at the beginning of the session and, except for the gaps during signal trials, remained on throughout the session.

A Sony E222 earphone was used to deliver sounds to all listeners. The frequency response of this earphone was relatively flat (i.e., it produced the same intensity) to about 6,000 Hz, with a gradual roll-off at higher frequencies. An equalizer was used to ensure that the spectrum of the noise delivered by the earphone was flat (±2 dB) to about 10,000 Hz. Calibrations were performed in a 6-cc coupler (meant to approximate the volume of the external ear) using a Hewlett Packard 3521A spectrum analyzer and routinely checked with a Bruel & Kjaer 2215 sound level meter (see Olsho et al., 1988, for details). The diameter of the earphone is approximately fi inch; it was placed in a foam cushion and held at the entrance to the ear canal with micropore tape. By taping the earphone cord to the back of the infant's shirt to reduce tension on the cord, we were generally able to maintain a stable earphone position throughout a session.

---

[1]Spectrum level is defined as the average intensity of sound in a 1-Hz band.

[2]The filter slope specifies the degree to which frequencies falling beyond the cutoff of the filter are attenuated. A filter slope of 96 dB/octave, for example, would mean that a frequency 1 octave below the filter cutoff would be attenuated by 96 dB relative to the cutoff frequency. The degree of attenuation provided by the filter may not actually be achieved since the noise level in the sound generation system can be higher than the level achieved by the filter; hence, the "nominal" filter slope is typically given.

Testing was conducted in a single-walled, sound-attenuating booth (IAC). The infant sat on a parent's lap, facing a window into an adjacent control room and a video camera in the test booth. There was a table directly in front of the parent and infant. An assistant was seated to the infant's left, and a smoked Plexiglas box containing lights and a mechanical toy, the "visual reinforcer," was placed to the infant's right at infant eye level.

Procedure. Infants were tested using the Observer-based Psychoacoustic Procedure (Olsho, Koch, Halpin, & Carter, 1987). In this procedure, an observer, blind to trial type, uses the infant's behavior on each trial to decide whether a signal or no-signal trial has occurred. In the current experiment, a signal trial was defined as a trial on which gaps were presented; a no-signal trial was a period of equal duration during which the stimulus was continuous.

The infant was seated on a parent's lap in the test booth, and the earphone was placed on the infant's right ear. An assistant was seated to the infant's left and manipulated toys to maintain the infant in a quiet, attentive state, facing forward. The parent and the assistant listened to masking sounds presented over circumaural headsets to prevent them from hearing the stimuli presented to the infant and inadvertently influencing the infant's responses. The parent heard music; the assistant monitored activity in the control room.

The observer watched the infant from the control room, either through the window or over a video monitor. The noise stimulus was presented continuously from the beginning of the session. The observer began a trial when the infant was quiet and attending at midline. Signal trials were presented to the infant with a probability of 0.65. A flashing LED indicated to the observer that a trial was in progress, but the observer did not know whether a signal (gap) or no-signal (continuous noise) trial was being presented. The observer used the infant's behavior to decide whether a signal or no-signal trial had been presented, and received feedback after each trial.

Each test session consisted of two phases, training and testing. During training, the duration of the gaps on signal trials was fixed at 100 ms. If the observer judged that a signal had occurred on a signal trial, the visual reinforcer was activated as soon as the observer recorded the judgment and continued for 4 sec after the end of the trial. If the observer judged that no signal had occurred on a signal trial, the reinforcer was activated for 4 sec at the end of the trial, and an error was scored. If the observer judged that no signal had occurred on a no-signal trial, a correct rejection was scored, and if the observer judged that a signal had occurred on a no-signal trial, an error (false alarm) was scored. In no case was the reinforcer activated during or after a no-signal trial. The purpose of this procedure was to encourage the infant to respond to the gaps in anticipation of the onset of the reinforcer. The observer could then use whatever response the infant made (e.g., head turning, eye widening, cessation of activity) as the basis of his or her judgment on each trial. The training phase continued until the observer had reached a criterion of four of the last five signal trials correct and four of the last five no-signal trials correct.

During the testing phase, the visual reinforcer was activated only when the observer judged that a signal had occurred when a signal trial had actually been presented. Gap duration was varied to estimate a threshold, following PEST rules (Taylor & Creelman, 1967; Spetner & Olsho, 1990, describe the threshold estimation procedure in detail). Briefly, these rules specify that if the observer is correct at a given gap duration, the gap should be made shorter, while if the observer is incorrect at a gap duration, the gap should be made longer. When the observer goes from being correct to being incorrect as the gap duration is changed (i.e., a reversal occurs), then the amount by which the gap duration changes (the step size) is halved. The effect is to generate a binary search for the threshold. In the current experiment, the observer was considered correct at a given gap duration if at least three of the last four signal trials at that duration were correct. The observer was considered incorrect if fewer than three of the last four signal trials at a given duration were correct. The observer was required to maintain a false alarm rate below 0.25 during testing. Testing was continued until 50 signal trials had been presented, or until the observer's false alarm rate exceeded 0.25, or until the infant's state precluded further testing. A typical test run lasted 20 min. An example of an infant test protocol is shown in Figure 1.

Thresholds were estimated as the gap duration at which the observer said "signal" 70% of the time. This duration was estimated by taking the proportion of "signal" judgments at each gap duration presented to an individual infant in a given condition and fitting a psychometric function to those data points using probit analysis (Finney, 1970). The fit of the function was assessed using a maximum likelihood criterion (Hall, 1968, 1981). The threshold for a session was used only if at least 30 signal trials were obtained, the false alarm rate did not exceed 0.25, and the slope of the best-fitting function was greater than zero. If a session was excluded, thresholds were obtained in subsequent visits if possible. If a condition was repeated, the entire training and testing procedure was completed on the return visit.

Adult thresholds were obtained using the same general procedure, except that the adults listened alone in the test booth and were asked to raise their hands when they heard gaps in the noise. An observer in the control booth recorded responses, and the reinforcer was activated as feedback to the adult following the same contingencies used in infant testing.

An attempt was made to test each subject under four conditions: no masker, high-pass masker with 500-Hz cutoff, high-pass masker with 2,000-Hz cutoff, and high-pass masker with 8,000-Hz cutoff. Thresholds in these four conditions were obtained in random order. All adults were able to complete the four thresholds within two 1-hour sessions. Infants were rescheduled as many times as possible to obtain four thresholds. However, only a few infants actually provided data in all four conditions; at least six infants at each age provided thresholds in each condition. The number of thresholds obtained in each condition are listed in Table 1.

RESULTS

The average gap detection threshold in each masking condition for listeners of various ages is shown in

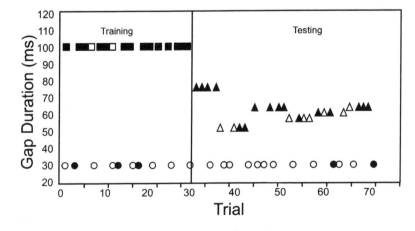

Figure 1. Example of a trial-by-trial protocol for a 12-month-old tested in the 8,000-Hz masker cutoff condition. Filled symbols represent trials on which the observer responded "signal"; circles are no-signal trials; squares are training signal trials; triangles are testing signal trials.

Figure 2. When adults were forced to use frequencies below 500 Hz to detect gaps, their gap detection thresholds averaged about 16 ms. Adult thresholds improved to about 5 ms when frequencies as high as 8,000 Hz were available. These average thresholds are consistent with those typically reported for adults (e.g., Fitzgibbons & Wightman, 1982; Irwin et al., 1981), and the improvement in performance with frequency has also been well documented in adults (e.g., Buus & Florentine, 1982; Fitzgibbons, 1983; Shailer & Moore, 1985).

Several aspects of infant performance are noteworthy. First, it is apparent that, in general, the infants do not perform as well as the adults do. Although that fact in itself is not startling, the size of the age effect is rather dramatic: 3- and 6-month-olds have average thresholds 40 to 60 ms higher than those of adults in all masking conditions. Compared to infants' fairly good pure tone thresholds and frequency difference thresholds (Olsho et al., 1988; Olsho, 1984), this is a large age difference. For example, in frequency discrimination, infant thresholds are roughly twice those of adults (e.g., Olsho, 1984; Sinnott & Aslin, 1985), while in gap detection, infant thresholds are at least four times those of adults. Second, the effect of frequency on the gap detection threshold is similar for 3-

month-olds, 6-month-olds, and adults: the threshold improves as higher frequencies are made available until the 8,000-Hz masker cutoff does not differ from the unmasked condition.

Third, the performance of the 12-month-olds appears to differ from that of both younger and older listeners. The 12-month-olds do no better than the 3- or 6-month-olds with 2,000- or 8,000-Hz masker cutoffs or in the unmasked condition. When the cutoff of the masker is as low as 500 Hz, the 12-month-olds' average gap detection threshold approaches that of the adults, but the variability in performance is extremely high. Examination of the individual thresholds in this condition (Table 2) suggests a bimodal distribution of thresholds. Two of the six subjects performed as poorly as the younger infants, while the other four performed as well as adults. There was no evidence of a bimodal distribution of thresholds in any of the other ages or conditions. This finding is discussed further below and led us to test a second group of 12-month-olds in this condition (Experiment 2).

Gap thresholds were transformed using the logarithmic function to make the variances more homogeneous before applying analysis of variance (Winer, 1971). Because of the extreme variability among 12-month-olds

Table 1. Means and Standard Deviations of Other Measures of Gap Detection Performance

Age	Masker Condition	N	False Alarm Rate	Trials to Training Criterion	Psychometric Function Slope (z/ms)
3	unmasked	9	.19 (.05)	22.11	5.83 (12.15)	(.21)
6	unmasked	12	.19 (.06)	17.25	3.31 (8.91)	(.35)
12	unmasked	6	.22 (.04)	24.17	4.48 (9.58)	(.25)
adult	unmasked	10	.00 (.00)	8.00	1.87 (1.33)	(.33)
3	500 Hz	6	.20 (.09)	29.00	3.43 (17.81)	(.50)
6	500 Hz	6	.21 (.03)	23.00	5.83 (15.40)	(.05)
12	500 Hz	6	.22 (.03)	25.33	1.69 (12.86)	(.49)
adult	500 Hz	10	.05 (.06)	10.30	.97 (1.49)	(.51)
3	2,000 Hz	6	.22 (.06)	17.67	3.38 (10.78)	(.16)
6	2,000 Hz	7	.22 (.02)	23.86	4.24 (10.82)	(.50)
12	2,000 Hz	6	.21 (.04)	25.83	4.26 (9.99)	(.41)
adult	2,000 Hz	11	.03 (.04)	9.09	2.06 (1.64)	(.35)
3	8,000 Hz	6	.18 (.06)	25.17	8.31 (18.60)	(.14)
6	8,000 Hz	9	.23 (.05)	18.22	4.05 (11.08)	(.27)
12	8,000 Hz	7	.23 (.02)	22.43	4.79 (10.05)	(.20)
adult	8,000 Hz	11	.04 (.07)	9.10	1.79 (1.64)	(.32)

Note. Standard deviations are in parentheses.

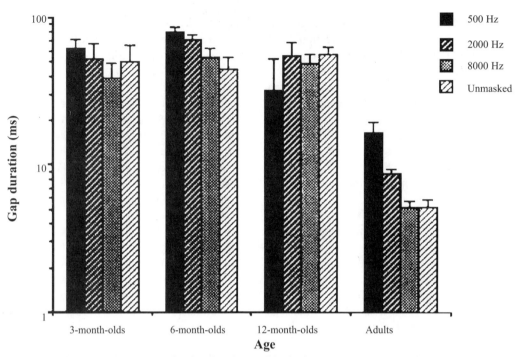

Figure 2. Average gap detection threshold (±1 SE) as a function of masker condition for four age groups. Note that a logarithmic scale is used on both axes.

at 500 Hz, this group was excluded from the analysis. An age (3) ˜ masking condition (4) analysis of variance[3] of the transformed thresholds showed a significant effect of age [$F(2,86) = 108.9, p < .001$], a significant effect of masking condition [$F(3,86) = 8.4, p < .001$], but no effect of the age ˜ masking condition interaction [$F(6,86) = .5, p = .8$]. One-way analysis of variance was used to examine the effect of age on the gap detection threshold in each masking condition. Twelve-month-olds were included in these analyses at 2,000 and 8,000 Hz and in the unmasked condition. The effect of age was significant at 500 Hz [$F(2,194) = 25.877, p < .001$], at 2,000 Hz [$F(3,26) = 27.867, p < .001$], at 8,000 Hz [$F(3,29) = 48.426, p < .001$], and in the unmasked condition [$F(3,33) = 16.583, p < .001$]; in each of these conditions Tukey HSD multiple comparisons indicated that 3-, 6-, and 12-month-olds (where included) did not differ from each other, but that each infant group had significantly higher thresholds than the adults. Thus, the statistical analyses confirmed the trends that appear evident in Figure 2.

In order to better understand the nature of the age differences in gap detection thresholds, three additional performance measures were examined: false alarm rate, number of training trials to criterion, and slope of the psychometric function used to calculate the threshold. The means and standard deviations of these measures for each age group are listed in Table 1. Differences among the age groups were tested using one-way analysis of variance in each masking condition.

All infant groups had higher false alarm rates than adults in all conditions. Thus, one factor contributing to the age difference in thresholds could be age differences in response bias. However, unless response bias varied in a systematic way with masker condition, it could not explain why the nature of the age difference in threshold varied with masker condition. False alarm rate was transformed using an arcsin transformation (Winer, 1971) for the statistical analysis. The effect of age was significant in each condition, unmasked [$F(3,33) = 18.456, p < .001$], 500 Hz [$F(3,24) = 7.918, p < .002$], 2,000 Hz [$F(3,26) = 34.457, p < .001$], and 8,000 Hz [$F(3,29) = 23.956, p < .001$]. In each case, though, post hoc analyses showed the same pattern of age differences, 3-, 6-, and 12-month-olds all having significantly higher false alarm rates than adults. Thus, differences in response bias cannot account for the difference between 500 Hz and the other masking conditions.

The number of training trials to criterion may reflect the difficulty experienced by listeners in learning the detection task under different masking conditions, and one might predict that thresholds would be higher for listeners and conditions under which the task is more difficult to learn. Again, infants generally required more trials

----

[3]The use of a factorial analysis was justified by the fact that none of the correlations between thresholds obtained from the same subjects in different masking conditions was significant after partialing out the effect of age.

Table 2. Individual Gap Detection Thresholds of 12-month-olds and Adults in the 500-Hz Masker Cutoff Condition

12-Month-Olds		Adults	
Subject Number	Gap Threshold (ms)	Subject Number	Gap Threshold (ms)
30019	6	32001	8
30018	15	32002	14
31013	10	32003	10
31018	18	32004	41
30020	74	32005	10
31015	94	32006	13
Mean	36.2	32007	19
SD	37.8	32009	24
		32010	19
		32011	8
		Mean	16.4
		SD	10.1

than adults to reach training criterion, as indicated in Table 1. The one-way analysis of variance showed a significant effect of age in all conditions, unmasked [$F(3,33)$ = 5.891, $p < .002$], 500 Hz [$F(3,24)$ = 3.94, $p < .028$], 2,000 Hz [$F(3,26)$ = 7.074, $p < .001$], and 8,000 Hz [$F(3,29)$ = 3.357, $p < .032$]. Newman Keuls analyses indicated that at 500 and 2,000 Hz and in the unmasked condition the infants all required significantly more trials to reach training criterion than the adults. At 8,000 Hz, only the 3-month-olds required more training trials than the adults. This suggests that the 8,000-Hz condition was relatively easier for the 6- and 12-month-olds to learn, but it is noteworthy that the three groups of infants had comparable thresholds in this condition nonetheless.

Finally, psychometric function slopes may affect threshold estimates in that thresholds estimated on shallower psychometric functions will be more variable than those estimated on steep psychometric functions (e.g., McKee, Klein, & Teller, 1985). The slopes derived from probit analysis (Finney, 1970) were transformed using a tan^{-1} transformation following Watson, Franks, and Hood (1972). Although examination of the average slopes listed in Table 1 suggests that the adults tended to have shallower psychometric functions than infants, one-way analysis of variance of the transformed slopes in each masking condition indicated no significant differences among the age groups in any masking condition. Thus, differences in gap detection thresholds do not appear to stem from differences in the accuracy of estimate for different age groups.

DISCUSSION

It was clear from the above results that infants generally have poorer gap detection thresholds than adults under all masking conditions, although the effect of masking condition is similar for younger infants and adults. If one considers just the 3- and 6-month-olds, the difference

between the infants and adults is difficult to interpret. The fact that restricting the frequency region in which gaps are heard has a similar effect on the performance of these infants and adults supports the interpretation that temporal coding operates in a similar way in the two groups. The dramatic difference between infant and adult gap thresholds according to this interpretation would result from other factors influencing performance, such as attention or motivation.

One result that argues against attention as an important factor is that infant and adult psychometric function slopes in gap detection did not differ. Inattentiveness would be expected to make the psychometric function slope shallower (Schneider, Trehub, Morrongiello, & Thorpe, 1989). This is a somewhat surprising result, because infant psychometric function slopes are typically shallower than those of adults, even when infant performance is fairly good (e.g., Olsho et al., 1987).

An alternate interpretation is that the age difference in thresholds results, at least partially, from immaturity of temporal coding. The finding that some 12-month-olds have adultlike gap detection thresholds at 500 Hz might be taken as support for this interpretation. If 12-month-olds are in a period of rapid development of temporal coding, then high variability in performance would not be unexpected. Given the small number of 12-month-olds who completed testing at 500 Hz, however, little faith can be put in the result. In Experiment 2 an additional group of 12-month-olds was tested with a 500-Hz masker cutoff to determine whether the result was replicable.

Experiment 2

METHOD

Subjects. The subjects were 11 12-month-old infants and five 20-30-year-old adults meeting the inclusion criteria described for Experiment 1. These subjects also passed tympanometry, a screening test for middle ear dysfunction, on the test date. An additional eight infants did not provide a threshold: four did not reach training criterion, and four did not complete enough test trials.

Stimuli and apparatus. The stimuli were the same as those used in the 500-Hz masker cutoff condition in Experiment 1. A General Radio 1381 noise generator produced the stimulus (gapped) noise. A Grason-Stadler 901B noise generator produced the masking noise. The masking noise was high-pass filtered using a Kemo VBF 25MD filter with a nominal slope of 90 dB/octave. Except for the earphone, the rest of the apparatus was the same as in Experiment 1.

An Etymotic insert earphone (ER-1) was used to deliver sounds to the listeners. This earphone has a flat frequency response over a broad frequency range, eliminating the need for equalization. The foam ear tips that held the delivery tube in place were trimmed to fit the infants' ear canals. Infants generally tolerate the insert earphones as well as or better than other earphones, and they deliver the stimulus at a more consistent intensity. Calibrations were performed in a Zwislocki coupler,[4] but in other respects as in Experiment 1.

Procedure. Each listener was tested in a single condition, the 500-Hz masker condition of Experiment 1. The test method, the Observer-based Psychoacoustic Procedure, was the same as in Experiment 1. General aspects of the procedure were the same, but several changes were made in the psychophysical procedure in an attempt to reduce the variability in infant performance.

Each session included two training phases. In the first training phase, signal trials were presented with a probability of 0.8 and the reinforcer was activated on signal trials, whether or not the observer responded correctly. Gap duration was 125 ms. This phase ended when the observer was correct on at least four of the last five consecutive trials as long as at least one of the correct trials was a no-signal trial. In the second training phase, the probability of a signal was 0.50, and the reinforcer was activated only when the observer correctly identified a signal trial. Gap duration was 125 ms. This phase continued until the observer was correct on at least four of the last five signal trials and on at least four of the last five no-signal trials.

During the test phase, threshold was estimated using a one-up, two-down adaptive method (Levitt, 1971). The probability of a signal trial was 0.50. Gap duration began at 125 ms. If the observer was correct on two consecutive trials (signal or no-signal), gap duration was reduced. If the observer was incorrect on one trial, gap duration was increased. The size of the step in gap duration was varied using PEST rules as in Experiment 1. The test phase con-

tinued until at least eight reversals had occurred. Threshold was defined as the average of the gap durations at which reversals occurred, excluding the first two reversals.

The advantage of this method over that used in Experiment 1 is that because responses on both signal and no-signal trials affect the threshold, the observer cannot obtain low thresholds simply by responding "signal" more often. Computer simulations indicate that this version of the one-up, two-down rule converges on approximately the 70% correct point on the psychometric function, and this test method and the method used in Experiment 1 produce the same average threshold for infants (Werner & Marean, 1991).

RESULTS

The average gap threshold of 12-month-olds in Experiment 2 was 62.2 ms (SEM = 9.0), while the average for the adults was 13.2 ms (SEM = 2.3). The 12-month-olds' average was much poorer than in Experiment 1; in fact, this mean would fall with those of 3- and 6-month-olds for Experiment 1. Thus, one might conclude that there is little evidence of improvement in gap detection between 3 and 12 months in any condition. The only hint that there is any difference here was the distribution of thresholds in the two age groups, shown in Figure 3. Although there is no overlap between the infants and adults in gap thresholds, the distribution of infant thresholds still appears to be bimodal. Six of the 11 infants had thresholds between 30 and 49 ms, and four had thresholds higher than 90 ms. Thus, although the best 12-month-olds in this sample were not as good at gap detection as adults, they are better than the 3- and 6-month-olds tested at 500 Hz in Experiment 1. It should be noted, moreover, that it was rare to find infants in any other condition in Experiment 1 whose thresholds fell within 10 ms of the worst adult in the same condition. This occurred four times in 80 thresholds, twice in the unmasked condition (a 3-month-old and a 6-month-old), once in the 500-Hz condition (a 3-month-old), and once in the 2,000-Hz condition (a 12-month-old). Finally, 12-month-olds' gap detection thresholds may have been somewhat poorer in Experiment 2 as a result of changes in procedure.

....

[4]An insert earphone fits into the listener's ear canal. The advantage of an insert is that there is little variability in the intensity of stimulus because the position of the delivery tube is less variable. Because the volume of the ear canal beyond the end of the delivery tube is smaller than the volume of the ear canal beyond an earphone that sits outside the ear canal, calibrations are performed in a smaller coupler. The Zwislocki coupler gives a more accurate calibration value than a 2-cc coupler at high frequencies.

Although the two procedures produce the same results in tone detection (Werner & Marean, 1991), it is possible that this would not be the case in gap detection. At this point, the safest conclusion may be that 12-month-olds are not different from younger infants in gap detection. That we continue to find 12-month-olds who perform fairly well at 500 Hz, however, suggests that improvement in the gap detection threshold may be occurring at this age.

GENERAL DISCUSSION

The major findings of this study are threefold. First, infants generally perform quite poorly in gap detection. Second, the effects of restricting the range of frequencies available for detecting gaps are qualitatively similar for infants and adults. Third, there is a suggestion that improvement in gap detection performance is occurring around 12 months of age and that this improvement occurs first in the case where only low frequency information is available for gap detection.

These results are consistent with Morrongiello and Trehub's (1987) finding that 6-month-olds required a greater change in the duration of repeated noise bursts to detect a change, and with Wightman et al.'s (1989) report that 3-year-olds had higher gap detection thresholds than adults. The 12-month-olds who performed well in gap detection at low frequencies here performed, on average, a little worse than Wightman et al.'s (1989) 3-year-olds did in their 400-Hz condition. Infants in all the other conditions in this study performed much worse than Wightman

et al.'s (1989) 3-year-olds. The psychophysical data thus suggest substantial improvement in auditory temporal resolution over the early years of life.

Numerous studies have demonstrated that infants as young as 1 month of age can discriminate between speech sounds that vary along a temporal dimension (reviewed by Aslin, Pisoni, & Jusczyk, 1983). Is the finding that infants have such poor gap detection thresholds inconsistent with that literature? In fact, it appears that when temporal information alone is provided, 6-8-month-olds may have difficulty discriminating speech stimuli (Eilers, Morse, Gavin, & Oller, 1981). Aslin et al. (1983) suggest that infants may have been using nontemporal cues to discriminate between sounds in earlier experiments. Thus, it appears that the poor gap detection performance reported here is not inconsistent with the infant speech perception literature.

There are at least three classes of factors that could contribute to age-related improvement in gap detection performance. The first is maturation of temporal coding in the primary auditory pathways. Brugge and his colleagues (Brugge, Javel, & Kitzes, 1978; Kettner, Feng, & Brugge, 1985) have shown that phase locking, the tendency of neurons to respond in a manner that is time-locked to a stimulus waveform, gradually improves following the onset of auditory function in kittens. Unlike absolute sensitivity and frequency resolution, which mature very quickly once the peripheral auditory system begins to function, temporal coding matures over a longer time course and appears to mature later at more central loci (Brugge et al., 1978; Kettner et al., 1985; Sanes & Rubel,

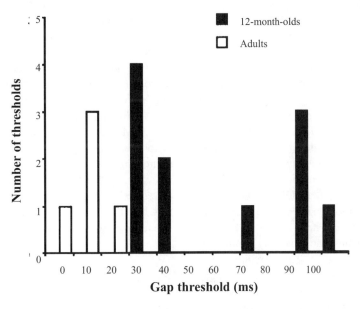

Figure 3. Frequency distribution of gap detection thresholds for 12-month-olds and adults in Experiment 2.

1988). Given the protracted time course of development in temporal coding and that the rate of development is slower in humans than in other mammals, it is possible that one would see continuing maturation of temporal coding during human infancy. In fact, the latency of the auditory brainstem response (ABR) continues to mature until some time after 12 months of age in humans, and this age-related change is usually attributed to increases in the synchrony of evoked neural activity (e.g., Eggermont, 1985). Since neural synchrony is a by-product of phase locking, one might conclude that maturation of temporal coding in humans continues at least until 12 months postnatal age. Finally, Brugge and his colleagues (Brugge et al., 1978; Kettner et al., 1985) have shown that the first neurons to achieve adultlike phase locking are those responding to low frequencies. The only infants we observed who approached adult performance in gap detection were 12-month-olds listening at 500 Hz. At the same time, the age differences in gap detection observed here are larger than would be predicted from the data on neural development, and it is not clear that one would predict a maturational course that exceeds 3 years in duration. It is also not obvious that one would expect to see an adultlike frequency effect in gap detection in infants if the infant system were substantially immature, since the variability in neural response resulting from immaturity would be likely to swamp the differences in variability associated with frequency.

Another factor that may contribute to the infant-adult performance difference in gap detection is the effective level of the stimulus. The stimuli here should have been well above threshold for all subjects at a spectrum level of 30 dB SPL, but since infants require higher intensities of sound for simple detection (e.g., Olsho et al., 1988; Trehub et al., 1980), and since the stimuli here were presented at a fixed intensity, the sensation level of the stimuli would be lower for the infants. Sensation level is known to affect gap detection threshold (e.g., Fitzgibbons, 1983), and it is likely that some of the difference between the younger infants and adults can be accounted for by sensation level differences. It is unlikely that sensation level can completely account for the observed age differences in gap detection performance for several reasons. First, infant-adult differences in sensation level on the order of those typically reported (e.g., Olsho et al., 1988) are far too small to account for the large age difference in gap detection performance (e.g., Fitzgibbons, 1983). Second, age differences in absolute sensitivity are frequency dependent (e.g., Olsho et al., 1988; Trehub et al., 1980), but for 3- and 6-month-olds, age differences in gap detection are constant across frequencies. To the extent that sensation level differences do contribute, however, it should be possible to show that infants improve more

rapidly than adults do as the level of the stimulus is increased beyond the level used here.

Clearly, nonsensory mechanisms that affect infant responses must be considered. At all ages, infants tend to require more trials to learn the task and to have a more liberal response bias during testing than adults do. This suggests a general inefficiency in infant processing of auditory information. More specifically, Werner and Bargones (1991) showed that 6-month-olds had difficulty detecting a sound in the presence of an irrelevant sound, even when the irrelevant sound was at a distant frequency, while adult performance was unaffected by the irrelevant sound. In other words, adults listened selectively for the target, while infants did not. The fact that adults in the present study achieved gap detection thresholds close to those reported in studies using narrow-band stimuli implies that they listened selectively for gaps in the optimal frequency region. If infants did not listen selectively, their performance would be relatively poor, since on many trials they would be listening in a nonoptimal frequency region. A frequency effect would still be predicted since the infants would happen to be listening in an optimal frequency region on some trials. This idea leads to the prediction that infants might do better in detecting gaps in a narrow band stimulus.

If anything, the finding that some 12-month-olds do relatively well in gap detection at 500 Hz suggests that temporal resolution is relatively mature. Why this only occurs in the 500-Hz condition is not clear, but it may involve some interaction between the factors described above. For example, 12-month-olds may have mature temporal resolution but only be able to listen selectively when gaps occur in a restricted frequency region. This hypothesis could be tested by examining infant gap detection when bandwidth and frequency are manipulated independently.

It is likely that some combination of factors—temporal coding, sensation level, general processing efficiency, or selective listening—is responsible for the large differences between infants and adults in gap detection performance. Moreover, it need not be the case that a single factor or even a single combination of factors accounts for improvement over the entire developmental course of gap detection. Studies that use similar stimuli and methods to assess performance over a broader age range, testing specific hypotheses about the nature of the age-related change in temporal processing, are clearly in order.

REFERENCES

Aslin, R.N., Pisoni, D.B., & Jusczyk, P. W. (1983). Auditory development and speech perception in infancy. In M.M.

Haith & J.J. Campos (Eds.), P.H. Mussen (Series Ed.), *Handbook of child psychology: Vol. 2. Infancy and developmental psychobiology* (4th ed., pp. 573-688). New York: Wiley.

Brugge, J.F., Javel, E., & Kitzes, L.M. (1978). Signs of functional maturation of peripheral auditory system in discharge patterns in anteroventral cochlear nucleus of kittens. *Journal of Neurophysiology, 41,* 1557-1579.

Buus, S., & Florentine, M. (1982). Detection of temporal gap as a function of level and frequency. *Journal of the Acoustical Society of America, 72,* S89.

Davis, S.M., & McCroskey, R.L. (1980). Auditory fusion in children. *Child Development, 51,* 75-80.

Dreschler, W.A., & Plomp, R. (1980). Relation between psychophysical data and speech perception for hearing-impaired listeners. *Journal of the Acoustical Society of America, 68,* 1608-1615.

Eggermont, J. (1985). Physiology of the developing auditory system. In S.E. Trehub & B.A. Schneider (Eds.), *Auditory development in infancy* (pp. 21-46). New York: Plenum.

Eilers, R.E., Morse, P.A., Gavin, W.J., & Oller, D.K. (1981). Discrimination of voice onset time in infancy. *Journal of the Acoustical Society of America, 70,* 955-965.

Finney, D.J. (1970). *Probit analysis.* Cambridge: Cambridge University Press.

Fitzgibbons, P.J. (1983). Temporal gap detection in noise as a function of frequency, bandwidth, & level. *Journal of the Acoustical Society of America, 74,* 67-72.

Fitzgibbons, P.J., & Wightman, F.L. (1982). Gap detection in normal and hearing-impaired listeners. *Journal of the Acoustical Society of America, 72,* 761-765.

Gottlieb, G. (1985). On discovering significant acoustic dimensions of auditory stimulation for infants. In G. Gottlieb & N.A. Krasnegor (Eds.), *Measurement of audition and vision in the first year of life: A methodological overview* (pp. 3-30). Norwood, NJ: Ablex.

Hall, J.L. (1968). Maximum likelihood sequential procedure for estimation of psychometric functions. *Journal of the Acoustical Society of America, 44,* 370.

Hall, J.L. (1981). Hybrid adaptive procedure for estimation of psychometric functions. *Journal of the Acoustical Society of America, 69,* 1763-1769.

Irwin, R.J., Ball, A.K.R., Kay, N., Stillman, J.A., & Rosser, J. (1985). The development of auditory temporal acuity in children. *Child Development, 56,* 614-620.

Irwin, R.J., Hinchcliffe, L.K., & Kemp, S. (1981). Temporal acuity in normal and hearing-impaired listeners. *Audiology, 20,* 234-243.

Kettner, R.E., Feng, J-Z., & Brugge, J.F. (1985). Postnatal development of the phase-locked response to low frequency tones of auditory nerve fibers in the cat. *Journal of Neuroscience, 5,* 275-283.

Levitt, H. (1971). Transformed up-down methods in psychoacoustics. *Journal of the Acoustical Society of America, 49,* 467-477.

McKee, S.P., Klein, S.A., & Teller, D.Y. (1985). Statistical properties of forced-choice psychometric functions: Implications

of probit analysis. *Perception & Psychophysics, 37,* 286-298.

Morrongiello, B.A., & Trehub, S.E. (1987). Age-related changes in auditory temporal perception. *Journal of Experimental Child Psychology, 44,* 413-426.

Olsho, L.W. (1984). Infant frequency discrimination. *Infant Behavior and Development, 7,* 27-35.

Olsho, L.W., Koch, E.G., Carter, E.A., Halpin, C.F., & Spetner, N.B. (1988). Pure-tone sensitivity of human infants. *Journal of the Acoustical Society of America, 84,* 1316-1324.

Olsho, L.W., Koch, E.G., & Halpin, C.F. (1987). Level and age effects in infant frequency discrimination. *Journal of the Acoustical Society of America, 82,* 454-464.

Olsho, L.W., Koch, E.G., Halpin, C.F., & Carter, E.A. (1987). An observer-based psychoacoustic procedure for use with young infants. *Developmental Psychology, 23,* 627-640.

Pisoni, D.B. (1977). Identification and discrimination of the relative onset of two component tones: Implications for voicing perception in stops. *Journal of the Acoustical Society of America, 61,* 1452-1461.

Sanes, D.H., & Rubel, E.W. (1988). The development of stimulus coding in the auditory system. In A.F. Jahn & J. Santos-Sacchi (Eds.), *Physiology of the ear* (pp. 431-456). New York: Raven.

Schneider, B.A., Trehub, S.E., & Bull, D. (1980). High-frequency sensitivity in infants. *Science, 207,* 1003-1004.

Schneider, B.A., Trehub, S.E., Morrongiello, B.A., & Thorpe, L.A. (1989). Developmental changes in masked thresholds. *Journal of the Acoustical Society of America, 86,* 1733-1742.

Shailer, M.J., & Moore, B.C.J. (1983). Gap detection as a function of frequency, bandwidth, and level. *Journal of the Acoustical Society of America, 74,* 467-473.

Shailer, M.J., & Moore, B.C.J. (1985). Detection of temporal gaps in bandlimited noise: Effects of variations in bandwidth and signal-to-masker ratio. *Journal of the Acoustical Society of America, 77,* 635-639.

Sinnott, J.M., & Aslin, R.N. (1985). Frequency and intensity discrimination in human infants and adults. *Journal of the Acoustical Society of America, 78,* 1986-1992.

Sinnott, J.M., Pisoni, D.B., & Aslin, R.M. (1983) A comparison of pure tone auditory thresholds in human infants and adults. *Infant Behavior and Development, 6,* 3-17.

Spetner, N.B., & Olsho, L.W. (1990). Auditory frequency resolution in human infancy. *Child Development, 61,* 632-652.

Taylor, M.M., & Creelman, D.C. (1967). PEST: Efficient estimates on probability functions. *Journal of the Acoustical Society of America, 41,* 782-787.

Trehub, S.E., Schneider, B.A., & Endman, M. (1980). Developmental changes in infants' sensitivity to octave-band noises. *Journal of Experimental Child Psychology, 29,* 283-293.

Watson, C.S., Franks, J.R., & Hood, D.C. (1972). Detection of tones in the absence of external masking noise: I. Effects of signal intensity and signal frequency. *Journal of the Acoustical Society of America, 52,* 633-643.

Werner, L.A., & Bargones, J.Y. (1991). Sources of auditory masking in infants: Distraction effects. *Perception & Psychophysics,* 50, 405-412.

Werner, L.A., & Marean, G.C. (1991). Methods for estimating infant thresholds. *Journal of the Acoustical Society of America,* 90, 1867-1875.

Wightman, F., Allen, P., Dolan, T., Kistler, D., & Jamieson, D. (1989). Temporal resolution in preschool children. *Child Development,* 60, 611-624.

Winer, B.J. (1971). *Statistical principles in experimental design.* New York: McGraw-Hill.

Developmental Changes in Speech Discrimination in Infants

Rebecca E. Eilers
University of Miami, Florida

Wesley R. Wilson and John M. Moore
University of Washington, Seattle

A visually reinforced infant speech discrimination (VRISD) paradigm is described and evaluated. Infants at two ages were tested with the new paradigm on the following speech contrasts: [sa] vs [va], [sa] vs [Ia], [sa] vs [za], [as] vs [a:z], [a:s] vs [a:z], [at] vs [a:d], [a:t] vs [a:d], [at] vs [a:t], [fa] vs [2a], and [fi] vs [2i]. The data reported are compared with data on the same speech contrasts obtained from three month olds in a high-amplitude sucking paradigm. Evidence suggesting developmental changes in speech-sound discriminatory ability is reported. Results are interpreted in light of salience of available acoustic cues and in terms of new methodological advances.

In recent years, detailed attention has been paid to the perceptual linguistic abilities of infants below four months of age. Employing either a paradigm in which infant sucking is monitored or a paradigm in which heart rate is monitored, researchers including Moffitt (1971), Eimas, Siqueland, Jusczyk, and Vigorito (1971), Eimas (1975), Trehub and Rabinovitch (1972), Trehub (1973), and Morse (1972) have reported on the infants's ability to discriminate among a variety of synthetically and naturally produced speech sounds. The overwhelming conclusion based on the first wave of evidence from the standard high-amplitude sucking paradigm and the heart-rate paradigm suggested that infants below four months of age could discriminate among many stop consonants and vowels, even when discrimination depended on very subtle acoustic cues. Some investigators (Eimas et al., 1971) even began to suggest that infants perceive speech in a manner approximating categorical perception, the manner in which adults perceive many speech sounds. Research suggested that the infant came "prewired" to make many, if not all, possible speech discriminations.

A second wave of evidence is now, however, accruing to indicate that some discriminations may be far more difficult than others for the infant. Employing both the standard and a modified high-amplitude sucking paradigm, Eilers and Minifie (1975) and Eilers (1977a, 1977b) were able to demonstrate discrimination among the fricative consonants [s] and [v], as well as [s] and [I], but in three attempts employing both the standard and modified high-amplitude sucking paradigm, they could find no evidence of discrimination between [s] and [z]. In addition, negative results were obtained in two attempts

using the standard paradigm for the pair [f] and [2]. Difficulty with [f] and [2] has been widely reported for older children as well (for example, Abbs and Minifie, 1969, for four and five year olds, and Eilers and Oller, 1976, for two year olds).

The inability to demonstrate discrimination of some fricative sounds by young infants raises the question of the role of development in speech-sound discrimination. At least for some speech sounds, infants may require some listening experience with the sounds to show evidence of discrimination. Our knowledge of the nature of this prerequisite experience or its effect on the schedule of acquisition of these sounds remains only speculative. To date, methodologies have been unavailable to study speech discrimination in infants between six months and two years of age. Consequently, the issue of developmental change has been largely ignored in the existing literature.

Procedural Rationale

To address the issue of developmental change in speech discrimination skills, an operant technique used successfully for assessment of hearing sensitivity in infants (Wilson, Moore, and Thompson, 1976) was modified to achieve the following goals: (1) to be capable of testing a single child's discrimination, (2) to be capable of evaluating multiple contrasts for each child tested, (3) to be applicable across a wide age range (six to 18 months of age), and (4) to employ a reinforcer that is independent of the stimuli to be discriminated, that is, the speech sounds themselves. In addition, if the procedure proved to be efficient—if the children could be tested in a few minutes—it would have broad applicability.

Reprinted by permission of authors and American Speech-Language-Hearing Association. Copyright 1977. *Journal of Speech and Hearing Research*, 20, pp. 766-780.

All of these goals seem to be met by the visually reinforced infant speech discrimination (VRISD) paradigm. In part, our goals were suggested by the shortcomings of the high-amplitude sucking technique, one of the two traditional methods for studying discrimination in infants below four months of age. Perhaps the most serious difficulty with the high-amplitude sucking technique (if one interprets the paradigm as an habituation-dishabituation paradigm) is that the speech sounds employed are both the discriminative stimuli and the reinforcers. In the high-amplitude sucking paradigm, negative results are very difficult to interpret, since one never knows whether the infant could not detect a change in sound or whether the particular detected change was not interesting or reinforcing. Our approach overcomes this problem by using a reinforcer (lighted, animated toy animal) that is independent of the speech contrasts being investigated, and that has been shown to be highly reinforcing for infants six to 18 months of age (Moore, Thompson, and Thompson, 1975; Moore, Wilson, and Thompson, 1977). Thus, even if the infant is not particularly interested in the sound change, he is extrinsically motivated to respond by the reinforcer. The second most serious problem with the high-amplitude sucking procedure, that of subject dropout rate, is also largely overcome by our approach. In our laboratory to date, over 90% of the infants who began the procedure could be tested, as opposed to approximately 40% of the infants tested with the high-amplitude sucking procedure. With the high-amplitude sucking procedure, one must test between 50 and 100 infants before a single speech contrast can be evaluated for experimental and control groups. Nothing can be firmly concluded about individual infants. With the procedure reported here, however, data from individual children can be analyzed and a firm statement concerning an individual child's ability to discriminate a given contrast can usually be made. Also, unlike the high-amplitude sucking procedure, the present technique can be used with the same child for a number of contrasts in a single session or over many months in multiple sessions, which allows developmental changes to be closely monitored. The present technique is reliably applicable over a much wider age range (six months to at least 18 months) than the high-amplitude sucking procedure, although the present paradigm cannot be employed with infants under five to six months of age. The upper age-range limit permitted by the present technique can be extended by changing the response mode to a bar press.

Method

Subjects

Subjects were nine six-month-old and eight 12-month-old normal infants, selected by mail solicitation from the greater Seattle area. Introductory letters explaining the nature and scope of a large research project were sent to parents of newborns. Parental response cards indicating a desire to participate were filed and parents were recontacted for this study as their infants reached six or 12 months of age. Infants were considered normal if experimenters, parents, and consulted medical personnel did not have any concerns about age of appearance of standard developmental milestones appropriate for the infant's status and if the infant's hearing was judged to be unimpaired. Infants were tested with the present technique only when no evidence of colds or abnormal middle-ear function (as measured by tympanometry) was present. No attempt was made to balance the experimental groups for sex because analyses of this factor in speech discrimination testing have not yielded significant sex-related differences (Spring, 1975; Eilers and Minifie, 1975). Three additional infants in each age group were not included in the analysis. In four cases (three six month olds and one 12 month old) parents were unable to return to the laboratory to finish testing. In the two remaining cases, the animated toy lost its reinforcing properties after several contrasts had been tested.

The experimental site consisted of a sound-treated booth with one-way observation window and an adjoining control room where Experimenter 2 was seated. The booth contained two chairs, one for parent/child and one for Experimenter 1, a small table, a loudspeaker, a visual reinforcer, and a two-way audio intercom for the experimenters (Figure 1 illustrates the layout). The reinforcer was housed in a smoked Plexiglas box directly in front of the loudspeaker, at a 45° angle to the child's left, and at eye level. The reinforcer consisted of a three-dimensional stuffed toy capable of movement when an electric circuit was activated. During activation of the toy, the box was back lighted, allowing the infant to see the reinforcer.

The reinforcer was activated by a logic circuit (see Figure 2). During stimulus-change intervals a timer provided preset appropriate response intervals (usually four sec) for the infant. If during an interval both experimenters observed a head turn toward the reinforcer and voted affirmatively, visual reinforcement (marking an appropriate discriminatory response) was supplied. If either or both experimenters failed to indicate an observed head turn within the limits of the response interval, the reinforcer was not activated.

The control room contained a clinical audiometer and four-channel tape deck. Taped stimuli were transmitted through the audiometer to the loudspeaker in the testing room and were controlled by Experimenter 2.

Stimuli

Ten stimulus pairs were selected from a stimulus pool of items prepared for use with one- to three-month-

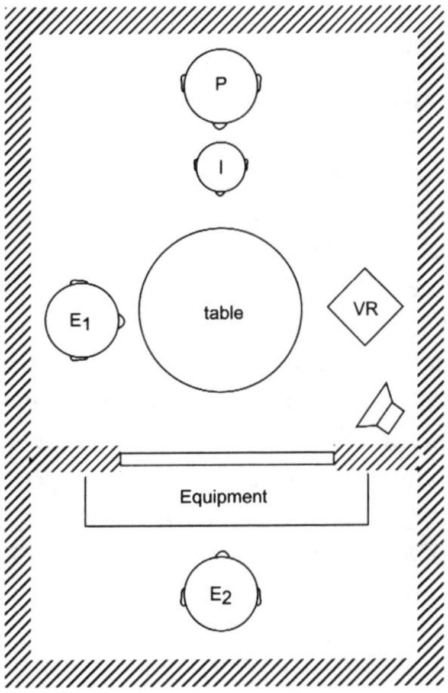

Figure 1. Arrangement of the experimental site. Legend: E_1 = Experimenter 1, E_2 = Experimenter 2, P = Parent, I = Infant, VR = Visual Reinforcer.

old infants on the high-amplitude sucking procedure. The pairs [sa] vs [va], [sa] vs [Ia], and [sa] vs [za], reported in Eilers and Minifie (1975), were from a set of naturally produced tokens matched for fundamental frequency, fundamental frequency contour, intensity, intensity contour, and total duration. Natural stimuli were used because of the poor quality of presently available synthetically produced fricative consonants, many of which were incorrectly identified by adult listeners. The remaining pairs [at] and [a:d], [a:t] and [a:d], [as] and [a:z], [at] and [a:t], [fi] and [2i] and [fa] and [2a] were also naturally produced and matched on the above criteria where appropriate. The discrimination data from the high-amplitude sucking procedure using these stimuli with one- to three-month-old infants (Eilers and Minifie, 1975; Eilers, 1977a, 1977b) will be included in the discussion section of this paper for comparison to the present discrimination data on both six- to eight- and 12- to 14-month-old infants. A more detailed description of each of the stimulus pairs follows.

Pair 1, [va] and [sa]. The stimuli differed along at least three major acoustic dimensions: amplitude, spectrum, and voicing. [s] has high-amplitude, high-frequency noise energy concentration (4000-7000 Hz) along the frequency spectrum. [v] is characterized by low-amplitude noise on which a harmonic series (due to voicing) is superimposed. Total duration and vowel duration for [va] and [sa], respectively, were 433 and 267 msec; 346 and 260 msec.

Pair 2, [sa] and [Ia]. These stimuli differed primarily in the spectral domain. [s] has the greatest concentration of noise energy above 4000 Hz while most of the aperiodic energy in [I] falls below 4000 Hz. [sa] and [Ia] had identical vowel and overall durations (165 and 299 msec, respectively) and had highly similar fundamental frequency contours, peak amplitude, and amplitude contours.

Pair 3, [sa] and [za]. This pair differed in voicing during noise generation and in fricative duration (152 msec for [s] and 102 msec for [z]). Voice-onset times for [z] and [s], respectively, were 0 and +95 msec from the beginning of frication. Both stimuli had fricative noise spectra concentrated between 4000 and 7000 Hz and had identical vowel durations (252 msec). Peak fundamental frequency and intensity contours were closely matched.

Pair 4, [as] and [a:z]. These syllables were matched for peak intensity, intensity contour, peak fundamental frequency, and fundamental frequency. The syllables differed in terms of final voicing during frication and in terms of vowel duration (323 msec for [a:z] and 197 msec for [as]). So that overall duration would not serve as a cue for discrimination, syllables were chosen with complementary fricative durations (299 msec for [as] and 181 msec for [a:z]). Therefore, overall duration differed only by eight msec. The syllables were judged to be natural-sounding tokens of normal adult speech and are represented here by the International Phonetic Alphabet symbology [as] and [a:z], the colon marking a long vowel.

Pair 5, [a:s] and [a:z]. These tokens were selected from several natural syllables so that they could be matched as closely as possible for peak fundamental frequency, fundamental frequency contour, and intensity and

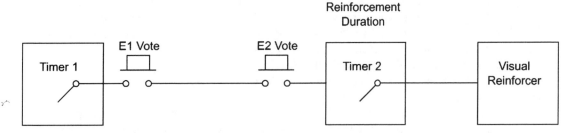

Figure 2. Visual reinforcement system flow chart. Timer 1 defines signal-change or control interval. If E_1 vote and E_2 vote are depressed during signal-change interval, Timer 2 initiates and controls duration of visual reinforcer.

intensity contour, as well as vowel duration and overall duration (556 msec for [a:s] and 551 msec for [a:z]).

Regulating the vowel duration of these syllables, however, proved extremely difficult, because of the natural tendency of the speaker to elongate the vowel before the voiced fricative. The best-matched syllables (which were comparable with regard to peak fundamental frequency, fundamental frequency contour, intensity, and so forth) still contained some vowel duration difference information. The vowel in [a:s] was 275 msec, while in [a:z] the duration was 354 msec. If, however, Stimulus Pair 5 is compared to Stimulus Pair 4, it can be seen that the vowel duration ratio (a:/a) in Pair 4 (1.54) is considerably greater than in Pair 5 (1.29). Also, the consonant duration ratio is larger in Pair 4 (1.65) than in Pair 5 (1.48). Thus, the availability of durational cues is much reduced though not eliminated in the [a:s] and [a:z] stimuli. The stimuli differed basically in final consonant voicing status.

Pair 6, [at] *and* [a:d]. These syllables differed principally on two parameters of interest—vowel duration (181 msec in [at] and 330 msec in [a:d]) and voicing during closure. Consonantal closure durations were 157 msec for [t] and 133 msec for [d]. The overall duration of [at] was 338 msec and [a:d] was 464 msec. Both consonants were released. The syllables were natural-sounding tokens of adult speech. The pair was matched for fundamental frequency, fundamental frequency contour, intensity, and intensity contour.

Pair 7, [a:t] *and* [a:d]. Stimuli were selected from natural syllables and matched as closely as possible on peak fundamental frequency, fundamental frequency contour, intensity, intensity contour, overall duration, and vowel duration. The overall vowel plus consonant closure duration were 488 msec for [a:t] and 456 msec for [a:d]. Vowel durations were 338 msec and 354 msec for [a:t] and [a:d], respectively. The vowel duration ratio of [a:t] and [a:d] was 1.05 as compared to a ratio of 1.82 for the naturally differing stimuli (Pair 6). The consonantal closure duration ratio was 1.46 in these stimuli as opposed to 1.18 for Pair 6. Thus, if the infant cues to the relative consonantal durations, in fact, there is a greater possibility for discrimination of Pair 7 stimuli than in Stimulus Pair 6.

Pair 8, [at] *and* [a:t]. The stimuli were selected from natural tokens so that they were matched on extraneous variables, including peak fundamental frequency, fundamental frequency contour, intensity, and intensity contour. The duration of the vowel in [at] was 189 msec, while the duration of the vowel in [a:t] was 299 msec. The consonantal closure durations were 165 msec and 142 msec for [at] and [a:t], respectively. The ratio of the two-vowel durations was 1.58 and of the consonant durations 1.16.

Pair 9, [fa] *and* [2a]. These stimuli were also selected from natural tokens so that they were matched for fun-

damental frequency, fundamental frequency contour, peak intensity, and intensity contour. Fricative and vowel durations for [fa] and [2a], respectively, were 110 and 212 msec; 118 and 228 msec.

Pair 10, [fi] *and* [2i]. Syllables were matched for fundamental frequency, fundamental frequency contour, peak intensity, and intensity contour. Fricative and vowel durations for [fi] and [2i], respectively, were 126 and 244 msec; 142 and 307 msec.

To test the validity of the exemplars chosen for each speech syllable, identification and discrimination tasks were completed with adult subjects. Ten adults (five with no background in phonetics or listening experiments and five with varying amounts of such experience) first completed an open-set consonant identification task requiring a written response. The adults then completed a discrimination task involving the same contrasts used with the infants. All stimulus pairs were correctly discriminated by all adult listeners. On the open-set identification task, the naive listeners and practiced listeners performed nearly equally well. Collectively, they made correct identifications 94% of the time. Identification errors occurred on the following syllables: [ad] 90% correct, [2i] 70% correct, and [va] and [2a] 60% correct. While 12 exemplars out of 200 possible (20 exemplars ˘ 10 subjects) were misidentified by adults, only three misidentifications could result in potential perceptual confusions. Nine of the 12 incorrect labels involved confusions with phonemes that were not stimulus members.

All stimuli were recorded on tape at one syllable/sec, allowing an interstimulus interval of approximately 500 msec. Stimulus 1 of the contrastive pair was recorded on Track 1 and Stimulus 2 on Track 2, with pairs being time locked. A silent switch allowed for easy selection of Stimulus 1 or 2 so that no audible cues signaled the change between stimuli.

The stimulus pairs were presented in different orders, as dictated by each infant's performance. Specifically, each infant was started on the [va]–[sa] comparison, which was proven discriminable on the basis of pilot data. Infants then received the other pairs in one of four orders, based on storage of stimulus pairs on four tapes. If an infant did not achieve success on a stimulus pair, he was resampled on that pair at the beginning of the next session to rule out fatigue as a cause for failure to discriminate. As a result, the individual presentation schedules varied considerably.

Procedure

Infants were seated on a parent's lap facing the one-way observation window. The speaker and reinforcer were approximately four feet from the infant and required at 45° left head turn to be directly in the infant's visual field. Experimenter 1 (equipped with headphones through which a tone signaling a response or control interval could be presented) was seated to the right of the infant (see Figure 1 for details). Experimenter 2 also wore headphones to receive from Experimenter 1. During the entire time the infant was in the booth, Experimenter 1 kept the infant visually stimulated by manipulating a series of toys at the child's visual midline. When the infant was looking at the toys, Stimulus 1 (for example, [sa]) was presented at the rate of one syllable/second at 50-dB sound pressure level (SPL). The circuit was calibrated using the standard procedure for speech audiometers (ANSI, 1969), except that dial readings were maintained in dB SPL. The procedure involves presentation of a 1 kHz warbled signal from a taped source through the audiometer and speaker, measured via a sound-level meter with the microphone at the infant's head. When the infant was observed to be in a ready state (calm and passively playing with or looking at the toys and his head facing forward), the syllable was changed to Stimulus 2 (for example [za]) for four sec at 65-dB SPL. After four sec, the signal was returned to Stimulus 1 at the original level. If the infant turned toward the speaker during the response interval, the toy animal was activated and lighted for two sec. A second shift, under the same conditions, followed. If the infant did not turn during the second trial, Experimenter 2 pointed to the reinforcer and said, "Look, look." After two or three training trials, most infants turned at the initiation of syllable change. The operant monitored was a complete 45° head turn to the left. Eye-movement only, even if in the correct direction, was considered no response. Over additional trials, the level difference between the stimuli was decreased in 5-dB steps. When both stimuli were at 50-dB SPL, the following vote procedure was initiated and the discrimination data were collected. Experimenter 2, while watching the infant through the glass, would decide when the infant was in a response-ready state (not crying, squirming, or vocalizing, and paying attention to toy presentation). At that time, the four-sec response interval tone (audible only to Experimenter 1 and Experimenter 2) was activated. During these four sec, the infant would receive either a change in syllables (change interval) or continue to hear the same stimulus (control interval). Experimenter 1 and Experimenter 2 would independently activate vote buttons if a head turn toward the visual reinforcer occurred during stimulus change. Voter disagreement or a vote outside of a four-sec interval would not result in presentation of the reinforcer, while activation of both vote buttons within the interval of a stimulus change resulted in two sec of reinforcement. (See Figure 2 for vote diagram.) Three change intervals and three control intervals were presented in random order to each child. Extraneous head turns, that is, turns outside of the four-sec response interval, were not scored as positive, and no

reinforcement was given. Data were collected over several visits, the exact number (Mean = 5) being determined by the individual infant's attention span. If an infant failed to give evidence of discrimination on a particular pair, the infant was retested during a subsequent visit. Thus, results indicating failure to discriminate were derived from at least two separate testings.

The statistical procedure used for defining presence of discrimination for a single subject on an individual contrast was a z test for the significance between two proportions (Bruning and Kintz, 1968). For this test, a comparison of the proportion of responses occurring during change intervals is compared with the proportion of responses occurring during control intervals. Using three control and three change (experimental) intervals, the analysis indicates significant discrimination if one of the following conditions are met:

(1) A subject may respond with a head turn during all three change intervals and not respond during any control intervals ($p < 0.01$).
(2) A subject may respond during all three change intervals and respond (that is, an inappropriate head-turn) during one of three control intervals ($p < 0.05$).
(3) A subject may respond to two change intervals and not respond during any control intervals ($p < 0.05$).

Results

Table 1a provides the results from this study for the six to eight month olds. Table 1b summarizes findings of high-amplitude sucking studies using these same stimuli with one- to three-month- old infants (Eilers, 1977a, 1977b). Each datum in 1b represents a study involving a large number of infants, 30 of whom successfully completed the procedure.

As is evident, [va] and [sa] were discriminable by infants at both age levels, that is, by six to eight month olds and the group of one to three month olds. The same is true for [sa] vs [Ia], [as] vs [a:z], and [at] vs [a:d] (in the latter two pairs, vowel duration differs as in Standard American English). Neither the one to three month olds nor the majority of the six to eight month olds showed evidence of ability to discriminate [a:t] and [at], where vowel duration was the only relevant parameter. Similar negative results were found for both age levels on the contrasts [fa] vs [2a] and [fi] vs [2i]. However, while all six month olds were able to discriminate [sa] from [za], the one-to-three- month-old infant group did not show discrimination for this pair. Similar positive results for the older group and negative results for the younger group are shown for the pair [a:s] and [a:z], where voicing is the relevant parameter. One reverse pattern was found (for [a:t] in opposition to [a:d]), where the younger infant group gave evidence of discrimination that was not obtained with the six month olds.

Results with 12- to 14-month-old infants are shown in Table 2. Most of these infants are able to discriminate [va] from [sa], [sa] from [Ia], [sa] from [za], [as] from [a:z], [a:s] from [a:z] and [at] from [a:d]. In addition, unlike the six month olds, half of the 12 month olds discriminate [a:t] and [a:d] as well as [at] and [a:t] and most discriminate [fi] from [2i]. Only one infant shows discrimination of [fa] and [2a].

Discussion

A proper perspective on the results reported here requires recognition not only of the importance of the substantive findings (that is, whether or not an infant discriminates between related speech sounds), but also of the merits of the methodological developments. In the long run, the methodological results may prove to be at least as important as the substantive findings.

On the methodological side, it has been shown that infants between six and 14 months of age can be tested for discrimination of subtle speech contrasts. Furthermore, it has been demonstrated that this testing can apply to individual infants (rather than groups), and that it can be applied repeatedly with the same infant to obtain information concerning discrimination of a variety of contrasts within or across time. But most significantly, even recognizing the limitations in scope and type of stimuli tested in the present work, it is still clear that extremely reliable and consistent differences occur and can be demonstrated between the discriminability of certain contrastive pairs as opposed to other pairs. Such results, while applying to a limited range of stimuli, suggest a potential for develop-

ment of a body of information concerning relative difficulty of various speech contrasts as well as changes in degree of discriminability of contrasts across time. Indeed, in the present study, there are significant developmental changes in the infants' ability to perceive some speech contrasts. It is precisely this sort of information that is needed to begin to understand the role of speech perception in young children's speech-sound production preferences.

The substantive results of this study, though of considerable interest, should be interpreted with caution. Cross-sectional developmental studies are normally fraught with interpretive difficulties stemming from the intrinsic confounding of age and subject variables. Adding an experimental paradigm variable, as in the present study, further complicates interpretation. Though we are now able to study speech perception throughout the first two years of life, we do not have a single technique that yields comparable data across the entire age range under investigation. It is essential, then, that these data be examined in light of the different limitations and assets of the high-amplitude sucking procedure and the visually reinforced infant speech discrimination paradigm. Because of the necessity to change from a high-amplitude sucking procedure to a visually reinforced infant speech discrimination paradigm after age four months, comparisons between one to three month olds and the groups of six to eight month olds and 12 to 14 month olds must be made with caution.

Yet if we do compare the data on the one- to three-month-old infants with the data on the six to eight month olds and 12 to 14 month olds, we can isolate two main discrimination patterns across ages. There are some contrasts that seem easily discriminable. On these contrasts evidence of discrimination can be obtained virtually from

Table 1a. Perception of speech contrasts by six- to eight-month-old infants.

Subject Number	Speech Contrast									
	va-sa	sa-Ia	sa-za	as-a:z	a:s-a:z	at-a:d	a:t-a:d	a:t-at	fa-2a	fi-2i
1	✿	✿	✿	✿	✿	✿	NS	NS	NS	NS
2	✿	✿	✿	✿	✿	✿	NS	NS	NS	NS
3	✿	✿	✿	✿	✿	✿	NS	NS	NS	NS
4	✿	✿	✿	✿	✿	✿	NS	NS	NS	NS
5	✿	✿	✿	✿	✿	✿	NS	NS	NS	NS
6	✿	✿	✿	✿	✿	✿	NS	NS	NS	NS
7	✿	✿	✿	✿	✿	NS	NS	NS	NS	✿
8	✿	✿	✿	✿	✿	✿	NS	NS	NS	NS

Table 1b. Perception of speech contrasts by three-month-old infants.

Infant Groups	va-sa	sa-Ia	sa-za	as-a:z	a:s-a:z	at-a:d	a:t-a:d	a:t-at	fa-2a	fi-2i
	✿	✿	NS	✿	NS	✿	✿	NS	NS	NS

✿   Indicates significant evidence of discrimination ($p < 0.05$).

NS   Indicates significant evidence of discrimination was not obtained.

birth onward. The pairs [sa] vs [Ia], [sa] vs [va], [as] vs [a:z], and [at] vs [a:d] are discriminated by one to three month olds, six to eight month olds, and 12 to 14 month olds. There are contrasts that seem difficult for very young children, but become easier as infants approach 14 months. These pairs include [a:s] vs [a:z], [fi] vs [2i], [at] vs [a:t], and [sa] vs [za]. Eight of the 10 stimulus pairs are accounted for by these two patterns. One additional pair, [fa] and [2a], seems difficult at all ages tested, although adult listeners had no difficulty discriminating the stimulus pair.

The final pair, [a:t] vs [a:d], shows a reverse pattern, that is, the youngest infants discriminate the pair while older infants show no evidence of the same discrimination. The question is, to what stimulus parameters can we attribute a backward developmental pattern? If this phenomenon is associated with listening experience, then it might be explained on the following grounds. In English, vowel duration cues are central in discrimination of voicing of consonants in VC syllables (Denes, 1955). It is possible that the infant learns this through experience with language and comes to disregard voicing differences in final-position stop consonants of relatively low amplitude and short duration. This inhibitory learning phenomenon may not occur with final fricatives because the longer duration and higher amplitude of the fricatives as opposed to the stops may provide a more salient framework within which to isolate the voicing cue. This explanation is very speculative, however.

Given that the high-amplitude sucking data on [a:t] vs [a:d] represent only one group experiment (as opposed to the eight or nine individual experiments from our visually reinforced infant speech discrimination data), we propose another way of looking at the phenomenon. Perhaps the single high-amplitude sucking experiment has yielded a false positive. Consider the subgroup of the data relating to final voicing and vowel duration cues as outlined in Table 3.

Several observations can be made. First, except for the pair [a:t] and [a:d], at one to three months, all the experimental data are consistent with the simple expectation that discrimination will improve with age. Second, discrimination of pairs where both duration and voicing differences occur seems easier than discrimination where only voicing or duration provides the cue. Third, voicing in final fricatives seems more salient than in final-stop consonants.

If we assume that the result for the one to three month olds with the high-amplitude sucking procedure is a false positive, the interpretive task is simplified immensely by eliminating the need to propose an elaborate explanation for the child's seeming loss of ability across time. In addition, such an assumption would simplify our interpretation from an acoustic point of view. Based on acoustic research, it is possible to argue that voicing should be more discernible in final fricatives than in final stops resulting from inherent differences in the duration of these elements (MacNeilage, 1963; Oller, 1973). Review of the present stimuli confirms that considerable durational differences exist between voiced and unvoiced final fricatives. The ratio of frication duration to stop duration was approximately two. Our reasoning suggests that acquisition of discrimination among these final fricatives and stop pairs may proceed in the following order:

(1) [as] vs [a:z] and [at] vs [a:d] (where both voicing and vowel duration differences are present).
(2) [a:s] vs [a:z] (here vowel durations are relatively equalized, but the long periods of voicing during final fricatives provides a basis for the discrimination).
(3) [a:t] vs [a:d] (where the stimuli differ in voicing only during the relatively short duration of the final stop).

Table 2. Perception of speech contrasts by 12- to 14-month-old infants.

| Subject Number | Speech Contrast | | | | | | | | | |
	va-sa	sa-Ia	sa-za	as-a:z	a:s-a:z	at-a:d	a:t-a:d	a:t-at	fa-2a	fi-2i
1	✿	✿	✿	✿	✿	✿	NS	NS	NS	✿
2	✿	✿	✿	✿	✿	NS	NS	NS	NS	✿
3	✿	✿	✿	✿	✿	✿	NS	✿	NS	✿
4	✿	✿	✿	✿	✿	✿	NS	✿	NS	✿
5	✿	✿	✿	✿	✿	✿	✿	✿	NS	✿
6	✿	✿	✿	✿	✿	✿	✿	✿	NS	✿
7	✿	✿	✿	NS	✿	✿	✿	NS	✿	✿
8	✿	NS	✿	✿	✿	✿	✿	NS	NS	NS

✿   Indicates significant evidence of discrimination ($p < 0.05$).
NS   Indicates significant evidence of discrimination was not obtained.

(4) [aːt] vs [at] (where stimuli differ only in vowel duration).

Although we prefer the second explanation as more defensible, our data do not specifically answer the question. Replication of the high-amplitude sucking data on [aːt] and [aːd] seem warranted. Certainly, the possibility of false positives or false negatives will always be problematic for infant-speech researchers. The primary safeguard against misleading results is increased numbers of subjects and replication in other laboratories. For researchers employing the high-amplitude sucking paradigm, either approach is an extremely costly procedure.

Another serious interpretive difficulty arises in the stimulus domain and relates to the acoustic nature of the stimuli employed in a given study, whether it be a high-amplitude sucking procedure, a heart-rate procedure, a visually reinforced infant speech discrimination paradigm, or other paradigms, and whether natural or synthetic stimuli are used. As in the present work, an individual syllable token used to represent a putative or actual linguistic category must be chosen with care —yet no amount of care can overcome the fact that selection itself eliminates from consideration the inherent variability within real linguistic categories. As a result, one cannot tell if the positive discriminations achieved by infants result from recognition of cues that are largely insignificant in real communicative situations. It is clear that future studies asking questions concerning discriminabilty of natural categories of speech sounds and using both high-amplitude sucking and visually reinforced infant speech discrimination paradigms will be required to move toward a form of natural stimuli that incorporates typical within-category variability. The multiple-token method successfully employed by Kuhl and Miller (1975) is an example of such an approach. By combining such improved methodologies in stimulus control and new operant methodologies such as visually reinforced infant speech discrimination, we should in the near future be able to make substantial advancements in our understanding of infant speech perception.

Acknowledgment

This research was supported by a contract from the National Institute of Child Health and Human Development (HD-3-2793) at the University of Washington and by Grant HD 09906-02 at the University of Miami. Requests for reprints may be directed to Rebecca E. Eilers, Mailman Center for Child Development, University of Miami, P.O. Box 520006, Biscayne Annex, Miami, Florida 33152.

References

Abbs, M.S., and Minifie, F.D., Effect of acoustic cues in fricatives on perceptual confusions in preschool children. *J. Acoust. Soc. Am.*, 46, 1535-1542 (1969).

American National Standards Institute, *Specifications for Audiometers*, ANSI S3.6-1969. New York: American National Standards Institute (1970).

Bruning, J.L., and Kintz, B.L., *Computational Handbook of Statistics*. Glenview, Ill.: Scott, Foresman (1968).

Denes, P., Effect of duration on the perception of voicing. *J. Acoust. Soc. Am.*, 27, 761-764 (1955).

Eilers, R.E., Context sensitivity perception of naturally produced stop and fricative consonants by infants. *J. Acoust. Soc. Am.*, 61, 1321-1336 (1977a).

Eilers, R.E., On tracing the development of speech perception. Paper presented to the Society for Research in Child Development, New Orleans (1977b).

Eilers, R.E., and Minifie, F.D., Fricative discrimination in early infancy. *J. Speech Hearing Res.*, 18, 158-167 (1975).

Eilers, R.E., and Oller, D.K., The role of speech discrimination in developmental sound substitutions. *J. Child Lang.*, 3, 319-329 (1976).

Eimas, P.D., Auditory and phonetic coding of the cues for speech: Discrimination of the [r-1] distinction by young infants. *Percept. & Psychophys.*, 18, 341-347 (1975).

Eimas, P.D., Siqueland, E.R., Jusczyk, P., and Vigorito, J., Speech perception in infants. *Science*, 171, 303-306 (1971).

Kuhl, P.K., and Miller, J.D., Speech perception by the chinchilla: Voiced-voiceless distinction in alveolar plosive consonants. *Science*, 190, 69-72 (1975).

Table 3. Perception of final voiced consonant distinctions at three ages. VRISD = visually reinforced infant speech discrimination; HAS = high-amplitude sucking.

Age	Contrast as-aːz	aːs-aːz	at-aːd	aːt-aːd	at-aːt
1-3 month (HAS) (one group)	☼	NS	☼	☼	NS
6-8 month (VRISD) (nine individuals)	+	+	+	−	−
12-14 month (VRISD) (eight individuals)	+	+	+	±	±

+   Indicates significant evidence of discrimination was obtained for most subjects.
−   Indicates significant evidence of discrimination was not obtained for most subjects.
±   Indicates half of the subjects discriminated and the other half provided no significant evidence of discrimination.
☼   Indicates significant evidence of discrimination for group data ($p < 0.05$).
NS Indicates no significant evidence of discrimination obtained for group.

MacNeilage, P.F., Electromyographic and acoustic study of the production of certain final clusters. *J. Acoust. Soc. Am.*, 35, 461-463 (1963).

Moffitt, A.R., Consonant cue perception by twenty- to twenty-four-week-old infants. *Child Dev.*, 42, 717-731 (1971).

Moore, J.M., Thompson, G., and Thompson, M., Auditory localization of infants as a function of reinforcement conditions. *J. Speech Hearing Dis.*, 40, 29-34 (1975).

Moore, J.M., Wilson, W.R., and Thompson, G., Visual reinforcement of head-turn responses in infants under 12 months of age. *J. Speech Hearing Dis.*, 42, 328-334 (1977).

Morse, P.A., The discrimination of speech and nonspeech stimuli in early infancy. *J. Exp. Child Psychol.*, 14, 477-492 (1972).

Oller, D.K., The effect of position-in-utterance on speech segment duration in English. *J. Acoust. Soc. Am.*, 54, 1235-1247 (1973).

Spring, D., Discrimination of linguistic stress location in one-to-four-month-old infants. Doctoral dissertation, University of Washington (1975).

Trehub, S.E., Infants' sensitivity to vowel and tonal contrasts. *Devl. Psychol.*, 9, 91-96 (1973).

Trehub, S.E., and Rabinovitch, M.S., Auditory-linguistic sensitivity in early infancy. *Devl. Psychol.*, 6, 74-77 (1972).

Wilson, W.R., Moore, J.M., and Thompson, G., Sound-field auditory thresholds of infants utilizing Visual Reinforcement Audiometry (VRA). Paper presented at the Annual Convention of the American Speech and Hearing Association, Houston (1976).

Received July 20, 1976
Accepted May 10, 1977

Linguistic Experience Alters Phonetic Perception in Infants by 6 Months of Age

Patricia K. Kuhl*
Department of Speech and Hearing Sciences, University of Washington (WJ-10), Seattle, WA 98195

Karen A. Williams and Francisco Lacerda
Institute of Linguistics, Stockholm University, S-106 91 Stockholm, Sweden

Kenneth N. Stevens
Research Laboratory of Electronics, Massachusetts Institute of Technology, Cambridge, MA 02139

Björn Lindblom
Department of Linguistics, University of Texas at Austin, Austin, TX 78712

Linguistic experience affects phonetic perception. However, the critical period during which experience affects perception and the mechanism responsible for these effects are unknown. This study of 6-month-old infants from two countries, the United States and Sweden, shows that exposure to a specific language in the first half year of life alters infants' phonetic perception.

At the beginning of life, human infants exhibit a similar pattern of phonetic perception regardless of the language environment in which they are born (*1*). They discern differences between the phonetic units of many different languages, including languages they have never heard, indicating that the perception of human speech is strongly influenced by innate factors. However, by adulthood, linguistic experience has had a profound effect on speech perception. Exposure to a specific language results in a reduction in the ability to perceive differences between speech sounds that do not differentiate between words in one's native language (*2,3*). Adult native speakers of Japanese, for example, have great difficulty in discriminating between words containing English /r/ and /l/, phonetic segments that belong to the same underlying category in Japanese (*2*). Adults thus exhibit a pattern of phonetic perception that is specific to their native language, whereas infants initially demonstrate a pattern of perception that is universal. At what point in development does linguistic experience alter phonetic perception, and what is the nature of the change brought about by experience with a particular language?

Previous studies suggested that the effects of linguistic experience on phonetic perception occur at about 1 year of age (*3*), coinciding with the age at which children begin to acquire word meanings (*4*). It was thus proposed that the change from a language-universal pattern of pho-

netic perception to one that is language-specific was brought about by the emergence of a milestone in the child's linguistic development, namely, the child's understanding that phonetic units are used contrastively to specify different word meanings (*3*).

We show here that by 6 months of age, well before the acquisition of language (*4*), infants' phonetic perception has been altered by exposure to a specific language. Infants in America and Sweden were tested with both native- and foreign-language vowel sounds. Infants from both countries exhibited a language-specific pattern of phonetic perception. Thus, linguistic experience alters phonetic perception at an unexpectedly early age, and this has implications for theories of speech perception and the development of language.

The present test focused on phonetic "prototypes," speech sounds that are identified by adult speakers of a given language as ideal representatives of a given phonetic category. Experiments with adults have shown that phonetic prototypes function like "perceptual magnets" in speech perception (*5*). The magnet effect causes other nonprototypic members of the category to be perceived as more similar to the category prototype than to each other, even though the actual physical differences between the stimuli are equal (*5*).

It has been shown that 6-month-old American infants tested with a prototype and a nonprototype of an American English vowel duplicate the magnet effect shown in adults (*5*). A critical question for theory is whether this infant effect reflects language-specific or language-universal perception. Is experience with a specific

Reprinted with permission from *Linguistic Experience Alters Phonetic Perception in Infants by 6 Months of Age Science*, 255, pp. 606-608. Copyright 1992. American Association for the Advancement of Science.

*To whom correspondence should be addressed.

language necessary, or would 6-month-olds show the magnet effect for all vowel prototypes regardless of language experience? We examined this question by conducting a cross-language study in 6-month-old infants from two countries using both native- and foreign-language sounds.

We tested infants in the United States and Sweden on two vowels. One vowel (American English /i/, the front unrounded vowel in the word "fee") constituted a native-language prototype for American adults and a nonprototype for Swedish adults; the other vowel (Swedish /y/, the front rounded vowel in the Swedish word "fy") constituted a native-language prototype for Swedish adults and a nonprototype for American adults (6). If experience with language in the first half year of life alters phonetic perception, a specific pattern is predicted in which the two groups of infants differ: (i) American infants would treat the American English /i/ as a prototype and the Swedish /y/ as a nonprototype, exhibiting a stronger magnet effect for American English /i/, (ii) Swedish infants would treat the Swedish /y/ as a prototype and the American English /i/ as a nonprototype, exhibiting a stronger magnet effect for Swedish /y/. However, if the results show any other pattern (if both groups of infants exhibit the magnet effect equally for both vowels or more strongly for the same one of the two vowels), then we would have no evidence that linguistic experience alters phonetic perception by 6 months.

We computer-synthesized prototypes of the American English /i/ and Swedish /y/ vowels (7). Each prototype was then modified to create 32 additional variants that were acoustically similar, but not identical, to each prototype (Fig. 1) (8). The magnet effect was assessed by testing infants' perception of the similarity between each prototype and its variants.

Infants sat on a parent's lap and watched an assistant, seated on the infant's right, manipulate silent toys. Each infant listened to one of the vowel prototypes (either American English /i/ or Swedish /y/), continuously repeated every 2 s from a loudspeaker located on the infant's left. In the training phase infants learned to produce a head-turn (HT) toward the loudspeaker when they heard the prototype vowel change (9). Two kinds of 6-s trials occurred. During change trials the prototype vowel was changed to one of its variants and infants' HT responses were rewarded by the activation of a toy bear that pounded a miniature drum. An equal number of control trials occurred in which the prototype vowel was not changed and infants' false-positive HTs were tabulated. Safeguards against bias on the part of the parent, the experimenter, and the assistant were stringent to ensure that these individuals did not influence infants' HTs (5). The test phase consisted of 64 trials, 32 change trials (one for each vari-

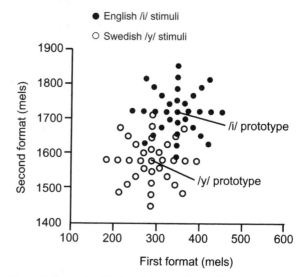

Figure 1. Six-month-old infants from America and Sweden were tested with two sets of vowel stimuli, American English /i/ and Swedish /y/. Each set included an exceptionally good instance of the vowel (the prototype) and 32 variants that formed four rings (eight stimuli each) around the prototype (8).

ant), and 32 control trials, presented in random order. The perceptual magnet effect was indicated by the degree to which infants responded to each prototype's variants as though they were identical to it, that is, trials in which infants did not detect a difference between a prototype and its variants.

Sixty-four 6-month-old infants were tested, 32 in the United States and 32 in Sweden. In each country, 16 infants were trained and tested with the American English /i/ prototype, and 16 were trained and tested with the Swedish /y/ prototype (10). Except for the critical variable of the language experience of the infants, all components of the experimental test remained the same in the two countries. The speech testing apparatus, computer equipment, and the three experimenters were physically moved from one site (the University of Washington, Seattle, Washington) to the other (Stockholm University, Stockholm, Sweden) for the duration of the tests. The same test protocol and stimuli were used.

The results confirmed that linguistic experience in the first half year of life alters infants' perception of speech sounds. Infants from both countries showed a significantly stronger magnet effect for their native-language prototype (Fig. 2). American infants perceived the American English /i/ prototype as identical to its variants on 66.9% of all trials; in contrast, they perceived the Swedish /y/ prototype as identical to its variants on 50.6% of the trials. Swedish infants perceived the Swedish /y/ prototype as identical to its variants on 66.2% of all trials; in contrast, they treated the American English /i/ prototype as identical to its variants on 55.9% of the trials. Infants' responses to the two

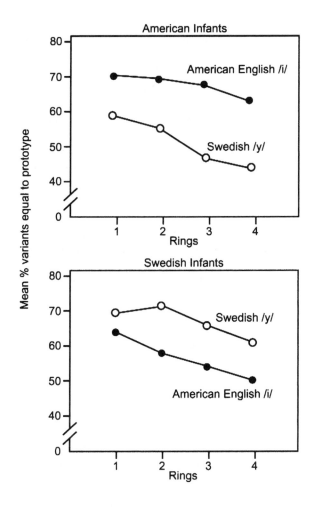

American Infants

Swedish Infants

Figure 2. Results showing an effect of language experience on young infants' perception of speech. Two groups of 6-month-old infants, (**A**) American and (**B**) Swedish, were tested with two different vowel prototypes, American English /i/ and Swedish /y/. The mean percentage of trials in which infants equated variants on each of the four rings to the prototype is plotted. Infants from both countries produced a stronger magnet effect (equated variants to the prototype more often) for the native-language vowel prototype when compared to the foreign-language vowel prototype. (Error bars = standard error.)

types have begun to function like nonprototypes in the native language (*12*). The results show that the initial appearance of a language-specific pattern of phonetic perception does not depend on the emergence of contrastive phonology and an understanding of word meaning. Rather, infants' language-specific phonetic categories may initially emerge from an underlying cognitive capacity and proclivity to store in memory biologically important stimuli (*13*) and from the ability to represent information in the form of a prototype (*5*).

The findings also suggest the process by which linguistic experience alters phonetic perception. Linguistic experience shrinks the perceptual distance around a native-language prototype, in relation to a nonprototype, causing the prototype to perceptually assimilate similar sounds (*5*). The native-language prototype's magnet effect may help explain why older children and adults fail to discriminate two speech sounds from a foreign language when both sounds resemble a native-language prototype for the subject (such as /r/ and /l/ for native Japanese speakers) (*2,3*).

Infants demonstrate a capacity to learn simply by being exposed to language during the first half year of life, before the time that they have uttered meaningful words. By 6 months of age, linguistic experience has resulted in language-specific phonetic prototypes that assist infants in organizing speech sounds into categories. They are in place when infants begin to acquire word meanings toward the end of the first year. Phonetic prototypes would thus appear to be fundamental perceptual-cognitive building blocks rather than by-products of language acquisition.

References and Notes

1. P.D. Eimas, J.L. Miller, P.W. Jusczyk, in *Categorical Perception*, S. Harnad, Ed. (Cambridge Univ. Press, New York, 1987), pp. 161-195; P.K. Kuhl, in *Handbook of Infant Perception*, P. Salapatek and L. Cohen, Eds. (Academic Press, New York, 1987), vol. 2, pp. 275-382.

2. H. Goto, *Neuropsychologia* 9, 317 (1971); K. Miyawaki et al., *Percept. Psychophys.* 18, 331 (1975); W. Strange and S. Dittmann, *ibid.* 36, 131 (1984).

3. J.F. Werker and R.C. Tees, *Infant Behav. Dev.* 7, 49 (1984); J.F. Werker and C.E. Lalonde, *Dev. Psychol.* 24, 672 (1988).

4. Many detailed studies of language acquisition have shown that infants first begin to comprehend and produce words after 9 months of age [E. Bates, I. Bretherton, L. Snyder, *From First Words to Grammar* (Cambridge Univ. Press, Cambridge, 1988)]. For word production, the mean age for acquiring ten words = 15.1 months (SD = 1.76), for 50 words = 19.6 months (SD = 2.89) [K. Nelson, *Monogr.*

sets of stimuli were submitted to a two-way analysis of variance to assess the effects of infants' language environment (American English versus Swedish) and the prototype vowel tested (American English /i/ versus Swedish /y/). The interaction between the two factors was highly significant [$F(1, 60) = 20.107$, $P < 0.0001$]; neither of the main effects was significant [language environment: $F(1, 60) = 0.526$, $P > 0.40$; vowel: $F(1, 60) = 0.978$, $P > 0.30$] (*11*).

The findings demonstrate that by 6 months infants exhibit a strong magnet effect only for native-language phonetic prototypes. By this age foreign-language proto-

Soc. Res. Child Dev. 38, 1 (1973)]; for word comprehension, the mean age for acquiring ten words = 10.5 months (SD = 0.92), for 50 words = 13.2 months (SD = 1.53) [H. Benedict, *J. Child Lang.* 6, 183 (1979)].

5.   D. Grieser and P.K. Kuhl, *Dev. Psychol.* 25, 577 (1989); P.K. Kuhl, *Percept. Psychophys.* 50, 93 (1991). For other work on speech prototypes see D.W. Massaro, *Speech Perception by Ear and Eye* (Erlbaum, Hillsdale, NJ, 1987); J.L. Miller and L.E. Volaitis, *Percept. Psychophys.* 46, 505 (1989); A.G. Samuel, *ibid.* 31, 307 (1982).

6.   The status of the two vowel prototypes in American English and Swedish was experimentally assessed. Adult native speakers of American English and Swedish were asked three questions about each prototype: (i) whether it was a sound used in their language, (ii) the category it belonged to, and (iii) its representativeness as a member of that category using a scale from "1" (poor) to "7" (good). American listeners unanimously judged the /i/ prototype as an English vowel, giving it an average rating of 5.4 as a member of the English /i/ category. They unanimously rated the Swedish /y/ prototype as not in their language. Swedish adults unanimously judged the /y/ prototype as a Swedish vowel, giving it an average rating of 4.7 as a member of the category /y/. They rated the American English /i/ prototype as present in the language but ambiguous with regard to category; /i/ was given an average rating of 2.6 as a member of the Swedish /e/ category and 1.8 as a member of the Swedish /i/ category. These ratings are typical of native-language nonprototypes *(5)*.

7.   The five formant frequencies of English /i/ were 270, 2290, 3010, 3300, and 3850 Hz; for Swedish /y/, 220, 1980, 2640, 3340, and 3720 Hz.

8.   Variants were created by manipulating the first two formant frequencies [scaled in mels *(5)*] in uniform, psychophysically equal steps. The variants formed four rings that were 30, 60, 90, and 120 mels, respectively, from each prototype.

9.   During change trials in training, the prototype vowel was changed to a variant from the fourth ring around the prototype and this stimulus change was paired with the reinforcer, causing infants to turn toward the reinforcer. Once infants were producing HTs reliably on change trials, control trials were introduced. Infants had to meet a criterion of seven out of eight consecutive correct trials (including both change and control trials) during training, and produce no more than 35% false-positive responses once the test started, to be included in the study.

10.   Mean age of infants: 6.5 months (range = 6.1 to 6.9) for American infants tested on /i/; 6.5 months (range = 6.0 to 7.0) for Swedish infants tested on /i/; 6.7 months (range = 6.2 to 7.1) for American infants tested on /y/; 6.6 months (range = 6.1 to 6.9) for Swedish infants tested on /y/.

11.   Follow-up tests indicated that for both the American and Swedish infants there was a significant difference between the vowels, $P < 0.05$.

12.   We have not yet determined whether prototypes for all vowels (or a subset of them) exist at birth and are modified by 6 months due to linguistic experience or whether prototypes are initially absent and subsequently formed by 6 months as a result of language experience.

13   Studies suggest that infants under 3 months are capable of remembering faces, voices, and certain acoustic characteristics of speech [M.E. Barrera and D. Maurer, *Child Dev.* 52, 714 (1981); A.J. DeCasper and W.P. Fifer, *Science* 208, 1174 (1980); J. Mehler et al., *Cognition* 29, 143 (1988); A.N. Meltzoff, P.K. Kuhl, M.K. Moore, in *Newborn Attention*, M.J.S. Weiss and P.R. Zelazo, Eds. (Ablex, Norwood, NJ, 1991), pp. 377-411].

14.   We thank S. Gordon and S. Smith for assistance in testing infants; D. Padden and E. Stevens for help on data analysis; and A. Meltzoff, A. Gopnik, C. Stoel-Gammon, E. Rubel, and L. Werner for valuable comments on the manuscript. Supported by grants to P.K.K. from NIH (DC 00520), the University of Washington Graduate School Research Fund, and the Bloedel Hearing Research Center.

14 August 1991; Accepted 19 November 1991

II. Behavioral Methodology

....

The series of articles included in this section traces the development of current audiometric and speech assessment procedures used by pediatric audiologists. The audiologic assessment of children can be thought of in two broadly different categories: procedures that rely on observing overt behaviors to sound (unconditioned responses) and those that rely on behavioral responses that are shaped through reinforcement (conditioned responses).

Historically, the behavioral evaluation of hearing sensitivity in infants and young children has been highly subjective. The clinicians considered the "best" pediatric audiologists were those with extensive experiences in the testing of young children. Their skills were honed by years of practice in observing the auditory responses of infants and young children with normal hearing or hearing loss. Testing usually involved two clinicians (both aware of the presence of a test signal) who observed an infant and agreed on whether a behavioral response had occurred during or immediately following the stimulus presentation.. Speech, environmental noises, and other familiar and novel sounds (e.g., music, whistles, bells, rattles) were often used as test stimuli. Acceptable behavioral responses included a change in facial expression, a startle response, the cessation of sucking activity, limb movement, an eye shift, or, depending on the age of the baby, an orientation (head turn) toward the source of the test stimulus. Because of state and developmental level, younger infants tended to be more variable in their responses and usually required louder test signals to elicit a response than older babies. Moreover, the likelihood of observing a response was directly related to the type of stimulus used; speech because it was inherently "interesting" and broad-band was more likely to elicit a response than less complex, frequency-specific test signals (Wilson & Thompson, 1984). This pattern of responsivity implied to some clinicians that hearing "improved" with age. Indeed, for their classic textbook *Hearing in Children,* Northern and Downs (1974) provided an "Auditory Behavior Index for Infants" that depicted expected behavioral responses for various test stimuli and intensities as a function of age. As a result, the concept of "normal response for age" evolved, and audiologists used these "normative data" to determine whether a child had normal hearing or a hearing loss. What commonly has been termed behavioral observation audiometry (BOA) became the accepted test strategy used in the audiologic assessment of infants and toddlers.

A new era in pediatric audiology was portended by the reports of Suzuki and Ogiba (1961) who developed conditioned orienting response (COR) audiometry and Liden and Kankkunen (1969). The latter investigators devised a modification of COR for use with preschool children, which they termed visual reinforcement audiometry (VRA). However, the catalyst for the present-day practice of behavioral pediatric audiometry (indeed, the practice we now refer to as VRA) was a series of studies in the 1970s completed at the University of Washington, Seattle. Wilson, Moore, Thompson (G), Thompson (M), and their students provided the solid foundation for our current approach to the audiologic assessment of infants and toddlers. These researchers demonstrated that the incorporation of operant conditioning techniques in the clinical setting provided a reliable, accurate, and efficient means for completing a behavioral assessment of hearing in infants and young children. Arguably, operant procedures used in conjunction with appropriate psychometric methods and computer/assisted test techniques have brought pediatric behavioral audiometry into an age of "objectivity (Widen, 1993)."

The classic 1974 article by Jerger and Hayes, was chosen to begin this section on Behavioral Methods, because the concept of cross-checking test results (first articulated by these authors) remains one of the maxims of pediatric clinical practice. Indeed, behavioral test methods used in conjunction with electrophysiologic test procedures constitute the standard audiologic battery for the assessment of the pediatric population across the age range.

The next two articles in this section examine the efficiency and accuracy of BOA. Thompson and Thompson examined responses obtained by unconditioned behavioral observation techniques in infants (7 to 12 months of age) and young children (22 to 36 months of age) and, in addition, COR and play audiometry in the older subjects. For infants, signal presentation intensity levels were varied and several types of auditory stimuli were used. Thompson and Thompson clearly demonstrated that response variability among infants with normal hearing was extreme as a function of both presentation intensity and signal type. Variability was reduced as both age increased and test methodology became more active than passive. The test stimuli most important for audiometric assessment, namely, frequency-specific signals (pure tones, FM tones, or narrow bands of noise), were the least effective in eliciting a response from the infants. Their work supports the conclusion that the accurate audiologic assessment of infants cannot be accomplished using unconditioned, observation methods.

Our current practice of VRA is supported by the outcomes of the three remaining studies in this section. Moore, Thompson, and Thompson systematically examined the head-turn response in infants as a function of reinforcer type.

These researchers demonstrated convincingly that the orientation response (head turn) could best be supported over repeated signal presentations by a complex reinforcer (animated, illuminated). Subsequently, Moore, Wilson, and Thompson found that complex visual reinforcement was effective in maintaining the head-turn response across numerous stimulus trials in infants 5 (but, not 4) months to 11 months of age. Thus, Moore and his colleagues demonstrated the importance of a highly complex visual reinforcer in maintaining strong response behavior. This response is necessary for threshold acquisition. Moreover, these researchers established the "lower age limit" for the effective use of visual reinforcement audiometry. Primus and Thompson found that variations in test stimulus parameters (bandwidth and starting intensity) did not influence the rate at which infants achieved a predetermined conditioning criteria for VRA.

In the second part of the Behavioral Methodology section, we present a series of studies on the assessment of speech detection and identification abilities in the pediatric population. Our ability to quantify the development of speech perception is important in both the assessment and the follow-up of children with hearing loss and in planning and validating management approaches.

The section on speech audiometry begins with the classic article, Developments in Speech Audiometry by Authur Boothroyd. Boothroyd delineates the problems associated with measuring speech discrimination and proposes a new speech discrimination test comprised of short isophonemic word lists. Scoring of this test is based on the percent of phonemes children identify correctly within monosyllabic words. Phonemic scoring offers several distinct advantages over word recognition tests including ease for phoneme recognition over complete words, improved test-retest reliability and improved validity. This important paper served as the basis for another seminal study by Boothroyd (1984) which examined phonemic identification in children with varying degrees of hearing loss and offered convincing evidence that children with hearing impairment have significant access to acoustic speech contrasts.

Speech audiometry in some form is one of the most commonly practiced test strategies in pediatric assessment. Speech audiometry (detection, threshold, and recognition) is often performed, however, using materials that may not be developmentally appropriate. Interestingly, one of the first pediatric speech recognition materials (PBK-50) was devised using children's vocabulary items, but the test material was not standardized on a pediatric population. Early measures of speech recognition ability required a verbal response from the child. Obviously, this response methodology precluded the test's use with younger children or those with speech production errors. The advent of picture identification speech materials such as the Threshold by Identification of Pictures (TIP), the Discrimination by Identification of Pictures (DIP), and the NUCHIPS (Northwestern University—Children's Identification of Pictures) provided both an appropriate response task and a reduced (closed-set) number of response choices. These tests were limited, however, by the restricted number of foil items, which increased the probability of chance performance and made the determination of any true test-retest differences problematic.

In their 1970 article, Ross and Lerman described the development of the Word Intelligibility by Picture Identification (WIPI) test, today, probably the most widely used pediatric speech recognition material. The WIPI was the first pediatric test to be normed on children with sensorineural hearing loss. The WIPI offered the advantage of a six-choice response task and foil items that allowed some analyses of phonemic errors made by the child. Sanderson-Leepa and Rintelmann were the first to provide critical information on the performance characteristics of three tests commonly used with children: the WIPI, the PBK-50, and the NU-6. The importance of this type of study to our understanding of the properties of these materials for the testing of speech recognition in children cannot be overemphasized.

Our appreciation of the need for appropriate speech materials for children with sensorineural hearing loss was furthered by the work of Norman Erber at the Central Institute for the Deaf (CID), St. Louis, Missouri. At CID, Erber conducted research into the auditory and visual speech recognition abilities of children with severe and profound hearing loss. In his 1974 classic article, Erber presents a systematic study of the relationship between a child's pure-tone thresholds and word recognition abilities.

Subsequently, sentence materials developed specifically for use with children with sensorineural hearing loss (Bench, Kowal, and Bamford, 1979) and monosyllabic and sentence identification materials useful for the differential diagnosis of various peripheral and central auditory dysfunctions (Jerger and Jerger, 1982) became available. The Pediatric Speech Intelligibility (PSI) test is the only standardized speech test useful for children as young as 3 years of age. The last two articles in our series present these well-devised and carefully studied speech materials that are extremely useful tools in the pediatric speech test armamentarium.

This section in Behavioral Methodology spans both audiometric assessment and speech audiometry and provides some of the fundamental literature for our day-to-day clinical practice.

References

Boothroyd, A. 1984. Auditory perception of speech contrasts by subjects with sensorineural hearing loss. *Journal of Speech and Hearing Research*, 27:134-144.

Liden, G., and Kankkunen, A. 1969. Visual reinforcement audiometry. *Acta Otolaryngologica* 67:281-292.

Northern, J.L., and Downs, M.P. 1974. *Hearing in children* (p. 138). Baltimore, MD: Williams and Wilkins.

Suzuki, T., and Ogiba, Y. 1961. Conditioned orientation audiometry. *Archives of Otolaryngology* 74:192-198.

Widen, J.E. 1993. Adding objectivity to infant behavioral audiometry. *Ear & Hearing* 14:49-57.

Wilson, W., and Thompson, G. 1984. Behavioral audiometry. In: J. Jerger (Ed.) *Pediatric Audiology* (pp. 1-44). San Diego, CA:College-Hill Press.

Additional Readings

Bernstein, R.S., and Gravel, J.S. 1990. A method for determining hearing sensitivity in infants: The interweaving staircase procedure (ISP). *Journal of the American Academy of Audiology* 1:138-145.

Eilers, R.E., Miskiel, E., Ozdamar, O., Urbano, R., and Widen, J.E. 1991. Optimization of automated hearing test algorithms: Simulations using an infant response model. *Ear & Hearing* 12:191-198.

Eilers, R.E., Widen, J.E., Urbano, R., Hudson, T., and Gonzalez, L. 1991. Optimization of automated hearing test algorithms: A comparison of data from simulations and young children. *Ear & Hearing* 12:199-204.

Tharpe, A.M., and Ashmead, D.H. 1993. Computer simulation technique for assessing pediatric auditory test protocols. *Journal of the American Academy of Audiology* 4:80-90.

The Cross-Check Principle in Pediatric Audiometry

James F. Jerger, Ph.D. and Deborah Hayes, M.A.

Department of Otorhinolaryngology and Communicative Sciences, Baylor College of Medicine,
Texas Medical Center, Houston

We discuss a method of pediatric audiologic assessment that employs the " cross-check principle. " That is, the results of a single test are cross-checked by an independent test measure. Particularly useful in pediatric evaluations as cross-checks of behavioral test results are impedance audiometry and brainstem-evoked response audiometry (BSER). We present five cases highlighting the value of the cross-check principle in pediatric audiologic evaluation. (*Arch Otolaryngol* 102:614-620, 1976)

Behavioral observation has been the traditional cornerstone of pediatric audiometry for many years. Some investigators enthusiastically report the success of this method for testing any child, regardless of his level of functioning:

> The trick, if there is any, is to become confidently familiar with the auditory behavior of normal-hearing children regardless of the integrity of their mental processing or central nervous system functioning. Once one knows the hearing level at which these children should respond, as well as the kind of response they will give, the deviation of the deaf child will become patently evident.[1]

We are not so sanguine. We have found that simply observing the auditory behavior of children does not always yield an accurate description of hearing loss. In our own experience, we have seen too many children at all levels of functioning who have been misdiagnosed and mismanaged on the basis of behavioral test results alone.

The mishandling of children based on the results of behavioral audiometry is an increasingly alarming problem. In our own audiology service we are evaluating children at much earlier ages than was common in the past. It is not unusual for us to evaluate infants as young as 5 weeks. Physicians and parents are becoming increasingly aware of the possibilities and implications of hearing loss in infancy. We are also seeing more multiply handicapped children. Special service agencies are requesting audiologic evaluations for these children to determine whether hearing handicap must be considered in planning the educational program. And it is just these two groups of children, very young infants and multiply handicapped

children, whom we have found are most often misdiagnosed by behavioral test results alone.

During the past decade two new techniques, uniquely suited to the evaluation of young children, have been made available to clinicians. The first, impedance audiometry, is not only sensitive to middle ear disorders,[2,3] but in the case of normal middle ear function permits quantification of sensorineural level.[4,5] The second technique, brainstem-evoked response (BSER)[6,7] audiometry, is an electrophysiologic technique that permits the clinician to estimate sensitivity above 500 hertz[8] by both air and bone conduction.

For the past three years, we have used these two techniques in combination with conventional behavioral audiometry as a pediatric test battery. Our fundamental approach has been to use either impedance audiometry or BSER audiometry as a "cross-check" of the behavioral test results.

We reasoned that, if behavioral test results obtained on a child could be confirmed by an independent test measure, then the errors made by behavioral testing alone would be substantially reduced, multiply handicapped children and very young infants could be more accurately tested, and configuration of audiometric contour could be more precisely defined. Impedance audiometry and BSER audiometry appear to be uniquely suited as cross-checks of behavioral test results. It is around these three test measures, behavioral audiometry, impedance audiometry, and BSER audiometry, then, that we have developed a test battery approach for evaluating children.

Test Battery

Behavioral audiometry is used at various levels in our service—from informal observation of a child's response to sound to conditioned play audiometry. Depending on the child's age and level of functioning, we determine the most appropriate behavioral procedure. For

Reprinted by permission of authors and American Medical Association. Copyright 1976. *Archives of Otolaryngology*, 102, pp. 614-620.

Reprint requests to Mail Station 009, Methodist Hospital, Texas Medical Center, Houston, TX 77030 (Dr Jerger).

Accepted for publication May 11, 1976.

very young children we present calibrated speech, toy noisemakers, white noise, or warble tones in the sound field and search for a behavioral response. For slightly older children, we pair the auditory signal with a visual stimulus in the performance of visual reinforcement audiometry. Finally, we use conditioned play audiometry whenever possible to test a child's hearing. Irrespective of the procedure used, however, our audiologic evaluation of the child does not stop with behavioral test results. We always insist that the behavioral result be confirmed by a cross-check.

We use impedance audiometry to confirm behavioral test results in two ways; first, to confirm middle ear disorders when behavioral test results suggest a conductive hearing loss; second, to obtain a rough prediction of the degree of sensorineural hearing loss by comparing the acoustic reflex thresholds for pure tones and for broadband noise. We have found this prediction of sensorineural hearing loss by the acoustic reflex (SPAR) to be remarkably accurate in children. It is a powerful technique for confirming behavioral test results.

A second test method useful in confirming behavioral test results is BSER audiometry. Evoked responses to rapidly presented clicks are recorded from nontraumatic scalp electrodes and processed by an average-response computer. The latency of the brain stem response ranges from 5 to 8 milliseconds and is age- and intensity-dependent.[6] We use BSER to cross-check behavioral test results whenever impedance audiometry is noncontributory in quantifying sensorineural level due to middle ear disorder. We also use BSER to cross-check the results of impedance audiometry when behavioral testing yields no useful information.

Irrespective of the test procedure used to gain an initial impression of a child's hearing—behavioral audiometry, impedance audiometry, or BSER audiometry—we always insist that the initial results be cross-checked by an independent measure. No one test or tester is infallible, and mistakes made with children can have devastating implications. Our experience has been that the confirmation of test results by an independent cross-check can substantially improve the audiological evaluation of children.

Report of Cases

The following five cases illustrate our experience with this cross-check principle in the evaluation of children.

Case 1. A 15-year-old boy was referred to our audiology service by the social worker in a community home where he lived. The child had been placed in this home at the age of 8 with the diagnosis of autism. According to the child's mother, he had been identified as deaf at the

age of 4. He was fitted with a body-borne hearing aid and placed in a preschool, hearing-impaired program. Noticing no improvement in the child's linguistic skills or behavior, the parents took him to a major university audiology service. The child was then 8 years old. Using psychogalvanic skin response (PGSR) audiometry, this service determined that the child had "normal hearing." Psychological evaluation following this determination of normal hearing resulted in a diagnosis of autism and the child was placed in a seemingly appropriate community center. The social worker at this center, however, did not think that this child's behavior was consistent with autism, and recommended further hearing tests.

The results of our audiologic evaluation are shown in Fig 1. The child's voluntary pure-tone audiogram, obtained by conditioned play audiometry, indicated a profound bilateral hearing loss. Speech awareness thresholds of 90 dB hearing level (HL) in the right ear, and 84 dB HL in the left ear were consistent with pure-tone results.

These behavioral test results were crosschecked by impedance audiometry. Tympanograms were type A bilaterally. Acoustic reflexes were present and elevated to pure-tone signals of 250 and 500 Hz in both ears. No reflexes could be elicited to either broad-band noise or pure-tone signals above 500 Hz. This reflex pattern is consistent with a severe bilateral sensorineural hearing loss.

In a nonverbal child with supposedly normal hearing, a diagnosis of autism is not unlikely. For this reason, it is imperative to be certain of the hearing level in children with behavior problems. We were "confident" of the results of our behavioral audiometry. Nonetheless, we demanded independent confirmation of these results by a cross-check. Impedance audiometry provided this confirmation.

It is unnecessary to dwell on the tragedy of this child. As long as audiologists are willing to accept the results of a single test measure they will continue to misdiagnose and mismanage some children. Perhaps this error might have been averted if the university audiologist had demanded an independent cross-check of the PGSR findings.

Case 2. This patient was a 2-year, 9-month-old boy. Although he had been under the care of an otologist for 18 months for recurrent ear infections, his mother thought that there was more hearing loss present than could be accounted for by simple middle ear disorder. Specifically, she did not notice any improvement in his speech or language after active medical management for middle ear disorder, including insertion of polyethylene tubes. This child's hearing had been tested three times by an audiologist at the physician's office. After each evaluation, the audiologist reported a bilateral moderate conductive hearing loss. Neither a hearing aid nor a preschool language

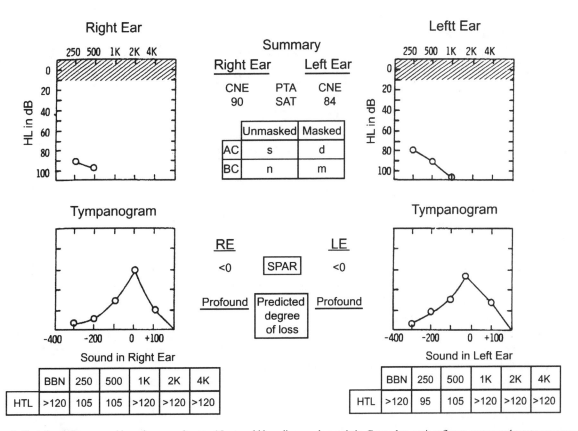

Figure 1. *Case 1*—audiogram and impedance results on a 15-year-old boy diagnosed as autistic. Crossed acoustic reflexes appear under tympanograms. The following abbreviations have been used in the figures. CNE, could not evaluate; PTA, pure-tone audiogram; SAT, speech awareness threshold; AC, air conduction; BC, bone conduction; RE, right ear; LE, left ear; HTL, hearing threshold level; BBN, broad-band noise; K, kilohertz.

stimulation program had been recommended. The last audiogram obtained at the otologist's office prior to evaluation by our audiology service is shown in Fig 2. These behavioral results indicate a moderate conductive hearing loss bilaterally.

Results of our audiologic evaluation are shown in Fig 3. These results indicated a severe bilateral mixed loss, greater in the right ear. Unmasked bone conduction thresholds indicated a substantial sensorineural component. Results of impedance audiometry were consistent with bilateral middle ear disorder—a flat, type B tympanogram in the right ear and a perforation in the left ear. Because acoustic reflexes were absent, impedance audiometry could not serve as a cross-check in confirming the degree of sensorineural hearing loss. For this reason, we carried out BSER audiometry. Air-conducted clicks at 80 dB HL failed to elicit responses from either ear. This finding was consistent with a bilateral air conduction hearing loss of at least 60 dB. Bone-conducted clicks, however, elicited slightly delayed responses at 45 and 55 dB HL. This finding was consistent with a high-frequency, sensorineural hearing loss in the better ear. Brainstem-evoked response audiometry, therefore, con-

firmed the results of both behavioral and impedance audiometry. All three measures were consistent with a bilateral, mixed hearing loss.

This case illustrates the use of BSER audiometry to confirm behavioral test results when impedance audiometry cannot contribute an effective cross-check of sensorineural level. This child's chronic middle ear disorder obscured the acoustic reflex, making prediction of sensorineural level impossible. It was essential, therefore, that the behavioral test results be confirmed by an independent procedure so that appropriate remediation could be initiated. By relying on the results of behavioral audiometry alone, the first audiologist unnecessarily delayed identification of this child's sensorineural hearing loss.

Case 3. A 4-year, 6-month-old boy was referred to our audiology service by an otologist. This child's hearing was first tested at the age of 3 years, 6 months. In the one year between his first hearing test and his evaluation at the Methodist Hospital, he had been tested by four different audiology facilities. The Table lists the results of these evaluations. The findings of the first evaluation suggested a severe hearing loss. The parents, seeking a second opinion, had the child tested by the second audiology service

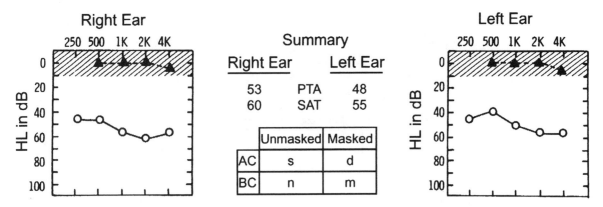

Figure 2. *Case 2*—audiogram obtained by audiologist at an otologist's office at age 2 years, 3 months, six months prior to his first visit to our audiology service.

one month later. This service found normal hearing. The parents then sought a third opinion at an audiology center in another city. This group found the child "untestable" and referred him to a fourth audiological facility. This facility reported a 60-dB loss in the right ear and a 95-dB loss in the left ear. They recommended the use of an ear-level hearing aid and a preschool educational program for the hearing-impaired.

After five months in the special school program, the teacher reported that she thought the child's hearing was normal. The parents then took the child to an otologist, who referred him to our service.

The results of our behavioral and impedance audiometry are shown in Fig 4. We were unable to obtain any consistent responses to either pure tones or speech by behavioral means. Impedance audiometry indicated normal middle ear function. We were able to predict cochlear sensitivity by comparing the acoustic reflex thresholds for pure tones with the reflex threshold for broad-band noise. The SPAR results indicated normal hearing in both ears.

Because of the long history of conflicting behavioral results on this child and our inability to obtain valid behavioral results, it was necessary to cross-check this SPAR prediction of normal cochlear sensitivity by BSER.

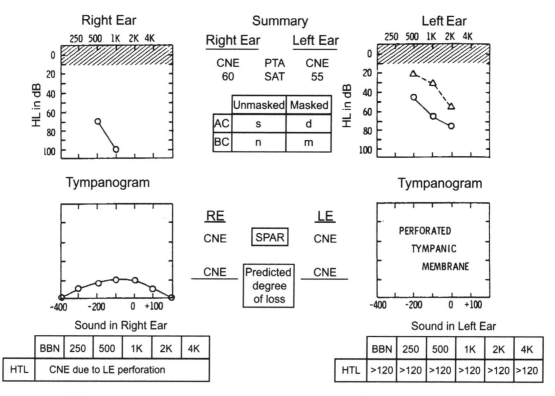

Figure 3. *Case 2*—audiogram and impedance results obtained by our audiology service when child was 2 years, 9 months old. Crossed acoustic reflexes appear under tympanograms.

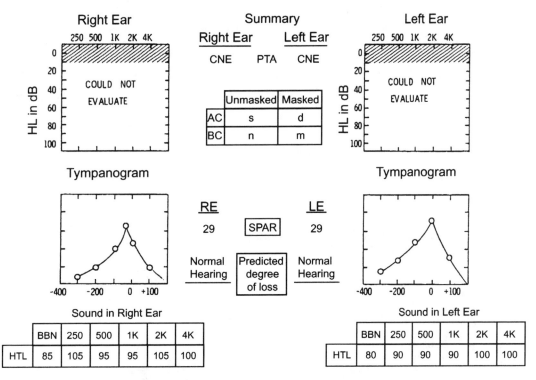

Figure 4. *Case 3*—audiogram and impedance results on 4-year, 6-month-old boy. Crossed acoustic reflexes appear under tympanograms. Valid behavioral audiogram could not be obtained.

The BSER results are shown in Fig 5. Air-conducted clicks evoked responses in the normal range of latencies at 30 dB HL in the left ear, and 40 dB HL in the right ear. These results are consistent with at most, only a mild sensorineural hearing loss. Thus, both impedance and BSER audiometry results are consistent with relatively little sensitivity loss in either ear.

This case illustrates how BSER audiometry can be used as a cross-check on impedance audiometry when behavioral audiometry fails to provide a coherent picture.

Case 4. A 5-year, 9-month-old girl was referred to our audiology service by a local otologist in consultation with a pediatric neurologist.

This child developed normally until age 2 years, 6 months, when she had a grand mal seizure of short duration associated with a high temperature. She had a left hemiparesis that lasted 24 hours. Seizure activity, characterized by twitching of the left side of the face, developed. The child was treated with phenobarbital, phenytoin, and diazepam until seizure activity subsided at age 3 years, 9 months. She was seen by an otolaryngologist at age 4 years, 6 months for possible hearing loss since she did not respond normally to verbal commands. Three audiograms, obtained in July 1973, December 1973, and March 1974 at the otolaryngologist's office are shown in Fig 6. These audiograms show a rapid progression in apparent hearing loss, from essentially normal sensitivity in July 1973, to a profound loss in March 1974.

Results of behavioral audiometry and impedance audiometry performed at our service in April 1974 are shown in Fig 7. Behavioral audiometry suggested a profound hearing loss. No consistent responses could be obtained to either pure-tone or speech signals. However, impedance audiometry suggested relatively normal hearing. Acoustic reflexes were present at normal levels to pure tones and broad-band noise in both ears. The SPAR prediction indicated normal sensitivity in the left ear, and, at most, only a mild sensitivity loss in the right ear.

In view of the discrepancy between behavioral and SPAR results, we turned to BSER audiometry as a cross-check. Results are shown in Fig 8. Well-formed responses at normal latencies were observed at 20 dB HL from both ears. This finding confirmed the overall picture of normal peripheral sensitivity predicted by SPAR.

This case again illustrates how BSER audiometry can be used as a cross-check when behavioral and impedance audiometry are discrepant. In view of this child's baffling history, appropriate diagnosis and management of the communication disorder depended on accurate estimation of auditory sensitivity. Following additional extensive testing of speech, language, and psychological and neurological behavior, a diagnosis of auditory agnosia was made, and appropri-

Results of Hearing Tests on Patient 3 at Four Different Audiology Centers*		
Audiology Center	Age	Result of Evaluation
1	3 yr, 6 mo	Severe hearing loss
2	3 yr, 7 mo	Normal hearing
3	4 yr	Child untestable
4	4 yr	60-dB loss in right ear; 45-dB loss in left ear

*All tests were given within the course of one year.

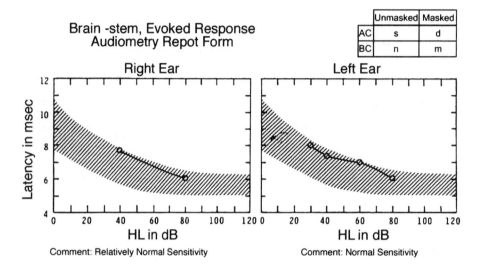

Figure 5. *Case 3*—results of BSER audiometry at age 4 years, 6 months.

ate therapy was initiated. Had this child been diagnosed as severely hearing-impaired, subsequent rehabilitation and educational management would have been inappropriate.

Case 5. A 6-month-old girl was referred to the audiology service by a local child care clinic. The child had first arch syndrome with bilateral atresia and left facial nerve palsy.

Behavioral audiometry suggested a severe, bilateral loss. The infant did not respond to any signal at equipment limits. In this ease, impedance audiometry could not be carried out due to the absence of ear canals. However, BSER audiometry could be performed by both air and bone conduction. Air-conducted clicks elicited a response only at 70 dB HL. Bone-conducted clicks, however, elicited responses at 20 and 30 dB HL. These results suggested

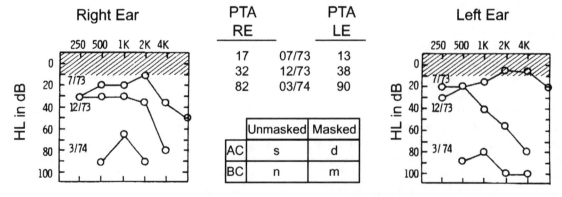

Figure 6. *Case 4*—three serial audiograms obtained at otolaryngologist's office in South America.

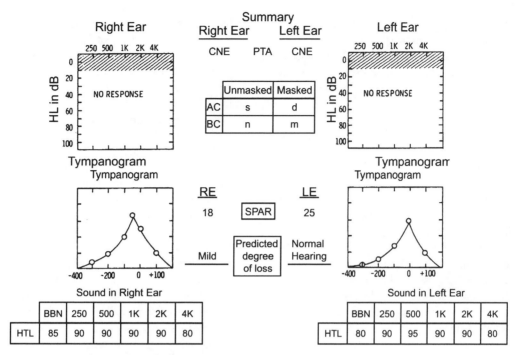

Figure 7. *Case 4*—audiogram and impedance results at age 5 years, 9 months. Crossed acoustic reflexes appear under tympanograms. No behavioral responses to either pure-tone or speech signals at equipment limits.

a large air-bone gap and were consistent with a substantial conductive hearing loss. In fact, comparison of air and bone levels yielding responses at equivalent latencies predicted an air-bone gap of approximately 40 dB. We therefore fitted the infant with a bone conduction hearing aid and recommended a parent-infant preschool program for hearing-impaired children.

In this case, BSER results could be cross-checked by neither behavioral audiometry nor impedance audiometry. For this reason, we closely monitored this child's progress

with her hearing aid. At age 23 months we were able to obtain a satisfactory behavioral audiogram. Unmasked bone conduction responses were between 20 and 30 dB HL from 500 to 2,000 Hz. Air conduction, warble-tone responses were noted at 60 to 70 dB HL across this same range. Thus, behavioral audiometry ultimately confirmed the BSER results obtained at age 6 months.

Figure 9 compares the BSER responses obtained at age 6 months with the behavioral audiogram obtained at age 23 months. Note that the actual air-bone gap (average

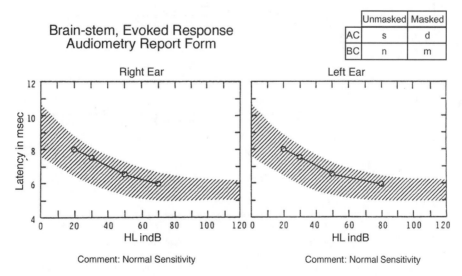

Figure 8. *Case 4*—results of BSER audiometry at age 5 years, 9 months.

of 500, 1000, and 2000 Hz) is within 2 dB of the air-bone gap predicted by BSER 17 months earlier.

This case illustrates the value of BSER audiometry for early identification when neither impedance audiometry nor behavioral audiometry can be carried out.

Comment

What we have attempted to highlight in this article is the value of the cross-check principle in the audiological evaluation of children. Whatever technique may be used in testing a child's hearing, it is important to confirm the result with an independent cross-check. Recent developments have made this principle clinically feasible. Both impedance audiometry and BSER audiometry are viable clinical techniques for cross-checking the result of conventional behavioral audiometry. In our experience, the application of this test battery cross-check principle represents a substantial advance over reliance on a single test approach.

In most instances, behavioral test results can be cross-checked by impedance audiometry alone. In conductive hearing losses, however, the absence of the acoustic reflex prevents the use of the SPAR technique for cross-checking sensorineural level. In such cases, however, BSER can serve as the cross-check measure. In still other cases, behavioral audiometry yields no useful data at all.

In these cases, impedance audiometry and BSER audiometry can serve as complementary cross-checks.

In order to implement this cross-check strategy successfully, it is important to recognize the appropriate test battery for a particular child. In so doing, however, one must understand the limitations of each test method.

Behavioral audiometry has several inherent limitations. It is least effective in testing very young children and "difficult-to-test" children. In many cases, the responses of these children are ambiguous and difficult to judge. Many do not give consistent responses to sound even though auditory sensitivity is normal. But these are the very children for whom accurate definition of peripheral sensitivity is often crucial to educational management. Since behavioral audiometry is more effective in older children, the accurate identification of hearing loss by this technique is often unnecessarily delayed.

Even under the best circumstances, mistakes are made when behavioral audiometry is the sole criterion. Observable responses often adapt quickly and are difficult to repeat. With very young infants and children, moreover, auditory signals may have to be considerably above threshold before responses are observed consistently. All of these factors increase the possibility of making a mistake in estimating auditory sensitivity by behavioral test results alone.

Impedance audiometry has its own unavoidable shortcomings. In children with conductive disorders,

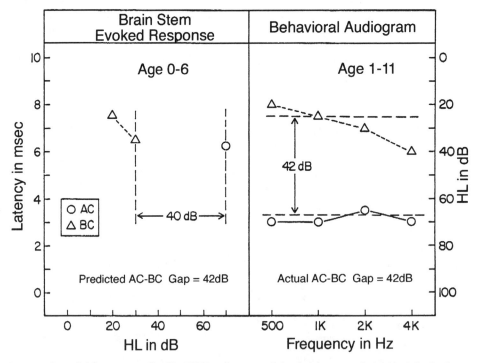

Figure 9. *Case 5*—comparison of air-bone gap predicted by BSER audiometry and actual air-bone gap obtained by behavioral means 17 months later. Predicted air-bone gap based on air and bone responses at comparable latencies.

impedance audiometry is certainly helpful in identifying the middle ear component, but absence of the acoustic reflex prevents the use of the SPAR technique for predicting sensorineural level. Similarly, central auditory disorders due to brain damage may abolish acoustic reflexes even though peripheral sensitivity is normal. Impedance audiometry also requires a relatively quiet child. Some children resist earphones and the probe tip to such a degree that impedance audiometry is not feasible without sedation.

The major problem with BSER audiometry is the need for sedation. To obtain satisfactory BSER responses from both ears over a full range of click intensities, the child must be relatively quiescent for about one hour. Infants and very young children can usually be tested in natural sleep. Children between ages 18 months and 4 years, however, often require sedation. In our experience, chloral hydrate in the dosage 50 mg/kg of body weight is usually satisfactory. In some cases, however, more effective sedation is required.

In summary, we believe that the unique limitations of conventional behavioral audiometry dictate the need for a "test battery" approach. The key concept governing our assessment strategy is the cross-check principle. The basic operation of this principle is that no result be accepted until it is confirmed by an independent measure. In most cases, impedance audiometry serves as an effective cross-check of behavioral audiometry. If they disagree, however, BSER audiometry can serve as a further cross-check. In cases in which behavioral audiometry fails, a consistent, cross-checked picture can still emerge from the combination of impedance and BSER audiometry. We believe that the application of the cross-check principle to our clinical population has had an appreciable effect on the accuracy with which we can identify and quantify hearing loss during the critical years for language-learning.

This study was supported by National Institutes of Health program project grant NS 10940. Toni Weaver, Francis Catlin, and Gail Neely provided assistance and encouragement throughout this research.

References

1. Northern J, Downs M: *Hearing in Children*. Baltimore, Williams & Wilkins Co, 1974, p. 137.

2. Jerger J: Clinical experience with impedance audiometry. *Arch Otolaryngol* 92:311-324, 1970.

3. Jerger S, Jerger J, Mauldin L, et al: Studies in impedance audiometry: II. Children less than six years old. *Arch Otolaryngol* 99:1-9, 1974.

4. Jerger J, Burney P, Mauldin L, et al: Predicting hearing loss from the acoustic reflex. *J Speech Hear Disord* 39:11-22, 1974.

5. Jerger J: Diagnostic use of impedance measures, in Jerger J (ed): *Handbook of Clinical Impedance Audiometry*. Dobbs Ferry, NY, American Electromedics Corp, 1975.

6. Hecox K, and Galambos, R: Brain stem auditory evoked responses in human infants and adults. *Arch Otolaryngol* 99:30-33, 1974.

7. Sohmer H, Feinmesser M, Bauberger-Tell L, et al: Routine use of cochlear audiometry in infants with uncertain diagnosis. *Ann Otol Rhinol Laryngol* 81:1-4, 1972.

8. Davis H, and Hirsh S: The audiometric utility of brain stem responses to low-frequency sound. *Int Aud* 15:181-195, 1976.

Response of Infants and Young Children as a Function of Auditory Stimuli and Test Methods

Marie Thompson and Gary Thompson
University of Washington, Seattle, Washington

Responses of infants and young children with normal hearing were assessed using five auditory stimuli at different hearing levels. The stimuli included broad-band and high-pass filtered signals and a 3-k Hz pure tone. The infants were tested with a behavioral observation test method. The young children were tested by either COR or play-audiometric test methods. The infants' responses varied as a function of the stimulus used. For this group, the 3-k Hz tone clearly produced fewer responses than did the other stimuli. This result is important for the assessment of high-frequency hearing loss in infants and young children. Differences between stimuli were not apparent for young children, although a comparison of test methods showed that play-audiometry resulted in more responses than COR audiometry, regardless of the stimulus used.

Hoversten and Moncur (1969) found that infants tend to respond more consistently to voice than to a 4000-Hz tone. Their data are consistent with clinical experience and, as a consequence, audiologists frequently employ speech and other wide frequency-band stimuli in preference to pure tones in audiologic assessment of infants and young children. While the use of speech and other wide frequency-band stimuli is clearly indicated in the assessment process, it also is clear that their exclusive use fails to identify children with frequency-selective hearing losses. For example, it is likely that a child with normal hearing for low frequencies but a severe hearing loss for high frequencies would, nevertheless, show normal awareness to a speech stimulus. As a consequence, such a child would be "passed" in any screening program which did not specifically assess his response to higher-frequency signals. The usual method for selective audiologic assessment is pure-tone testing. But since infants and young children tend to respond poorly to pure tones, particularly those in the high-frequency range, the choice of pure tones as test stimuli is questionable.

There is some evidence (for example, Eisenberg, 1965; Ling, Ling, and Doehring, 1970) that newborn infants are more responsive to narrow bands of noise than they are to pure tones. Hoversten and Moncur's (1969) data show that infants in the three- to eight-month range respond better to speech and white noise than to a 4000-Hz pure tone. Furthermore, Mendel (1968) found that responses of four- to eight-month-old infants were related to stimulus band width. More responses occurred to broad-band stimuli than to narrow-band noise or a warbled tone. If filtered speech and noise are similar to unfiltered speech and noise in alerting or producing responses in young children, then their use would provide an alternative to pure-tone assessment of high-frequency hearing loss in infants.

It is likely that the difference in response to filtered complex stimuli and pure tones observed in infants is not apparent for slightly older children for whom play-audiometric techniques are appropriate. In play audiometry, the child is taught to perform a motor act (for example, putting a ring on a spindle, dropping a block into a box, pushing a button) in response to an auditory stimulus. Inherent in this procedure is the child's ability to "attend" to the stimulus. When the child has been taught to listen and respond to an auditory stimulus, there is no reason to suppose that one could become more conditioned to one stimulus than another. Consequently, it would be anticipated that pure tones and filtered speech and noise would be equally effective as test stimuli in play audiometry.

We studied responses of infants and young children to auditory signals of various band widths. The purpose was to explore the general hypothesis that their responses vary as a function of age and test method and have implications for high-frequency hearing-loss assessment.

Method

Subjects

The subjects were 45 infants and young children between seven and 36 months of age. Group 1 ($N = 15$) included infants between seven and 12 months of age. At this age, normally-developing babies ordinarily localize the direction of sound but are not sufficiently mature to be taught play audiometry. Group 2 ($N = 30$) was composed of children between 22 and 36 months of age. At this age, many normal youngsters respond to play-audiometric techniques, but do not respond well to conventional assessment procedures, such as raising their hands in response to auditory signals.

Reprinted by permission of authors and American Speech-Language-Hearing Association. Copyright 1972. *Journal of Speech and Hearing Research*, 15, pp. 699-707.

Subjects in Groups 1 and 2 were drawn from the Well-Baby Clinic of the Child Development and Mental Retardation Center, University of Washington. Medical records indicated that each child was the product of normal pregnancy and birth, was showing normal development growth, had not had an ear infection for at least three months prior to audiometric evaluation, and did not have a cold at the time of audiometric evaluation. These criteria helped to insure that our sample represented a population of infants and young children with normal hearing and normal developmental growth.

Test Stimuli and Instrumentation

Test stimuli included broad-band noise, speech, high-pass filtered noise, high-pass filtered speech, and a 3000-Hz pure tone. The broad-band noise was the masking white noise from an Allison 22 audiometer. The speech stimulus was the phrase "Hi (child's name), look at me." Filtered speech and noise were these same two stimuli passed through a Krohn-Hite Model 3202R Filter set to reject frequencies below 2 k Hz at the rate of 24 dB per octave. Measurements with a Bruel and Kjaer Sound Level Meter (Type 2203), Octave Band Filter (Type 1613), and Condenser Microphone (Type 4132) indicated that the acoustic filtering was approximately 28 dB for the first octave below 2 k Hz and approximately 20 dB for the second octave.

All stimuli were presented "live" (not recorded). While it is recognized that recorded presentations allow for precise stimulus control, we felt that by careful use of the VU meter, variability of signal presentation could be kept to a minimum. Furthermore, live presentation affords greater flexibility in testing and is the method most often used in clinical assessment of young children.

An Allison Model 22 Audiometer was used to deliver test stimuli to one of two Electro-Voice SP12 loudspeakers located in the test room. The Krohn-Hite Filter was inserted into one of the audiometer channels to provide high-pass filtering when needed. All testing was done in a two-room IAC test suite.

Calibration

Prior to collecting data, it was necessary to equate test stimuli to 0 dB HL for awareness. This was accomplished by obtaining sound-field thresholds on 10 normal adult listeners. Each subject was seated in the test room equidistant and approximately five feet from two loudspeakers. Stimuli were delivered through one of the loudspeakers on a random schedule. The testing plan basically was that described by Carhart and Jerger (1959). Threshold for each stimulus was defined as the lowest level which produced two responses out of three presentations. Averages of these threshold values were calculated and converted to 0 dB HL for each stimulus. Sound pressure level measurements were made with a Bruel and Kjaer Sound Level Meter (Type 2203) and Condenser Microphone (Type 4132). Average peak linear scale readings were observed for each stimulus at 60 dB HL and converted to sound pressure levels corresponding to 0 dB HL (Table 1). Differences between the two loudspeakers were no greater than 3 dB for any stimulus, indicating a reasonable match in output.

Test Procedures

Group 1. The testing plan for Group 1 (seven to 12 month infants) was similar to that described by Hoversten and Moncur (1969). The child was placed on his or her mother's lap in the test room. Soft colorful toys were available to occupy the child during the test, which took approximately 30 minutes. The mother was instructed not to respond in any way to test stimuli and to be completely quiet during the test session.

Stimuli were presented on a random basis through two loudspeakers which were placed at a 45 degree angle from the child's front line of vision. Each of the five test stimuli was presented twice at 15, 30, 45, and 60 dB HL for a total of 40 stimulus presentations. Stimulus order was randomized for each child, but all stimuli were presented in an ascending intensity order (15 dB first, 30 dB second).

Two examiners independently judged whether a response occurred following each stimulus presentation. One examiner was located in the test room with the child. The other observed the child's behavior from the control room. Response criteria included localization and awareness to sound. Localization was defined as a head turn in the direction of the sound source. Awareness was defined as either a movement of the eyes in the direction of the sound source, or looking up, usually at the examiner or the mother. In order for a response to be counted, both examiners had to agree, that is, if one examiner judged

Table 1. Average sound-pressure-level values required to produce 0 dB HL for five test stimuli. $N = 10$ normal adult listeners.

Stimuli	Sound Pressure Level (dB re 0.0002 dy/cm≈)	
	Loudspeaker 1	Loudspeaker 2
White noise	8	9
Speech	9	10
Filtered noise	8	9
Filtered speech	5	8
3000 Hz	4	7

that a response occurred and the other did not, the trial was counted as no response.

Stimulus duration was maintained as closely as possible at two seconds. This was accomplished by the experimenter's practicing, prior to seeing subjects, until each stimulus could be presented consistently with the aid of a stop watch. The minimum interstimulus interval was 10 seconds. Stimuli were presented when the child was relatively quiet, not engaged in excessive motor activity, and visually oriented to a midline position.

Group 2. The testing plan for Group 2 (22 to 36 month children) followed one of two courses: play audiometry, or a variation of conditioned orientation reflex audiometry (COR) (Suzuki and Ogiba, 1961).

Play audiometry proceeded as follows: The child was seated in the test room with an examiner. The stimulus was a moderate level complex noise (60-dB HL) presented through a loudspeaker. The examiner attempted to condition the child to perform a motor task (such as putting a ring on a stick or dropping a block into a box) whenever the stimulus was presented. Initially the examiner helped the child perform the task by demonstration and by physical assistance. Three successive appropriate responses without help were taken as evidence that the child had learned the conditioning task. Testing proceeded using a descending intensity plan. Each of the five test stimuli was presented twice at 45, 30, and 15 dB HL for a total of 30 stimulus presentations. Stimulus order was randomized for each child.

Responses were judged independently by two examiners, one in the control room and the other in the test room with the child. In order for a response to be counted, the examiners' judgements had to be in agreement. Social reinforcement (good, that's nice, you're doing fine, pat on the back) was used throughout the test as needed to maintain cooperation from the child.

Conditioned orientation reflex (COR) audiometry was used for children who failed to condition to play audiometry. The essence of this method involves the use of visual reinforcement for appropriate localization behavior. The procedure was carried out by having the child sit at a table and play quietly with toys. Each time the child localized (turned in the direction of the auditory stimulus), a light mounted on the loudspeaker was flashed. Presentation of stimuli, method of response scoring, and social reinforcement schedule followed the same plan as outlined previously for the play audiometry procedure.

Thirty-six children were initially screened for inclusion in Group 2. Six children were eliminated from the study because we were unable to obtain their cooperation for a sufficient length of time to complete testing. Of the remaining 30 subjects, 19 were tested using play audiometry and 11 were tested with COR audiometry.

Results

Results for the seven- to 12-month-old infants (Group 1) and 22- to 36-month-old children (Group 2) are displayed in Figures 1 and 2, respectively. The data represent percent judged response to five stimuli at different hearing levels. The design of this experiment limited the application of conventional statistical analyses in that each child had the opportunity to give only zero, one, or two responses. However, by performing an arcsin transformation of the data (Walker and Lev, 1953, pp. 423, 424, and 479), it was considered appropriate to test differences among groups, stimuli, and hearing levels by analysis of variance (Winer, 1962, p. 320).

A comparison of Figures 1 and 2 shows several patterns of response. First, young children responded more frequently than infants ($F = 42.16$; $df = 1, 43$; $p < 0.01$), but regardless of age, both groups responded more frequently as the hearing level increased ($F = 78.87$; $df = 2, 86$; $p < 0.01$).[1] Responses also varied as a function of the stimulus ($F = 26.23$, $df = 4, 172$; $p < 0.01$) but this effect was only apparent for the infant group. That is, there was a significant interaction between groups and stimuli ($F = 15.20$; $df = 4, 172$; $p < 0.01$). For the infant group, speech and high-pass filtered speech produced the most responses and 3 k Hz the least responses, regardless of hearing level. In contrast, the stimulus effect was negligible for the group of young children. This can be observed by noting the clustering of response curves in Figure 2.

It will be recalled that children in Group 2 were tested by one of two methods, play audiometry ($N = 19$) or COR audiometry ($N = 11$). Results, as a function of test method, are shown in Figure 3. Children in the play-audiometry group gave a significantly greater number of responses than those in the COR group ($F = 69.95$; $df = 1, 28$; $p < 0.01$). There was, however, a significant interaction of hearing levels and groups, in that the difference between the two groups was greatest at 15 dB HL and least at 45 dB HL ($F = 41.59$; $df = 2, 56$; $p < 0.01$).

Discussion

Results of this study clearly support previous research (Eisenberg, 1965; Hoversten and Moncur, 1969; Ling et al., 1970), which indicated that the auditory responses of infants vary as a function of the test stimulus. These studies also showed that for newborn infants and babies up to about one year old, pure tones consistently produced fewer responses than speech or other complex stimuli, regardless of the intensity level at which the stimuli were compared.

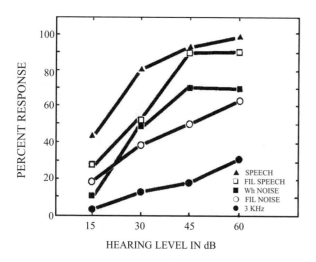

Figure 1. Percent response to five stimuli at four hearing levels for normal infants seven to 12 months of age (*N* = 15).

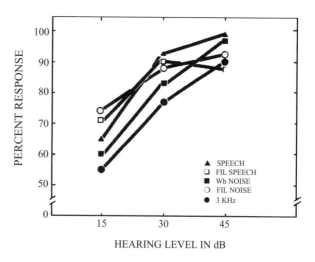

Figure 2. Percent response to five stimuli at three hearing levels for normal young children 22 to 36 months of age (*N* = 30).

A number of factors may contribute to make complex stimuli more effective than pure tones and, furthermore, to make some complex stimuli more effective than others. Band width probably is a significant variable (Mendel, 1968), although as band width is expanded beyond 200 Hz, other factors are likely to predominate (Eisenberg, 1965). For example, given band widths of at least 200 Hz, the frequency characteristics of the band may assume importance. Eisenberg (1965) and Ling et al., (1970) report that newborn infants tend to respond better to stimuli associated with the speech-frequency region than to stimuli with primary energy in higher-frequency regions. Eisenberg has speculated ". . . that increased sensitivity to a critical band of speech-frequencies may be present at birth."

Whether infants are born with a tendency to respond to speech-frequency signals or not, the results of Hoversten and Moncur's study (1969) and this study clearly indicate that speech is an effective stimulus for older infants in the age range of three to 12 months. Whether speech is effective primarily because of linguistic or learning factors or simply because of its spectral characteristics is unclear.

The clinical implication of these findings is that the use of pure tones is not suitable for assessing responses of infants to high-frequency stimuli. In the present study, for example, the infants in Group 1 (seven to 12 months old) responded to 3 k Hz only 30% of the time at 60 dB HL.[1] If normal infants fail to respond consistently to 3 k Hz, it is evident that this stimulus, and probably other high-fre-

quency pure tones as well, cannot be used effectively to identify infants with hearing loss.

In contrast, high-pass filtered speech resulted in a relatively high response rate (80%) at both 45 and 60 dB HL. These data support the use of filtered speech (or perhaps other filtered bands of noise) in place of pure tones for selective high-frequency assessment of infants.

We anticipated that the difference in response to filtered complex stimuli and 3 k Hz, apparent in infants under one year of age, would not occur for slightly older children for whom COR audiometry and play-audiometric test methods are appropriate. The data for children in Group 2 (22 to 36 months of age) support this expectation. Figure 2 shows no clear advantage for one stimulus over the others. Furthermore, all stimuli produced relatively high response rates (roughly 80% or higher) at 30 and 45 dB HL.

Subjects in Group 2 were tested by play audiometry if possible, and if not, by a version of COR audiometry. The results displayed in Figure 3 show clearly that, regardless of stimulus used, play audiometry led to more responses than COR audiometry, particularly when stimuli were presented at low hearing levels (15 and 30 dB HL). These results are not surprising when one considers the nature of these procedures. In play audiometry, the child is taught to listen and perform a motor task in response to auditory signal. In contrast, this attending feature is not present in COR audiometry. In COR audiometry, the child is allowed to play quietly or be occupied by the examiner in some way. Since auditory signals must compete with the ongoing play activities of the child (as is the case with behavioral observation audiometry) it would be expected that COR audiometry would produce less precise estimates of threshold than does the play-audiometric method.

---

[1]Children in Group 2 were tested at three hearing levels and infants in Group 1 were tested at four hearing levels. Because the statistical analysis required an equal number of hearing levels across the two groups, data for the infant group at 60-dB HL were not included in the analysis of variance.

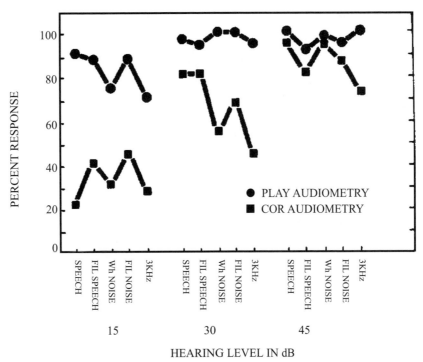

Figure 3. Percent response to five stimuli at three hearing levels as a function of test method for normal young children 22 to 36 months of age. N for play audiometry = 19. N for COR audiometry = 11. Combined N = 30.

In summary, the results suggest that when the auditory responses of young children can be brought under stimulus control through play-audiometric test methods, pure tones are as effective as complex stimuli in determining hearing threshold. It follows that for these children, pure tones are appropriate test stimuli in high-frequency hearing-loss assessment. In contrast, infants tested by behavioral observation methods tend to respond more frequently to complex stimuli than to pure tones. The assessment of high-frequency hearing loss in this group is better accomplished through the use of high-pass filtered speech or noise.

Acknowledgment

This study was supported in part by Contract 71-2446 from the National Institutes of Health, National Institute of Child Health and Human Development. Requests for reprints should be directed to Marie Thompson, Communication Disorders Program, Child Development and Mental Retardation Center, University of Washington, Seattle, Washington 98195.

References

Carhart, R., and Jerger, J., Preferred method for clinical determination of pure-tone thresholds. *J. Speech Hearing Dis.,* 24, 330-345 (1959).

Eisenberg, R., Auditory behavior in the human neonate: 1. Methodologic problems and the logical design of research procedures. *J. Aud. Res.,* 5, 159-177 (1965).

Hoversten, G., and Moncur, J., Stimuli and intensity factors in testing infants. *J. Speech Hearing Res.,* 12, 687-702 (1969).

Ling, D., Ling, A., and Doehring, D., Stimulus, response, and observer variables in the auditory screening of newborn infants. *J. Speech Hearing Res.,* 13, 9-18 (1970).

Mendel, M., Infant responses to recorded sounds. *J. Speech Hearing Res.,* 11, 811-816 (1968).

Suzuki, T., and Ogiba, Y., Conditioned orientation reflex audiometry. *Arch. Otolaryng.,* 74, 192-198 (1961).

Walker, H., and Lev, J. *Statistical Inference.* New York: Holt (1953).

Winer, B., *Statistical Principles in Experimental Design.* New York: McGraw-Hill (1962).

Received February 25, 1972

Responses of Infants and Young Children to Behavior Observation Audiometry (BOA)

Gary Thompson and Bruce A. Weber
Child Development and Mental Retardation Center, University of Washington, Seattle, Washington

One-hundred and ninety children, ranging from three to 59 months of age, were tested by behavior observation audiometry (BOA) in an attempt to formulate a guide for clinical interpretation of BOA thresholds. The results showed that BOA thresholds are influenced by chronological age. Children who could be tested by both BOA and play audiometry consistently demonstrated lower thresholds on the latter procedure.

Normal hearing is relatively well defined for older children and adults. For this group, responses in the 0-20-dB hearing level (HL) range are typically considered to be evidence of normal hearing. Such thresholds are readily attainable because older children and adults can be taught to listen actively for the test stimuli in conventional or play audiometry. In contrast, definitive responses in the 0-20-dB HL range cannot be expected from infants and young children whose immature development generally precludes the use of conventional audiometric techniques. As an alternative, such children are usually tested behaviorally by some observational technique. This form of testing relies on the onset of the stimulus to elicit some detectable change in the child's behavior. Generally, behavior observation audiometry (BOA) yields threshold values somewhat above the 20-dB level. A number of factors such as preoccupation of the child at the time of stimulus onset, motor activity that obscures a behavioral response, and response habituation contribute to the elevated thresholds. The age of the child being tested is also an important variable. That neonates give detectable behavioral responses only to rather intense stimuli is well documented (Wedenberg, 1956; Ling, Ling, and Doehring, 1970). Older infants demonstrate head-turning responses to sounds of lower intensity, but the intensity levels at which the response occurs are also influenced by the age of the child (Hoversten and Moncur, 1969; Thompson and Thompson, 1972). As a result, the audiologist testing the hearing of a young child by means of BOA is likely to encounter threshold values above 20 dB HL. Because such elevated thresholds may be obtained from normal-hearing children, interpretation of the test results must be based to a large degree on values expected from normal children of comparable age and development. Unfortunately, such information is available only in scattered investigations which have used varying testing protocols. Accordingly, this paper presents descriptive audiometric data on infants and children from three to 59 months of age. Though the number of children tested in each age group is not sufficiently large for the results to be viewed as definitive normative data, it does permit the results to be viewed as a guide for the audiometric evaluation of infants and young children which has not been heretofore available.

Method

Subjects

Subjects were available for this study largely through a series of normative language studies conducted at the Child Development and Mental Retardation Center at the University of Washington from 1971 to 1973. There were five criteria for inclusion in the study: normal development according to parental report; no unusual medical history; language development at least grossly within normal limits; no known ear infection during the past three months; and no evidence of a cold on the test day. These criteria were applied to help insure that the sample represented a population of infants and young children with normal hearing and development.

A total of 289 infants and young children were screened using the criteria outlined above. Ninety-nine were eliminated because they failed to meet one or more of the criteria. The 190 subjects included in this study were divided into nine age categories: 3-5 months (14 subjects), 6-11 months (12 subjects), 12-17 months (17 subjects), 18-23 months (14 subjects), 24-29 months (33 subjects), 30-35 months (31 subjects), 36-41 months (27 subjects), 42-47 months (25 subjects), and 48-59 months (17 subjects). The unequal range size was selected to conform closely with the known slowing of development with increasing age.

Reprinted by permission of authors and American Speech-Language-Hearing Association. Copyright 1974. *Journal of Speech and Hearing Disorders*, 39, pp. 140-147.

Auditory Stimuli

Several investigators (for example, Hoversten and Moncur, 1969; Thompson and Thompson, 1972) have shown that broad-band stimuli are more effective than pure tones in eliciting auditory responses from infants. Speech and noise were used as auditory stimuli in this study. Speech was the live voice phrase "Hi, [child's name], look at me." The noise was complex noise generated by an Allison Model 22 audiometer and presented through a loudspeaker (Electro Voice SP 12). Both stimuli were shaped by a Krohn-Hite filter (Model 3202R) set to pass the frequencies 500-2000 Hz. The resulting filtered stimuli were matched in energy level as measured by a Bruel and Kjaer sound-level meter (Type 2203) and octave-band analyzer (Type 1613) positioned 5 ft from the loudspeaker. Prior to the testing of each subject, the examiner practiced saying the speech phrase until he could consistently peak the VU meter of the audiometer to 0 dB. Adjustment of the complex noise stimulus to peak at 0 dB was readily accomplished. Stimulus intensity was recorded in terms of sound pressure level (SPL). (Because the speech circuit of a clinical audiometer was used to present the stimuli, zero on the hearing loss dial was based on the normal speech intelligibility threshold rather than the standard 0.0002 dynes/ cm≈ sound pressure level reference. The conversion from HL to SPL was made by adding a constant value to all hearing loss dial readings. This conversion value equaled the SPL output of the speech circuit at 0 dB HL.) Periodic calibration checks confirmed that the intensity levels for each stimulus varied no more than ±2 dB throughout the course of the study.

Test Procedures: Behavior Observation Audiometry

Each subject sat on a chair or on his mother's lap, approximately 5 ft from a loudspeaker placed at a 45° angle from the subject's front line of vision. Two examiners were present for all testing. One was in the test room of a two-room IAC sound suite and occupied subjects with "non-noisy" toys and games appropriate to the age level of the subject. A second examiner, in the control room of the suite, presented stimuli to subjects through the audiometer, filter, and loudspeaker.

The duration of each stimulus presentation was approximately 2 sec. The interval between stimuli varied between approximately 10 and 20 sec, depending on the activity of the subject. Stimuli were presented only when subjects were relatively quiet and when their attention was focused on the toys and games in front of them.

Three threshold assessment trials, each using a single stimulus, were administered to each subject. The stimuli were alternated across trials in an effort to reduce

response habituation over three test trials. The two sequences (speech-noise-speech or noise-speech-noise) followed a random schedule for all subjects. The intensity of the stimulus was varied using an ascending technique, the first stimulus being presented at 0 dB HL. If a response was not observed, the intensity of the stimulus was increased in successive 10-dB increments until a response was observed, which terminated Trial 1. Trials 2 and 3 proceeded in the same manner.

Both the examiner with the subject and the examiner in the control room observed the subjects' behavior after the onset of the stimulus. Each judge had a score sheet for each subject on which he could independently record a plus, zero, or question mark after each presentation of a stimulus. The judges scored a plus if they observed (1) localization (head turn) in the direction of the loudspeaker; (2) looking up at the parent or examiner; (3) a verbal utterance directly related to the stimulus, such as "What was that?" or (4) an eye blink or whole-body startle. A "response" was defined as both judges scoring a plus or one scoring a plus and the other a question mark. Two zeros, two question marks, or a plus and a zero constituted a "no response." After each presentation, the two examiners independently recorded their judgments of the response and then checked with each other through an intercommunication system to determine whether they were in agreement. This process was necessary in order to determine when to terminate each threshold trial.

No systematic reinforcement of responses was employed. The examiner in the test room interacted with subjects, but only to the degree necessary to maintain general cooperation so that the three test trials could be employed.

Test Procedures: Play Audiometry

Subjects 18 months of age and older were tested by play audiometry upon completion of BOA. They were taught to perform a motor task (for example, putting a ring on a stick or dropping a block in a box) in response to the complex noise stimulus. Initial conditioning trials in play audiometry were conducted at a level above the BOA threshold. The test room examiner took an active role in the conditioning process. This included demonstrating appropriate responses, physically helping subjects to perform the desired behavior, and socially reinforcing appropriate responses (such as "That's good listening," or a pat on the back). If a subject failed to learn the task after several conditioning trials, testing was discontinued. Subjects who learned the task, as evidenced by three consecutive correct responses, were tested for threshold to the complex noise stimulus. The stimulus was presented in 10-dB decrements. Threshold was defined as the lowest level at which the subject responded correctly twice out of the three descending trials.

Results and Discussion

Because there are no recognized hearing level (HL) calibration standards for the type of sound field measurements obtained in this study, results for both BOA and play audiometry are presented in sound pressure level (SPL). Conversion of these data to HL values would require adjustments based on empirically determined calibration data for individual sound suites.

When the subjects' responses were studied initially as a function of stimuli, no significant differences between the thresholds were obtained for speech and complex noise (sign test: $p > 0.05$, NS). Accordingly, the results for speech and complex noise were combined and are displayed in Figure 1. There is a systematic reduction in threshold for all three trials as a function of age, but only for the younger groups. At about age two the curves flatten out, suggesting no age effect for the older groups. Examination of the separate threshold curves shows no practical difference between Trials 1 and 2, with the exception of the two youngest and two oldest groups, where lower thresholds were obtained in Trial 1. In contrast, thresholds for Trial 1 tend to be lower than for Trial 3 across the entire age range tested.

These results might be explained on the basis of a general reduction in responsiveness encompassing fatigue, loss of attention, restlessness, and other factors. In addition, the manner in which the stimuli were presented could have influenced the results. A different stimulus

(speech or complex noise) was presented for Trials 1 and 2. In Trial 3 the stimulus used in Trial 1 was repeated. This meant that speech and complex noise provided novel stimuli only during the first two trials. Had a third novel stimulus (for example, music, or an animal sound) been used for Trial 3, it might have had the effect of generally lowering the response curve for Trial 3.

While the trend favored lower thresholds for Trial 1 than for Trial 3, a number of subjects reversed this trend. For example, 28 subjects (15%) produced lower thresholds in Trial 3 than in either Trial 1 or 2. With respect to consistency of response, 89 subjects (47%) showed no more than 10 dB of variation across the three test trials, and 127 subjects (67%) varied by no more than 20 dB for the three trials. Of the remaining 63 subjects, who varied by more than 20 dB across the trials, the range of responses was wide, including a few that varied by as much as 80 dB.

In a clinical assessment, the audiologist would prefer to estimate hearing status on the basis of several threshold attempts. This is a reasonable strategy for infants who give relatively consistent responses to successive presentations of a stimulus. In contrast, if an infant varies markedly in his response to repeated threshold attempts, rather than averaging his responses, it may be more appropriate to accept one response (often the first) as the best estimate of threshold.

Figure 2 shows the intersubject variability of responses obtained on Trial 1, as a function of age. The variability is reflected in the separation between the percentile lines. Greatest variability is found in the lowest age groups, with the oldest group also showing a few

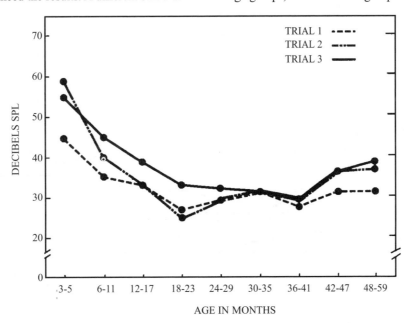

Figure 1. Median response curves in decibels sound pressure level for three test trials as a function of age.

children with thresholds much higher than the rest. The middle age groups show much less intersubject variability, as seen by the closeness of the percentile curves.

The results displayed in Figures 1 and 2 are a guide for interpreting BOA responses as a function of age. They provide at least a rough yardstick for comparing the responses of an individual infant with those obtained from a group of normally developing infants of comparable age. Caution must be exercised, however, if the threshold data from this study are used as a gauge for interpreting clinical BOA test results. First, the number of subjects in each age group does not permit the values to be treated as definitive normative data. In addition, the nature of the BOA procedure enhances the likelihood that the child will not respond until the stimulus is presented somewhat above his "true threshold." Just as neonatal screening uses the Moro response that occurs clearly above the infant's threshold, the arousal response obtained in BOA is unlikely to occur consistently near threshold. As a result, BOA thresholds may well tend to underestimate the extent of a child's hearing. That is, the child who does not respond below 50 dB HL may well have a "true threshold" somewhat below this level. Unfortunately, there is no way to determine an appropriate correction factor for an individual child. Put in proper perspective, BOA is probably best viewed as a screening assessment procedure. Sometimes, the information obtained from the test is sufficient to conclude that the infant's peripheral hearing status is at least grossly within normal limits and certainly adequate for language acquisition. In these cases, there may be no need for further clinical disposition in regard to hearing. In other cases, the audiologist will need to apply all available information—including the developmental level and medical status of the child and the results of additional hearing tests (when feasible to administer)—toward arriving at the best estimate of hearing status.

Play Audiometry

The subjects' performance for play audiometry is shown in Table 1. The thresholds are consistently much lower than those shown for BOA in Figure 1. Of the 122 children who satisfactorily performed both BOA and play audiometry, only one yielded a lower BOA threshold. Three additional children demonstrated the same threshold level for both procedures. Thus, play audiometry, when successful, clearly is more likely to yield lower thresholds than BOA. Unfortunately, with the play technique used in this study, little success (2%) was experienced with children under 24 months of age.

Conclusions

Hearing assessment of infants and young children dictates a clinical strategy aimed at obtaining relevant information within as short a time as possible. BOA, with or without the use of a visual reinforcer for appropriate behavioral responses (COR audiometry: Suzuki and Ogiba, 1961), provides an efficient assessment tool. The procedure is quick to administer, the results can often rule out significant peripheral hearing loss, and sometimes there is no satisfactory behavioral alternative to the test's use. At minimum, BOA results can help determine an

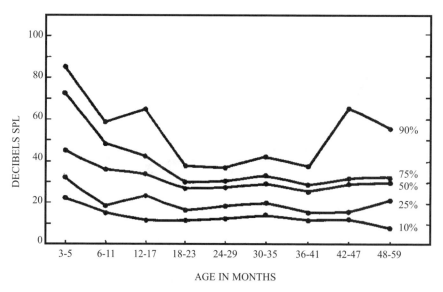

Figure 2. Percentile response curves in decibels sound pressure level for Test Trial 1 as a function of age.

Table 1. Median threshold values in decibels of sound pressure level and the percentage of success for play audiometry as a function of age.

	3-5	6-11	12-17	18-23	24-29	30-35	36-41	42-47	48-59
Median Threshold	—	—	—	—	26 dB	13 dB	14 dB	12 dB	12 dB
Percentage Success	—	—	—	—	70	90	96	100	100

appropriate intensity conditioning level for follow-up tests including play audiometry and TROCA (Lloyd, 1966). For these reasons, a strong case can be built for using BOA as the initial test procedure for any child whose chronological age or developmental level raises doubts about successful completion of other test procedures.

Acknowledgment

The authors are indebted to Dona Hedrick and Elizabeth Prather, University of Washington, and to Annette Tobin, Seattle Public Schools, who in developing normative standards for the Sequenced Inventory of Language Development (SILD) provided many subjects for this study. The authors are also indebted to Peggy Williams, Mary Abbs, Annette Tobin and Marilyn Hamilton for their assistance in collecting data. Requests for reprints should be directed to Gary Thompson, Child Development and Mental Retardation Center, WJ-10, University of Washington, Seattle, Washington 98195.

References

Hoversten, G., and Moncur, J., Stimuli and intensity factors in testing infants. *J. Speech Hearing Res.,* 12, 687-702 (1969).

Ling, D., Ling, A., and Dochring, D., Stimulus, response, and observer variables in the auditory screening of newborn infants. *J. Speech Hearing Res.,* 13, 9-18 (1970).

Lloyd, L.L., Behavioral audiometry viewed as an operant procedure. *J. Speech Hearing Dis.,* 31, 128-136 (1966).

Suzuki, T., and Ogiba, Y., Conditioned orientation reflex audiometry. *Arch. Otolaryng.,* 74, 192-198 (1961).

Thompson, M., and Thompson, G., Response of infants and young children as a function of auditory stimuli and test methods. *J. Speech Hearing Res.,* 15, 699-707 (1972).

Wedenberg, E., Auditory tests on newborn infants. *Acta Otolaryng.*, 46, 446-461 (1956).

Received December 6, 1973
Accepted January 8, 1974

Auditory Localization of Infants as a Function of Reinforcement Conditions

John M. Moore, Gary Thompson, and Marie Thompson
Child Development and Mental Retardation Center, Seattle, Washington

The influence of four reinforcement conditions on the auditory localization behavior of normal infants was studied. Forty- eight infants 12 to 18 months of age were assigned to one of four groups of 12 subjects each. All received 30 presentations of complex noise at suprathreshold level. After each response to the stimulus, Group 1 received no reinforcement, Group 2 received social reinforcement, Group 3 received " simple " visual reinforcement (a blinking light), and Group 4 received " complex " visual reinforcement (an animated toy animal). The two visual reinforcement conditions produced the most localization responses, followed in order by the social reinforcement and no reinforcement conditions. These results indicate that auditory localization behavior of infants is influenced by reinforcement and that the extent of this effect is related to the type of reinforcement employed.

Conditioned orientation reflex (COR) audiometry was developed by Suzuki and Ogiba (1961) and is based on the idea that a visual stimulus can reinforce (increase) auditory localization behavior in infants and young children. Suzuki and Ogiba indicated that, if properly conditioned, a child will turn toward the sound source after each auditory presentation to receive a visual reward (an illuminated doll).

COR audiometry, or variations of it, has become a common procedure for assessing children two years of age and younger who cannot readily be conditioned to play audiometry (performing motor tasks, such as dropping a block in a box in response to the auditory stimulus). It has been assumed that the visual stimulus does in fact reinforce auditory localization behavior, thereby increasing the probability of getting a satisfactory hearing test on infants. This is a reasonable assumption. However, it lacks empirical support, because Suzuki and Ogiba did not report using a control group in their study. More specifically, they did not report comparative results with and without the visual stimulus. Accordingly, the specific reinforcing value of the visual stimulus remains unknown.

Furthermore, if it can be shown that visual stimuli reinforce localization behavior, can it also be shown that the strength of reinforcement varies, depending on the type of stimulus employed? Suzuki and Ogiba (1961) proposed the use of an illuminated doll. The Houston Speech and Hearing Center *(Asha,* 1964) suggested that a simple blinking light can be effective. Hodgson (1972, p. 506) said that stimuli involving animation may be appropriate. It is possible, of course, that the reinforcing value of a visual stimulus is not related to complexity. A simple light

may be as effective as a colorful animated doll in strengthening localization behavior of infants. It is also possible that social reinforcement (verbal praise, a pat on the back) is as effective as visual stimuli.

When assessing the hearing of infants, who often demonstrate a limited attention span, it is essential that the audiologist elicit as many responses as possible within the shortest time possible. Appropriate reinforcement techniques may help to increase the number of responses obtained while the infant's attention is maintained. Accordingly, we investigated the auditory localization behavior of infants as a function of reinforcement. Specifically, localization behavior was examined under the following conditions: no reinforcement, social reinforcement, "simple" visual reinforcement (a blinking light), and "complex" visual reinforcement (an animated toy animal).

Method

Subjects and Instrumentation

The subjects were 48 infants between 12 and 18 months of age. The criteria for selection were no suspicion of hearing loss, normal development according to a parental report, no evidence of a cold on the test date, and no indication of an ear infection for three months before the test date. Each infant also had to show a localization response to the initial auditory presentation during testing to be included as a subject.

There is evidence (Hoversten and Moncur, 1969; Thompson and Thompson, 1972) that broad- band stimuli are more effective than pure tones in eliciting auditory responses from infants. Complex noise generated by an Allison Model 22 audiometer was selected as the auditory stimulus for this study. Octave-band analysis (Bruel and

Kjaer sound pressure level meter Model 2203, octave band filter Model 1613, with condenser microphone Model 4132) showed energy present across a wide frequency spectrum, with primary energy between 1000 and 4000 Hz.

Testing was done in a two-room IAC sound suite. The Allison audiometer was used to deliver the auditory signal to the subjects through an Electro-Voice SP-12 loudspeaker in the test room. All stimuli were presented at 70 dB SPL. This was accomplished by adjusting the hearing level dial on the audiometer (before testing each subject) to produce a peak linear scale reading of 70 dB on the Bruel and Kjaer sound level meter. Measurements were made in the position where the subjects' ears would be during testing.

Procedures

Each subject sat on his mother's lap 5 ft. from the loudspeaker. The loudspeaker was situated at a 45-degree angle to the left of the subject's front line of vision. Parents were instructed not to respond in any way during testing and to remain quiet. One examiner was in the test room with the parent and child and attempted to keep each subject's attention focused to the midline with soft, colorful toys. A second examiner presented auditory stimuli from the audiometer in the control room. Stimuli were presented only when subjects were relatively calm and when their attention was directed to the toys in front of them. Each subject received 30 stimuli. The duration of each stimulus was 2 sec. The interstimulus interval varied according to the readiness of the subjects, but the minimum was 10 sec.

The two examiners made independent judgments whether or not a response occurred after each presentation of a stimulus. A response was defined as a head turn in the direction of the loudspeaker during or immediately after each presentation. For a response to be counted, the examiners had to agree.

In addition to 30 test trials, each child received 10 control trials. Each control trial lasted 4 sec., during which the two examiners recorded whether or not the infant turned his head toward the loudspeaker in the absence of an auditory stimulus. The control trials were interspersed among the test trials on an assigned basis and provided a measure of false-positive responses.

The 48 infants were divided into four groups of 12 each. Group 1 (the control group) received no reinforcement after responses to auditory stimuli. Group 2 received social reinforcement after each response. Social reinforcers included a smile from the examiner in the test room, verbal praise, and a pat on the head or shoulders.

Group 3 received visual reinforcement in the form of a flashing light that followed each response. The light, mounted on the loudspeaker at the subject's eye level, was 5" ~ 8" and was powered by a 100-watt bulb through a red-jeweled cover. The light was considered to be a simple visual stimulus because it was only one color (red), had no movement, was two-dimensional (had length and height), and was rectangular. Group 4 also received visual reinforcement—in this case an animated toy animal—after each appropriate localization response. The toy was a colorful bear, 10 in. high, that moved in place when activated by a switch. The toy was enclosed in a clear plastic box mounted adjacent to the loudspeaker at the subjects' eye level. The toy was considered to be a complex visual stimulus because it consisted of several colors, had movement, was three-dimensional (had length, height, and depth), and contained a multitude of contour lines. For Groups 3 and 4, the visual stimulus was presented for approximately 3 sec. after each appropriate localization response.

Results

Table 1 shows the mean, standard deviation, and range of auditory localization responses to 30 stimuli for each group. An analysis of variance (Winer, 1962, p. 320) indicated significant differences among the group means ($F = 25.8$, $df = 3, 44$, $p < 0.01$). Mean comparisons were tested for significance by the critical d test (Lindquist, 1953, p. 93). A difference of 5.67 between any pair of means was required for significance at the 0.01 level, and a difference of 4.24 was required at the 0.05 level. Complex visual reinforcement (the animated toy animal) resulted in more localization responses than simple visual reinforcement (the flashing light), social reinforcement, and no reinforcement ($p < 0.01$). Simple visual reinforcement produced more responses than social reinforcement ($p < 0.05$) and no reinforcement ($p < 0.01$). Social reinforcement resulted in more responses than no reinforcement ($p < 0.05$).

Figure 1 shows the cumulative responses of the four groups in blocks of stimulus trials. The group that received no reinforcement essentially failed to respond after the twentieth stimulus presentation. The group averaged less than one positive response over the last 10 presentations. In contrast, the group that received complex visual reinforcement continued to show a high rate of response over the full 30 presentations. Subjects in this group averaged eight responses during the last 10 presentations. To a lesser degree, subjects in the simple visual and social reinforcement groups continued to respond over the full 30 stimulus presentations, averaging three to four responses during the last 10 presentations.

Table 1. Mean, standard deviation, and range of auditory localization responses of infants 12-18 months old, as a function of four reinforcement conditions (*N* = 12 in each group).

Groups	Mean	Standard Deviation	Range
No Reinforcement	9.7	3.4	5-16
Social Reinforcement	15.2	4.8	9-27
Simple Visual Reinforcement	20.5	7.1	9-28
Complex Visual Reinforcement	27.3	4.7	13-30

Subjects randomly looked toward the sound source only 4.8% of the time when no auditory stimulus was presented (during control trials). Therefore, random behavior (looking toward the sound source) can be ruled out as a major factor accounting for the number of positive responses obtained during test trials. The agreement of the judges was reliable; the two examiners recorded the same responses 98.6% of the time after stimulus presentations and 98.9% of the time during control periods.

We infer from these data that the auditory localization behavior of 12-18-month-old infants is indeed influenced by reinforcement and that the extent of this effect is related to the type of reinforcement employed.

Discussion

There is some indication that infants' responses to visual stimuli are related to the complexity of the stimuli (Cohen, 1969; Frantz and Nevis, 1967). Meyers and Cantor (1967) speculated that complex visual stimuli require additional response time (increased looking

behavior) because the infant requires more time to retain the stimulus mentally. The complexity factor may explain why the "complex" visual stimulus (the animated toy animal) was a stronger reinforcer than the "simple" visual stimulus (the blinking light) in this study. On the other hand, these results might be explained on the basis of the familiarity of the stimulus. The infants' learning history may have included pleasurable experiences with animals and toys. If so, the reinforcing attributes of the dancing toy bear may have been associated more with these pleasant experiences than with complexity per se. In any event, our results suggest that colorful, toy-like visual stimuli that include movement are apt to be more effective than blinking lights as reinforcement for localization behavior.

While infants in the 12-18-month age range are visually responsive (Mussen, Conger, and Kagan, 1969, p. 159), they are relatively immature in social development (Doll, 1953, pp. 231-259). Accordingly, it is not surprising that social reinforcement was less effective than either of the two visual reinforcers in producing localization responses. In a clinical situation it would be uncommon for the audiologist to employ visual reinforcement without also employing social reinforcement. The combined use of visual and social reinforcement was not investigated in this study, but it is reasonable to expect that the two forms would complement each other. In fact, the data argue against the exclusive use of social reinforcement. Although all measurements were made at suprathreshold level, it is reasonable to assume that the results have implication for threshold assessment.

Acknowledgment

This study was supported by Contract 71-2446 from the National Institutes of Health, National Institute of Child Health and Human Development. Marie Thompson is currently affiliated with the Seattle Public Schools. Requests for reprints should be directed to John (Mick) Moore, Communication Disorders Program, Child Development and Mental Retardation Center, CTU/WJ -10, University of Washington, Seattle, Washington 98195.

References

Asha, Clinical and Educational Materials: Audiometric assessment technique. 6, 261 (1964).

Cohen, L., Observing responses, visual preferences, and habituation to visual stimuli in infants. *J. Exp. Child Psychol.,* 7, 419-433 (1969).

Doll, E.A., *The Measurement of Social Competence: A Manual for the Vineland Social Maturity Scale.* Minneapolis: Educational Test Bureau (1953).

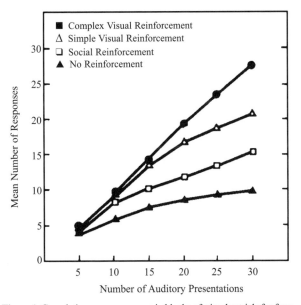

Figure 1. Cumulative mean responses in blocks of stimulus trials for four reinforcement conditions *(N* = 12 in each group).

Frantz, R., and Nevis, S., Pattern preference and perceptual cognitive development in early infancy. *Merrill-Palmer Quart.,* 13, 77-108 (1967).

Hodgson, W., Testing infants and young children. In J. Katz (Ed.), *Handbook of Clinical Audiology,* 498-519 (1972).

Hoversten, G., and Moncur, J., Stimuli and intensity factors in testing infants. *J. Speech Hearing Res.,* 12, 687-702 (1969).

Lindquist, E., *Analysis of Experiments in Psychology and Education.* Boston: Houghton Mifflin (1953).

Meyers, W., and Cantor, G., Observing and cardiac responses to human infants to visual stimuli. *J. Exp. Child Psychol.,* 5, 16-25 (1967).

Mussen, P., Conger, J., and Kagan, J., *Child Development and Personality.* New York: Harper (1969).

Suzuki, T., and Ogiba, Y., Conditioned orientation reflex audiometry. *Arch. Otolaryng.,* 74, 192-198 (1961).

Thompson, M., and Thompson, G., Response of infants and young children as a function of auditory stimuli and test method. *J. Speech Hearing Res.,* 15, 699-707 (1972).

Winer, B., *Statistical Principles in Experimental Design.* New York: McGraw-Hill (1962).

Received March 18, 1974
Accepted May 15, 1974

Visual Reinforcement of Head-Turn Responses in Infants Under 12 Months of Age

John M. Moore, Wesley R. Wilson, and Gary Thompson

University of Washington, Seattle

The effect of complex visual reinforcement (animated toy animal) on auditory localization responses of infants below 12 months of age was studied. Sixty infants served as subjects and each subject received 30 presentations of complex noise at suprathreshold level. After each response to an auditory signal, one-half of the infants (experimental group) received complex visual reinforcement and the other half (control group) received no reinforcement. The experimental and control groups were further subdivided into three age groups: four months, five and six months, and seven to 11 months. Visual reinforcement produced significantly more responses (head turn) than no reinforcement for the two older age groups. There was no significant difference between the experimental and control conditions at four months of age.

Normal infants begin to localize toward a sound source at four to six months of age and this process develops throughout the first year of life (Ewing and Ewing, 1944; Murphy, 1962; Wolski, Wiley, and McIntire, 1964; Watrous, McConnell, Sitton, and Fleet, 1975). Observation of localization responses to controlled auditory stimuli forms the basis for hearing assessment of infants up to about two years of age or until other behavioral test procedures can be successfully employed. It is a relatively common audiological practice to present a visual stimulus following each appropriate localization response, under the assumption that the visual stimulus will reinforce (increase) localization behavior and lead to a more accurate clinical assessment (Suzuki and Ogiba, 1960, 1961; "Audiometric Assessment Technique," 1964; Haug, Baccaro, and Guilford, 1967; Liden and Kankkunen, 1969; Warren, 1972).

Suzuki and Ogiba (1961) reported that use of a visual stimulus as a reward for appropriate auditory localization responses was successful in testing children between one and three years of age, but only partially successful for infants under one year of age. Haug et al. (1967) reported clinical success with a visual reinforcement technique on subjects under three years of age, including a small number of infants in the five- to 12-month age range. These studies suggest that use of visual reinforcement is a powerful addition to the clinical assessment process, possibly even for infants below one year of age. However, since control (no reinforcement) groups were not included for comparison, the specific reinforcing value of the visual stimulus remained uncertain.

Moore, Thompson, and Thompson (1975) studied localization responses as a function of visual reinforcement, social reinforcement, and no reinforcement (control group). They found that a visual stimulus which contained movement and color (that is, an electrically animated toy animal) was a strong reinforcer for auditory localization responses (head-turn) of infants 12 to 18 months of age. Since these infants demonstrated a high rate of response, it seemed logical to investigate this visual reinforcer with younger infants to define the lower boundary of the paradigm's effectiveness.

Accordingly, the present study was designed to investigate visual reinforcement (animated toy animal) of auditory localization responses to infants under 12 months of age.

Method

Subjects

Sixty infants between four and 11 months of age were selected from a list of infants available for participation in university research studies. Subject selection was based on the following criteria: (1) no suspicion of hearing impairment; (2) normal development as reported by the parents; (3) no colds on the test date; and (4) no ear infections for the three months prior to the test date. These criteria were verified by an interview with the parents of the infants on the day of the hearing investigation.

Auditory Stimulus

Complex noise was used in this study, as well as by Moore et al. (1975), because it consists of a wide frequency band and can be easily calibrated in a sound field. Also, broadband stimuli have been shown to be more effective than pure tones in eliciting responses from

Reprinted by permission of authors and American Speech-Language-Hearing Association. Copyright 1977. *Journal of Speech and Hearing Disorders*, 42, pp. 328-334.

infants (Eisenberg, 1965; Mendel, 1968; Hoversten and Moncur, 1969; Ling, Ling, and Doehring, 1970; Thompson and Thompson, 1972). It should be recognized that broad-band stimuli do not provide predictive information relative to slope of loss. However, since the focus of the study was on reinforcement characteristics, no additional signal forms were employed.

A spectral analysis of the complex noise indicated that the major concentration of energy was between 1000 and 4000 Hz with decreasing energy in the higher and lower frequencies. The level of the signal was maintained at 70 dB SPL (measured at the position of the infant's head) for all presentations. Electroacoustic calibration was checked before each test session with a Bruel and Kjaer sound pressure level meter (Model 2203).

Apparatus

An Allison audiometer (Model 22) was used to produce the auditory signal and was located in one room of a two-room IAC sound-treated audiometric test suite. A one-way mirror-window allowed the tester to observe the infants in the adjacent sound-treated room. Electrical switches allowed the tester to activate the animated toy animal. In the test room, a single loudspeaker (Electro-Voice SP-12) was located at ear level, approximately five feet from the infant and at a 45-degree angle to the right of the infant's midline of vision. The visual reinforcer was located at, or slightly below, the infant's eye level near the loudspeaker. A small table was located in front of the infant. The assistant used a signal-button and microphone talk-back with earphones (Phonic Ear HC 214) to communicate with the tester. To avoid confusion in differentiating a localization response from a random look toward the assistant, the assistant was located to the infant's left side, while the response monitored was a localization to the right side only.

The term *localization,* as used in this study, requires discussion. If the primary intent of a procedure is to determine localization to both sides, it follows that two loudspeakers are required for a signal delivery. Clinically, one often elects to do this, but the process was considered unnecessary and perhaps even inappropriate under the design of this experiment. We were interested in the effect of visual reinforcement on head-turn responses and the least complicated method for studying this question is through use of a single loudspeaker.

Procedures

Each mother was instructed to sit in a chair located in the sound suite. She was asked to hold her child in her lap or in an infant seat on the table and not to react or to show interest in the auditory presentation.

The assistant encouraged the infant to observe or play with soft toys passively. The assistant cued the tester, using the signal-button, to present an auditory stimulus when the infant was in a ready state (that is, calm, playing with toys, and head facing forward). Auditory stimuli were not presented if the infant was crying, fretting, vocalizing, looking at the assistant or loudspeaker, in a state of preoccupation with himself, or moving excessively.

The auditory stimulus was presented 30 times to each subject. Stimulus duration was approximately two seconds and the interstimulus interval was varied with a minimum interval of 10 seconds.

The assistant and the tester independently recorded the infant's responses as positive or no response. A positive response was defined as a complete head turn toward the loudspeaker within four seconds of the initiation of the auditory signal. Eye movement only was scored as no response. A timer indicated the four-second period to the examiners. Disagreement between judges was scored as no response.

Ten control trials were randomly interspersed among the 30 auditory presentations to determine whether the positive responses might be the result of random behavior. Each control period lasted four seconds as defined by the timer, and the assistant and tester independently recorded whether or not the infant turned his head toward the sound source (a false-positive response) when no auditory stimulus had been presented.

The 60 infants were equally divided into three groups based on age. Group 1 contained four month olds (three months, 16 days through four months, 15 days). Group 2 contained five- and six-month-old infants (four months, 16 days through six months, 15 days) and Group 3 contained infants who were seven through 11 months of age (six months, 16 days through 11 months, 15 days). Each group contained 20 subjects; 10 served as control subjects (no reinforcement), and 10 served as experimental subjects (visual reinforcement). The visual reward was an animated toy animal—a colorful bear—enclosed in a clear plastic box, which moved in place when activated. The toy animal was activated for approximately three seconds following each appropriate localization (head-turn) response.

Results

Figures 1a, b, and c present cumulative mean results for the visual reinforcement and control groups at seven to 11, five to six, and four months of age, respectively. Tables 1 and 2 present means, standard deviations, and ranges for the experimental and control groups. Analysis of variance (Winer, 1962, p. 228) indicated that the visual reinforcement and control groups responded differently (F = 43.0; df = 1, 54; $p < 0.01$) and that infants responded differently as a function of age (F = 15.9; df = 2, 54; $p <$ 0.01). In addition, there was a significant interaction between reinforcement conditions and age (F = 12.3; df = 2, 54; $p < 0.01$). The interaction suggests that while the visual stimulus served to reinforce (increase) localization behavior, the effect was not the same for all age groups. Specific mean comparisons were made using the Sheffe procedure (Winer, 1962, pp. 85-86). Results indicated that for the seven- to 11- and five- to six-month groups, the visual reinforcement (experimental) groups responded more frequently than the control groups ($p < 0.01$). There was no difference between the experimental and control

groups at four months of age ($p > 0.01$ NS). The inference from these data is that a complex visual stimulus can be used to reinforce localization behavior of infants as young as approximately five months of age.

Infants randomly looked toward the sound source an average of 6.2 percent of the time during the control trials (that is, when no auditory stimulus was presented). It was concluded that random head turns toward the sound source can be ruled out as a major factor accounting for the number of positive responses obtained during the test sessions.

Judge reliability was high. The examiner and assistant independently recorded the same responses 98.6% of the time immediately following an auditory presentation, and 96.0% of the time during the control periods.

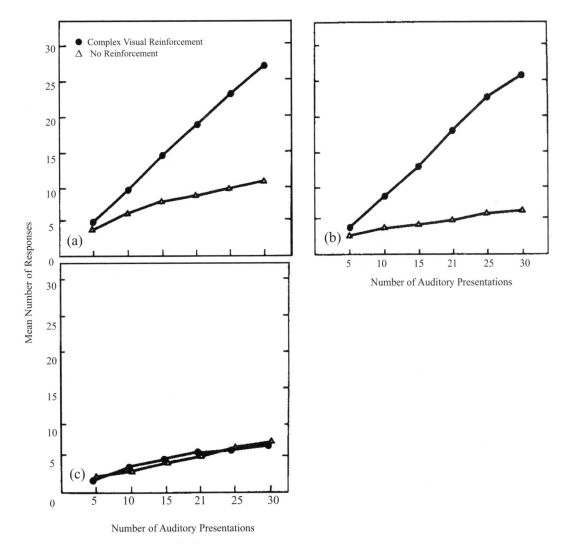

Figure 1. Cumulative mean responses in blocks of stimulus trials as a function of visual reinforcement and age—(a) seven to 11 months *(N* = 20), (b) five and six months *(N* = 20), and (c) four months of age *(N* = 20).

Table 1. Means, standard deviations, and ranges of auditory localization responses to 30 signals for experimental groups ($N = 10$ in each group).

Age (Months)	Mean	Standard Deviation	Range
Seven to 11	26.6	4.1	19-30
Five to six	25.5	3.8	17-30
Four	6.4	12.4	0-26

Table 2. Means, standard deviations, and ranges of auditory localization responses to 30 signals for control groups ($N = 10$ in each group).

Age (Months)	Mean	Standard Deviation	Range
Seven to 11	10.7	7.9	3-25
Five to six	5.5	6.5	1-19
Four	7.0	8.5	0-23

Discussion

Moore et al. (1975) showed that complex visual stimuli can be used to reinforce auditory localization responses of infants 12 to 18 months of age. The present study extends this finding downward in age to a level of five months. Analysis of individual performance showed that very little overlap occurred across experimental and control subjects. Of the 20 experimental subjects in the two older age groups, the least responsive subject responded 17 times out of 30 stimulus trials. Among the 20 control subjects, only three responded more often than 17 times. Thus, only a few of the most responsive members of the control groups responded more frequently than the least responsive member of the experimental groups. Further, the response-to-stimulus functions (Figures 1a and b) illustrate that responses of the five- to 11-month-old experimental subjects had not begun to habituate within the 30 presentations of the study. Had there been more trials, it is likely there would have been an even greater difference between the control and experimental groups. The clinician desiring to assess an infant's response to more than a very limited number of auditory presentations would find these differences important.

It is apparent that, at least for normally developing infants, the lower age limit for this operant conditioning approach is not 12 months as suggested by Suzuki and Ogiba (1960, 1961) and Motta, Facchini and D'Auria (1970), but closer to five months as implied by Haug et al. (1967). There is reason to believe that with modifications of Suzuki and Ogiba's (1961) conditioned orientation reflex (COR) audiometry approach, it may be possible to establish reliable thresholds on many infants under 12 months of age.

Acknowledgment

This research was supported by a contract from the National Institute of Child Health and Human Development (HD-3-2793) entitled, "An Investigation of Certain Relationships between Hearing Impairment and Language Disability." Requests for reprints should be directed to John M. Moore, Child Development and Mental Retardation Center (WJ-10), University of Washington, Seattle, Washington 98195.

References

Audiometric assessment technique, Clinical and Educational Materials, *Asha,* 6, 261 (1964).

Eisenberg, R., Auditory behavior in the human neonate. I. Methodological problems and the logical design of research procedures. *J. Aud. Res.,* 5, 159-177 (1965).

Ewing, I.R., and Ewing, A.W.G., The ascertainment of deafness in infancy and early childhood. *J. Lar. Otol.,* 59, 309-333 (1944).

Haug, O., Baccaro, P., and Guilford, F.R., A pure-tone audiogram on the infant: The PIWI technique. *Archs Otolar.,* 86, 435-440 (1967).

Hoversten, G.H., and Moncur, J.P., Stimuli and intensity factors in testing infants. *J. Speech Hearing Res.,* 12, 687-702 (1969).

Liden, G., and Kankkunen, A., Visual reinforcement audiometry. *Acta Oto-lar.,* 67, 281-292 (1969).

Ling, D., Ling, A.H., and Doehring, D.G., Stimulus, response, and observer variables in the auditory screening of newborn infants. *J. Speech Hearing Res.,* 13, 9-18 (1970).

Mendel, M.I., Infant responses to recorded sounds. *J. Speech Hearing Res.,* 11, 811-816 (1968).

Moore, J.M., Thompson, G., and Thompson, M., Auditory localization of infants as a function of reinforcement conditions. *J. Speech Hearing Dis.,* 40, 29-34 (1975).

Motta, G., Facchini, G.M., and D'Auria, E., Objective conditioned-reflex audiometry in children. *Acta Oto-lar.,* Suppl. 273, 1-49 (1970).

Murphy, K.P., Development of hearing in babies. *Child Family,* 1, 16-20 (1962).

Suzuki, T., and Ogiba, Y., A technique of pure tone audiometry for children under three years of age: Conditioned orientation reflex (C.O.R.) audiometry. *Rev. Lar.,* 81, 33-45 (1960).

Suzuki, T., and Ogiba, Y., Conditioned orientation reflex audiometry. *Archs Otolar.,* 74, 192-198 (1961).

Thompson, M., and Thompson, G., Responses of infants and young children as a function of auditory stimuli and test methods. *J. Speech Hearing Res.,* 15, 699-707, (1972).

Warren, V.G., A comparative study of the auditory responses of normal and "at risk" infants from twelve to twenty-four months of age using COR audiometry. Doctoral dissertation, Univ. of Southern California (1972).

Watrous, B.S., McConnell, F., Sitton, A.B., and Fleet, W.F., Auditory responses of infants. J. *Speech Hearing Dis.*, 40, 357-366 (1975).

Winer, B.J., *Statistical Principles in Experimental Design.* New York: McGraw-Hill (1962).

Wolski, W., Wiley, J., and McIntire, M., Hearing testing in infants and young children. *Medical Times*, 92, 1107-1110 (1964).

Received June 22, 1976
Accepted September 17, 1976

Response Strength of Young Children in Operant Audiometry

Michael A. Primus
University of *Wyoming, Laramie*

Gary Thompson
University of Washington, Seattle

An operant conditioning discrimination paradigm was evaluated in terms of relationships between response behavior of young children and two stimulus components of the paradigm, the discriminative stimulus (DS) and the reinforcing stimulus (RS). Experiment I measured response performance in normal 1-year-old subjects as a function of differences in intensity and/or complexity among three DSs. Results showed no significant differences in conditioning rate, habituation, or consistency of the conditioned response relative to variable properties of the DS. Experiment II examined response performance of normal 2-year-old children as a function of two modifications in the RS, reinforcement schedule and reinforcement novelty. Subjects reinforced on a variable-ratio schedule of intermittent reinforcement and subjects reinforced on a 100% schedule demonstrated equivalent response habituation and consistency. In the second part of the experiment, subjects receiving novel RSs showed significantly greater response recovery than subjects reinforced with familiar RSs. Comparison of normal 1- and 2-year-old children revealed similar rates of conditioning and response consistency. However, 2-year-olds habituated more rapidly than 1-year-olds.

Operant conditioning is a valuable instrument for the behavioral assessment of auditory function in infants and young children and other difficult-to-test populations. In an operant procedure, a specific behavior of the subject is strengthened (i.e., its probability of occurrence is increased) by making it a contingency for presentation of a positive reinforcer. The operant discrimination paradigm represents one application of operant conditioning. In this paradigm, a test (discriminative) stimulus signals the availability of the reinforcer.

The operant discrimination paradigm has three primary elements: the discriminative stimulus (DS), the response, and the reinforcing stimulus (RS). The DS is typically selected on the basis of specific experimental or clinical objectives. For example, pure-tone stimuli are employed to establish frequency-specific auditory thresholds; speech stimuli are used to assess more complex processing skills. The final two components of the paradigm, the subject's response mode and the RS, are selected to facilitate the evaluative process, to maximize test efficiency and test validity for a particular subject or group of subjects.

Visual Reinforcement Audiometry

Moore, Thompson, and Thompson (1975) described an operant discrimination procedure that utilizes a single reinforcer, an animated toy animal, and defines a single distinct response criterion, a head turn toward the reinforcer. This procedure was termed Visual Reinforcement Audiometry (VRA), after Liden and Kankkunen (1969). In the initial experiment with the VRA paradigm, Moore et al. (1975) demonstrated robust responsivity in 12 to 18 month-old infants. Subsequently, Moore, Wilson, and Thompson (1977) determined that VRA is an effective technique for assessing skills in infants over 5 months of age. Additional studies have used the VRA paradigm and modifications of the procedure to evaluate normal auditory processes in infants, including sensitivity thresholds (Nozza & Wilson, 1984; Schneider, Trehub, & Bull, 1980; Trehub, Schneider, & Endman, 1980; Wilson & Moore, 1978; Wilson, Moore, & Thompson, 1976), speech discrimination abilities (Eilers, Wilson, & Moore, 1977), binaural fusion (Diefendorf & Wilson, 1980), and frequency selectivity (Nozza & Wilson, 1984). VRA has also been adapted to assess visual abilities in infants (Mayer, 1980; Mayer & Dobson, 1980), and to substantially expand the data base in the study of infant speech perception (Hillenbrand, Minifie, & Edwards, 1979; Holmberg, Morgan, & Kuhl, 1977; Kuhl, 1979a, 1979b).

In seeking to improve the effectiveness with which children can be audiometrically evaluated, there is substantial justification for working within the VRA paradigm. First, VRA represents a procedure with an extensive experimental background and therefore a strong

Reprinted by permission of authors and American Speech-Language-Hearing Association. Copyright 1985. *Journal of Speech and Hearing Research*, 28, pp. 539-547.

data base on which to make modifications. Second, many auditory laboratories and clinics are already equipped to use the VRA procedure. Instruments for implementing VRA are relatively few and are simple to obtain. Third, the VRA animated-doll reinforcer demonstrates a strong initial influence on the response behavior of children, even though some habituate rapidly in the task. Classical psychological research describes a number of techniques to delay habituation through modification of the reinforcer (Morse, 1966; Skinner, 1938, 1970).

Experiment I

Experiment I used the VRA technique to examine conditioned response behavior of young children as a function of intensity and complexity of the auditory DS. The relationship between qualitative aspects of the DS and response is important to the design of assessment procedures. If the relationship is independent, response reflects only the auditory skill under evaluation (e.g., detection, discrimination). However, if response is influenced by the child's interest in qualitative properties of the signal, audiometric findings cannot be interpreted with confidence. In the operant discrimination paradigm, the DS is characterized as a cue that signals the availability of a reinforcer (Cairns & Butterfield, 1975; Fulton, 1974, 1978; Lancioni, 1980). Generally, response strength is assumed to be a product of reinforcer potency with little consideration of effect by the DS. Experiment I examined the effect of DS intensity and complexity in the operant paradigm. These signal features have been shown to influence response behavior when systematic reinforcement is not employed (Eisenberg, 1976; Hoversten & Moncur, 1969; Thompson & Thompson, 1972).

Experiment II

Experiment II investigated two methods for increasing the power of the RS in VRA based on principles of reinforcement outlined in the operant literature. First, experiments have shown that the reinforcement schedule can be manipulated to maximize the efficiency of an operant conditioning procedure. In general, evidence reveals that a 100% schedule—reinforcement for every appropriate response—results in more rapid conditioning and habituation. Conversely, an intermittent reinforcement schedule produces slower conditioning and a slower rate of habituation. Accordingly, investigators recommend a protocol that begins with a 100% reinforcement schedule and then gradually shifts to an appropriate intermittent reinforcement schedule (Lancioni, 1980; Morse, 1966; Seward, 1970; Sulzer-Azaroff & Mayer, 1977).

Performance varies as a function of the manner in which the schedule is applied. Variable-ratio schedules, which designate reinforcement for a select proportion of trials randomly interspersed among all trials, produce both the highest rate of response and the most consistent response over trials (Lancioni, 1980).

Secondly, operant experiments indicate that the use of novelty in the reinforcement protocol is an effective technique for improving response. Evidence shows that infants and young children attend more to novel versus familiar stimuli, and are more willing to work (emit a response behavior) to elicit novel stimuli (Caron & Caron, 1968, 1969; Caron, Caron, & Caldwell, 1971; Fantz, 1964; Lewis & Goldberg, 1969; Lipsitt & Werner, 1981). Change in reinforcement during the test session introduces novelty as a property of reinforcement. Novelty is a unique attribute of reinforcement because in addition to slowing a decline in response rate, it can renew a subject's interest in the experimental task and revive response behavior (Bond, 1972; Lipsitt & Werner, 1981; Saayman, Ames, & Moffitt, 1964).

Experiment II applied a modified schedule and novelty to the VRA reinforcement protocol with attention to the effectiveness of these techniques in prolonging response behavior of a young child in a single test session.

Method

Subjects

Subjects were 1-year-old (11 to 13 months of age) and 2-year-old (22 to 26 months of age) children selected from a subject pool established for perceptual research at the University of Washington. The pool is maintained through letters of inquiry sent to parents listed in the birth announcements of local newspapers. Children whose parents respond to the letter become members of the subject pool.

The following criteria were met for inclusion in the study (on the basis of parental report): observed-normal hearing and visual skills; no major medical or developmental problems; no history of chronic middle-ear pathology or surgical insertion of pressure-equalization tubes; limited research and clinical exposure to an operant assessment procedure that uses an animated toy animal as reinforcer. Limited exposure was defined as no exposure in the previous 5 months (1-year-olds) or 11 months (2-year-olds) and no more than a single exposure prior to these time periods. Each subject was also required to demonstrate bilaterally normal tympanograms following the test protocol. Tympanograms with compliance peaks at negative middle-ear pressure values ≤ 200 daPa were accepted as normal for this study.

Discriminative Stimuli

Two signal spectra were used as discriminative stimuli: a 1500-Hz warble tone and a complex noise band pass (CNBP). The CNBP was the filtered product of a complex noise with a fundamental frequency of 60 Hz. Band-pass filtering yielded a signal with primary energy between 500 and 2000 Hz and approximate roll-off values of 40 dB and 30 dB in the octaves below and above the band, respectively. The CNBP was selected for use in this study because of its past success in eliciting response from young children in this clinic. Prior to subject evaluation, an average sensitivity threshold of 8 normally hearing adults (0 dBnHL) was obtained for each of the two stimuli. Calibration checks were completed prior to test sessions daily with a Bruel & Kjaer model 2203 sound level meter. Measurements were performed with the SLM held at the subject's position in the test area, and with its microphone at a 90 degree angle of incidence to the sound source.

Instrumentation and Procedures

Test procedures employed in this study have been described previously (Moore et al., 1975, 1977). Signals were controlled by a standard audiometer (Madsen Electronics model OB 77) and presented in the sound field through a single loudspeaker. The reinforcer was a lighted, animated toy animal converted to receive examiner-controlled electrical current (see Wilson, Lee, Owen, & Moore, 1976, for a description of reinforcer instrumentation). The toy was housed in a black Plexiglas box and was not apparent to the child except during specified reinforcement periods. A logic instrument processed votes by two examiners, E1 and E2, through an AND-gate, and during stimulus trials activated the reinforcer   for 2 s if both votes occurred within a 4-s poststimulus-onset response window. A vote was an indication that a head-turn response toward the reinforcer had been observed.

Figure 1 is a diagram of the experimental test suite. From the control room E1 initiated trials, voted for observed responses, and recorded the result of each trial. In the test room, E2 attempted to keep the child passively attending, face-forward, by manipulating pictures or quiet toys on a table in front of the child. In an attempt to produce uniformity across subjects with respect to these distracting stimuli, a specified sequence of presentation of distracting stimuli was employed. The stimuli used with the 1-year-old children, however, differed from those presented to the 2-year-olds, because of their different inter-

ests and behaviors. Masking noise (the CNBP signal) transmitted during trials to E2 via earphones signaled trial onset and made E2 blind to differentiation of stimulus and control trials. Measurement of false-positive responding during control trials was based on E2's voting record alone, since E1 was aware of the trial type presented. Children whose false-positive rate exceeded 25% were disqualified from participation in the study. E2 was trained in VRA protocol but was blind to the conceptual design of the study and experimental questions posed by the study. The use of a trained examiner as E2 is critical to efficient evaluation of young children with this procedure.

Schedule of Trials

The basic schedule of trials is shown in Table 1. The first phase of the trial schedule was the conditioning process. Trials 1 and 2 were training trials; following an approximately 1-s lead by the DS, the subject experienced simultaneous presentation of both DS and the reinforcer. After two training trials, a series of randomized stimulus and control trials began. One control trial (no signal) was randomly included in each set of three stimulus trials. The DS was presented in stimulus trials, and the reinforcer was activated if the subject demonstrated a criterion response. The subject was required to achieve a conditioning criterion of three consecutive correct responses to

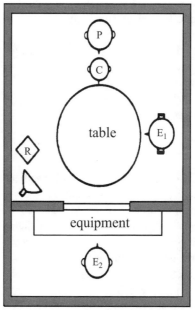

E_1-Examiner 1
E_2-Examiner 2
P - Parent
C - Child
R - Reinforcer

Figure 1. Diagram of the two-room test suite.

Table 1. Basic schedule of trials.

Phase I		Phase II	
Training trials	Reinforcing & control trials	Reinforcing & control trials	
TT	RRCR ...	RRRC RCRR CRRR RCRR ...	
	Conditioning criterion		Habituation criterion

Note. T = DS & RS simultaneously; R = DS, RS contingent upon response; and C = No DS or RS.

advance to Phase II of the experiment. Following each no-response trial prior to criterion, two training trials were again presented. Children were disqualified if conditioning was not accomplished with a maximum of ten training trials. Phase II of the schedule consisted of those trials occurring subsequent to conditioning trials and prior to a habituation criterion of four no-response trials among five consecutive stimulus trials.

Experiment I

Experiment I examined response behavior with respect to the discriminative stimuli that precede it in an operant discrimination paradigm. Subjects were 36 one-year-old children arbitrarily assigned to one of three groups (12 subjects per group). Each group received a different DS. Stimulus conditions were divided among subject groups as follows: Group 1, 50 dBnHL CNBP; Group 2, 25 dBnHL CNBP; Group 3, 50 dBnHL 1500-Hz warble tone. The three stimuli represented differences of intensity and complexity in the DS. Hoversten and Moncur (1969) and Thompson and Thompson (1972) have shown that these stimulus parameters affect response behavior in procedures where response strength is closely tied to the test stimulus (i.e., in nonconditioned procedures). Accordingly, these parameters offered a reasonable means by which to investigate a relationship between the DS and response strength in an operant discrimination procedure. The experiment measured the rate of conditioning of the criterion response, response habituation, and response consistency across the three conditions.

Experiment II

Experiment II investigated the influence of specified modifications in reinforcement protocol on response behavior. The experiment focused on means to increase response strength in the VRA operant procedure. A slightly older age group was selected for this part of the study because older children tend to habituate more rapidly (Lewis, Goldberg, & Campbell, 1969). Thus, the need to increase response strength was expected to be greater in 2-year-old children than in 1-year-olds. In this experiment, 45 two-year-old children were divided into four groups: Groups 4, 5, 6, and 7. Each group consisted of 12 subjects (the design of the experiment allowed use of data of 3 subjects for both groups 4 and 6, thus reducing the required number of subjects from 48 to 45). A 50 dBnHL CNBP signal was used as the DS for all four groups in Experiment II.

The first portion of Experiment II examined effects of modification of the reinforcement schedule. Group 4 subjects were reinforced on a 100% schedule and operated as controls to children in Group 5, who were reinforced on a variable-ratio schedule of intermittent reinforcement (Table 2). Group 5 subjects received reinforcement according to the following schedule: 100% reinforcement in Phase I stimulus trials; 67% reinforcement in the first six stimulus trials of Phase II; and 50% for remaining trials. RS trials and no-reinforcing-stimulus (NRS) trials were combined according to the schedule in a quasi-random manner, so that no more than three NRS trials occurred consecutively. As in Experiment I, one control trial was randomly included in each set of three stimulus trials. Scoring was terminated following habituation (four no-responses in five consecutive stimulus trials). The effect of the intermittent reinforcement schedule on response behavior was measured in terms of response habituation and response consistency.

The second part of Experiment II investigated a modification in RS familiarity. A series of additional trials, Phase III trials, was presented to each subject in Groups 6 and 7 following habituation of response (Table 3). During these trials, responses by subjects in Group 6 were reinforced with the same toy animal seen in prior trials, whereas responses by Group 7 subjects elicited novel reinforcers. Both groups received six sets of experimental trials. Each set included three stimulus trials and one control trial, and in addition, an initial training trial that introduced the reinforcer assigned to that set.

The presentation schedule of reinforcers is shown in Table 4. In Phases I and II of the trial schedule, familiarization trials, Groups 6 and 7 were rewarded for responses with the same reinforcer (R1). Experimental treatment of groups occurred in Phase III, where novel reinforcers (R2, R3, and R4) became available to Group 7, while Group 6 continued to receive the familiar reinforcer. Group 7 saw a new reinforcer for each set of trials.

Four different toy animals served as R1, R2, R3, and R4: a standing golden bear that beats on a drum; a bunny

Table 2. Typical schedule of trials in Experiment II: Reinforcement schedule.

| | Phase I | | Phase II |
	Training trials	Reinforcing & control trials	Reinforcing, nonreinforcing, & control trials
Group 4	TT	(100%) RRRC ...	(100%) CRRR RRCR RCRR CRRR RCRR RRRC ...
Group 5	TT	(100%) RCRR ...	(67%) (50%) RCNR NRCR NRNC RRCN RCNR RCNN ...

<table>
<tr><td></td><td></td><td style="text-align:center">Conditioning
criterion</td><td style="text-align:right">Habituation
criterion</td></tr>
</table>

Note. T = DS & RS simultaneously; R = DS, RS contingent upon response; C = no DS or RS; and N = DS; no RS.

Table 3. Typical schedule of trials in Experiment II: Novelty.

| | Familiarization Trials | | | Experimental Trials |
	Phase I Training trials	Reinforcing & control trials	Phase II Reinforcing & control trials	Phase III Training, reinforcing, & control trials
Group 6	TT	RRRC ...	RRCR CRRR ...	(Familiar RS) TRRCR TRCRR ... TRCRR
Group 7	TT	RCRR ...	CRRR RRCR ...	(Novel RSs) TRCRR TRRCR ... TCRRR

<table>
<tr><td></td><td></td><td style="text-align:center">Conditioning
criterion</td><td style="text-align:center">Habituation
criterion</td><td></td></tr>
</table>

Note. T = DS & RS simultaneously; R = DS, RS contingent upon response; C = no DS or RS.

that plays a drum set; a panda that plays a drum set; and a pup that moves its legs, sits up, and barks. The reinforcers were presented in a counter-balanced manner across subjects in each of the two groups to minimize any difference in reinforcement value among the toy animals. Thus, each toy animal was designated as R1 for 3 subjects in Groups 6 and 7. The remaining toy animals were available to the 3 subjects in Group 7 during experimental trials as novel reinforcers.

The influence of novel reinforcement was evaluated in experimental trials in terms of the difference between Groups 6 and 7 in number of responses emitted. In effect, this measure indicates not only the extent to which response behavior of a particular subject can be prolonged, but also whether or not response behavior can be revived following habituation.

Results

Experiment I

Variation in DS properties had no effect on the rate of conditioning. Conditioning rate was measured as the number of training trials required to achieve conditioning. Analysis of variance showed that differences among the three group means of training trials were not significant $[F(2, 33) = 0.26, p > .05]$. Thirty-two of the 36 subjects satisfied the conditioning criterion immediately following the initial two training trials. The remaining 4 subjects, 2

in Group 1 and 1 each in Groups 2 and 3, required four training trials prior to reaching the conditioning criterion.

Nine 1-year-olds were disqualified from the study because they failed to condition to the task within 10 training trials. Six of the 9 children demonstrated bilateral flat tympanograms, and thus were highly suspect for hearing loss. Two additional children resisted placement of the tympanometric probe, and the procedure could not be completed. The final child who failed to reach the conditioning criterion exhibited normal middle-ear function and was the only child for whom conductive hearing loss did not provide a plausible explanation for failure.

Response habituation over the sequence of experimental trials is shown in Figure 2. Performance was initially high among the 12 infants in each of the three groups, and then decreased gradually as the trial sequence progressed. The rate of habituation, reflected in the slope of the curves, was similar across groups, although separation of the curves is apparent.

Table 4. Schedule of reinforcers presented to control subjects (Group 6) and experimental subjects (Group 7). Each designated reinforcer (e.g., R1) was available in three consecutive stimulus trials. In Familiarization Trials all subjects were exposed to R1. In the 18 Experimental Trials the familiar reinforcer (R1) was available to Group 6, and novel reinforcers (R2, R3, R4) were available to Group 7.

	Familiarization trials (Phases I & II)	Experimental trials (Phase III)
Group 6	R1, R1, R1 ...	R1, R1, R1, R1, R1, R1
Group 7	R1, R1, R1 ...	R2, R3, R4, R2, R3, R4

The habituation score was calculated as the number of responses (Phases I and II) provided by each child prior to the habituation criterion or a maximum of 75 Phase II stimulus trials. Analysis of variance revealed no significant difference in habituation among groups [$F(2, 33) = 3.23, p > .05$]. It should be mentioned, however, that the variation in means approached significance at the $p = .05$ level, and in contrast to the pattern of unconditioned response, the more intense and complex signal yielded the fewest responses. Average habituation scores were 31.3 ($SD = 15.09$) for Group 1 (50 dB CNBP); 40.4 ($SD = 13.06$) for Group 3 (50 dB warble); and 47.1 ($SD = 17.46$) for Group 2 (25 dB CNBP). Three subjects, all in Group 2 (25 dB CNBP), reached the designated maximum number of trials before habituation.

Modification of properties of the DS also had no effect on the proportion of trials in which the subjects responded. Response consistency is represented by the number of responses as a percentage of the number of stimulus trials presented. Analysis of variance showed no significant difference in consistency among groups [$F(2, 33) = 0.641, p > .05$]. Groups 1, 2, and 3 produced consistency scores of 88%, 89%, and 86%, respectively. The high rate of response demonstrated by the infants reflects the efficiency of this operant technique. The average subject, for example, provided 36 responses in 41 stimulus trials (88%). Most of the individual ratios in all three groups show performance above 80%. Response consistency was highest during initial trials when interest in the reinforcer was high, and lowest toward the end of the trial sequence.

Experiment II

In the first part of Experiment II, reinforcement schedule demonstrated no effect on response habituation or consistency in normal 2-year-old children. Subjects in Group 4 were reinforced for every appropriate response in the procedure, while Group 5 subjects were treated with a prescribed, variable-ratio schedule of intermittent reinforcement. Figure 3 shows the course of response emission over the sequence of stimulus trials, and demonstrates that group response curves essentially overlap. Performance for both groups decreased sharply after approximately five trials.

The mean number of responses provided by subjects was 20.0 ($SD = 10.99$) for Group 4 and 21.6 ($SD = 10.94$) for Group 5. Statistical analysis showed no significant difference between groups on the basis of habituation [$t(22) = 0.353, p > .05$; all t tests in this study were nondirectional]. Thus, even though Group 4 subjects received a considerably greater number of exposures to the RS, they habituated at the same rate as Group 5. Analysis of indi-

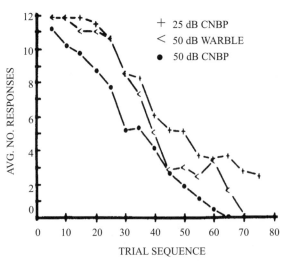

Figure 2. Response performance for three groups of 1-year-olds as a function of the DS employed. Each data point shows the average number of responses across five trials for the 12 subjects in each group.

vidual response consistency rates also revealed no significant difference between groups [$t(22) = 0.514, p > .05$]. Groups 4 and 5 responded in 85% and 88% of stimulus trials, respectively. No subject in either group produced a consistency score less than 70%. As in Experiment I, subjects in both groups conditioned rapidly. All achieved the conditioning criterion following the initial two training trials.

The second part of Experiment II revealed a significant effect of novel reinforcement on response behavior. Figure 4 shows the performance of two groups of normal 2-year-old children, Groups 6 and 7, across the trial sequence. Each group was exposed to the same reinforcer through familiarization trials, and subjects performed similarly. The mean number of responses to habituation was, respectively, 21.0 and 19.3 for Groups 6 and 7. Response recovery in experimental trials demonstrated the effect of RS novelty following habituation. Children who received a series of three new reinforcers (Group 7) substantially outperformed subjects who were reinforced with the familiar RS (Group 6). The graph shows that Group 7 produced eight to nine responses for each experimental trial compared to two responses by Group 6. The slope of the novelty response curve shows little habituation across experimental trials and suggests that even more responses could have been obtained with the three novel reinforcers. The limited response recovery among Group 6 subjects appeared to be the result of reintroduction of training trials in the experimental set.

Each child in Group 6 responded an average of 2.8 times ($SD = 2.04$) in the 18 experimental trials. Group 7 subjects, reinforced with novel stimuli, averaged 12.8 responses ($SD = 4.52$) subsequent to habituation. The dif-

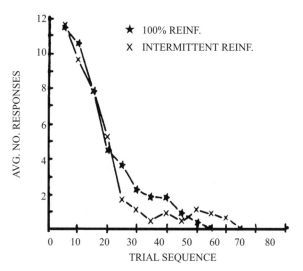

Figure 3. Response performance for two groups of 2-year-olds as a function of the schedule of reinforcement.

ference in response recovery between groups is significant [$t(22) = 6.937, p < .001$]. Strong response recovery was fairly uniform among the Group 7 2-year-olds, 11 of 12 subjects providing at least eight responses. In contrast, only 1 subject in Group 6 responded more than four times.

Most children in both groups conditioned rapidly at the onset of the experiment, consistent with subject performance in previous portions of the study. Three children who were tympanometrically normal failed to condition. Testing was terminated with one of these children because of the child's fear of the test situation. The other two children seemed to respond appropriately, but apparently with insufficient interest to achieve conditioning.

Age

An investigation of response performance across age was made by comparing 1-year-olds in Group 1 with 2-year-olds in Group 4. The data show no difference in the rate of conditioning [$t(22) = 1.482, p > .05$] or in response consistency [$t(22) = 0.585, p > .05$] between the two groups. A difference was apparent, however, in response habituation. Figure 5 shows that 2-year-olds exhibited a steeper rate of habituation than 1-year-olds. Eleven of the 12 two-year-old subjects habituated in the first 30 stimulus trials. A single subject responded through the 65th trial, reflected in the tail of the 2-year-old curve in Figure 5. One- year-olds, in contrast, demonstrated a more gradual rate of habituation and 50% more responses in an identical experimental protocol. The difference in mean responses between 1-year-olds (31.3) and 2-year-olds (20.0) was significant [$t(22) = 2.087, p < .05$].

Additional Performance Measures

Observer agreement exceeded 98% for all groups in Experiments I and II, consistent with the high values recorded in previous studies employing the same procedure (Moore et al., 1975, 1977). Strong observer agreement in this paradigm further demonstrates its efficiency in assessing young children and reflects the distinctive nature of the single, time-locked (head turn) response brought under operant control. The rate of false-positive responding was comparable among all groups (mean rate 6%). Only one child exceeded the allowable rate of false-positives (25%), and this child also failed tympanometry. Overall, 35 one-year-old and 25 two-year-old children

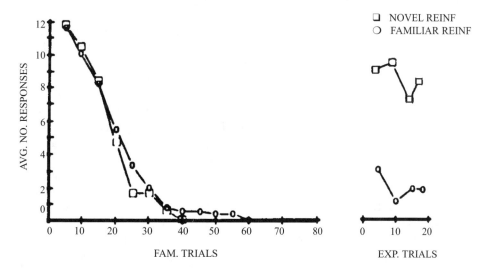

Figure 4. Response performance for two groups of 2-year-olds. Both groups were exposed to the same RS during familiarization trials. In the subsequent 18 experimental trials, one group received the familiar RS, and the second group received novel RSs.

were disqualified from the study, primarily on the basis of failed tympanometry.

Discussion

The Discriminative Stimulus

Complex signals (e.g., bands of noise or speech) are commonly employed in the clinical assessment of young children because their use often elicits "natural" or unconditioned head-turn responses to initial auditory presentations. While the use of broad-band stimuli provides valuable diagnostic information, their exclusive use fails to identify frequency-specific hearing loss. Accordingly, it becomes important to determine whether frequency-specific auditory signals (warble tones) can be used with the same degree of effectiveness as complex stimuli during VRA. Experiment I showed that properties of the DS had no influence on conditioning rate, habituation, or consistency of response in normal infants. This finding is consistent with results of a recent VRA study (Thompson & Folsom, 1985) in which stimuli with differing band widths (2000 Hz warble tone, 2000 Hz tone pips, and a 2000-4000 Hz noise band) had no effect on response behavior of infants under conditions of suprathreshold and threshold-level stimulation. Taken together, these findings provide evidence that examiners need not compromise signal parameters in the assessment of young children so long as the children condition well to the VRA task.

A second aspect of Experiment I dealt with the sound pressure level (SPL) at which stimuli were presented. Results indicated that low to moderate SPL stimuli (25 and 50 dBnHL) had no effect on response behavior. A similar study by Thompson and Folsom (1984) looked at

VRA performance as a function of different methods of conditioning. Results of both studies lead to the inference that the SPL used for conditioning probably has no effect on response performance. If this observation is accurate, there is reason to initiate testing with a relatively "soft" auditory stimulus (e.g., 25-30 dBnHL). If high SPLs are employed in initial trials, the child may habituate before response to lower SPLs can be investigated. In addition, clinical observation suggests that high-intensity signals suppress nonconditioned response to subsequent lower-intensity levels. Since successful conditioning cannot be predicted for each individual child, it is more useful, clinically, to have obtained a few unconditioned responses at relatively soft as opposed to relatively intense levels. When a child fails to respond, as in the case of a hearing loss, the examiner can quickly introduce SPL increments until a response is observed or elect to go immediately to a high level of stimulation for conditioning trials to establish the desired response behavior.

In the current study, normal 1-year-olds were brought under operant control rapidly. This finding suggests that normal 1-year-old children are immediately available for evaluation without the need for a lengthy conditioning protocol. Considering the time constraints involved in behavioral assessment of infants and young children, rapid operant control of behavior is a notably positive element in this assessment paradigm. A particular child's failure to condition rapidly should alert the examiner to a potential auditory problem or other factors (e.g., physical, cognitive, social problems) that affect the child's behavior.

Schedule of Reinforcement

A reduced schedule of reinforcement had no impact on response performance of normal 2-year-old children. These results depart from evidence that demonstrates a slower rate of habituation for intermittent versus 100% reinforcement (Sulzer-Azaroff & Mayer, 1977). The willingness of 2-year-olds to sit agreeably in a controlled experiment and the reinforcing quality of the test procedure itself as a game may have influenced response behavior. In addition, failure of the current reinforcement schedule to enhance response performance does not rule out a potential effect by alternative schedules of reinforcement or alternative test procedures.◊

The experimental findings support use of a conservative reinforcement strategy in clinical evaluation. An occasional delayed or otherwise ambiguous response presents a dilemma for the examiner: Should the behavior be reinforced? Reinforcing a false-positive response or failing to reinforce an appropriate response may confuse the child. According to the present data, the latter alternative does not degrade performance.

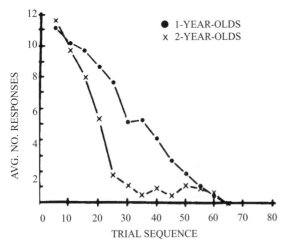

Figure 5. A comparison of response performance between 1-year-olds (11-13 months) and 2-year-olds (22-26 months).

Novel Reinforcement

Experimental findings demonstrated a strong influence of novel reinforcement in eliciting conditioned responses from normal 2-year-old children. Following habituation to an initial reinforcer, subjects receiving novel reinforcement responded an average of 13 times in 18 stimulus trials. The 2-year-olds averaged only 20 responses prior to habituation; thus, the number of responses was substantially increased with a small number of novel reinforcers. The data also show that attempts to recover response were universally unsuccessful among subjects receiving the familiar RS. Once habituated to a reinforcer, the 2-year-olds could not be retrained with the same reinforcer.

Novel reinforcement is easily implemented with on-line decisions by the examiner relative to the child's behavior. The primary benefit of novel reinforcement is its ability to increase the amount of information that can be obtained in a single test session, an especially valuable advantage when a child is unable to return for multiple visits.

Age

The two age groups conditioned at the same rate and responded with equal consistency. One-year-old children, however, provided significantly more responses than 2-year-olds. This finding agrees with other research that indicates an increase in habituation rate with increasing age (Fantz, 1964; Lewis, 1969; Lewis et al., 1969). Experiment II addresses the problem of rapid habituation in 2-year-olds in the operant procedure, demonstrating that habituation can be delayed with the introduction of novel reinforcers. Additional techniques to prolong responsivity are needed. In general, an examiner can increase test effectiveness for a certain child by anticipating the rate of habituation, and planning the evaluation accordingly. Age provides an important clue to the capabilities and responding potential of a particular child.

Acknowledgments

This report was based on a doctoral dissertation by the first author at the University of Washington. The study was conducted at the Child Development and Mental Retardation Center, University of Washington.

References

Bond, E.K. (1972). Perception of form by the human infant. *Psychological Bulletin, 77,* 225-245.

Cairns, G.F., & Butterfield, E.C. (1975). Assessing infants' auditory functioning. In B.Z. Friedlander, G.M. Sterritt, & G.E. Kirk (Eds.), *Exceptional Infant* (Vol. 3, pp. 84-108). New York: Brunner/ Mazel.

Caron, R.F., & Caron, A.J. (1968). The effects of repeated exposure and stimulus complexity on visual fixation in infants. *Psychonomic Science, 10,* 207-208.

Caron, R.F., & Caron, A.J. (1969). Degree of stimulus complexity and habituation of visual fixation in infants. *Psychonomic Science, 14,* 78-79.

Caron, R.F., Caron, A.J., & Caldwell, R.C. (1971). Satiation of visual reinforcement in young infants. *Developmental Psychology, 5,* 279-289.

Diefendorf, A.O., & Wilson, W.R. (1980). *Auditory fusion in infants: One aspect of central auditory function.* Paper presented at the American Speech and Hearing Association annual convention, Detroit.

Eilers, R.E., Wilson, W.R., & Moore, J.M. (1977). Developmental changes in speech discrimination in infants. *Journal of Speech and Hearing Research, 20,* 766-780.

Eisenberg, R.B. (1976). *Auditory competence in early life: The roots of communicative behavior.* Baltimore: University Park Press.

Fantz, R.L. (1964). Visual experience in infants: Decreased attention to familiar patterns relative to novel ones. *Science, 146,* 668-670.

Fulton, R.T. (1974). *Auditory stimulus-response control.* Baltimore: University Park Press.

Fulton, R.T. (1978). *Pure-tone tests of hearing—Age one year through five years.* In F.N. Martin (Ed.), *Pediatric Audiology* (pp. 201-235). Englewood Cliffs, NJ: Prentice-Hall.

Hetsko, R.J., & Gans, D.P. (1981). Maintaining conditioning in young children with varied schedules of reinforcement. *Human Communication/Communication Humaine, 6,* 35-40.

Hillenbrand, J., Minifie, F.D., & Edwards, T.J. (1979). Tempo of frequency change as a cue in speech-sound discrimination by infants. *Journal of Speech and Hearing Research, 22,* 147-165.

Holmberg, T.L., Morgan, K.A., & Kuhl, P.K. (1977). Speech perception in early infancy: Discrimination of fricative consonants. *Journal of the Acoustical Society of America, 62,* (Suppl. 1), 599(A).

....

◊Since completion of this study, results from another study of reinforcement schedules has come to our attention. Hetsko and Gans (1981) measured the number of responses produced by groups of 12- to 24-month-old children receiving 100% or 50% reinforcement in conditioned orientation reflex (COR) audiometry. They found no difference in performance prior to a response decrement criterion of 80%. In the ten trials following this criterion, however, the group receiving 50% reinforcement provided more responses than the continuously reinforced group. Precriterion response consistency was similar to that determined in the present study.

Hoversten, G.H., & Moncur, J.P. (1969). Stimuli and intensity factors in testing infants. *Journal of Speech and Hearing Research,* 12, 687-702.

Kuhl, P.K. (1979a). The perception of speech in early infancy. In N.J. Lass (Ed.), *Speech and language: Advances in basic research and practice* (Vol. 1, pp. 1-47). New York: Academic Press.

Kuhl, P.K. (1979b). Speech perception in early infancy: Perceptual constancy for spectrally dissimilar vowel categories. *Journal of the Acoustical Society of America,* 66, 1668-1679.

Lancioni, G.E. (1980). Infant operant conditioning and its implication for early intervention. *Psychological Bulletin,* 88 (No. 2), 516-534.

Lewis, M. (1969). Infants' responses to facial stimuli during the first year of life. *Developmental Psychology,* 1, 75-86.

Lewis, M., & Goldberg, S. (1969). The acquisition and violation of expectancy: An experimental paradigm. *Journal of Experimental Child Psychology,* 7, 70-80.

Lewis, M., Goldberg, S., & Campbell, H. (1969). A developmental study of information processing within the first three years of life: Response decrement to a redundant signal. *Monographs of the Society for Research in Child Development,* 34 (9, Serial No. 133), 1-41.

Liden, G., & Kankkunen, A. (1969). Visual reinforcement audiometry. *Archives of Otolaryngology,* 89, 865-872.

Lipsitt, L.P., & Werner, J.S. (1981). The infancy of human learning processes. In E.S. Gollin (Ed.), *Developmental plasticity: Behavioral and biological aspects of variations in development* (pp. 101-133). New York: Academic Press.

Mayer, D.L. (1980). *Operant preferential looking: A new technique provides estimates of visual acuity of infants and children.* Unpublished doctoral dissertation, University of Washington, Seattle.

Mayer, D.L., & Dobson, V. (1980). Assessment of vision in young children: A new operant approach yields estimates of acuity. *Investigative Ophthalmology and Visual Science,* 19, 566-570.

Moore, J.M., Thompson, G., & Thompson, M. (1975). Auditory localization of infants as a function of reinforcement conditions. *Journal of Speech and Hearing Disorders,* 40, 29-34.

Moore, J.M., Wilson, W.R., & Thompson, G. (1977). Visual reinforcement of head-turn responses in infants under twelve months of age. *Journal of Speech and Hearing Disorders,* 42, 328-334.

Morse, W.H. (1966). Intermittent reinforcement. In W.K. Honig (Ed.), *Operant behavior: Areas of research and application* (pp. 52-108). New York: Appleton-Century-Crofts.

Nozza, R.J., & Wilson, W.R. (1984). Masked and unmasked pure-tone thresholds of infants and adults: Development of auditory frequency selectivity and sensitivity. *Journal of Speech and Hearing Research,* 27, 613-622.

Saayman, G., Ames, E.W., & Moffett, A. (1964). Response to novelty as an indicator of visual discrimination in the human infant. *Journal of Experimental Child Psychology,* 1, 189-198.

Schneider, B.A., Trehub, S.E., & Bull, D. (1980). High-frequency sensitivity in infants. *Science,* 207, 1003-1004.

Seward, J.P. (1970). Conditions of reinforcement. In M.H. Marx (Ed.), *Learning: Theories* (pp. 67-79). London: MacMillan.

Skinner, B.F. (1938). *The behavior of organisms.* New York: Appleton-Century-Crofts.

Skinner, B.F. (1970). Operant conditioning. In W. Sahakian (Ed.), *Psychology of learning: Systems, models, and theories* (pp. 185-204). Chicago: Markham.

Sulzer-Azaroff, B., & Mayer, G.R. (1977). *Applying behavior-analysis procedures with children and youth.* New York: Holt, Rinehart, & Winston.

Thompson, G., & Folsom, R.C. (1984). A comparison of two conditioning procedures in the use of Visual Reinforcement Audiometry (VRA). *Journal of Speech and Hearing Disorders,* 49, 241-245.

Thompson, G., & Folsom, R.C. (1985). Reinforced and nonreinforced head-turn responses of infants as a function of stimulus bandwidth. *Ear and Hearing,* 6, 125-129.

Thompson, M., & Thompson, G. (1972). Responses of infants and young children as a function of auditory stimuli and test methods. *Journal of Speech and Hearing Research,* 15, 699-707.

Trehub, S.E., Schneider, B.A., & Endman, M. (1980). Developmental changes in infants' sensitivity to octave-band noises. *Journal of Experimental Child Psychology,* 29, 282-293.

Wilson, W.R., Lee, K., Owen, G., & Moore, J.M. (1976). *Instrumentation for operant infant auditory assessment.* (Paper developed for distribution to persons requesting information on instrumentation. Department of Speech and Hearing Sciences, University of Washington, Seattle.)

Wilson, W.R., & Moore, J.M. (1978). *Pure-tone earphone thresholds of infants utilizing visual reinforcement audiometry (VRA).* Paper presented at the American Speech and Hearing Association annual convention, San Francisco.

Wilson, W.R., Moore, J.M., & Thompson, G. (1976). *Soundfield auditory thresholds of infants utilizing visual reinforcement audiometry (VRA).* Paper presented at the American Speech and Hearing Association annual convention, Houston.

Received August 27, 1984
Accepted June 27, 1985

Requests for reprints should be sent to Michael A. Primus, University of Wyoming, P.O. Box 3311, 30 Ross Hall, Laramie, WY 82071.

Developments in Speech Audiometry

Arthur Boothroyd
The University of Manchester, Manchester, United Kingdom

Introduction

All tests of hearing in which speech is used as a stimulus may be grouped under the heading of speech audiometry. There is no unique function of such tests. The may, for example, be used to test various factors involved in speech perception, to detect the presence of malingering or to compare the effectiveness of different hearing aids. Among these tests are those whose basic functions is to measure a subject's ability to make correct phonemic classifications on the basis of acoustical information, i.e. to recognize the sounds of speech. These are collectively known as speech discrimination tests, and it is the purpose of this paper to describe a form of speech discrimination test which has been used by the author for clinical and research work during the past three years. The test was designed to solve some of the problems inherent in the measurement of speech discrimination.

Problems in the Measurment of Speech Discrimination

One of the problems lies in the dependence of speech discrimination score on intensity. As Carhart[1] has said:

"...the clinician who tests at only one presentation level can be sure that he has a valid estimate of a person's maximum discrimination score only if the score approximates 100%. If the score is lower than this there is no way of knowing whether it represents the patient's best performance..."

To obtain a complete assessment of a subject's discrimination ability requires the measurement of discrimination at several intensities and the plotting of a discrimination curve or articulation function, but time limitations make this impracticalbe as a routine clinical procedure with conventional speech discrimination tests.

A second problem is the influence of language skills on the results of discrimination tests. In spite of the use of relatively non redundant test material it is not possible completely to eliminate this influence. As Hirsh[2] has put it, the present tests combine the effects of discrimination with those of recognition. One approach to this problem is to design tests whose vocabulary contents are appropriate to the language skills of various populations. There are obvious advantages, however, in having a test whose results are relatively independent of language ability.

Discrimination scores are subject to a number of sources of variation. These may originate from the word lists used, the test method, or the patient himself. If a discrimination score is to have any value it is essential to know its limits of uncertainty. This is particularly true when making comparisons between hearing aids or assessing the benefits of some training procedure. The only way to be sure of the confidence limits of a particular discrimination score is to repeat the measurment several times and calculate the standard error, a procedure advocated by Lafon[3]. Once again this becomes impracticable as a routine clinical procedure with conventional speech discrimination tests.

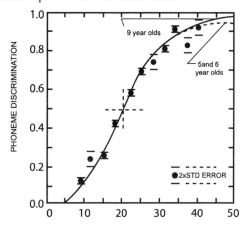

Figure 1. The normal phoneme discrimination curve dervied from the results of tests wth normally hearing children

The Discrimination Test

Basic Features

Two features are basic to the test of speech discrimination to be described:

(i) The use of very short word lists.
   This permits the rapid determination of a discrimination score making it possible to plot complete discrimination curves and, where necessary, to calculate confidence limits.

(ii) The use of phonemic scoring.
   By scoring in terms of the number of phonemes correct instead of the number of words correct, the number of test items is increased, giving a reduction in test score variability. In addition it will be shown that the influences of language factors and inter list differences are reduced.

No originality is claimed for this method of testing which is based on the tests used by Professor J.J. Groen of Utrecht and used for example in the research by Groen and Hellema[4] on binaural speech audiometry.

The Word Lists

The word lists are given in Appendix 1. There are fifteen different lists, each containing the same thirty

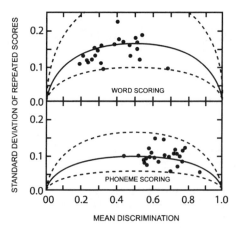

Figure 2. The normal phoneme discrimination curve derived from the results of tests wth normally hearing children

phonemes arranged to form ten consonant-vowel words. The only constraints placed on vocabulary are the exclusion of first names and obscenities. In such short lists it is not possible to represent all English phonemes, the ones used being the ten vowels and twenty consonants occurring most frequently in the author's vocabulary of consonant-vowel-consonant words. A close examination of the lists will reveal the influence of the Northern English accent, in which no distinction is made between the vowels in "bat" and "bath", "could" and "come" or "shoot" and "shook". Except in respect of list length the lists are similar in design to the N.U. auditory test No. 4 of Tillman and others[5].

Test Method

The author prefers to present the word lists from a tape recording via an attenuator and headset. Among other things this permits the measurement of discrimination scores at very low intensities without the need for a two-room arrangement, an advantage for anyone wishing to carry out the test in makeshift clinical surroundings.

On the tape recording the words occur at regular five-second intervals without an introductory phrase. The absence of such a phrase has not been found to be a disadvantage, and it is quite possible that the rhythmic occurrence of the words partly replaces the normal function of an introductory phrase.

Subjects are asked to repeat what they hear and are scored on the percentage of phonemes correctly repeated. In establishing the discrimination curve it is usually sufficient to make discrimination measurements at 10 dB intervals though 5 dB intervals may be used for greater precision. A reasonable minimum aim is to obtain three scores on the slope of the discrimination curve and three scores on the plateau, a procedure which takes just under six minutes of testing time.

Table 1. Test lists utilized during the preliminary phase.

Age in years	Mean phoneme score in percent	Sample standard deviation	No. in sample
9	97.8	2.7	10
5 and 6	92.4	4.7	15

Norms

Normal Discrimination Curve

The normal discrimination curve obtained with the test and method described above is shown in Fig. 1. The measurements used for producing this curve were carried out with a group of children attending a normal school in the Manchester area. Ten of the children were nine years old and 15 were five or six years old. Twenty decibels was the model value of discrimination threshold (the intensity giving a 50% phoneme score) and individual results were corrected to this value in order to calculate the mean scores on which the curve is based. The maximum gradient of the curve is 4% per decibel.

Age was not found to be a factor influencing discrimination threshold, but it had a significant effect on the maximum discrimination score, as shown in Table 1.

Although this curve was established with normally hearing children, subsequent use with adults has shown no marked variations. The chief difference to be expected would be an increased gradient due to the greater redundancy of the test material when used with adults.

Reliability of Near Threshold Discrimination Scores

Short-term test-retest reliability was assessed by testing the normally hearing sample with ten consecutive lists at a near threshold intensity. The standard deviations of repeated scores were 10.1 percentage points for phoneme scores and 15.3 percentage points for word scores. However, an analysis of variance showed significant differences between lists, and when this was allowed for, the standard deviations fell to 9.3 and 13.7 percentage points respectively.

Thus, without allowing for inter list differences, the 95% confidence limits of a single near threshold, phoneme discrimination measurement are + 20% (approx.). This appears at first sight to be a wide margin of uncertainty, but since the gradient of the normal discrimination curve is four percent per decibel, an error of 20% in discrimination represents an error of only 5 dB in threshold. In addition, a single score would not be used for determining discrimination threshold. It was suggested earlier that a minimum of three scores should be obtained on the sloping part of the discrimination curve. This should reduce the uncertainty in threshold by a factor of 1.73 (the square root of 3). In other words, use of the test as described permits the measurement of discrimination threshold to within + 3 dB, these being the 95% confidence limits.

It can also be shown from the above results that to obtain the same precision with word scoring requires list length to be increased by a factor of 2.3. In other words, for near threshold discrimination measurements a 10-word list, scored by phonemes, gives the same precision as a 23-word list scored by words. This conclusion strictly applies only to this particular test.

Reliability and Sampling Theory

It is interesting to compare the measured standard deviations of test scores with those predicted from random sampling theory. The equations used are given in Appendix II, and the comparisons between the individual measured standard deviations and those predicted from these equations are shown in Fig. 2. The agree-

Table II. Mean scores of lists 1 to 10 heard at a constant, near-threshold intensity

List No.	1	2	3	4	5	6	7	8	9	10	Grand Mean
Mean phoneme score (%)	68.5	68.7	66.9	64.7	67.6	69.7	58.1	69.1	59.9	59.9	65.1
Difference from grand mean (%)	1.4	3.6	1.8	−0.4	2.5	4.6	−7.0	4.0	−5.2	−5.2	—
Mean word score (%)	42.8	44.4	38.4	38.8	38.4	40.8	31.6	40.8	26.8	22.8	36.6
Difference from grand mean (5)	6.2	7.8	1.8	2.2	1.8	4.2	−5.0	4.2	−9.8	−13.8	—

ment is very good and gives support to the hypothesis that the reduced variability of phoneme scores is a function of increased sample size.

This procedure is open to the objection that the lists are not random samples of phonemes since each list must contain the same phonemes. However, the exact acoustical properties of a speech sound depend on its relation to the rest of the word and it would appear that the repeated rearrangement of phonemes leads effectively to random sampling. If the same lists were used repeatedly the sampling would no longer be random and the variability of scores would be considerably reduced.

Inter List Differences

Although statistically significant, the inter list differences were not large, being of the same order of magnitude as the variability of a single subject's scores. Since the analysis of variance showed that removal of inter list differences would have only a small effect on the reliability of discrimination scores it was not felt at this stage to be a worthwhile procedure. The mean scores obtained with lists one to ten are shown in Table 2, and it will be noticed that the use of phoneme scoring reduced the magnitude of these differences. Whether these differences are inherent in the lists or are a function of the tape recording has not, as yet, been investigated.

Reliability of Maximum Discrimination Scores with the Partially Hearing

A group of partially hearing children were given repeated discrimination tests at intensities giving maximum discrimination. The standard deviations of repeated discrimination scores were a little less than those of the near-threshold measurements with the normally hearing, but were still in approximate agreement with the predictions of sampling theory. The reduction of variability may be attributed to the differential effect of the hearing losses on the recognition of various phonemes. Thus if a patient consistently fails to recognize a particular sound regardless of its position in different words, this sound cannot contribute to variability of test scores.

Validity

As was stated earlier, the language ability of a subject has an influence on his discrimination score when measured with meaningful monosyllabic words. It is

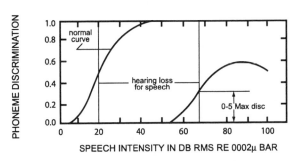

Figure 3. Showing the method used by the author for measuring hearing loss from a discrimination curve

pertinent, however, to inquire about the magnitude of this influence. If language factors are removed from a test score of 50% will it fall to 50% or to 10%? The following results indicate that the influence of language factors on phoneme scores is small compared with their influence on word scores:

(i) Fourteen of the words used in the test were unknown by five or more of the nine-year-old children. The mean near threshold phoneme score for these words was 54% as compared with 65% for the complete test. The mean, near-threshold word score was 20%, as compared with 37% for the complete test.

(ii) A statistical theory has been developed by the author which, by making certain assumptions, permits real discrimination scores to be obtained if each sound had to be determined on the basis of its intrinsic acoustical properties. This theory has been applied to the discrimination measurements described above, and the results, which have been reported elsewhere[6], indicate that the phoneme score gives a more valid measure of the ability to make phonemic classifications on the basis of acoustical information than does the word score.

(iii) Stitt[7] has compared the near-threshold scores obtained by children and adults when listening to nonsense and meaningful monosyllables. Her results show clearly that the change from nonsense words to meaningful words has a greater effect on word score than on phonemic score.

Examples of Clinical Applications

Measurement of Hearing Loss

In addition to the information it provides about supra-threshold hearing ability, the discrimination curve, when compared with the pure tone audiogram

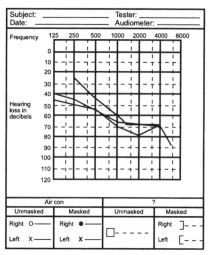

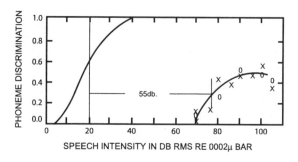

Figure 4. An example of correlation between speech and pure tone measures of hearing loss

increases the confidence with which audiological diagnosis can be made. For example the extent of a hearing loss may be measured as the shift of discrimination threshold from its normal value.

In order that this quantity shall remain meaningful for patients with severe discrimination losses, it has been found useful to define discrimination threshold as the intensity at which a subject scores 50% of his maximum. For example, if a subject has a maximum discrimination of 60%, his discrimination threshold is the intensity at which he scores 30%. This is illustrated in Fig 3.

The hearing loss measured in this way should be within 15 dB of the pure tone hearing loss measured at 1 kHz, providing the subject has a reasonably "flat" pure tone audiogram. See for example Fig. 4. When the hearing loss decreases at higher frequencies the hearing loss given by the discrimination curve is generally closer to the pure tone loss at 2 or 4 kHz. With a steeply falling pure tone audiogram the two measures of hearing loss seldom agree, but the slope of the discrimination curve for such cases is reduced, as shown in Fig. 5. Subjects with a high frequency plateau in their pure tone audiograms frequently have "two stage" discrimination curves of the type shown in Fig. 6. Filtering experiments with

the partially hearing have shown that this is due to the differential sensitivity for high and low frequencies.

Lack of correlation between the hearing losses as measured by pure tone and speech audiometry occurs with disturbingly high frequency among children and can often be traced to a failure to respond appropriately to the pure tone stimulus. Sometimes the discrimination curve shows a patient to have no hearing loss at all, and at other times an apparently mixed hearing loss is found to be purely conductive in nature. An example of the latter is shown in Fig. 7. In the author's experience this phenomenon has always been associated with either emotional disturbance, brain injury, or a history of middle ear disorders. It is quite different from malingering in that there is no attempt on the part of the patient to falsify the speech results, and it may be associated with the low arousal value of pure tones. It is true that the astute clinician is usually aware when a pure tone audiogram fails to correlate with a patient's apparent communication ability. However, unless some alternative measure of hearing loss is made, he is then left simply with a pure tone audiogram which he knows to be invalid. It is also true that some children may never see an astute clinician. It is not unknown for normally

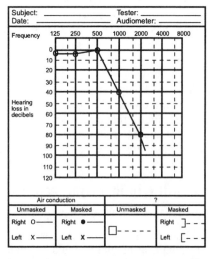

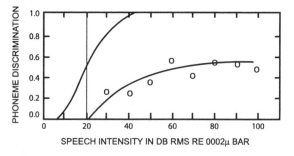

Figure 5. Showing the reduced gradient of the discrimination curve when a patient has a steeply falling pure tone audiogram

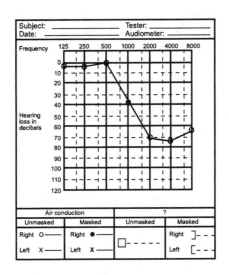
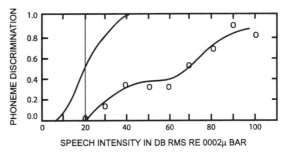

Figure 6. The "two stage" discrimination curve of a patient with a high frequency plateau in his pure tone audiogram

hearing children to be fitted with hearing aids on the basis of invalid pure tone audiograms.

All the comments made above apply equally well to the speech reception threshold as measured with spondaic words, and, of course, the relation between pure tone hearing loss and speech reception threshold has been thoroughly investigated[9]. It is, however, useful and time saving, to determine hearing loss and maximum discrimination with the same test.

Potential Value of Amplification

The discrimination curve can be used to determine the intensity required for maximum discrimination. If this intensity is above the levels of normal conversational speech, this is a good indicator of the potential value of amplification. Adding 10 dB to the intensity required for maximum discrimination gives an estimate of the maximum output required from a hearing aid. It is also possible to see when discrimination falls at high intensity and thus avoid over amplification.

It is wrong to assume that a discrimination curve such as that of Fig. 5, which does not rise beyond the intensity levels of normal conversational speech, contraindicates the value of amplification. This could be due to the lack of experience of higher intensity levels and does not automatically imply an inability to learn the use of the additional clues provided by amplification. This comment applies mainly to cases with high frequency hearing losses.

Hearing Aid Evaluation

By replaying the word lists through a loudspeaker (or hearing aid test box) and permitting a patient to listen through a hearing aid it is possible to plot an aided discrimination curve. This may be compared with the curve obtained when using the headphones. In addition to confirming that the aid provides adequate discrimination it is possible to ensure that it has sufficient gain to give maximum discrimination score with speech inputs at normal conversation levels.

It is assuming too much to make fine distinctions between hearing aids on the basis of this type of test, as there are too many important factors not accounted for. However, it does permit one to discard certain undesirable instruments.

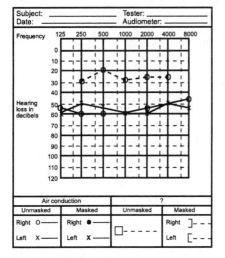
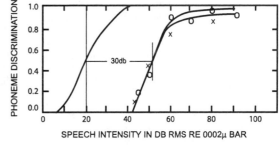

Figure 7. Lack of correlation between pure tone audiogram and discrimination curve implying that the patient has only a conductive loss of hearing

Conclusions

There are several problems associated with the measurement of speech discrimination which the test described above does nothing to solve. Examples are the influence of the individual characteristics of the person making the test recordings, variations in the judgment of the tester, and the interference of speech defects with test scores. However, providing these limitations are recognized and due allowance made for the limited precision of speech discrimination measurements, the use of short word lists and phonemic scoring permits the clinician to obtain much useful information in a relatively short time.

Acknowledgements

Thanks are due to Professor Taylor of the Department of Audiology and Education of the Deaf, Manchester University, for providing the clinical and research facilities without which the discrimination test would not have been developed, and to the various school authorities, staff and children who cooperated in the standardization tests. The contribution of Professor J. J. Groen has already been mentioned and is gratefully acknowledged.

Summary

A speech discrimination test is described, which uses short, isophonemic word lists. With these lists a discrimination measurement occupies one minute of testing time, and it is therefore possible to plot complete discrimination curves and to calculate confidence limits. Scoring is based on the number of correctly recognized phonemes. This increases the reliability of discrimination measurements, and also reduces the influence of language factors on test scores. Norms are given for children, together with the results of repeatability tests and examples of clinical applications.

References

Carhart, R. (1965). Problems in the measurement of Speech Discrimination, Archives of Otolaryngology, 82, 253-260.

Hirsh, I.J. (1964). Clinical audiometry and the perception of speech and language, Rev. de Laryngol. Otol. Rhinnl., 85, 453-464.

Lafon, J.C., Morgan, A., Gauthier, J. (1965). L'intervalle de confiance des mesure audiometriques vocales', Int. Audiol., 4, 94-96.

Groen, J.J., Hellema, A., C. (1960). Binaural speech audiometry, Acta. Oto., 52, 397-414.

Tillman, T.W., Carhart, R., Wilber, L. (1963). A test for speech discrimination composed of CNC monosyllabic words, report No. SAM-TDR-62-135 USAF, Brooks Air Force Base.

Boothroyd, A. (1967). Theoretical aspects of auditory training, Proceedings of the International Conference on Oral Education of the Deaf, 705-729.

Stitt, E. (1967). The significance of transition probabilities, Diploma Dissertation, Manchester University (Unpublished).

Boothroyd, A. (1967). The discrimination by partially hearing children of frequency distorted speech, Int. Audiol. 6, 136-145.

Carhart, R. (1964). Speech reception in relation to pattern of pure tone loss, J. Speech Dis., 11, 97-108.

Appendix I

Short Isophonemic Word Lists

1.	2.	3.	4.	5.
ship	fish	thud	fun	fib
rug	duck	witch	will	thatch
fan	gap	wrap	vat	sum
cheek	cheese	jail	shape	heel
haze	rail	keys	wreath	wide
dice	hive	vice	hide	rake
both	bone	get	guess	goes
well	wedge	shown	comb	shop
move	tooth	bomb	job	June

6.	7.	8.	9.	10.
fill	badge	bath	hush	jug
catch	hutch	hum	gas	match
thumb	kill	dip	thin	whip
heap	thighs	five	fake	faith
wise	wave	ways	chime	sign
rave	reap	reach	weave	bees
goat	foam	joke	jet	hell
shone	goose	noose	rob	rod
bed	not	got	dope	vote
juice	shed	shell	lose	shook

11.	12.	13.	14.	15.
man	have	kiss	wish	hug
hip	whiz	buzz	dutch	dish
thug	buff	hash	jam	ban
ride	mice	thieves	heath	rage
siege	teeth	gate	laze	chief
veil	gauge	wife	bike	pies
chose	poach	pole	rove	wet
shoot	rule	wretch	pet	cove
web	den	dodge	fog	loose
cough	cosh	moon	soon	moth

Appendix II

Random Sampling Theory

If the probability of success in a single trial is p, the mean number of successes in a series of n trials is equal to np, with a standard deviation of (np(1-p)) fi.

Considering a success as the recognition of a phoneme and a word list as 30 trials, the expected standard deviation of repeated discrimination measurements will be given by:

{30p(1-p)} fi where p is the phoneme discrimination.

in percentage points this will be

100{p(1-p)/30} fi.

For example for a phoneme discrimination score of 50% or 0.5, the expected standard deviation scores will be

{(0.5 x 0.5)/30} fi which equals

0.091 or 9.1%.

Similarly, the expected standard deviation of word scores is given by

100 {w(1-w)/10} fi percentage points, where w is the word discrimination.

A Picture Identification Test for Hearing-Impaired Children

Mark Ross and Jay Lerman
University of Connecticut, Storrs, Connecticut

A picture identification test for measuring speech discrimination ability in hearing-impaired children was developed in two phases. In the first phase the word stimuli were evaluated to determine whether they were within the recognition vocabulary of the children and whether the pictorial representations of the words were adequate. Before the second phase, the test was revised to consist of 25 plates with 6 pictures on each plate, with only 4 of the pictures on each plate used as test stimuli. These 4 lists were given to 61 hearing-impaired children on two separate occasions. The results indicate reliability coefficients in excess of 0.87 for all four lists, with mean differences of less than 3% and correlation coefficients between lists greater than 0.84. The test appears to be a potentially valuable clinical tool in pediatric audiology. We call it the Word Intelligibility by Picture Identification test (WIPI).

One of the unmet needs of pediatric audiology is a test which can be used to assess the speech discrimination ability of hearing-impaired children. It is not possible to use conventional speech discrimination tests with these children for several reasons: (1) because of the children's probable retardation in language development, the test words are unfamiliar and thus the task cannot be considered one of auditory discrimination; (2) children with a long-standing or congenital hearing loss usually exhibit articulatory problems which frequently make their oral response to a word unintelligible to the examiner; and (3) because of their ages, written responses are not feasible. Thus it has been the unfamiliarity of the stimuli and the inability to make suitable responses which have prevented the development of a speech discrimination test with young hearing-impaired children. In order to construct a workable speech discrimination test for use with these children, stimuli have to be selected which are within their recognition vocabulary, and the response must require neither speech nor writing.

The response criterion can be met with a picture identification task. In such a task the child simply points to one of several pictures upon hearing the associated word, instead of repeating or writing the word. The major difficulty in devising such a test has centered around the selection of a sufficient number of stimulus words. The hallmark of this population is retarded and/or deviant language development and it is no easy task to find words which can be recognized by this population and also be adequately portrayed pictorially. The inclusion of any stimulus item has to be considered tentative until its suitability for a hearing-impaired population is confirmed by direct investigation. If the probability of chance selections is to be reduced, a sufficient number of appropriate stimuli should be included on each picture matrix from which the child makes a selection; and if the test is to provide a range of auditory discrimination difficulty, then an adequate number of matrices must be developed.

Although there have been many previous attempts to develop a useful test (Dale, 1962, p. 33), these difficulties are no doubt responsible for the fact that to date there is no widely accepted picture identification speech discrimination test for use with young hearing-impaired children.

The test developed by Siegenthaler and Haspiel (1966) represents the most recent of these attempts. Their test, Discrimination by Identification of Pictures (DIP), consists of 48 cards with 2 pictures on each card. The test was administered to 295 normal-hearing children, ages 3 to 8, at sensation levels of 0, 5, and 10 dB. Three test lists were constructed from the two-picture matrix. Reliabilities of the three test lists at the three sensation levels ranged from 0.36 to 0.50, with an error of measurement of five items (approximately 10%). Chance selections would produce a 50% score since only two choices are involved in any one matrix. An interesting feature of this test is the selection of test words based on contrasting acoustic dimensions rather than on a phonetic balance (PB) concept. In a follow-up study these authors administered the test to a large number of young hearing-impaired children with satisfactory reliability coefficients (0.60 to 0.84), recognition of the stimulus words, and articulation-gain function.

Our own attempt to develop a suitable test dates from 1965, when we revised a test which had been developed with normal-hearing and mentally retarded children (Myatt and Landes, 1963), and administered it to a group of hearing-impaired children. Our results (Lerman, Ross, and McLauchlin, 1965) indicated that the test could be a

Reprinted by permission of authors and American Speech-Language-Hearing Association. Copyright 1970. *Journal of Speech and Hearing Research*, 13, pp. 44-53.

useful clinical tool, but also that revisions would be necessary before its maximum potential could be realized. Specifically, we found that some of the words were too difficult, some of the pictures were poor representations of the words, and chance scores were too high in a four-picture matrix. The study reported here represents a revision and extension of this previous study, with the goal of developing a clinically useful picture-pointing speech discrimination test.

Preliminary Evaluation

Selection of Stimulus Words. Children's books and word-count lists were perused in order to select simple monosyllabic words which could be adequately represented pictorially. Questionable choices were shown to experienced kindergarten and nursery school teachers for their judgments regarding inclusion. The words on our previous test which had proved to be satisfactory were included whenever possible. The remaining words were then arranged in 26 sets of 6 words each, with some of the matrices arranged to present a gross discrimination task and others arranged to present a fine discrimination task. The limited number of suitable words which could be used with this population sometimes severely restricted the possible choices. On an a priori basis, each of the six 26-word lists were equalized to present the same number of difficult and easy discrimination tasks (Table 1).

Pictorial Representations. A commercial artist drew pictorial representations of each word after lengthy consultations with the authors. Pictures which were ambiguous, poorly drawn, or confusing in terms of foreground-background differentiation were redrawn. Six color pictures were placed on 8 ˘ 10 drawing paper and photographed. The 26 sets of 8 ˘ 10 glossy color photo reproductions were placed in a loose-leaf binder to form a test book.

Subjects. Fifteen hearing-impaired children were used as subjects during the preliminary stage of the study. The children ranged in age from 6 through 12, with 3 of the children 6 years old, 2 children 7 years old, 2 children 8 years old, 1 child 9 years old, 1 child 10 years old, 4 children 11 years old, and 2 children 12 years old. Twelve of the children had bilateral sensorineural hearing losses, while 3 had bilateral mixed or conductive hearing losses. Their loss in the test ear exceeded 30 dB (1964 ISO standard) at one of the speech frequencies. The test ear was selected arbitrarily, provided it met the above criterion. Where both ears met this criterion, the better ear was selected as the test ear.

Test Procedures. Air-conduction thresholds were determined at 250, 500, 1000, 2000, 4000, and 8000 Hz for both ears. Bone-conduction thresholds were obtained

in all cases which presented diagnostic questions (i.e. no consistent previous results). The two best of the three speech frequencies were averaged to obtain the pure-tone average (PTA). This figure was used in lieu of the speech reception threshold (SRT) as the base from which the sensation level was computed.

The six test lists were delivered by live voice through a calibrated GS162 speech audiometer by one examiner exclusively. The list order was rotated among the subjects, with subject one receiving lists one, two, three, four, five, and six in that order, while subject two received lists two, three, four, five, six, and one in that order, and so on. The lists were delivered at a sensation level of 40 dB re the PTA; limitations imposed by a child's uncomfortable loudness listening (UCL) level necessitated delivering the lists to seven of the children at a lower sensation level, which ranged from 20 to 36 dB. This level was maintained for all six of the lists. Each test word was preceded by either the carrier phrase "show me" or "point to." Testing was accomplished in a two-room sound-treated audiometric testing suite. The child was seated in the test room with his back to the examiner in the control room. A test assistant faced the child in the test room and was also in visual contact with the examiner. The test assistant turned the page after the child made a selection, and also attempted to maintain the child's interest in the task. Each child was given verbal and/or pantomime instructions for the test, by being told or shown to point to a picture as he heard a word through the earphones.

Scoring. For scoring, the six pictures were considered to be numbered from one to six, with number one at the upper left-hand corner and number six at the lower right-hand corner. As the examiner read a test word, he would check the appropriate column on his score sheet if the child selected the correct picture. If the child erred, the examiner would note the error by indicating the number of the incorrect choice. After delivering all 6 lists of 26 words each, the examiner entered the test room and faced the child. If the child had a hearing aid, he was asked to adjust it for normal listening. Then in a "moderately loud" voice the examiner would read each of the words from each of the lists the child had missed previously. If, in this "look and listen" situation, the child corrected his previous error, the examiner so noted it by checking an appropriate column on his score sheet. If the child still made an incorrect choice, the examiner noted the number of the error. After the "look and listen" stage had been completed, the examiner went through all the lists again, this time asking the child to name all the pictures which were missed on the previous occasions. If the child made a correct choice at this point, it was so noted. The purpose of this elaborate scoring procedure was to determine if the word used to name the picture was within the child's

Table 1. Test lists utilized during the preliminary phase.

A	B	C	D	E	F
bowl	bow	bell	boat	belt	ball
coat	coke	cone	comb	goat	smoke
horn	door	fork	house	floor	corn
clock	box	socks	blocks	rocks	fox
bath	bag	flag	hat	black	match
bat	cat	cap	glass	rat	grass
can	fan	man	hand	sand	pan
bed	head	sled	bread	red	thread
leg	neck	nest	egg	desk	dress
pear	hair	chair	bear	stair	ear
tie	fly	pie	eye	kite	pipe
tree	bee	key	knee	bean	tea
meat	feet	street	teeth	beet	leaf
king	ring	spring	swing	wing	string
moon	spoon	broom	school	boot	shoe
house	mouse	mouth	clown	crown	cow
shirt	church	girl	bird	skirt	dirt
duck	truck	thumb	gun	gum	sun
cup	rug	bug	bus	book	nut
plate	plane	train	snake	cake	lake
star	car	barn	arm	heart	farm
fish	dish	stick	milk	ink	chick
bib	lip	crib	ship	hill	pig
wheel	queen	sheep	green	seal	screen
wall	ball	straw	dog	frog	saw
pail	nail	mail	tail	jail	sail

recognition vocabulary. In addition, to determine if the picture was a good representation of the word, consistent confusions, the child's spontaneous comments, and the examiner's on-the-spot judgments were recorded.

Results. Most of the errors which the children made in the "listen" condition were corrected in either the "look and listen" or "naming" conditions. Only three of the children (two of them six years old) made more than two errors on any list after all the conditions were completed, and only three of the plates had two pictures which were consistently confused (i.e., stimulus word *egg* would elicit pointing response to picture of the *nest*; stimulus word *plate* elicited *cake*; and *farm* elicited *barn)*. Thus it appeared that in our task of constructing the final test version, we were able to consider most of the original stimuli for inclusion. We had very early decided not to be bound by the limitations imposed by the phonetic balance (PB) concept in the construction of our test lists, but rather to focus on the development of four reliable and comparable test lists which would be sensitive to different discrimination abilities of different individuals.

Each six-picture matrix was analyzed in conformance with our results and four pictures were selected as the final test stimuli. The other two pictures remained in the final matrix as additional foils, which served to increase the difficulty of the discrimination task from the subject's point of view. That is, upon hearing a word the subject would have to select the appropriate picture from a matrix of six rather than four pictures. To simplify scoring, one entire matrix of six pictures was omitted from the test. The result was twenty-five matrices in which four pictures in each matrix would be utilized as test stimuli. Only one of these four pictures was included in a particular test list, and thus we were able to construct four completely different test lists of twenty-five words each (Table 2). The equalization of the test lists was accomplished partly on the basis of our experience, partly on the basis of acoustic phonetic considerations (Liberman et al., 1967), and partly on an a priori basis. In the final evaluation phase our judgments underwent empirical verification.

Final Evaluation

Subjects. Sixty-one subjects, none of whom was used during the preliminary phase, were tested for the final evaluation phase of the project. Their ages ranged from 4 years, 7 months, to 13 years, 9 months, with a mean of 10 years, 2 months. The hearing level in the better ear for all subjects exceeded 30 dB (1964 ISO standard) at one or more of the speech frequencies. The better ear was used as the test ear in all cases except when the degree and configuration of the hearing loss were bilaterally similar; in these cases the test ear was selected arbitrarily. The average two-frequency PTA in the test ear was 52.2 dB, with a range from 5 to 90 dB. Fifty-eight of the

Table 2. Final 4 test lists of 25 words each.

I	II	III	IV
school	broom	moon	spoon
ball	bowl	bell	bow
smoke	coat	coke	goat
floor	door	corn	horn
fox	socks	box	blocks
hat	flag	bag	black
pan	fan	can	man
bread	red	thread	bed
neck	desk	nest	dress
stair	bear	chair	pear
eye	pie	fly	tie
knee	tea	key	bee
street	meat	feet	beet
wing	string	spring	ring
mouse	clown	crown	mouth
shirt	church	dirt	skirt
gun	thumb	sun	gum
bus	rug	cup	bug
train	cake	snake	plane
arm	barn	car	star
chick	stick	dish	fish
crib	ship	bib	lip
wheel	seal	queen	green
straw	dog	saw	frog
pail	nail	jail	tail

subjects had congenital sensorineural hearing losses and the remaining three had long-standing conductive or mixed hearing losses. Twenty-four were students enrolled in a school for the deaf. Their age range was 9 years, 5 months, to 13 years, 9 months, with a mean of 11 years 7 months.

Test Procedures. Air-conduction thresholds were obtained at 250, 500, 1000, 2000, 4000, and 8000 Hz for both ears. Bone-conduction thresholds were determined in all cases which presented diagnostic questions (i.e., no consistent previous results). All discrimination tests were administered live-voice by the same examiner at a 40 dB sensation level (SL) re the PTA. When the difference between the PTA and uncomfortable loudness level (UCL) was less than 40 dB, the test was delivered at a level 5 dB below the UCL. Four lists were administered to each subject. The order of presentation was rotated between lists. Testing arrangements were similar to those accomplished in the preliminary phase. The child was seated in the test room with his back to the examiner in the control room. A test assistant faced the child and also maintained visual contact with the examiner. The child was given verbal and/or pantomime instructions in the task. No practice list was given. Each word was preceded by the carrier phrase "show me." After the child's selection, the test assistant would name the picture pointed to by the child and turn the page in preparation for the next selection.

One to three weeks after the initial presentation, the subjects were recalled and the same four lists were read-ministered with the test order again rotated during this second testing session. The same examiner administered the lists at the same sensation level as on the previous occasion.

Results

Reliability. The test-retest reliability coefficient and the error of measurement of each of the four lists are shown in Table 3. The reliability coefficients range from 0.87 to 0.94, and the errors of measurement range from 4.7 to 7.7. These results indicate that all four lists of the test are highly reliable, with comparable reliabilities for all four lists.

Equivalence. The equivalence of the four lists was evaluated by assessing the mean differences and the correlations between lists. Table 4 shows the means and the standard deviations of the two presentations of each list (A and B) as well as the average means and standard deviations.

The differences between the A and B presentations indicate that a learning effect took place between the first and second presentation of each list. These differences were evaluated by a standard sign test (Ostle, 1963, pp. 471-472) and, except for list III, were significant beyond the 0.01 level. The learning effect for list III was significant at the 0.06 level. Since the order of presentation of the four lists was rotated and all four of the lists show the learning effect, this effect would still have been present even if a practice list had been utilized. In any event, the differences are no more than the equivalent of one extra word correct (4% per word) during the second presentation of each list and should not be clinically significant.

Table 4 also shows means and standard deviations of the four lists, with presentations A and B averaged. A comparison of the means and standard deviations of the four lists indicates that the average level and range of difficulty are comparable. The only significant mean difference was at the 0.05 level and occurred between lists III and IV. However, this difference of 2.8% is less than a one-word variation and, as in the learning effect, cannot be considered to be clinically significant.

Table 5 gives the Pearson product-moment correlation coefficients of the four lists (A and B presentations collapsed). They range from 0.84 to 0.95, with five of the six correlations being 0.92 or higher. Taken together with the negligible mean difference lists, these results indicate that the four lists are highly equivalent.

Relationships between the discrimination scores and the PTAs: Table 6 shows the Pearson product-moment correlation coefficients between the list scores and the

Table 3. Reliability and standard error of measurement of the four lists.

Lists	Reliability	Standard Error of Measurement
I	0.89	6.59
II	0.94	4.74
III	0.87	7.74
IV	0.88	7.61

Table 5. Intercorrelations between collapsed lists.

	II	III	IV
I	0.84	0.96	0.95
II	—	0.95	0.92
III	—	—	0.92

Table 6. Correlations between list scores and the two-frequency pure-tone averages.

I	II	III	IV
−0.65	−0.63	−0.64	−0.60

PTAs. These correlations range from 0.60 to 0.65, and they are negative, indicating the more severe the hearing loss the poorer the list scores. These results agree with similar findings obtained from testing adults with conventional speech discrimination lists (Ross et al., 1965).

Discussion

The purpose of the present study was to develop a picture identification test for the measurement of speech discrimination ability in hearing-impaired children. The results of the study indicate that we have been successful in developing a reliable test of four equivalent lists. The words used were within the recognition vocabulary of the subjects, and the pictures appear to be adequate representations of the words.

The study would have been strengthened if a larger number of younger hearing-impaired children had been utilized as subjects. However, the practical problems of securing this type of subject precluded this desirable goal. Considering our experiences with the children of varying ages and hearing losses who were utilized as subjects, it appears that the test is suitable for children with moderate hearing losses from ages five or six and for children with severe hearing losses from ages seven or eight. These age limitations include a large number of hearing-impaired children for whom conventional speech discrimination testing is not possible. We have little information which indicates whether the test can be successful with children younger than five years of age. Below this age, it should be used cautiously.

Speech discrimination scores obtained with the use of this test cannot be considered equivalent to the scores obtained with conventional speech discrimination lists, and cannot be interpreted in the same way. In the present test, the subject is confronted with a closed-set discrimination task with chance scores ranging around eighteen percent, while conventional discrimination lists present to the listener an open-ended discrimination task with chance scores that are essentially zero percent. In addition, an acoustic analysis of the type and proportion of perceptual clues presented to listeners with both types of tests would undoubtedly show significant differences, and therefore differences in the scores obtained by the listeners would also be expected. Based on theoretical expectations and the limited data we do have, discrimination scores obtained with the picture identification test should exceed conventional test scores by approximately 25%. A direct evaluation comparing scores obtained on the present test with scores obtained on different types of tests would be a useful project for a future investigator to undertake.

The design of the study did not permit the determination of articulation-gain functions. These data would permit a more complete description of the properties of the test, and it would be useful to obtain this information in future research. In using the test, however, it is still possible to run these functions with specific individuals in order to evaluate their optimal listening levels. Such information can be utilized, for example, in determining the gain level at which to set a hearing aid.

The test can be used in the same manner as conventional speech discrimination tests. Scores obtained with this test can be used to compare an individual's discrimination ability to scores obtained by a similar population.

Table 4. Means and standard deviations of forms A and B of each list.

Lists		Means	Standard Deviations	Average Means	Standard Deviations
I	A	74.89	19.00	76.36	19.93
	B	77.84	20.70		
II	A	74.75	19.16	77.11	19.10
	B	79.48	18.74		
III	A	74.49	21.38	75.67	21.86
	B	76.85	22.27		
IV	A	76.66	18.32	78.43	18.78
	B	80.20	19.06		

The relative difference in discrimination ability between a subject's two ears can be evaluated, as well as the relative difference between hearing aids and/or acoustical changes in the same hearing aid. The results of an auditory training program can be assessed by a longitudinal evaluation of the scores. In this respect the test has a sufficient number of simple discrimination tasks to permit the measurement of a base speech discrimination score among a population of children from a school for the deaf. With this kind of information a meaningful evaluation of auditory training programs in schools for the deaf can be accomplished. The test will undoubtedly be too easy for a large number of hearing-impaired children. These children, perhaps with conductive or minimal sensorineural type hearing losses, will consistently obtain scores at or close to 100% with the test. Since the test ceiling is too low for these children, differences in discrimination ability among them cannot be meaningfully evaluated. It is probable that most of the children who fall into these categories can be tested with conventional speech discrimination tests. Those who cannot, that is those who have good discrimination ability but still cannot give valid oral or written responses, are not suitable subjects for either the conventional or picture-pointing type of discrimination test. In order to test their discrimination ability, it would be desirable to develop new norms with the present test based on scores obtained when some type of noise is introduced into the listening situation.

Our experience with the test indicates that it is a simple and rapid test to administer, and that the children have little difficulty in comprehending the nature of the task. When a test assistant is unavailable, we have found that parents can quickly be taught to act as test assistants. In many instances, we have administered the test without a test assistant by having the child turn the page after he makes a choice.

Finally, in order to develop a distinguishable acronym for the test based on its function and the nature of the task involved, we propose to call the test the WIPI test.

Acknowledgment

This research was supported by Grant No. OEG-1-7-008038-0504 from the Office of Education, U.S. Department of Health, Education, and Welfare. We are grateful to Robert M. McLaughlin, James E. Peck, and staff members at the American School for the Deaf for their assistance during this study. Information regarding the availability of the WIPI test can be obtained from Stanwix House, Inc., 3020 Chartiers Avenue, Pittsburgh, Pennsylvania, 15204.

References

Dale, D.M.C., *Applied Audiology with Children.* Charles C. Thomas, Ill.: Springfield (1962).

Lerman, J.W., Ross, M., and McLaughlin, R.M., A picture-identification test for hearing-impaired children. *J. Aud. Res.,* 5, 273-278 (1965).

Liberman, A.M., Cooper, F.S., Shankweiler, D.P., and Studdert-Kennedy, M., Perception of the speech code. *Psychol. Rev.,* 74, 431-461 (1967).

Myatt, B.D., and Landes, B.A., Assessing discrimination loss in children. *Arch. Otolaryngol.,* 77, 359-362 (1963).

Ostle, B., *Statistics in Research.* Downstate Univ. Press (1963).

Ross, M., Huntington, D.A., Newby, H.A., and Dixon, R.F., Speech discrimination of hearing-impaired individuals in noise: its relationship to other audiometric parameters. *J. Aud. Res.,* 5, 47-72 (1965).

Siegenthaler, B.M., and Haspiel, G.M., *Development of Two Standardized Measures of Hearing for Speech by Children.* Pennsylvania State Univ. (1966).

Siegenthaler, B.M., and Haspiel, G.M., Evaluation of two measures of speech hearing for hearing-impaired children. Final Report, Project No. R6-1159, U.S. Dept. HEW, Off. Educ., Bureau of Research (1968).

Received January 2, 1969

Articulation Functions and Test-Retest Performance of Normal-Hearing Children on Three Speech Discrimination Tests: WIPI, PBK-50, and NU Auditory Test No. 6

Mary E. Sanderson-Leepa
Lansing School District, Michigan

William F. Rintelmann
University of Pennsylvania School of Medicine, Philadelphia

This study investigates the performance of normal-hearing children on three types of speech discrimination tasks: (1) a multiple-choice, closed-message set test requiring no verbal response, the WIPI; (2) an open-message set test constructed for use with children, the PBK - 50; and (3) a standardized, open set test for adults, Northwestern University Auditory Test No. 6 (NU-6). Versions of these tests tape-recorded by a single male talker were administered to 60 normal-hearing children, divided equally between the ages three-and-one-half, five-and-one-half, seven-and-one-half, nine-and-one-half, and 11-and-one-half years. The number of tests and sensation levels administered varied by age. The WIPI test yielded the highest discrimination scores, the PBK - 50 was intermediate, and the NU-6 was most difficult. A small number of items on the WIPI test accounted for a large percentage of the errors. For three-and-one-half year olds, the WIPI appears to be the instrument of choice. For children aged five-and-one-half years, both the WIPI and the PBK - 50 appear to be appropriate clinical tools. Children aged seven-and-one-half scored similar to children aged nine-and-one-half on the WIPI and to children aged nine-and-one-half and 11 and-one-half on the PBK -50 and NU-6. Test-retest differences were small on all three tests.

Young children represent a substantial portion of the population for whom audiological services are usually provided. In one university hearing clinic during a 10-week period, over one-third of the case load was 11 years of age or younger. Audiological methods that accurately assess the hearing of children in this age-group have long been sought.

Standardization of tests of speech discrimination on populations of normal-hearing children has received little attention. In fact, one of the most commonly used speech discrimination tests for children, the Phonetically Balanced Kindergarten Word Lists (PBK-50), was developed by Haskins (1949) using normal-hearing adults. Haskins's goal was to construct a test which would be useful for measuring discrimination ability of not only hearing-impaired children, but also adults with limited language background. Also, the Word Intelligibility by Picture Identification (WIPI) test was constructed by Ross and Lerman (1970) for assessing speech discrimination ability of hearing-impaired children. Therefore, they employed hard- of-hearing children as subjects in the development of the WIPI test.

As a consequence, there is need for normative data on tests commonly employed for assessing discrimination ability of both normal-hearing and hearing-impaired children. Fortunately, a few studies have been conducted using normal-hearing children as subjects. Siegenthaler and Haspiel (1966) administered the Discrimination by Identification of Pictures (DIP) to young normal-hearing children; Schwartz (1971) employed two lists of the WIPI to test preschool normal-hearing children; and Hodgson (1973) compared the performance of normal-hearing children in two age-groups on the WIPI, a closed-message set test, and with the PBK-50, an open-message set test. The WIPI was also given as an open set test. All three tests were given at a single intensity level, 70 dB SPL. Hodgson found that the children in both age-groups attained significantly higher scores when the WIPI was given as a picture test, compared to the other two conditions (open-message set).

In order to establish clinically useful data on speech discrimination tests for children, articulation functions should be generated for each of the tests and test-retest comparisons should be made. Further, there is need to obtain data on children using adult discrimination tests such as the Northwestern University Auditory Test Number Six (NU-6) to determine the lowest chronological age for its appropriate use. Finally, it is important to establish how children ranging from preschool through school age respond to various types of speech discrimination tests. In other words, what is the relationship of different types of speech discrimination tests when administered to the same sample of subjects?

For audiologists attempting to determine the speech discrimination ability of a young child, three types of materials are currently available: (1) multiple-choice discrimination tests requiring no verbal response on the part of the child, (2) conventional discrimination tests which have been modified for use with children, and (3) standardized discrimination tests for adults. The purpose of this study was to investigate the performance of a group of preschool through school-age normal-hearing children on one test representative of each of these three types of materials. The goal of the investigation was to provide data to assist clinicians in selecting a test(s) appropriate for a particular age-group(s). The particular tests chosen were the Word Intelligibility by Picture Identification test (WIPI), the Phonetically Balanced Kindergarten Word Lists (PBK-50), and the Northwestern University Auditory Test No. 6 (NU-6). The three tests were given at several sensation levels so that articulation functions could be generated, and test-retest measures were obtained.

In spite of the large number of studies reported in the literature concerning speech discrimination testing, to date evidence does not exist to demonstrate that particular speech discrimination tests are superior to others in either assessing normal discrimination ability or in measuring the everyday significance of hearing impairment. The selection of the three specific tests we chose to investigate was essentially based on our empirical judgment of their clinical and research utility. As stated earlier, such comparative information should be clinically useful.

Method

Subjects

The subjects were 60 normal-hearing children, 12 from each of the following age-groups: three-and-one-half, five-and-one-half, seven-and-one-half, nine-and-one-half, and 11 and-one-half years. These ages were chosen to represent age levels of clients frequently tested in hearing clinics and for whom little normative speech discrimination data has been established. All children were within three months of the age level of the group they represented. Twenty-six of the subjects were male and 34 were female. Each subject was judged by one of the investigators to have speech within normal limits for his age-group.

Instrumentation

Equipment for sound-field speech testing included a speech audiometer (Grason-Stadler, Model 162) that amplified and attenuated the electrical output of a tape recorder (Ampex, Model 500) used to present the stimulus items. The output of the speech audiometer drove a loudspeaker (Grason-Stadler, Model 162-400). All testing was conducted in a prefabricated double-walled IAC test room, with the subject seated at a zero degree angle of incidence from the loudspeaker. The ambient noise level in the test room was sufficiently low, 42 dBC, so as not to interfere with the test results.

The speech audiometer was calibrated so that audiometric zero was 13 dB above 0.0002 dynes/cm≈. "Speech noise" was used for calibration, in the manner described by Tillman, Johnson, and Olsen (1966), who reported that the spectral configuration of "speech noise" is closer to the spectrum of speech produced by male speakers than is a 1000-Hz tone.

Calibration of the loudspeaker was accomplished by placing the condenser microphone (Bruel and Kjaer, Type 4131) four feet from the face of the loudspeaker at a height of 42 inches. The condenser microphone was positioned so that its diaphragm was perpendicular to the floor and ceiling of the test chamber at a zero degree angle of incidence from the loudspeaker. The intensity of the speech spectrum noise generated by the speech audiometer at a 60-dB attenuator setting was then recorded. All measurements were made without the presence of an observer in the field; however, the location of the condenser microphone was approximately where the center of the subject's head would be when he was seated in the test chamber. A piston-phone (Bruel and Kjaer, Type 4220) was used to set the meter needle of the audio frequency spectrometer (Bruel and Kjaer, Model 2112) from which the intensity of the sound field was read directly in decibels re 0.0002 dynes/cm≈. Measurements of the overall SPL of the speech noise were made on all days that subjects were tested, and adjustments made so that the readings were within ±1 dB of 13 dB re 0.0002 dynes/cm≈. Attenuator linearity was also checked throughout the experiment.

Speech Stimulus Materials

The WIPI was selected to represent the multiple-choice type of picture discrimination test (Myatt and Landes, 1963; Lerman, Ross, and McLauchlin, 1965; Ross and Lerman, 1970). The WIPI is composed of four lists of 25 monosyllabic words. Each page of this test contains six pictures. One word from each of the four lists is represented, together with two additional pictures which are not stimulus items but act as foils.

The PBK-50 test represents conventional discrimination tests modified for use with children. Haskins (1949) constructed this test in an attempt to simplify, yet maintain the design of the PB-50 lists. Originally, the test was composed of four lists; however, using normal-hearing adults as subjects, Haskins found List 2 to be easier than the other lists. Subsequently, List 2 was deleted, and what were formerly Lists 3 and 4 are referred to as Lists 2 and 3.

The NU-6, composed of four phonemically equivalent consonant-nucleus-consonant (CNC) lists, represents the third type of test, namely, standardized CNC monosyllabic discrimination tests for adults (Lehiste and Peterson, 1959; Peterson and Lehiste, 1962; Tillman, Carhart, and Wilber, 1963; Tillman and Carhart, 1966; Rintelmann and Associates, 1974).

All stimulus materials were recorded in our laboratory by the same experienced male speaker with a General American dialect. Using a microphone (Electrovoice 635A), the speaker monitored his vocal intensity to 0 dB on a VU meter. During the recording of the Utley Children's Spondees (1951), both syllables of the stimulus words were monitored. For the PBK-50 and NU-6 the final word of the carrier phrase "You will say _____" was monitored with the test item allowed to fall naturally. The monitored carrier phrase for the WIPI test was "Show me _____" with the stimulus item again permitted to follow naturally. The initial recordings were made on a tape recorder (Ampex, Model AG 500) with the speaker in a single-walled, sound-treated booth (IAC, Series 400). The tapes of these recordings were balanced utilizing a level recorder (Bruel and Kjaer, Model 2305) and dubbed onto another tape. The output of the spondee words and the last word of each carrier phrase were equated to within ±2 dB of the level of a 1000-Hz calibration tone spliced to the beginning of each tape. Two Ampex tape recorders (Models AG 500 and 602) were used for this purpose. An additional form of all lists was created by copying the original tape and splicing the words into a different scrambling in an order determined by a table of random numbers.

Procedure

Initially, a pure-tone air-conduction screening test was administered to every subject at a 20-dB hearing level re ANSI, 1969. Speech audiometric tests were administered to each subject on either two or three separate days depending upon the number of tests given according to age-group (see Table 1). At the beginning of each test session a sound-field speech reception threshold

(SRT) was obtained (via a taped version of the Utley Children's Spondee List, 1951) and was used as the basis for administering the speech discrimination tests in that session.

In determining the articulation function for each of the three speech discrimination tests, each successive presentation was given at a higher intensity, with a different list of the test given at each sensation level re SRT. Because of the age range of the subgroups tested, the number of tests and sensation levels employed varied by age-group. For all subjects discrimination tests were followed by a retest, approximately 10 minutes after the test session. For the retest, the alternate randomization of the same list of words was presented at each sensation level. The specific sensation levels used as well as the tests administered to each age-group are indicated in Table 1. The decision to limit the number of sensation levels tested for the younger children was based on the necessity of maintaining interest in the task and minimizing fatigue. The order of test administration as well as the order of list presentation within each test was rotated.

Results

WIPI

Table 2 displays the data obtained on the WIPI test for the subjects during the test and retest sessions. In this table the means and standard deviations are indicated for each age-group at every sensation level (SL) in the test and retest.

Table 2 reports that the differences in the mean number of items correct between adjacent age-groups were small, with an improvement in scores positively related to age. Two-way analysis of variance indicated that the main

Table 1. Sensation levels at which children of each age-group were administered the WIPI, PBK-50, and NU-6 speech discrimination tests.

Age	Test	Sensation Level 8	16	24	32
3½	WIPI	—	x	x	x
	PBK-50	—	—	—	x
5½	WIPI	x	x	x	x
	PBK-50	—	x	x	x
7½	WIPI	x	x	x	x
	PBK-50	—	x	x	x
	NU-6	x	x	x	x
9½	WIPI	x	x	x	x
	PBK-50	—	x	x	x
	NU-6	x	x	x	x
11½	PBK-50	—	x	x	x
	NU-6	x	x	x	x

effect associated with sensation level was statistically significant ($p < 0.01$) but the main effect for age was not significant ($p > 0.01$). The three-and-one-half year olds were not tested at the 8-dB sensation level and therefore were excluded from this analysis.

The Tukey post hoc method of multiple comparisons was used to test the significance of individual treatment means for sensation level. The mean percentage of correct responses made at the 8-dB sensation level was significantly lower than the mean percentages of correct responses made at the three higher sensation levels ($p \leq 0.05$). No other paired contrasts of means on sensation level were significant ($p > 0.05$). In the separate analysis of data for the three-and-one-half-year-old group, however, a change in sensation level from 16 to 24 dB demonstrated a marked improvement (9.6%) in discrimination score.

Further examination of Table 2 reveals that the variability of scores, as exhibited by the standard deviations, decreased rather systematically with higher sensation levels. At a given sensation level, variability appears to bear an inverse relationship to the age of the subjects, although it is quite similar between adjacent age-groups except between the three-and-one-half- and five-and-one-half-year-old age levels where the greatest difference in variability occurred.

Differences between the mean scores of the subjects from test to retest were small. They differed by more than

one item only at the 8-dB sensation level of the five-and-one-half-year-old age-group. This is in essential agreement with Ross and Lerman (1970), who found WIPI test-retest scores among hearing-impaired children to differ by no more than the equivalent of one word, or 4%.

The WIPI test appears to have gained widespread clinical and research use for testing both normal-hearing and hearing-impaired children. Hence, as part of our investigation of the WIPI, we decided that an item analysis for each of the four lists would be useful clinical information especially for testing preschool-age children. A similar item analysis was not accomplished for the PBK-50 and NU-6 tests. Simply for the sake of brevity, the detailed item analysis was restricted to the single test (WIPI) from among the three we investigated which appears most appropriate for testing the youngest children in our sample. The results reported below for each of the three tests support our rationale for choosing the WIPI for this item analysis. These data are presented in Tables 3, 4, and 5.

Table 3 displays the mean percentage of items correct and the standard deviation for each WIPI list, with all sensation levels combined, for the test session. Each age-group is shown separately. The mean scores were highly similar from list to list, at all age levels. The maximum difference in mean scores between lists was between List 2 and List 4 among three-and-one-half-year-old subjects (2.7 items, or 10.7%). In no other age-group did the mean scores between test lists differ by more than one item, or 4%. This generally substantiates the findings of Ross and Lerman (1970) who reported mean list differences to be less than one word among hearing-impaired children.

Table 4 exhibits the range of difficulty of items on the WIPI test with all lists combined. Only errors from the first test session were included. It can be observed from Table 4 that 21 of the 100 items of the WIPI test were not missed by any subject at any sensation level. Twenty-four words were missed only once. Therefore, the easiest 45 words of the WIPI test accounted for only 7% of the total errors made; further, 60 words were responsible for only 17% of the total test errors. Of the more difficult words, four items of the 100-word WIPI test were responsible for almost 20% of the total test errors.

Table 5 displays the number of times each individual word in the four WIPI lists was missed. The total pool of each list is divided into subgroups on the basis of the number of times the words were missed. This table indicates that the three most difficult words of List 1 (*pan, fox, bread*) accounted for 41% of the total number of errors made by all subjects on this 25-item word list. When the two next most difficult words of the list (*knee, pail*) are included, 56% of the total number of errors of the list are accounted for. Of the easiest items, 10 of the

Table 2. Means and standard deviations in percent correct of 12 normal-hearing children from each of the age-groups 3½, 5½, 7½, and 9½ years on the WIPI as a function of sensation level (SL) during the test and retest sessions. Dash indicates not tested at this sensation level.

Age	SL in dB	Mean		Standard Deviation	
		Test	Retest	Test	Retest
3½	8	—	—	—	—
	16	78.7	—	10.14	—
	24	88.3	87.7	10.85	12.58
	32	91.7	—	6.26	—
5½	8	83.0	87.7	8.20	11.37
	16	94.0	95.7	7.91	5.25
	24	95.7	95.3	3.17	7.20
	32	97.3	98.3	2.16	3.17
7½	8	89.3	90.3	8.56	8.44
	16	95.3	97.3	4.56	1.97
	24	97.3	98.7	2.61	2.61
	32	98.7	99.0	2.61	2.49
9½	8	89.3	90.3	7.88	5.25
	16	96.3	97.3	3.17	2.61
	24	98.7	99.0	1.97	1.81
	32	99.0	99.3	1.80	1.56

Table 3. Mean percentage of items correct and standard deviation of each WIPI list for the test session (sensation levels combined) for children aged 3½, 5½, 7½, and 9½ years.

Age	List	Mean %	Standard Deviation
3½	1	90.2	6.64
	2	91.1	7.96
	3	83.1	12.92
	4	80.4	11.20
5½	1	93.7	7.52
	2	93.7	6.32
	3	93.7	7.52
	4	90.0	11.00
7½	1	96.3	5.24
	2	93.3	6.64
	3	96.6	7.96
	4	94.3	4.32
9½	1	95.3	8.16
	2	95.7	3.60
	3	96.3	5.24
	4	96.0	6.16

Table 4. Range of difficulty of words on the WIPI test, all lists combined.

Number of Words	Number of Times Each Word Was Missed	Column 1 × Column 2	Accumulative %age of Errors (Easy to Difficult)
21	0	0	—
24	1	24	0.07
15	2	30	0.17
8	3	24	0.24
8	4	32	0.34
5	5	25	0.42
3	6	18	0.48
7	7	49	0.63
3	8	24	0.70
2	10	20	0.76
1	14	14	0.81
1	19	19	0.87
1	21	21	0.93
1	22	22	1.00
Σ = 100		Σ = 322	

25 words were responsible for only 9% of the errors made on the word list.

In List 2, four words (*bowl, tea, coat, fan*) were responsible for 63% of the errors. In contrast, the easiest 15 words were responsible for only 6% of the errors.

In List 3, six words of the 25-item word list accounted for 50% of the total list errors, while 11 words were responsible for only 7%.

In List 4, three words accounted for 47% of the list errors, and 11 items produced only 8%.

PBK-50

Table 6 displays the data obtained on the PBK-50 test during both the test and retest sessions. The means and standard deviations are reported for the three PBK-50 lists combined for each age-group.

The F statistic for the main effect of sensation level was significant ($p < 0.01$), but the main effect for the age factor was not significant ($p > 0.01$). Tukey post hoc analysis of sensation level demonstrated that all possible paired contrasts between the sample means were significant ($p < 0.01$).

It can be observed from Table 6 that, as the sensation level increased, the variability of scores, as indicated by the standard deviations within age-group, systematically decreased. In contrast to the WIPI test, variability does not appear to be inversely related to the age of the subjects at a given sensation level. However, by far the most variability in test scores was found for the three-and-one-half-year-old subjects, with a standard deviation of 15.75% at the only sensation level tested (32 dB).

Variability of test and retest scores was generally similar and was not consistently lower for either the test or retest sessions.

Absolute differences between mean performances of the subjects on test and retest were small. Only with the three-and-one-half-year-old subjects did these mean scores differ by more than one item, or 2%.

In terms of list equivalency, the mean scores of the three PBK-50 lists generally did not vary by more than two items, or 4%, indicating that the lists are of similar difficulty.

NU-6

Table 7 presents data obtained for NU-6 during the test and retest sessions. The means and standard deviations are indicated for each age-group at every sensation level tested. In the first test session there were only minimal differences in mean scores as a function of age; however, in the retest mean scores were ordered by age-group. Perhaps this difference between test and retest was due to a slight learning effect for the older children (11-and-one-half-year group) and a slight reduction in task motivation on the part of the younger children (seven-and-one-half-year group).

For the test session the mean scores of the seven-and-one-half- and nine-and-one-half-year-old groups differed by two items, or 4% at only 8 dB SL. At higher sensation levels smaller mean differences between age-groups were found. Performance of the 11-and-one-half-year-old children on this test closely approximates the findings of

Table 5. Analysis of words missed on the WIPI test: Lists 1, 2, 3, and 4.

Words	Number of Times Word Was Missed	%age of Total Errors	Accumulative %age of Errors	Words	Number of Times Word Was Missed	%age of Total Errors	Accumulative %age of Errors
List 1				**List 2**			
bus	0	0	—	cake	0	0	—
hat	0	—	—	church	0	—	—
smoke	0	—	—	clown	0	—	—
train	0	—	—	dog	0	—	—
crib	1	—	—	door	0	—	—
eye	1	—	—	flag	0	—	—
mouse	1	—	—	seal	0	—	—
neck	1	—	—	ship	0	—	—
shirt	1	—	—	socks	0	—	—
stair	1	0.09	0.09	stick	0	—	—
arm	2	—	—	bear	1	—	—
ball	2	—	—	broom	1	—	—
floor	2	—	—	nail	1	—	—
gun	2	—	—	rug	1	—	—
straw	2	—	—	string	1	0.06	0.06
street	2	—	—	red	2	—	—
wheel	2	0.21	0.30	thumb	2	0.05	0.11
chick	3	—	—	barn	3	—	—
school	3	—	—	desk	3	0.08	0.19
wing	3	0.14	0.44	meat	7	—	—
knee	5	—	—	pie	7	0.18	0.37
pail	5	0.15	0.59	fan	8	0.10	0.47
bread	6	0.09	0.68	coat	10	—	—
fox	7	0.11	0.79	tea	10	0.25	0.72
pan	14	0.21	1.00	bowl	22	0.28	1.00
List 3				**List 4**			
bell	0	0	—	man	0	0	—
chair	0	—	—	star	0	—	—
cup	0	—	—	tie	0	—	—
snake	0	—	—	dress	1	—	—
car	1	—	—	fish	1	—	—
dirt	1	—	—	goat	1	—	—
dish	1	—	—	thumb	1	—	—
feet	1	—	—	horn	1	—	—
sun	1	0.07	0.07	plane	1	—	—
can	2	—	—	spoon	1	—	—
key	2	—	—	tail	1	0.08	0.08
queen	2	0.08	0.15	bed	2	—	—
bib	3	—	—	bug	2	—	—
nest	3	0.08	0.23	frog	2	0.06	0.14
bag	4	—	—	ring	3	0.03	0.17
box	4	—	—	green	4	—	—
coin	4	—	—	lip	4	—	—
fly	4	—	—	skirt	4	0.12	0.29
saw	4	0.27	0.50	black	5	0.05	0.34
crown	5	—	—	pear	6	0.06	0.40
jail	5	0.13	0.63	blocks	7	—	—
coke	6	0.08	0.71	mouth	7	0.14	0.54
moon	7	—	—	bee	8	0.08	0.62
thread	7	0.19	0.90	beet	19	0.19	0.81
spring	8	0.11	1.00	bow	21	0.20	1.00

Table 6. Means and standard deviations in percent correct of 12 normal-hearing children from each of the age-groups $3\frac{1}{2}$, $5\frac{1}{2}$, $7\frac{1}{2}$, $9\frac{1}{2}$, and $11\frac{1}{2}$ years on the PBK-50 test as a function of sensation level (SL) during the test and retest sessions. Dash indicates not tested at this sensation level.

Age	SL in dB	Mean		Standard Deviation	
		Test	Retest	Test	Retest
$3\frac{1}{2}$	16	—	—	—	—
	24	—	—	—	—
	32	71.7	69.5	15.75	14.48
$5\frac{1}{2}$	16	85.8	86.3	4.86	4.89
	24	92.8	92.5	3.66	4.36
	32	95.8	95.7	2.48	3.49
$7\frac{1}{2}$	16	89.5	89.3	4.68	3.94
	24	95.0	93.2	2.36	4.39
	32	97.5	97.7	1.51	1.67
$9\frac{1}{2}$	16	89.2	89.2	4.13	6.06
	24	95.8	96.3	2.89	3.17
	32	98.5	98.3	1.24	1.67
$11\frac{1}{2}$	16	89.2	89.7	7.51	6.87
	24	97.0	97.3	2.89	3.65
	32	98.8	99.3	1.80	1.30

Tillman and Carhart (1966) and Rintelmann and Associates (1974) with normal-hearing adults at 32 dB SL.

Two-way analysis of variance revealed that the F statistic for the sensation level main effect was significant ($p < 0.01$), but again, the main effect for the age factor was not significant ($p > 0.01$). Tukey post hoc results showed that the paired contrasts between the mean scores obtained at every sensation level were significantly different from each other ($p \leq 0.05$).

In general, variability of test scores during the test session was not consistently related either to age level or to sensation level except for the seven-and-one-half-year-old group. However, as expected, the smallest standard deviations were found for all age-groups at 32 dB SL. Standard deviations for the retest became progressively lower with added intensity at all three age levels.

Differences between test and retest mean scores varied by less than two items, or 4%, except at 8 dB SL.

The mean scores between lists were quite similar in most instances. This is in agreement with the findings of Tillman and Carhart (1966) and Rintelmann and Associates (1974) who reported that the NU-6 lists are essentially equivalent. However, at low sensation levels (8 and 16 dB), there was a slight tendency for List 1 to be the most and List 4 to be the least difficult with Lists 2 and 3 of intermediate difficulty. The range in mean scores, between lists, never exceeded 6% and in most cases was within ±2%.

Discussion

For purposes of comparing results of the tests within each age-group, the mean scores of the test sessions were plotted separately for each age-group.

Figure 1 displays the results of the WIPI and the PBK-50 test administered to subjects three-and-one-half years old during the test session. The numbers in parentheses indicate the observed standard deviations in percent.

For assessing speech discrimination ability of children in this age-group, the 25-item multiple-choice WIPI test appears to be a suitable instrument. The mean score of normal-hearing children in this age-group is close to 92% at 32 dB SL. The mean score at 24 dB SL is almost as high, but the standard deviation increased to over 10%.

On the PBK-50 test at a 32 dB SL, the mean score of these children was considerably lower. Further, the variability of scores was greater than on the WIPI suggesting that factors other than hearing may be influencing test scores. Such factors may include speech problems, short attention span, open- versus closed-message set, and vocabulary variables. For children aged three-and-one-half years, the WIPI test administered at a 32 dB SL appears to have the double advantage of allowing normal-hearing children to obtain high scores, and of having less variability among scores. A further advantage of the WIPI is that the closed set of the test allows scores to be obtained even from children who, because of personality factors or speech inadequacies, find it difficult to respond to more conventional speech tests. This notion is supported by the findings of Hodgson (1973). Also, token reinforcement (for example candy, toy, money) was found to be an effective method of maintaining interest of young children in the PBK-50 test by Smith and Hodgson (1970).

Table 7. Means and standard deviations in percent correct of 12 normal-hearing children from each of the age-groups $7\frac{1}{2}$, $9\frac{1}{2}$, and $11\frac{1}{2}$ years on NU-6 as a function of sensation level (SL) during the test and retest sessions.

Age	SL in dB	Mean		Standard Deviation	
		Test	Retest	Test	Retest
$7\frac{1}{2}$	8	56.3	51.83	13.15	11.42
	16	81.3	78.20	5.00	6.63
	24	88.8	88.20	5.36	6.24
	32	92.8	92.50	3.66	3.63
$9\frac{1}{2}$	8	62.0	61.50	5.85	10.59
	16	79.8	80.70	6.35	7.78
	24	89.3	91.50	4.92	4.68
	32	93.5	95.33	2.97	3.75
$11\frac{1}{2}$	8	62.7	67.70	6.84	8.22
	16	82.3	84.20	6.37	6.58
	24	88.8	92.33	6.90	4.74
	32	96.5	96.00	2.71	2.09

Figure 2 shows the mean articulation scores and standard deviations (in parentheses) of five-and-one-half-year-old children, for the test sessions of the WIPI and the PBK-50. For children aged five-and-one-half years it also appears that the WIPI is an appropriate clinical tool. The mean score of normal-hearing children at a 32 dB SL was 97.3% with a standard deviation of 2.16%. The small standard deviation and the small difference in mean test-retest scores (1.0%) suggest that the test is a reliable one at this age level. On the PBK-50 test, the mean score for five-and-one-half-year-old children at a 32 dB SL was 95.8%. This test also appears appropriate for children aged five-and-one-half, provided these children have normal speech and language development. Taking into consideration the formats of the tests, the WIPI test might be preferred on the grounds that it is shorter, it is not limited by speech and language dissimilarities, and simply because it is an intrinsically more interesting task for children of this age-group.

The test results of children aged seven-and-one-half and nine-and-one-half years will be discussed together, because of the similarities in response patterns of the two age-groups. Figure 3 reveals the mean articulation scores and the standard deviations (in parentheses) for children aged seven-and-one-half years on the test session of the WIPI, the PBK-50, NU-6. Figure 4 presents the same information for children aged nine-and-one-half years. It

can be observed that these age-groups achieved high mean scores on the WIPI test at both the 24 and 32 dB SLs, with little variability of scores. Of the two open-message set speech discrimination tests used in this study (PBK-50 and NU-6), the PBK-50 is the easier for these age- groups as evidenced by substantially higher mean discrimination scores at every sensation level, by less variability of test scores, and by smaller differences in test-retest mean scores (see Tables 2, 6, and 7).

Figure 5 shows the articulation function of the 11 and-one-half-year-old children on the PBK-50 and the NU-6. The WIPI was not administered to this age-group. Observation of the articulation functions of the two tests again demonstrates that NU-6 is the more difficult task for children.

In conclusion, it appears that the multiple-choice, closed set WIPI test is the preferred test for children aged three-and-one-half years because mean scores are higher and less variable than those obtained with the PBK-50 test. For children aged five and one-half, both the WIPI and the PBK-50 appear to be appropriate tools, provided the children have good speech and normal language development. For children aged seven-and-one-half, nine-and-one-half, and 11 and-one-half, the NU-6 is more difficult than the PBK-50 test, as evidenced by lower discrimination scores at all sensation levels, and greater variability of test scores. It can be presumed that the larger number of errors is due to the fact that the words on this test were not selected on the basis of familiarity to children.

As pointed out by Carhart (1965), the intended purpose of the discrimination test should dictate the selection of the specific test to be administered. If the purpose of the test is to determine whether the hearing of the child falls within normal limits, the WIPI and the PBK-50 appear to be the tests of choice, allowing high scores among normal-hearing children of these age-groups, with little dispersion of test scores. However, if testing is to be done for purposes of evaluating a hearing aid or of determining differences in auditory discrimination ability between ears, it is suggested that the more difficult Northwestern University Auditory Test No. 6 be used, where a wider dispersion of speech discrimination scores can be obtained.

Acknowledgment

This investigation was supported, in part, by a Traineeship Award from the Rehabilitation Services Administration, U.S. Department of Health, Education, and Welfare, and was based upon the first author's doctoral dissertation completed in the Department of Audiology and Speech Sciences at Michigan State

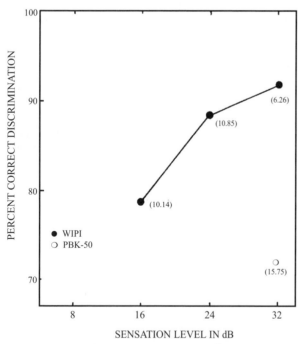

Figure 1. Mean discrimination scores and standard deviations (in parentheses) of 12 normal-hearing children aged three and one-half years on the WIPI and the PBK-50 during the test session.

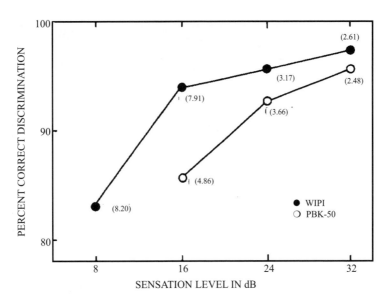

Figure 2. Mean discrimination scores and standard deviations (in parentheses) of 12 normal-hearing children aged five and one-half years on the WIPI and the PBK-50 during the test session.

University under the direction of William F. Rintelmann. Appreciation is expressed to Judith P. Frankmann for her assistance with the statistical analysis and for her critique of the manuscript. Requests for reprints should be directed to William F. Rintelmann, Department of Otorhinolaryngology and Human Communication, University of Pennsylvania School of Medicine, 3400 Spruce Street, Philadelphia, Pennsylvania 19104.

References

Carhart, R., Problems in the measurement of speech discrimination. *Archs Otolar.,* 82, 253-260 (1965).

Haskins, H., A phonetically balanced test of speech discrimination for children. Master's thesis, Northwestern Univ. (1949).

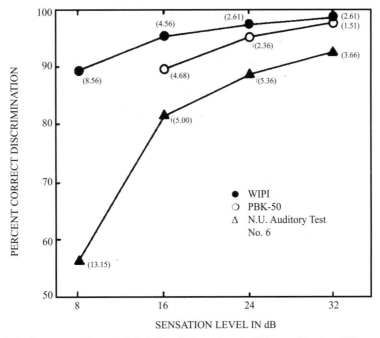

Figure 3. Mean discrimination scores and standard deviations (in parentheses) of 12 normal-hearing children aged seven and one a half years on the WIPI, the PBK-50, and the Northwestern University Auditory Test No. 6 during the test session.

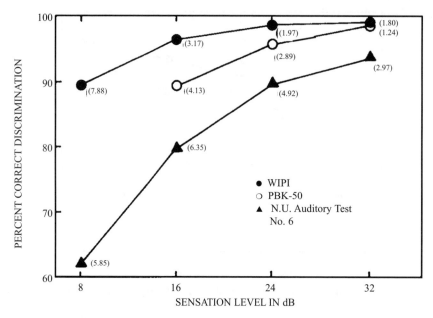

Figure 4. Mean discrimination scores and standard deviations (in parentheses) of 12 normal-hearing children aged nine and one-half years on the WIPI, the PBK-50, and the Northwestern University Auditory Test No. 6 during the test session.

Hodgson, W., A comparison of WIPI and PB-K discrimination test scores. Paper presented at the Annual Convention of the American Speech and Hearing Association, Detroit (1973).

Lehiste, I., and Peterson, G., Linguistic considerations in the study of speech intelligibility. *J. Acoust. Soc. Am.*, 31, 280-286 (1959).

Lerman, J., Ross, M., and McLauchlin, R., A picture-identification test for hearing-impaired children. *J. Aud. Res.,* 5, 273-278 (1965).

Myatt, B., and Landes, B., Assessing discrimination loss in children. *Archs Otolar.*, 77, 359-362 (1963).

Peterson, G., and Lehiste, I., Revised CNC lists for auditory tests. *J. Speech Hearing Dis.*, 27, 62-70 (1962).

Rintelmann, W., and Associates, Six experiments on speech discrimination utilizing CNC monosyllables: Northwestern University Auditory Test No. 6. *J. Aud. Res.,* Suppl. 2, 1-30 (1974).

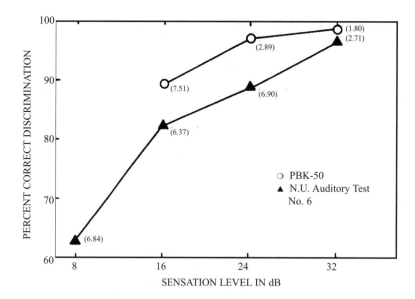

Figure 5. Mean discrimination scores and standard deviations (in parentheses) of 12 normal-hearing children aged 11 and-half years on the PBK-50 and the Northwestern University Auditory Test No. 6 during the test session.

Ross, M., and Lerman, J., A picture identification test for hearing-impaired children. *J. Speech Hearing Res.*, 13, 44-53 (1970).

Schwartz, D., The usefulness of the WIPI—A speech discrimination test for pre-school children. Master's thesis, Central Michigan Univ. (1971).

Siegenthaler, B., and Haspiel, G., Development of two standardized measures of hearing for speech by children. U.S. Department of Health, Education, and Welfare, Project No. 2372, Contract No. OE-5-10-003 (1966).

Smith, K., and Hodgson, W., The effects of systematic reinforcement on the speech discrimination responses of normal and hearing-impaired children *J. Aud. Res.,* 10,110-117 (1970).

Tillman, T., and Carhart, R., An expanded test for speech discrimination using CNC monosyllabic words (Northwestern Univ. Auditory Test No. 6). *SAM-TR-66-55* (1966).

Tillman, T., Carhart, R., and Wilber, L., A test for speech discrimination composed of CNC monosyllabic words (Northwestern Univ. Auditory Test No. 4). *SAM-TDR-62-135* (1963).

Tillman, T., Johnson, R., and Olsen, W., Earphone versus sound-field threshold sound-pressure levels for spondee words. *J. Acoust. Soc. Am.,* 39, 125-133 (1966).

Utley, J., *What's Its Name*. Urbana, Ill.: Univ. of Illinois Press (1951).

Received June 6, 1975

Accepted January 19, 1976

The BKB (Bamford-Kowal-Bench) Sentence Lists for Partially-Hearing Children[*]

John Bench

School of Communication Disorders, Lincoln Institute, Victoria 3053, Australia

Åse Kowal and John Bamford

Audiology Unit, Royal Berkshire Hospital, Reading, Berkshire, England

Abstract

Linguistic guidelines for the design of sentences for speech audiometry with children are described, and new lists of test sentences which are based on such guidelines—the Bamford-Kowal-Bench Sentence Lists for Children—are introduced. Audiometric data relating to the use of the new lists are presented and discussed.

Introduction

At present, comparatively little work is being done in speech audiometry with sentences, largely because the main audiometric emphasis is on the assessment of the end organ/brain relationship and hence test material has been influenced more by a consideration of phonemic than of linguistic aspects. Thus for the most part, speech audiometry is conducted with lists of phonemically balanced words, or more recently, with computer-synthesised 'phonemes', reflecting the current interest stemming from recent work in acoustic phonetics (Lehiste, 1967). Moreover, most of the experimentally rigorous work, as in the standardisation of speech audiometric tests, has been conducted on adults (Coles, et al.,1973).

Our approach is rather different (Bamford and Bench, 1979). Firstly, we are particularly interested in work with partially-hearing (PH) children; secondly, we have some concern for the more linguistic problems which are associated with hearing loss (though such problems are not discussed more than briefly in this paper); and thirdly, we are concerned with the reception of speech in natural settings, although we are aware that this area is fraught with arbitrary assumptions as to 'naturalness' since natural conditions are so variable, and that whatever material one produces is open to criticism on almost innumerable counts. However, as more fully described in Bench and Bamford (1979), we are attempting, at least in part, to look the bogey of natural usage in the face, rather than to rely solely on tests which are technically excellent though they may not be very natural.

One of our first problems, therefore, has been to acquire speech audiometric tests which reflect natural language usage for children, and consist of connected-speech. On examining published tests containing connected-speech in the form of short sentences (The Sentence Lists of Watson (1967) and The Fry (1961) Sentence Lists), we find that the vocabulary is too advanced; or the sentences, even though relatively short, are too long for our purpose; or the grammar is too complex; or the sentence lists have not been standardised; or they are too time-consuming; or the scoring criteria are not specified; or there are not enough lists for rehabilitative work (because it takes 5-7 lists to define a speech audiometric curve reliably, and several curves are needed to cover various test conditions); and so on (Bench and Bamford, 1979).

In short, a strong case can be made for arguing that published tests which might be thought to represent natural language samples do not properly do so, nor have they been tried and evaluated in a systematic way. We thus felt that we had no option but to design and evaluate our own material.

This paper deals mainly with the method employed for the construction of the sentences used in our new BKB speech audiometric sentence tests, together with two small-scale validation studies and conclusions.

Method of Sentence List Construction

We began by taking natural language samples from the kind of children for whom we were designing our tests. Thus, we visited schools for the deaf and PH units in Berkshire and surrounding counties, and tape-recorded the utterances of over 240 children aged eight to fifteen years. The children were asked to describe a set of

[*]This article is based on a paper presented to the British Society of Audiology Meeting: 'The Development of Language in Hearing-Impaired Children', September 1978.

coloured drawings which depicted scenes and events from commonplace play or family environments. The recordings were subsequently transcribed and subjected to a grammatical analysis using the LARSP (The Language Acquisition Remediation and Screening Procedure) profile of Crystal et al. (1976), a parsing for each word, and a vocabulary count. At the same time, careful note was made of each child's pure tone hearing loss, non-verbal I.Q. (W.I.S.C. performance scales), age, educational background and medical history. These data are currently being analysed in detail, but a provisional analysis was sufficient for us to identify three main groups of PH children for whom different speech audiometric material may well be necessary. These groups were:

(1) PH children whose language ability was so   poor that they seemed unlikely to cope even with very short and simple sentences;

(2) PH children who could cope with sentences if the vocabulary was relatively simple and if they were given additional contextual information, e.g. from looking at corresponding pictures while listening to the speech audiometric material; and

(3) PH children who probably could cope with the sentences while listening only.

We proceeded to ignore group (1) for the time being, and to draw up rules for designing test sentences for groups (2) and (3). The basic approach was to use vocabulary and grammar which we knew were familiar to the children (and were thus 'natural' to them because the vocabulary and grammar had been produced by the children themselves). We limited ourselves to orthodox vocabulary and grammar. The data which we had obtained on the spoken vocabulary and grammar of our large sample of PH children was assessed in detail (Bamford and Bench, 1979) to allow us to draw up criteria for the construction of our lists of sentences. Those items were used which, within the criteria, showed the most common spoken usage. Thus, for grammar, subject–verb–complement/object, subject–verb–adverb, and subject– verb sentences were allowed at the clause level; the ten phrase structures most frequently elicited were used at the phrase level; and the seven most frequent morphological structures were allowed at the word level. For vocabulary, we attempted to include those words which had an overall high frequency of occurrence with preference given to the words produced by the younger and more impaired children. The minimum requirement was that any word used in sentence list construction had to appear at least twice in the total collected vocabulary. Further, the sentence length could not exceed seven syllables. The permissible grammar and the first word of the sentences were balanced across the lists of sentences. The

following is an example of a list of sentences thus constructed (BKB Standard List No 14, copyright Academic Press Ltd). Key words, which can be used for scoring purposes, are underlined.

> The <u>angry</u> <u>man</u> <u>shouted.</u>
> The <u>dog</u> <u>sleeps</u> in a <u>basket.</u>
> <u>They're</u> <u>drinking</u> <u>tea.</u>
> <u>Mother</u> <u>opens</u> the <u>drawer.</u>
> An <u>old</u> <u>woman</u> was at <u>home.</u>
> <u>He</u> <u>dropped</u> his <u>money.</u>
> <u>They</u> <u>broke</u> <u>all</u> the <u>eggs.</u>
> The <u>kitchen</u> <u>window</u> was <u>clean.</u>
> The <u>girl</u> <u>plays</u> with the <u>baby.</u>
> The <u>big</u> <u>fish</u> <u>got</u> <u>away.</u>
> <u>She's</u> <u>helping</u> her <u>friend.</u>
> The <u>children</u> <u>washed</u> the <u>plates.</u>
> The <u>postman</u> <u>comes</u> <u>early.</u>
> The <u>sign</u> <u>showed</u> the <u>way.</u>
> The <u>grass</u> is <u>getting</u> <u>long.</u>
> The <u>match</u> <u>fell</u> on the <u>floor.</u>

At present, the 21 lists, each of sixteen sentences and containing 50 'key' words, which make up the 'Standard BKB Sentence Lists for Children',* and the eleven lists, each of which also have sixteen sentences and 50 'key' words, which make up the 'Picture-related BKB Sentence Lists for Children'—designed for the second group of children mentioned above—have been tape-recorded, and are being standardised on a further large sample of PH children. It should be noted that each sentence is preceded on the tape by a low-pass filtered white noise warning signal, recorded at the same level as the speech peaks.

Validation

Instead of presenting what at this stage can only be preliminary findings from this standardisation work we shall in the remainder of this paper deal: I. with work in which our Standard BKB speech audiometric test employing connected-speech is compared with a speech audiometric test consisting of the same vocabulary items (key words) presented as lists of unconnected words; and II. with an assessment of our Standard BKB Test against measures from the Illinois Test of Psycholinguistic Abilities (ITPA).

Validation Exercise I

We have maintained as a fundamental argument that the use of sentences rather than unconnected words for

---
*The senior author of this article is currently adapting the Standard BKB Sentence Lists for use with hearing-impaired children in Australia.

our speech audiometric test will give a more valid indication of how a child copes during natural communication with others. However, we recognise that although this argument has a high face validity there is little supporting evidence available in the literature. An experiment was consequently conducted by one of us (Å. Kowal) in which selected sentence lists from the BKB Standard Sentence Test and lists consisting of the randomised key words from the same selected sentence lists were compared in a speech audiometry task. That is, the 50 key words from a given list were taken and presented one at a time in random order. Thus the scored elements (key words) in the two conditions were the same, but in one condition they were embodied in a linguistic context (sentence), in the other they were isolated units. The object of the experiment was to discover whether a test such as our Standard BKB Sentence Test is a more sensitive test than the equivalent word test, in that the percentage of correct responses (intelligibility score) would be expected to increase more rapidly as the relative hearing level is increased in the case of sentences than for unconnected words. Thus the speech audiograms for the sentence test should exhibit steeper slopes than those from a test using the key words from the same sentences presented in random order. Since the intelligibility of natural connected-speech, with its high levels of redundancy, gives rise to very steep intelligibility curves, it can be argued that within limits the steeper is the slope of the curve, the more valid is the material for assessing the hearing for natural speech. Furthermore, it is generally agreed that 'a test should produce large differences in per cent correct for small differences of signal-to-noise ratio . . . in a listener's hearing mechanism' (Haggard and Summerfield, 1978).

Sixteen PH children aged 11 to 13 years, with pure tone hearing losses (averaged over 0.5, 1 and 2 KHz) of between 30 and 80 dB (ISO) and an average WISC performance IQ of 90-120 points were assessed by speech audiometry. Five BKB sentence lists were presented to the child (better ear) one sentence at a time from a tape-recorder through headphones at selected relative hearing levels, and the corresponding five randomised key word lists were administered one key word at a time at the same relative hearing levels as the sentence lists from which they were derived. In both cases the method of scoring was to measure the percentage of correctly repeated key words for each list. Logit indices were calculated for the data of each child. This procedure involves the calculation of a regression on the natural logarithms of the intelligibility scores. The logit transformation assumes an underlying cumulative logit distribution. It is particularly appropriate for dealing with two-parameter data of which one parameter consists of proportions (or percentages), where the proportions extend over a wide range of values. It has the advantage of producing a curve which lies within the 0-100% (intelligibility) scale as distinct from the theoretical possibility in the case of a straight regression line of obtaining a negative intelligibility score at one end of the scale, or a score greater than 100% at the other end of the scale. The slope index derived from the regression on the logits indicates the steepness of the slope, so that the larger the logit index number, the steeper the slope (see Table I).

A sign test was carried out on the logit slope index for the data from each of the two tests with the exception of the results from three children whose data in the opinion of three independent and experienced judges could not be assumed to have a cumulative logistic distribution. The sign test showed that the slopes for the sentences were significantly steeper ($p < 0.002$, one tailed) than the slopes for the randomised words.

Table I also shows that a similar result was obtained for eleven normally-hearing children aged from 10 years 6 months to 15 years 3 months (mean age 12 years 10 months) and selected to be of average to above average IQ. A sign test on their data showed the sentences to be significantly better repeated than the randomised key words (p equal to 0.006, one tailed).

As the scored items (key words) were the same in both cases these results must primarily indicate the extent to which the child's linguistic knowledge impinges on his hearing.

The results from our samples of children support our general argument that the BKB Standard Sentence Test is appropriate for assessments which relate to natural listening conditions. In passing it may be noted that the test using the randomised key words represent 'natural' vocabulary better than do tests of phoneme-balanced words, not only in the sense that they are well known to the children, but also because they are not of uniform length, which is an unnatural feature of PB word lists.

Validation Exercise II

The sample of PH children was assessed with the (ITPA) Illinois Test of Psycholinguistic Abilities (auditory/verbal subtests only), spoken by the same speaker as for the BKB Sentences and BKB randomised words.

When the results were correlated with the children's performance on the BKB Sentence Test, as indicated by the logit indices for the slopes, none of the correlations was statistically significant (Table II).

Bench and Cotter (1978), in a similar study of another 20 PH children, compared the scores from the same sub-tests of ITPA with the scores on Fry's Sentence Test. These latter children were comparable in age, hearing loss and IQ to Kowal's sample of children. Bench and Cotter plotted a line of best fit to the speech audiogram points to

Table I. Slope indices derived from speech intelligibility scores from words in isolation and the same words embedded in sentences.

	N = 13 PH Children			N = 11 Normally Hearing Children	
S	Logit of Sentence Data	Logit of Randomised Words Data	S	Logit of Sentence Data	Logit of Randomised Words Data
1	.3089	.1283	1	.3535	.3074
2	.1980	.0886	2	.1698	.2374
3	.2010	.2450	3	.3679	.1402
4	.1435	.1320	4	.3281	.2359
5	.2308	.0233	5	.8036	.2505
*6	.0283	.0039	6	.4120	.2902
7	.0872	.0696	7	.4387	.3150
8	.2007	.1444	8	.3258	.1579
9	.0630	.0595	9	.2680	.2071
10	.2387	.0644	10	.2124	.1519
11	.1755	.0572	11	.2483	.1789
12	.1225	.0813		Sign Test: Significant at 0.006 level (one tailed).	
13	.1303	.0568			
*14	.0992	.0269			
15	.2182	.1563			
*16	.0627	.1148			

Sign Test: Significant beyond 0.002 level (one tailed).

*Excluded from analysis (do not appear to conform to cumulative logit distribution).

measure the slope in degrees at the 50% intelligibility score, and proceeded to correlate these slopes with the children's ITPA scores. Bench and Cotter obtained four out of five significant correlations with Fry's Sentence scores. When Kowal's results were re-analysed using Bench and Cotter's method, there were still no significant correlations between ITPA sub-test scores and slopes from the BKB Sentence Lists. The difference in results between the two studies may thus reflect a difference in the level of linguistic difficulty between the two sentence tests used. Performance levels using the Fry Sentence Lists would seem to be related to linguistic ability, whereas hearing performance on the BKB Sentence Lists is unaffected by the child's linguistic ability.

From the above comparison we might conclude that as a hearing test for children the BKB Sentence Test is more valid than Fry's sentence test, since audiometric variables were more closely correlated with ITPA scores for the Fry than for the BKB sentences. On the other hand, if the object is to assess impairments involving linguistic ability as well as hearing, then Fry's test may be more suitable. However, our intention when constructing our sentence test was to ensure that the test would give a good indication of the child's hearing for speech rather than his linguistic ability, and the two validation studies would seem to indicate that our new test will meet this goal.

N.B. Anyone wishing to pursue in further detail the background to the BKB Sentence Lists is referred to Bench and Bamford (1979). Those wishing to purchase printed copies (Copyright Academic Press) and/or tape-recorded copies of the

Table II. The correlation coefficients obtained between some ITPA subtests and the slopes of speech intelligibility curves from two different studies.

	ITPA SUBTESTS				
	Auditory Reception	Auditory Association	Auditory Sequential Memory	Grammatical Closure	Verbal Expression
Bench and Cotter (Fry Sentences)	44	.54	.62	.69	.41
Correlation	p < .05	p < .05	p < .01	p < .001	NS
Kowal (BKB Sentences)	.30	−.10	.33	.02	.12
Correlation	NS	NS	NS	NS	NS

lists should write to: The Audiology Unit (Tape-Recordings), Royal Berkshire Hospital, Reading, Berkshire, RG1 5AN.

Acknowledgments

The work on which this paper is based was funded by the Medical Research Council (G 975/245/N). The authors are grateful to Mr. Ian Wilson, Department of Applied Statistics, University of Reading, for his statistical advice, and to the County Education Officers, Head Teachers and Teachers of the Deaf in Berkshire, Hampshire, Surrey, Sussex, Oxfordshire, Hertfordshire, Buckinghamshire, London and Birmingham for access to hearing-impaired children.

References

Bamford, J.M. and Bench, J. (1979). A grammatical analysis of the speech of partially-hearing children. In Crystal, D. (ed.) *Working with LARSP: Methods and Applications.* London: Edward Arnold. In press.

Bench, J. and Cotter, S. (1978). Psycholinguistic abilities and hearing for speech. *Brit. J. Disord. Comm.* In press.

Bench, J. and Bamford, J.M. (1979). (Eds). *Speech-Hearing Tests and the Spoken Language of Hearing-Impaired Children.* London and New York: Academic Press. In press.

Coles, R.R.A., Markides, A. and Priede, V.M. (1973). Uses and abuses of speech audiometry. In Taylor, W. (ed.) *Disorders of Auditory Function.* London and New York: Academic Press, 181-202.

Crystal, D., Fletcher, P. and Garman, M. (1976). *The Grammatical Analysis of Language Disability: A Procedure for Assessment and Remediation.* London: Edward Arnold.

Fry, D.B. (1961). Word and sentence tests for use in speech audiometry. *Lancet, 2:*197-199.

Haggard, M. and Summerfield, Q. (1978). *On realising the multiple possibilities in speech audiometry.* Paper to the Brit. Soc. Audiol., Jan 1978.

Lehiste, I. (1967). (Ed.) *Readings in Acoustic Phonetics.* Cambridge, Mass. and London: M.I.T. Press.

Watson, T.J. (1967). *The Education of Hearing Handicapped Children.* London: Univ. Lond. Press.

Pediatric Speech Intelligibility Test: Performance-Intensity Characteristics*

Susan Jerger and James Jerger
Department of Otorhinolaryngology and Communicative Sciences
Baylor College of Medicine, Houston, Texas

Abstract

Performance-intensity (PI) functions for Pediatric Speech Intelligibility (PSI) test materials were obtained in 40 normal-hearing children between 3 and 6 yrs of age. PSI messages were monosyllabic words and sentences presented in quiet and in the presence of a competing speech message. The message-to-competition ratio was constant across intensity levels: +4 dB (words) and 0 dB (sentences). Maximum speech intelligibility scores were 100% correct in all children for all conditions. The steepness of the PSI-PI functions, defined by the intensity range yielding performance between 20 and 80%, ranged from 8 to 12 dB. Threshold levels (50% correct) ranged from 21 to 26 dB SPL. With one exception, chronological age did not significantly influence the steepness of PSI-PI functions. The exception was the increasing steepness with increasing age noted for sentences in competition. A significant chronological age developmental trend was noted for all speech threshold results.

During the past 10 yrs, certain dimensions of speech audiometry have gained increasing importance as diagnostic tools for the evaluation of both peripheral and central auditory function in adults. For example, previous investigators[5,9,19,23,36] have reported that valuable diagnostic information can be obtained not only from maximum scores for monosyllabic phonetically balanced (PB) words, but also from the shape of the performance versus intensity (PI) function for PB words. In patients with retrocochlear disorder, an unique "rollover" configuration of the PI-PB function occurs. As the intensity of speech signals is increased above the level yielding maximum performance, there is a paradoxical reduction in performance, often to an astonishing degree.

In 1976, we[25] attempted to extend the clinical utility of PI-PB functions by demonstrating that a speech threshold, defined as the 50% correct intelligibility level, can be derived from the function. In a series of 1672 patients with varying types and degrees of hearing loss, we showed that the PI-PB speech threshold can be used interchangeably with the more conventional spondee word threshold, thereby reducing the need for a separate speech threshold procedure.

In 1977, Jerger and Hayes[22] noted that comparison of PI functions for PB words and synthetic sentence identification (SSI) materials enhances the differentiation of peripheral and central sites of auditory disorder. The direction and magnitude of any discrepancy between PB and SSI functions appears to provide an estimate of the relative contributions of peripheral versus central components to a patient's total auditory impairment. Clinical experience in patients with a wide variety of central auditory pathologies has documented the sensitivity of the word-sentence relation in detecting the presence of central auditory dysfunction.[26,38]

The success of diagnostic speech audiometry in adults has encouraged efforts to apply the same principles in the evaluation of young children. A variety of pediatric speech audiometric procedures have been developed, either by (1) scaling down adult materials or (2) devising new materials uniquely suited to children's interests and abilities. Both approaches to developing pediatric speech tests encountered major problems, however, due to the contaminating influence of receptive language (RL) skills on test performance.

A major concern in pediatric test development is to obtain test materials that are not influenced by normal developmental differences in RL ability. The contaminating influence of variable RL skills on speech audiometry in children has been emphasized by several investigators.[12,31] Previous attempts to control the effect of developmental RL differences on speech intelligibility performance primarily involved (1) confining testing to older children and (2) confining test materials to word items. However, the importance of testing younger children and of using speech materials, such as sentences, that are more sensitive to the presence of central auditory disorder has been consistently recognized.

Reprinted by permission of authors and Williams & Wilkins. Copyright 1982. *Ear & Hearing*, 3, pp. 325-334.

*This study was supported by Public Health Service Clinical Research Center Grant NS-10940 from the National Institute of Neurological and Communicative Disorders and Stroke. In response to inquires, the PSI test will be commercially available within 1 year.

In an attempt to meet these problems, we recently developed a new Pediatric Speech Intelligibility (PSI) test. The PSI test consists of word and sentence materials generated by normal children between 3 and 6 yrs old. In an initial report on the PSI test,[28] we showed that the word materials generated by the children did not differ as a function of chronological age (CA) or RL ability. The sentence materials, however, did reflect differences in CA and RL age. For example, younger children responded by omitting the auxiliary verb "be" in forming the verb tense of the sentence (e.g., "A bear combing his hair"). In contrast, older children responded with complete, adult-like sentences (e.g., "A bear is combing his hair"). To represent the differences in the children's responses, two different types of test sentences, subsequently referred to as format I and format II sentences, were formed. An example of a format I sentence is "Show me a bear combing his hair." An example of a format II sentence is "A bear is combing his hair." The two different types of test sentences were constructed in an attempt to control the influence of RL skills on speech audiometry results. Individual sentence and word items comprising the PSI test are published elsewhere.[28]

In a second study[27] on the PSI test, the effects of RL ability and CA on PSI performance were explored in normal children between 3 and 6 yrs old. Performance for format I and format II sentences differed significantly as a function of RL ability. On the basis of these results, we constructed an algorithm that determines the appropriate sentence format for speech audiometry from a child's RL age. Performance based on the algorithm yielded "language equivalent" norms, that is, equivalent performance in children with varying RL skills. Performance for PSI word materials was not influenced by differences in RL ability. However, CA developmental trends were noted for all speech materials.

The purpose of the present study was to define normal characteristics of PI functions for PSI word and sentence materials presented in quiet and in the presence of a competing speech message. In this paper, we attempt to construct a normal foundation for the subsequent interpretation of PI functions in children with peripheral and central auditory disorders.

Method

Materials and Instrumentation

Format I and format II sentence lists, word lists, and competing sentences were recorded onto a dual-track magnetic tape recorder (Ampex, 351). Channel 1 contained the PSI test sentences and words. Format I sentences and word items were preceded by an introductory carrier phrase,

"Show me." Format II sentences were not preceded by a carrier phrase. Channel 2 contained competing sentences. The competing sentence messages, test sentences, and test words were composed by the same children. The test items (words and sentences) and the competing sentences were recorded by different male talkers with general American dialect. The interitem interval was 10 sec for the sentence test and 7.5 sec for the word test. Speech level was defined as the sound pressure level (SPL) of a 1000 Hz sinusoid recorded at the average level of frequent peaks of the speech as monitored on a VU meter. The tape playback system consisted of a multichannel recorder (Sony TC-788-4) fed through a speech audiometer (Grason Stadler model 162) to either a loudspeaker (Phillips, type 22RH544/64R) or to an earphone (Telephonic, TDH- 39) mounted in a circumaural cushion (CZW-6).

Procedure

Subjects were tested inside a sound-treated booth in a single test session of approximately 45 min. Testing included a pure-tone audiogram, the Northwestern Syntax Screening test (NSST),[29] and the PSI test. Each child was seated at a table containing a picture identification response card (a 36.5 ˇ 39.0 cm card with five pictures arranged in a truncated horseshoe configuration). After each sentence or word had been presented, the child responded by pointing to the picture corresponding to the sentence or word that he heard.

PI functions were constructed by presenting blocks of words or sentences at several suprathreshold intensity levels. The initial test intensity was 50 to 60 dB SPL. Intensity was then reduced in 10 dB steps until the "knee" of the PI function (i.e., the point of inflection below which performance decreased rapidly with further decrease in intensity) had been defined. Below this knee-point, intensity was decreased in 5 dB steps until a 0 to 20% performance level had been reached. Finally, intensity was raised to either 100 dB SPL (for loudspeaker condition) or 110 dB SPL (for earphone condition) to define the high-intensity region of the PI function.

PI functions were obtained for speech messages presented in quiet and in competition. The message-to-competition ratio (MCR) was constant across intensity levels: 0 dB for sentences (format I and format II) and +4 dB for words. The basis for selecting these standard MCR test conditions has been explained previously.[27] For sentence results, PI functions were obtained with list A in one-half of the children and with list B in one-half of the children. The equivalence of PSI sentence and word lists has been established previously in a group of normal listeners between 3 and 6 yrs of age.[27] The order of administration of word and sentence materials, and quiet versus competing message conditions, was counterbalanced among subjects.

At any given intensity level, a listening trial consisted of the presentation of each of the five alternative sentences or words of a list. If performance on this trial was 80 to 100% correct (at least four out of five) or 0 to 20% correct (at most one out of five), only one trial (five items) was presented at that SPL. If performance on the first trial was between 21 and 79% correct, then a second trial was presented at that SPL. For sentence materials, successive trials represented the same five sentences presented in different random orders. For word materials, listening trials progressed through each word list (with one replication in a different random order) until all four lists (20 word items) had been presented. At this time, if necessary, the five words of a list(s) were presented again in a different random order.

All children were tested with the same corpus of word materials. However, sentence materials were varied according to the child's RL ability as measured by the NSST. The criteria for the selection of the sentence format, either format I or format II, from the NSST-RL score has been detailed previously.[27] In brief, children with NSST scores of less than 32 were tested with format I sentences; children with NSST scores of greater than or equal to 32 were tested with format II sentences. The purpose of the sentence selection criteria is to minimize the influence of RL skills on sentence intelligibility performance. As previously discussed,[27] PSI word intelligibility performance is not influenced by differences in RL ability.

Subjects qualifying for format I sentence materials were routinely tested in the sound field. For these data, a loudspeaker was placed opposite the test ear at a distance of 20 cm. The speaker distance was selected from results of a pilot study evaluating MCR functions obtained via earphone and via loudspeaker at various distances from the child's ear. Results showed that earphone results and sound field results were equivalent at a speaker distance of 20 cm.

Subjects qualifying for format II sentence materials were routinely tested via earphone. In children tested under earphones, PI functions were obtained on only one ear of each subject. Whenever the speech signal to the test ear was sufficiently intense to cross over to the nontest ear, a white noise masking signal was delivered to the nontest ear at a level 20 dB less than the test signal SPL. The selection of the test ear or the ear facing the loudspeaker was counterbalanced among the subjects.

Subjects

Subjects were 40 children, 21 girls and 19 boys, ranging in age from 3 yrs 1 mo to 6 yrs 10 mos. Of the 40 subjects, 17 had participated in previous PSI studies.[27] Seven children were 3 yrs old; 8 children were 4 yrs old; 14 children were 5 yrs old; and 11 children were 6 yrs old. The mean CA was 5 yrs 2 mos; the mean RL (NSST) age was 5 yrs 2 mos. All children had normal hearing [less than or equal to 20 dB hearing level (HL)] for pure-tone signals at octave intervals between 500 and 4000 Hz on both ears. Average pure-tone sensitivity (PTA) for 500, 1000, and 2000 Hz was 5.9 dB HL on the right ear and 4.6 dB HL on the left ear. Subjects represented a middle-income socioeconomic level and diverse cultural levels.

The children were divided into two groups depending on whether they qualified for format I or format II sentences. Children qualifying for format I sentences are subsequently referred to as the receptive language level I (RLL I) group; children qualifying for format II sentences are termed the RLL II group. Children in both groups, however, were tested with the same word materials. Each group contained 20 children. The average CA in the two groups of children differed by 1 yr 6 mos. The mean CA was 4 yrs 5 mos in the RLL I group and 5 yrs 11 mos in the RLL II group. The range of ages showed overlap between the two groups. Ages ranged from 3 yrs 1 mo to 6 yrs 4 mos in the RLL I group and from 4 yrs 10 mos to 6 yrs 10 mos in the RLL II group. The average RL age differed by 2 yrs 4 mos between the two groups. The average RL (NSST) age was 3 yrs 11 mos in the RLL I group and 6 yrs 3 mos in the RLL II group. The NSST scores ranged from 19 to 30 in the RLL I group and from 32 to 37 in the RLL II group. The average PTA score differed by 2.3 dB between the two groups. Average PTAs were 6.8 dB HL in the RLL I group and 4.5 dB HL in the RLL II group. PTA scores ranged from 4 to 11 dB HL in the RLL I group and from −1 to 9 dB HL in the RLL II group. Differences in CA ($t = 6.08$, corrected $p < 0.01$), RL (NSST) ability ($t = 9.14$, corrected $p < 0.01$), and pure-tone sensitivity ($t = 2.67$, $p < 0.05$) between the two groups were significant. (See Technical Appendix, item 2, for an explanation of corrected critical probability values.)

Results

Steepness of PI Function for Words

Figure 1 shows average performance as a function of speech intensity for PSI monosyllabic word materials in quiet and in the presence of a competing speech message (+4 dB MCR). Data are organized into two groups depending on whether the child qualified for format I or format II sentences (RLL I or RLL II groups). In both groups, individual maximum speech intelligibility scores were 100% correct in all subjects for both quiet and competing message conditions.

Table I lists the steepness characteristics of the word functions in the RLL I and RLL II subject groups. For comparative purposes, data for other pediatric audiometric word materials are summarized. Other procedures include the Gottinger test,[8] the A. B. test,[7] the Northwestern University-Children's Perception of Speech (Nuchips) test,[14] the Discrimination by Identification of Pictures (DIP) test,[39] and the PB-Kindergarten (PB-K) test.[20] Results for these latter tests are grouped according to CA, instead of RL ability.

In Table 1, entries represent the intensity range in decibels corresponding to the performance range from 20 to 80%. To quantify the steepness of PI functions, data were plotted on normal probability paper and a best-fit linear function was visually determined. Steepness characteristics are summarized by the decibel range yielding 20 to 80%, rather than the conventional percentage per decibel approach, because we did not want the steepness estimates from other investigations to be subjected to an additional transformation.

In Figure 1 and Table 1, the performance range defining 20 to 80% correct was 8 to 10 dB for PSI words in quiet and 10 to 12 dB for PSI words in competition. Standard deviations were 2.0 dB (RLL I) and 1.7 dB (RLL II) for words in quiet and 3.7 dB (RLL I) and 2.5 dB (RLL II) for words in competition. The degree of steepness of a PI function may be quantified by computing the "h" statistic[18]

$$h = 1 / F \, p2b$$

where F refers to the standard deviation of the underlying distribution. This statistic considers the steepness of an entire normal integral, rather than just the midregion from 20 to 80%. The value of h approaches unity as steepness increases. The h values for PSI words were 0.14 (RLL I) and 0.19 (RLL II) in quiet and 0.13 (RLL I) and 0.15 (RLL II) in competition. These results are consistent with expectation. The degree of steepness is relatively increased for words in quiet (easy listening condition) in the RLL II group and is relatively decreased for words in competition (difficult listening condition) in the RLL I group.

Although average performance showed systematic differences between RLL I and RLL II groups, the steepness of the PI functions in the two subject groups was not statistically different for words in quiet (t = 0.63, $p >$ 0.50) or in competition (t = 0.46, $p >$ 0.50). Within each subject group in Table 1, the PI function in quiet was steeper than the corresponding PI function in competition. The difference between the quiet and competing message conditions for word materials was significant for the RLL I group (t = 3.19, $p < 0.005$, one-tailed test) and for the RLL II group (t = 3.34, $p < 0.005$, one-tailed test).

In comparison to PI functions for other pediatric word materials shown in Table 1, PSI-PI functions are steeper. With one exception the performance range between 20 and 80% correct for other materials is between 10 and 15 dB. The exception involves the Nu-chips word materials. The steepness of PI functions for the Nu-chips materials appears to be more gradual than the steepness of other pediatric word tests. For the Nu-chips test, the performance range between 20 and 80% is

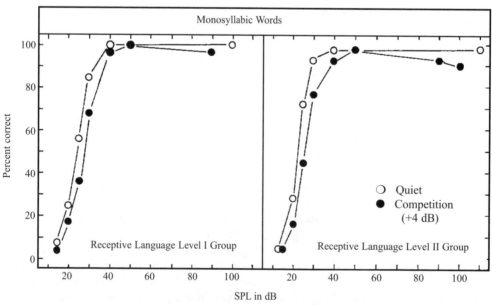

Figure 1. PI functions for PSI word materials in quiet and in the presence of a competing speech message (+4 dB MCR) in 40 normal-hearing children between 3 and 6 yrs of age.

Table 1. Steepness index in decibels: words[a]

	Word Materials	Groups	
		RLL I	RLL II
Present study	PSI-Q	10	8
	PSI-CM	12	10
		3-4 yr olds	5-6 yr olds
Previous studies	PB-K test-Q[b]		14
	A. B. test-Q[c]		15
	DIP-Q[d]	14	12
	Gottinger test-Q[e]	14	10
	Nu-Chips-Q[f]	21	18
	Adult words-Q:[g]		
	11-15		

[a]Steepness characteristics of normal performance-intensity functions for PSI monosyllabic words presented in quiet (Q) and in the presence of a competing message (CM) at a message-to-competition ratio of +4 dB. Table entries represent the intensity range in decibels corresponding to the performance range from 20 to 80%. For comparative purposes, normal data for other word materials are presented in Table 1. Data from the present investigation are grouped according to receptive language level (RLL I vs. RLL II). Data from other studies are grouped according to chronological age (3 to 4 yrs vs. 5 to 6 yrs).
[b]Personal unpublished data.[24]
[c]Boothroyd.[17]
[d]Siegenthaler.[39] Data obtained by plotting author's results from about 40 to 80% on normal probability paper and extrapolating down to 20%.
[e]Chilla et al.[8]
[f]Elliott and Katz.[13,14] Data obtained by plotting authors' results from about 50 to 80% on normal probability paper and extrapolating down to 20%.
[g]For References, see text.

21 dB in 3-yr-olds and 18 dB in 5-yr-olds. In adults, the intensity range corresponding to 20 to 80% correct for a variety of monosyllabic word materials ranges from about 11 to 15 dB.[34] The h statistic reported for PAL-PB words in adults is 0.10.[41] Relative to the steepness of adult word materials, the steepness of pediatric PI functions is slightly increased for the PSI test, is comparable for the Gottinger test, the A. B. test, the DIP test, and the PB-K test, and is flatter for the Nu-chips test. Differences in the steepness of PI functions may be due to a variety of auditory and nonauditory factors, such as differences (1) in the homogeneity of test items, (2) in the scoring techniques (e.g., words versus phonemes), (3) in the influence of cognitive skills on the task, (4) in the perceptual salience of the verbal materials, and (5) in the number of test items per trial, etc. Some of these factors have been discussed previously by Bench and Bamford and their colleagues.[3]

Steepness of PI Function for Sentences

Figure 2 shows average performance as a function of speech intensity for PSI sentence materials in quiet and in the presence of a competing message (0 dB MCR). Data are organized into two groups depending on whether the child was tested with format I or format II sentences (RLL I or RLL II groups). In both groups, all children achieved maximum intelligibility scores of 100% correct for both quiet and competing message conditions.

Table 2 tabulates the steepness characteristics of PI functions for the RLL I and RLL II subject groups.

Results for other sentence materials—the Fry test,[17] Manchester test,[45] Bamford-Kowal-Bench (BKB) picture-related test,[3] and the SSI test[42]—are presented for comparative purposes. The latter results are grouped according to CA. Data were determined from the line of best fit for PI functions as plotted on normal probability paper. In Table 2, notice that PSI materials differ from other sentence procedures relative to the appropriate age range for the test. The PSI test was successfully administered to 3- to 6-yr-olds, whereas other sentence tests have been administered to children in the 10- to 15-yr age range.

As shown in Figure 2 and Table 2, the intensity (decibels) range yielding 20 to 80% correct performance for PSI sentences was 8 to 9 dB in quiet and 10 to 11 dB in competition. Standard deviations were 1.9 dB (RLL I) and 2.1 dB (RLL II) for sentences in quiet and 2.8 dB (RLL I) and 1.8 dB (RLL II) for sentences in competition. The h values for PSI sentences were 0.18 (RLL I) and 0.14 (RLL II) in quiet and 0.15 (RLL I) and 0.12 (RLL II) in competition. This finding is somewhat unexpected. Apparently, average performance in the RLL I group for both quiet and competing conditions was slightly steeper than the corresponding performance condition in the RLL II group. The steepness of the functions in the RLL I and RLL II groups was statistically equivalent for sentences in quiet (t = 1.37, $p > 0.10$). However, the steepness of the PI functions for sentences in competition was significantly different between the two groups (t = 2.90, corrected $p < 0.05$). (Please see Technical Appendix, item 3, for explanation of corrected probability value.) Within each RLL group, the PI function in quiet was significantly

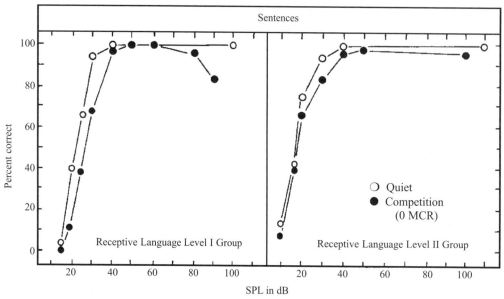

Figure 2. PI functions for PSI sentence materials in quiet and in the presence of a competing speech message (0 dB MCR) in 40 normal-hearing children between 3 and 6 yrs of age.

steeper than the corresponding PI function in competition (for RLL I group, t = 3.47, $p < 0.005$, one-tailed test; for RLL II group, t = 1.99, $p < 0.05$, one-tailed test). This finding is consistent with expectation.[44]

In comparison to results for 10- to 15-yr-olds obtained by other investigators and summarized in Table 2, PI functions for PSI sentence materials are steeper. The intensity range defining 20 to 80% correct for other sentence tests varied from 12 to 13 dB for the Fry and Manchester sentence materials to 15 to 17 dB for the BKB picture test and the SSI materials in the presence of a competing message at 0 dB MCR. One comment concerning the BKB picture test is that subsequent testing in children with hearing loss[4] yielded a steeper function, about 13 dB. If one assumes that the PI function in normal listeners should theoretically be steeper or at least as steep as PI functions in children with hearing loss, then the normal data of Bamford and Wilson[1] reported in Table 2 may be somewhat spurious.

In adults, the intensity range yielding 20 to 80% is 5 to 7 dB for SSI sentences in quiet, first-order approximations,[41,43] and third-order approximations,[24,44] 7 dB for German sentences in quiet,[32] and 19 dB for SSI materials (third-order approximations) in competition (0 dB MCR).[24] The h values for adult SSI sentences in quiet are 0.22 to 0.26.[41,43,44] Relative to PI functions for adult sentence materials, results for pediatric PI functions in quiet are more gradual. In contrast, PI functions for PSI sentence materials in competition are relatively steeper. The steepness of SSI functions (0 dB MCR) is comparable in older children and adults. In general, the h values for the PSI-PI

functions for sentences, 0.12 to 0.18, are similar to the h value observed for adult spondee words, 0.15.[41]

Effect of Chronological Age

The steepness of PI functions for PSI word materials was not influenced by age. The correlation between age and the steepness of PI word functions was not significant for the quiet condition (r = 0.052, $p > 0.05$, one-tailed test) or for the competing message condition (r = –0.054, $p > 0.05$, one-tailed test). For PSI sentence materials, the steepness of the PI function in quiet was not related to age (r = –0.143, $p > 0.05$, one-tailed test). However, the steepness of the PI sentence function in competition was significantly, but weakly, related to age (r = –0.265, $p < 0.05$, one-tailed test). For the latter condition, the steepness of the PI function increased significantly with increasing age. For example, the intensity range defining 20 to 80% correct was 12 dB in the 3-yr-olds, but only 9 dB in the 6-yr-olds. In no case, however, was a strong correlation coefficient obtained.

Speech Thresholds for Word Materials

Table 3 and Figure 1 show the SPLs corresponding to the threshold, or 50% correct level, of PSI word materials in quiet and in competition. In Table 3, speech thresholds for other pediatric word materials are also shown. PSI results are grouped according to RL ability (RLL I and RLL II groups); data for other word tests are grouped according to CA.

Table 2. Steepness index in decibels: sentences[a]

	Sentence Materials	Groups	
		RLL I	RLL II
Present study	PSI-Q	8	9
	PSI-CM	10	11
			10-15 yr olds
Previous studies	Fry test-Q[b]		12
	Manchester test-Q[b]		13
	BKB Picture test-Q[b]		15
	SSI-CM[c]		17
	Adult sentences-Q:[d] 5-7		
	Adult sentences-CM[c]		
	19		

[a]Steepness characteristics of normal performance-intensity functions for PSI sentences presented in quiet (Q) and in the presence of a competing message (CM) at a message-to-competition ratio of 0 dB. Table entries represent the intensity range in decibels corresponding to the performance range from 20 to 80%. For comparative purposes, normal data for other sentence materials are presented in Table 2. Data from the present investigation are grouped according to receptive language level (RLL I vs. RLL II). Data from other studies are grouped according to chronological age (10 to 15 yrs).
[b]Bamford and Wilson.[1]
[c]Personal unpublished data.[24]
[d]For References, see text.

The thresholds for PSI word materials were 23 dB SPL (RLL I) and 22 dB SPL (RLL II) in quiet and 26 dB SPL (RLL I) and 25 dB SPL (RLL II) in competition. Standard deviations were 5.1 dB (RLL I) and 3.5 dB (RLL II) for words in quiet and 6.5 dB (RLL I) and 4.2 dB (RLL II) for words in competition. Speech thresholds in the RLL I versus RLL II subject groups were equivalent for words in quiet ($t = 0.68$, $p > 0.50$) and in competition ($t = 0.65$, corrected $p > 0.50$). (Please see Technical Appendix, item 4.) Failure to observe a significant difference between word thresholds in the two subject groups is in contrast to the slight, but statistically significant, difference between the two groups for pure-tone thresholds (see subject description). Within each subject group, threshold results for words in quiet were characterized by lower SPLs than corresponding threshold results for words in the presence of a competing message. Word thresholds in quiet versus in competition were significantly different in the RLL I group ($t = 2.69$, $p < 0.01$, one-tailed test) and in the RLL II group ($t = 4.32$, $p < 0.001$, one-tailed test). This finding is consistent with expectation.[12]

Speech thresholds for PSI words are comparable to threshold levels for other word materials. With two exceptions, speech thresholds for other pediatric materials range from 18 to 29 dB SPL. The exceptions are the unusually sensitive threshold, 14 dB SPL, observed for Threshold by Identification of Pictures (TIP) monosyllabic words in 5- to 6-yr-olds and the unusually poor speech threshold, 37 dB SPL, observed for PB-K words in the same age group. A difference of about 20 dB between PB-K speech thresholds and other speech thresholds suggests that the PB-K word test is a more difficult

listening task for children. However, as shown in Table 1, the steepness of the PI function for PB-K words was not unusually flat relative to other pediatric monosyllabic word materials. Bench and Bamford[3] suggest that a threshold difference without a steepness difference does not indicate a more difficult speech task, but simply indicates a calibration error. However, the PB-K threshold reported in Table 3 is consistent with extrapolated results for previous PB-K threshold estimations in 5- and 6-yr-old children.[2,14,37] With the exception of PB-K and TIP results, the speech thresholds reported in Table 3 are in agreement with the speech thresholds observed for monosyllabic word materials in adults, about 24 to 31 dB SPL.[21,25,32,41]

Speech Thresholds for Sentence Materials

Table 4 and Figure 2 show speech thresholds for PSI sentence materials presented in quiet and in competition. Data for other older child-adult sentence materials are also shown. Thresholds for PSI sentence materials were 21 dB SPL (RLL I and RLL II) in quiet and 26 dB SPL (RLL I) and 21 dB SPL (RLL II) in competition. Standard deviations were 3.7 dB (RLL I) and 4.6 dB (RLL II) for sentences in quiet and 4.2 dB (RLL I) and 4.1 dB (RLL II) for sentences in competition. Speech threshold results in the two subject groups were equivalent for sentences in quiet ($t = 0.57$, $p > 0.50$). However, speech thresholds for sentences in competition were significantly different between the two RLL groups ($t = 3.92$, $p < 0.001$). Within the RLL I group, sentence thresholds obtained in quiet versus in competition were significantly different ($t = 6.94$, $p < 0.001$, one-tailed test). However, in the RLL II group, sentence thresholds in quiet versus competing conditions did not significantly differ (t = 0.57, $p > 0.10$, one-tailed test). This latter result is not consistent with expectation.[44]

Relative to results for other sentence materials in children 10 to 15 yrs of age, PSI speech thresholds are more comparable to sentence threshold results in adults. Speech thresholds for other sentence materials in older children ranged from 30 to 34 dB SPL. In adults, thresholds are about 16 to 18 dB SPL for sentences in quiet[24,32,41] and 31 dB SPL for SSI sentences (third-order approximations) in competition (0 dB MCR).[24]

Effect of Chronological Age

The correlation between age and each of the pure-tone and speech thresholds was weak, but statistically significant. Correlations (one-tailed test of significance) were as follows: age versus pure-tone sensitivity (r = –0.50, $p < 0.005$); age versus word thresholds in quiet (r = –0.46, $p < 0.005$); age versus sentence thresholds in quiet (r = –0.41, $p < 0.005$); age versus word thresholds in competition (r = –0.49, $p < 0.005$); and age versus sentence thresholds in competition (r = –0.72, $p < 0.0005$).

Improvement in pure-tone sensitivity and speech thresholds with increasing age has been reported previously.[11,13,15,35] In the present study, the degree of improvement with increasing age from 3 to 6 yrs was 4 dB for pure-tone thresholds, 3 dB (sentences) to 4 dB (words) for speech thresholds in quiet, and 6 dB (words) to 9 dB (sentences) for speech thresholds in competition.

Rollover Effect

To provide a normative framework for evaluation of the rollover effect in children with auditory disorder, we quantified the degree of performance decrement at high speech intensity levels characterizing PI functions in the normal children. Performance decrement was defined as the difference between the maximum speech intelligibility (max) score and the minimum speech intelligibility (min) score. The max score is the maximum intelligibility score at any speech level; the min score is the lowest intelligibility score at any speech level above the level yielding the max score. The maximum speech intensity level was 110 dB SPL for the earphone condition (RLL II group) and 100 dB SPL for the loudspeaker condition (RLL I group).

Derived indices (max score minus min score) in the 40 children used in this study were not normally distributed. Instead, the form of the distribution was markedly skewed. A large number of observations clustered at 0% (no decrement). For this reason, data are described by distribution-free, nonparametric statistical measures.

In both the RLL I and RLL II groups, the median decrement was 0% for words in quiet, 0% for words in competition, and 0% for sentences in quiet. For sentences in competition, the median decrement was 10% (RLL I) and 0% (RLL II). Performance decrements in the two subject groups were equivalent for words in competition (Mann-Whitney $U = 146.5$, $p > 0.10$),[10] but not for sentences in competition ($U = 89.5$, $p < 0.05$). For the latter condition, the degree of decrement was significantly greater in the RLL I group than in the RLL II group. The absolute degree of performance decrement encompassing 95% of observations in the present normal subjects was 0 to 10% (words in quiet, RLL I and RLL II groups), 0% (sentences in quiet, both groups), 0 to 40% (words in competition, both groups), 0 to 40% (sentences in competition, RLL I group), and 0 to 10% (sentences in competition, RLL II group). These findings agree with the results of Shirnian and Arnst[38] in aged listeners. These data provide a framework against which to detect significant rollover effects in children with suspected retrocochlear disorders.

Discussion

Words versus Sentences

In Tables 1 to 4, performance for PSI word versus sentence materials may be contrasted. Comparison of the steepness of word versus sentence functions (Tables 1 and 2) within each subject group shows that results are statistically equivalent for the quiet condition (for RLL I group, t = 1.58, $p > 0.10$; for RLL II group, t = 0.58, $p > 0.50$) and for the competing condition (for RLL I group, t = 1.52, $p > 0.10$; for RLL II group, t = –0.52, $p > 0.50$). This finding is not consistent with previous results on adult speech materials (summarized at the bottom of Tables 1 and 2). In adults, PI functions for sentences are characteristically steeper than PI functions for words.[3,34,41]

In general correspondence with steepness results, threshold results for PSI word versus sentence materials (tables 3 and 4) were also statistically equivalent within each subject group except for the competing condition in the RLL II group [for quiet condition, t = 1.93, $p > 0.05$ (RLL I) and t = 2.04, $p > 0.05$ (RLL II); for the competing message condition, t = 0.001, $p > 0.10$ (RLL I) and t = 3.83, $p < 0.002$ (RLL II)]. In the RLL II group, a lower threshold SPL was observed for sentences than for words in the presence of competing speech. Only this latter finding is consistent with previous results obtained with word and sentence materials in adults.[30,32,40,41]

In relating performance for words versus sentences on the PSI test to previous findings in adults, it should be remembered that word and sentence performance in

Table 3. Threshold in decibels SPL: words[a]

	Word Materials	Groups	
		RLL I	RLL II
Present study	PSI-Q	23	22
	PSI-CM	26	25
		3-4 yr olds	5-6 yr olds
Previous studies	PB-K test-Q[b]		37
	A. B. test-Q[c]		20
	TIP-Q[d]	18	14
	Gottinger test-Q[e]	26	20
	Nu-Chips-Q[f]	29	24
	Adult words-Q[g]		
	24-31		

[a]Normal threshold values (50% correct level) in sound pressure level (decibels SPL) for PSI monosyllabic words presented in quiet (Q) and in the presence of a competing message (CM) at a message-to-competition ratio of +4 dB. For comparative purposes, normal data for other word materials are presented. Data from the present study are grouped according to receptive language level (RLL I vs. RLL II). Data from other studies are grouped according to chronological age (3 to 4 yrs vs. 5 to 6 yrs).

[b]Personal unpublished data.[24]

[c]Boothroyd.[7]

[d]Siegenthaler.[39]

[e]Chilla et al.[8]

[f]Elliott and Katz.[13,14] Data obtained by converting sensation level results to hearing level (HL) by adding mean spondee word threshold for group, then converting HL to SPL (0 dB HL = 20 dB SPL).

[g]For References, see text.

adults has traditionally been studied with one or both of the speech materials presented in an open, rather than a closed, message set. Consequently, results based on adult speech materials may not be applicable to PSI results in children. This viewpoint is supported by Wilson and Antablin's[46] recent demonstration that a closed message set paradigm noticeably increased the slope and improved the threshold of monosyllabic word PI functions in adults.

Clinical Feasibility of PI Functions in Children

Is it possible to carry out diagnostic speech audiometry in children in addition to the basic requirements of any pediatric audiological evaluation, e.g., pure-tone audiometry and immittance audiometry? Can children be motivated to cooperate for a sufficient length of time to permit completion of pure-tone, immittance, and diagnostic speech audiometric procedures? In this study, every child completed pure-tone audiometry, the NSST test, and PI functions for PSI words and sentences. In subsequent studies, we added immittance audiometry to the protocol. Our experience suggests that young children can easily complete this test battery. The time required is approximately 1 hr.

Three strategies may underlie success with pediatric audiological testing. First, in relatively younger (RLL I) children, we routinely administered speech audiometry in the sound field. The information gained by PSI speech functions seems to justify the sacrifice of ear-specific

information. To date, the only circumstance in which we have altered this strategy concerns children with markedly asymmetric hearing sensitivity. In these children, we always attempt to obtain PI functions on each ear. However, in young children, complete PSI results may require two separate test sessions.

A second strategy that seems helpful in young children concerns a flexible number of test items (5 versus 10) for individual test conditions. Our theoretical goal is to base percent correct scores (1) on 5 items for performance levels at the ceiling (80 to 100%) and the floor (0 to 20%), and (2) on 10 items for midrange performance levels (21 to 79%). We also try to apply this goal in a practical manner. For example, if initial performance for five items in a very young hearing-impaired child is 60% at 70 dB SPL and 60% at 80 dB SPL, we frequently do not obtain five more items at each test SPL. The percent correct levels for the two intensity levels are consistent and cross-check each other.

Finally, a third important strategy concerns goal-reinforced behavior. We encourage mothers to bring young children to the test session slightly hungry and to allow us to give children candy. Alternatives to candy, such as raisins and cereal, do not aid testing in our experience. A reward for desired behavior is not necessary for each child and, in fact, may be too distracting in some very young children. However, this strategy has allowed us to test several children that seemed uncooperative initially. In short, flexible testing techniques may enable testers,

Table 4. Threshold in decibels SPL: sentences[a]

	Sentence Materials	Groups	
		RLL I	RLL II
Present study	PSI-Q	21	21
	PSI-CM	26	21
			10-15 yr olds
Previous studies	Fry test-Q[b]		31
	Manchester test-Q[b]		32
	BKB Picture test-Q[b]		30
	SSI-CM[c]		34
	Adult sentences-Q:[d]		
	16-18		
	Adult sentences-CM:[c]		
	31		

[a]Normal threshold values (50% correct level) in sound pressure level (decibels SPL) for PSI sentences presented in quiet (Q) and in the presence of a competing message (CM) at a message-to-competition ratio of 0 dB. For comparative purposes, normal data for other sentence materials are presented. Data from the present study are grouped according to receptive language level (RLL I vs. RLL II). Data from other studies are grouped according to chronological age (10 to 15 yrs).
[b]Bamford and Wilson.[1]
[c]Personal unpublished data.[24]
[d]For References, see text.

mothers, and young patients to benefit maximally from pediatric diagnostic audiological evaluations.

Summary

1. The steepness of PSI-PI functions, as defined by the intensity range between 20 and 80% correct performance, was 8 to 10 dB for words in quiet, 10 to 12 dB for words in competition, 8 to 9 dB for sentences in quiet, 10 to 11 dB for sentences in competition.

2. The threshold, or 50% correct level, was 22 to 23 dB SPL for words in quiet, 25 to 26 dB SPL for words in competition, 21 dB SPL for sentences in quiet, and 21 to 26 dB SPL for sentences in competition.

3. In the RLL I versus RLL II groups, the steepness and threshold results for PSI-PI functions were equivalent for sentences and words in quiet and for words in competition (+4 MCR).

4. In the two subject groups, the steepness and threshold results were significantly different for sentences in competition (0 dB MCR).

5. With one exception, CA did not influence the steepness of PSI-PI functions. The exception concerned the increasing steepness with increasing age for sentences in competition.

6. CA did significantly affect threshold results for all PSI speech materials.

7. In relation to other sentence and pediatric word tests, PSI-PI functions were generally steeper and threshold values were generally at lower SPLs.

8. Within each subject group, the steepness and threshold values of PSI-PI functions for words versus sentences were equivalent with one exception. The exception concerned the competing condition in the RLL II group. In this latter group, a lower threshold SPL was observed for sentences than for words in the presence of a competing speech message.

9. Within each subject group, the steepness and threshold values of PSI-PI functions in quiet versus in competition were significantly different with one exception. The exception concerned the sentence materials in the RLL II group. In this latter group, sentence thresholds in quiet versus in competition were equivalent.

10. The median performance decrement at high speech intensity levels for PSI-PI functions in quiet and in competition was 0% (no decrement) for words and sentences with one exception. In the RLL I group, a median decrement of 10% occurred for sentences in competition. For this latter condition, the degree of decrement was significantly greater in the RLL I group than in the RLL II group. The range of performance decrement encompassing 95% of observations in the present normal children was 0 to 10% (words in quiet, RLL I and RLL II groups), 0% (sentences in quiet, both groups), 0 to 40% (words in competition, both groups), 0 to 40% (sentences in competition, RLL I group), and 0 to 10% (sentences in competition, RLL II group).

References

1. Bamford, J., and I. Wilson, 1979. Methodological considerations and practical aspects of the BKB sentence lists. pp.

147-187. in J. Bench, and J. Bamford, eds. *Speech-Hearing Tests and the Spoken Language of Hearing-Impaired Children*. Academic Press, London.

2. Beasley, D., J. Maki, and D. Orchik. 1976. Children's perception of time-compressed speech on two measures of speech discrimination, *J. Speech Hear. Disord.* 41, 216-225.

3. Bench, J., and J. Bamford. 1979. *Speech-Hearing Tests and the Spoken Language of Hearing-Impaired Children*. Academic Press, London.

4. Bench, J., J. Bamford, I. Wilson, and L. Clifft. 1979. A comparison of the BKB sentence lists for children with other speech audiometry tests. *Aust. J. Audiol.* 1, 61-66.

5. Bess, F., A. Josey, and L. Humes. 1979. Performance intensity functions in cochlear and eighth nerve disorders. *Am. J. Otol.* 1, 27-31.

6. Boneau, C. 1971. The effects of violations of assumptions underlying the t test. pp. 357-369. in B. Lieberman, ed. *Contemporary Problems in Statistics. A Book of Readings for the Behavioral Sciences.* Oxford University Press, New York.

7. Boothroyd, A. 1968. Developments in speech audiometry. *Sound* 2, 3-11.

8. Chilla, R., P. Gabriel, P. Kozielski, D. Bansch, and M. Kabas. 1976. Der Gottinger kindersprachverstandnistest. I. Sprachaudiometrie des "kindergarten"—und retardierten kindes mit einem einsilber-bildtest. *H.N.O.* 24, 342-346.

9. Dirks, D., C. Kamm, D. Bower, and A. Betsworth. 1977. Use of performance intensity functions for diagnosis. *J. Speech Hear. Disord.* 42, 408-415.

10. Downie, N.M., and R.W. Heath. 1974. *Basic Statistical Methods.* Ed. 4. Harper & Row, New York.

11. Eagles, E., S. Wishik, L. Doerfler, W. Melnick, and H. Levine. 1963. Hearing sensitivity and related factors in children. *Laryngoscope* 73, 78-104.

12. Elliott, L., S. Connors, E. Kille, S. Levin, K. Ball, and D. Katz. 1979. Children's understanding of monosyllabic nouns in quiet and in noise. *J. Acoust. Soc. Am.* 66, 12-21.

13. Elliott, L., and D. Katz. 1980. Children's pure-tone detection. *J. Acoust. Soc. Am.* 67, 343-344.

14. Elliott, L., and D. Katz. 1980. Development of a new children's test of speech discrimination. Auditec, St. Louis.

15. Fior, R. 1972. Physiological maturation of auditory function between 3 and 13 years of age. *Audiology* 11, 317-321.

16. Fleming, S., J. McClung, and D. Allen. 1977. Sentence and spondee stimuli: responses of hearing impaired children. *Am. Ann. Deaf* 122, 553-556.

17. Fry, D. 1961. Word and sentence tests for use in speech audiometry. *Lancet* 22, 197-199.

18. Guilford, J. 1954. *Psychometric Methods.* McGraw-Hill, New York.

19. Hannley, M., and J. Jerger. 1981. PB rollover and the acoustic reflex. *Audiology* 20, 251-258.

20. Haskins, H. 1949. A phonetically balanced test of speech discrimination for children. M.S. thesis, Northwestern University, Evanston, IL.

21. Hirsh, I., H. Davis, S. Silverman, E. Reynolds, E. Eldert, and R. Benson. 1952. Development of materials for speech audiometry. *J. Speech Hear. Disord.* 17, 321-337.

22. Jerger, J., and D. Hayes. 1977. Diagnostic speech audiometry. *Arch. Otolaryngol.* 103, 216-222.

23. Jerger, J., and S. Jerger. 1971. Diagnostic significance of PB word functions. *Arch. Otolaryngol.* 93, 573-580.

24. Jerger, S. 1980. Unpublished data. Baylor College of Medicine, Houston, TX.

25. Jerger, S., and J. Jerger. 1976. Estimating speech threshold from the PI-PB function. *Arch. Otolaryngol.* 102, 487-496.

26. Jerger, S., and J. Jerger. 1981. *Auditory Disorders. A Manual for Clinical Evaluation.* Little, Brown, and Company, Boston.

27. Jerger, S., J. Jerger, and S. Lewis. 1981. Pediatric speech intelligibility test. II. Effect of receptive language age and chronological age. *Int. J. Pediatr. Otorhinolaryngol* 3, 101-118.

28. Jerger, S., S. Lewis, J. Hawkins, and J. Jerger. 1980. Pediatric speech intelligibility test. I. Generation of test materials. *Int. J. Pediatr. Otorhinolaryngol.* 2, 217-230.

29. Lee, L. 1971. *The Northwestern Syntax Screening Test.* Northwestern University Press, Evanston, IL.

30. Miller, G., G. Heise, and W. Lichten. 1951. The intelligibility of speech as a function of the context of the test materials. *J. Exp. Psychol.* 41, 329-335.

31. Mills, J. 1977. Noise and children: a review of literature. *J. Acoust. Soc. Am.* 58, 767-779.

32. Niemeyer, W. 1965. Speech audiometry with phonetically balanced sentences. *Audiology* 4, 97-101.

33. Norton, D. An empirical investigation of some effects of non-normality and heterogeneity on the F-distribution. Summarized in Lindquist, E. 1971. The Norton study of the effects of non-normality and heterogeneity of variance. pp. 348-356. in B. Lieberman, ed. *Contemporary Problems in Statistics. A Book of Readings for the Behavioral Sciences.* Oxford University Press, New York.

34. Olsen, W., and N. Matkin. 1979. Speech audiometry. pp. 133-206. in W. Rintelmann, ed. *Hearing Assessment.* University Park Press, Baltimore.

35. Palva, A., and K. Jokinen. 1975. Undistorted and filtered speech audiometry in children with normal hearing. *Acta Otolaryngol.* 80, 383-388.

36. Sanders, J., A. Josey, and M. Glasscock. 1974. Audiologic evaluation in cochlear and eighth nerve disorders. *Arch. Otolaryngol.* 100, 283-289.

37. Sanderson-Leepa, M., and W. Rintelmann. 1976. Articulation functions and test-retest performance of normal-hearing children on three speech discrimination tests: WIPI, PBK-50, and NU auditory test no. 6. *J. Speech Hear. Disord.* 41, 503-519.

38. Shirnian, M., and D. Arnst. 1982. Patterns in the performance-intensity functions for phonetically balanced word lists and synthetic sentences in aged listeners. *Arch. Otolaryngol.* 108, 15-20.

39. Siegenthaler, B. 1969. Maturation of auditory abilities in children. *Audiology* 8, 59-71.

40. Silverman, S., and I. Hirsh. 1955. Problems related to the use of speech in clinical audiometry. *Ann. Otol. Rhinol. Laryngol.* 64, 1234-1244.

41. Speaks, C. 1967. Performance-intensity characteristics of selected verbal materials. *J. Speech Hear. Res.* 10, 344-347.

42. Speaks, C., and J. Jerger. 1965. Method for measurement of speech identification. *J. Speech Hear. Res.* 8, 185-194.

43. Speaks, C., J. Jerger, and S. Jerger. 1966. Performance-intensity characteristics of synthetic sentences. *J. Speech Hear. Res.* 9, 305-312.

44. Speaks, C., J. Karmen, and L. Benitez. 1967. Effect of a competing message on synthetic sentence identification. *J. Speech Hear. Res.* 10, 390-396.

45. Watson, T. 1957. Speech audiometry for children. pp. 278-296. in A. Ewing, ed. *Educational Guidance and the Deaf Child.* The Volta Bureau, Washington, DC.

46. Wilson, R., and J. Antablin. 1980. A picture identification task as an estimate of the word-recognition performance of nonverbal adults. *J. Speech Hear. Disord.* 45, 223-238.

Technical Appendix

1. **Procedure.** In a series of 35 normal-hearing children, the correlation between performance scores based on 5 items versus 10 items was 0.90 (RLL I) and 0.92 (RLL II) for words in competition (+4 dB MCR) and 0.56 (RLL I) and 0.89 (RLL II) for sentences in competition (0 dB MCR).

2. **Subjects.** Sample variances were not homogeneous for CA ($F = 2.56$, $p < 0.05$) nor for NSST scores ($F = 8.97$, $p < 0.01$). Consequently, the interpretation of the t ratios reported in the text was corrected according to Norton.[6,33] Standard deviations were 11.1 mos (RLL I) and 7.0 mos (RLL II) for CA and 3.7 (RLL I) and 1.2 (RLL II) for NSST. Sample variances were homogeneous for PTA scores ($F = 1.54$, $p > 0.05$). Standard deviations were 2.4 dB (RLL I) and 3.0 dB (RLL II) for PTA measures.

3. **Steepness characteristics.** For word materials, sample variances for RLL I and RLL II groups were equivalent in quiet ($F = 1.40$, $p > 0.05$) and competing ($F = 2.13$, $p > 0.05$) conditions. For sentence materials, sample variances were equivalent between groups in quiet ($F = 1.17$, $p > 0.05$), but were not homogeneous between groups in competition ($F = 2.43$, $p < 0.05$). For the latter condition, the interpretation of the t ratio was corrected according to Norton.[6,33] The standard error of estimate, corrected for $N < 50$, for predicting the steepness of PSI performance from age was 1.84 dB (words-Q), 3.15 dB (words-CM), 2.06 dB (sentences-Q), and 2.48 dB (sentences-CM). The 95% confidence intervals for r in the population ranged from -0.26 to $+0.35$ (words-Q), -0.35 to $+0.26$ (words-CM), -0.27 to $+0.18$ (sentences-Q), and -0.65 to -0.13 (sentences-CM).

4. **Threshold characteristics.** For word materials, sample variances for RLL I and RLL II groups were homogeneous in quiet ($F = 2.12$, $p > 0.05$), but not in competition ($F = 2.46$, $p < 0.05$). For the latter condition, the interpretation of the t ratio was corrected.[6,33] For sentence materials, sample variances between groups were equivalent in quiet ($F = 1.53$, $p > 0.05$) and in competition ($F = 1.10$, $p > 0.05$). The standard error of estimate, corrected for $N < 50$, for predicting PSI speech thresholds from age was 2.3 dB (PTA), 3.8 dB (words-Q), 4.7 dB (words-CM), 3.8 dB (sentences-Q), and 3.3 dB (sentences-CM). The 95% confidence intervals for r in the population range from -0.70 to -0.22 (PTA), -0.68 to -0.18 (words-Q), -0.69 to -0.21 (words-CM), -0.64 to -0.11 (sentences-Q), and -0.84 to -0.53 (sentences-CM).

Acknowledgments

We thank Sue Abrams and Susan Lewis for assistance in data collection.

Address reprint requests to Susan Jerger, 11922 Taylorcrest, Houston, TX 77024.

Received January 14, 1982
Accepted June 15, 1982

III. Electrophysiologic/Physiologic Methodology

The articles included in this section provide the reader with background on three of the most commonly used procedures to detect auditory dysfunction and to assess auditory system integrity in infants and young children. These measures (aural acoustic immittance, the auditory brainstem response [ABR], and evoked otoacoustic emissions [EOAEs]) have rapidly become incorporated into the pediatric test armamentarium. Although these procedures are sometimes considered "objective" measures (primarily because they require no response from the child), "subjective" decisions are made routinely by audiologists during response interpretation. Thus, appreciating the application and limitations of these procedures is fundamental to pediatric audiology practice. Moreover, the critical importance of developing norms specifically for infants and children, and studying the techniques directly in those who have normal and impaired hearing is highlighted in the series of studies we have chosen to include here.

As clinical tools, aural acoustic immittance, ABR, and EOAEs can be used to evaluate auditory sensitivity in infants and young children who would otherwise be considered "untestable." When an infant is too young, or when a child has neurodevelopmental deficits that preclude reliable behavioral hearing evaluation, electrophysiologic measures become the audiologist's primary assessment tools. However, regardless of the age or developmental level, direct observations of the child's behavioral response to auditory stimuli should always be incorporated into the comprehensive audiologic evaluation (JCIH, 2000). Overall impressions of the child's hearing status gained through behavioral observations (and parent/caregiver report) should be in accord with the outcomes of all physiologic and electrophysiologic tests performed, and vice versa. Indeed, one or more of these measures should routinely be used as a means of cross-checking the validity of behavioral test results (see Jerger and Hayes, 1976; Section II). When the findings lack agreement, suspicion is raised as to the true auditory status of the child. In some circumstances, the outcomes suggested by various procedures will be discordant. In such cases, the findings of one test (behavioral or electrophysiologic/physiologic) should not be dismissed as inconsequential; neither should one measure be deemed "wrong" or "right." Rather, lack of agreement among the test outcomes should be regarded as a provocative clinical challenge. The use of these test procedures provides the pediatric audiologist the opportunity to provide valuable differentiation of heretofore elusive auditory pathologies and to develop the intervention/management strategies necessary for each child's unique auditory disability.

The readings selected for the section on aural acoustic immittance highlight the development of tympanometry and acoustic reflex assessment procedures in the pediatric population. The advent of clinical "impedance" measurement heralded a new and exciting opportunity for pediatric audiologists to "objectively" determine middle ear status in infants and young children, which could not be determined adequately with the use of traditional bone-conduction audiometry. Jerger's 1970 classic description of five tympanogram "types" (A, B, C, As, and Ad) became the most widely used method for classifying middle ear findings in both adults and children. However, currently, the study of aural acoustic immittance (a term used to describe clinical impedance and acoustic admittance assessment) has evolved from simple qualitative tympanogram typing to the more accurate quantification of the features of acoustic admittance (e.g., tympanometric width or gradient, equivalent ear canal volume, peak admittance, and tympanometric peak pressure). Moreover, use of a high probe frequency may be useful for tympanometry in younger infants, allowing clinicians to more fully appreciate subtle changes in middle ear function.

Studies in impedance audiometry in both infants and children proliferated in the early 1970s. In the pediatric population, tympanometry rapidly became the primary means of detecting middle ear dysfunction (otitis media) in young children with and without normal cochlear function. Indeed, there was such excitement about the use of impedance measures that many vigorously advocated for routine tympanometric screening of preschool and school-age children for otitis media (Northern, 1980). However, it was soon apparent that large numbers of children with normal middle ear function and/or transient otitis media were being referred for medical examination based on "abnormal" impedance findings, and critics cautioned about the negative repercussions of such a practice (Bess, 1980). Although several guidelines (e.g., ASHA, 1997) have been proffered regarding the use of acoustic immittance in the screening of young children, the field has yet to fully agree on the protocols.

Impedance technology was also applied to infants in the newborn nursery. Results revealed that with use of the 220-/226-Hz probe frequency, conventional as well as unexpected (W-configuration) tympanogram shapes and absent acoustic reflexes typified this population (Keith, 1973). In 1976, Paradise, Smith, and Bluestone directly examined the efficiency of tympanometry in the detection of middle ear effusion in children 10 days to 5 years of age. Paradise and his colleagues devised seven general tympanogram types and examined them against the only acceptable "gold standard": findings at surgery. Paradise and coworkers found flat (low compliance) tympanograms were highly correlated with the presence of middle ear effusion, but other patterns (neither "normal" nor "flat") lacked reasonable accord with surgical findings. In this study, conventional tympanometry was often not sensitive to the presence of middle ear effusion in infants less than 7 months of age. Infants with confirmed middle ear fluid demonstrated "normal" tympanograms (a false negative finding). The result was attributable to the highly distensible ear canals of infants. This finding led some clinicians to abandon impedance testing in infants below the age of 7 months. Later studies by Marchant and his colleagues (1986), among others, demonstrated the usefulness of a higher, 660-Hz probe frequency for detecting middle ear effusion in infants 4 months of age and younger for both tympanometry and acoustic reflex assessment.

The quantification of tympanometric gradient in preschool-age children is described by Koebsell and Margolis. This study serves as the normative data base by which we have come to judge the normality of the tympanogram. Toward a similar goal, Nozza, Bluestone, Kardatzke, and Bachman examined the sensitivity, specificity, positive and negative predictive value of various acoustic admittance features (e.g., tympanometric width, peak admittance, peak pressure, equivalent volume), the acoustic reflex, and pneumatic otoscopy for the detection of middle ear effusion. Individual acoustic admittance features and their combination were examined against pneumatic otoscopy as well as findings at myringotomy (the gold standard). Three populations of children were studied: One group had normal middle ear histories and were selected to represent the general population, a second group had documented histories of chronic middle ear disease, and a third cohort of children were awaiting myringotomies with tubes for relief of middle ear effusion. Nozza and his coworkers found that the efficiency of acoustic admittance features and pneumatic otoscopy were highly dependent on the characteristics of the population studied. Because the sensitivity and the specificity of each of the features are systematically detailed in this study, clinicians may determine the accuracy that is most acceptable for their own clinical purpose. The paper by Roush, Drake, and Sexton compares two screening protocols that are used regularly for the detection of middle ear dysfunction in young school-age children. The findings of this study underscore the responsibility that the pediatric audiologist must assume for fully appreciating the consequence of selecting a screening protocol. Finally, in this section a paper by Keefe and colleagues describes the usefulness of a new middle ear measurement technique—wide-band reflectance in a newborn hearing screening protocol. In this report, reflectance measures revealed inadequate probe fitting in the ear canal during OAE screening, which could have accounted for some of the test failures. This new technique, although not currently available clinically, shows great promise for delineating middle ear function in the pediatric population more efficiently than has been previously possible.

The importance of ABR in the pediatric audiology setting cannot be overemphasized. This electrophysiologic procedure has made it possible for audiologists to estimate hearing sensitivity and determine the integrity of the auditory pathway to the level of the brainstem. Again, the studies presented here are representative of the numerous studies that exist on the application of ABR in the pediatric population. In their classic 1977 paper, Starr and colleagues detail the now familiar maturation of the ABR in infants 25 to 44 weeks of age. Importantly, they also present atypical patterns of the ABR which were documented in several cases of infants with cochlear and brainstem dysfunction. These authors were among the first to predict the great clinical utility of the ABR for assessing very young and difficult-to-test children. Gorga and colleagues further describe developmental changes in the ABR in infants from 3 months to 3 years of age. Because of the large number of children studied (over 500) and the strict data inclusion criteria utilized, their data are extremely valuable toward our appreciating the maturation of absolute ABR wave latencies, interwave latency differences, and interaural symmetry of the response. The study by Hyde, Riko, and Malizia describes the relationship of ABR thresholds obtained in the newborn period to conventional audiometric test findings from the same children at later ages. Although the ABR was found to be very useful in the identification of children with sensorineural hearing loss, a limitation of the conventional click-ABR was the lack of frequency-specific audiometric information. The study by Stapells, Gravel, and Martin demonstrates that one frequency-specific ABR technique (tones-in-notched noise) provides valid information on audiometric configuration in infants and children with normal hearing and with sensorineural hearing loss. Then Yang and colleagues describe the use of bone-conducted ABR threshold assessment for differentiating conductive from cochlear hearing loss. When the goal of the ABR assessment is to provide information similar to that available through conventional audiometry, the utility of these latter procedures is obvious. The last paper in this section on auditory evoked potentials presents findings from Australian researcher Field Rickards and his colleagues who describe the application of the auditory steady state response (ASSR) for screening hearing in neonates. The advent of ASSR technology portends a measurement technique useful for identification and assessment in the pediatric population, particularly because of its inherent frequency-specificity. More research on the performance characteristics of the ASSR is needed, however, before its use in the pediatric clinical setting is fully delineated.

The last series of articles focuses on studies of both transient- (click-) evoked otoacoustic emissions and distortion product otoacoustic emissions in the assessment of infants and children at risk for peripheral hearing impairments. The various applications of otoacoustic emissions in the pediatric population are overviewed by Norton and Widen. Next,

Smurzynski and his colleagues present a systematic and detailed analysis of the properties of both distortion-product and transient-evoked otoacoustic emissions in both premature and full-term infants. Their study provides valuable normative data for these populations.

All of these techniques provide pediatric audiologists the opportunity to gain new and unique insights into the integrity of the cochlea and portions of the central auditory pathway. Electrophysiologic/physiologic test procedures are intregal components of the audiologic test battery for the determination of the type and degree of hearing loss. Moreover, their usefulness for screening assessment and follow-up of infants and children who have or are suspected of having permanent or transient hearing loss cannot be overemphasized.

References

ASHA. 1997. Guideline for audiologic screening. *American Speech-Language-Hearing Association Panel on Audiologic Assessment* Rockville, MD: Author.

Bess, F.H. 1980. Impedance screening for children: A need for more research. *Annals of Otology, Rhinology and Laryngology* 89(3)(Suppl. 68):228-232.

Jerger, J. 1970. Clinical experience with impedance audiometry. *Archives of Otolaryngology* 92:311-324.

Joint Committee on Infant Hearing (JCIH). 2000. *Position Statement and Guidelines* (www.jcih.org).

Keith, R.W. 1973. Impedance audiometry with neonates. *Archives of Otolaryngology* 96:465-467.

Marchant, C., McMillan, P., Shurin, P., et al. 1986. Objective diagnosis of otitis media in early infancy by tympanometry and ipsilateral acoustic reflex thresholds. *Journal of Pediatrics* 109:390-395.

Northern, J.L. 1980. Impedance screening: An integral part of hearing screening. *Annals of Otology, Rhinology and Laryngology* 89(3)(Suppl. 68):233-235.

Additional Readings

Bergman, B.M., Gorga, M.P., Neely, S.T., Kaminski, K.L., and Peters, J. 1995. Preliminary descriptions of transient-evoked and distortion-product otoacoustic emissions from graduates of an intensive care nursery. *Journal of the American Academy of Audiology* 6:150-162.

Despland, P., and Galambos, R. 1980. The auditory brainstem response (ABR) is a useful diagnostic tool in the intensive care nursery. *Pediatric Research* 14:154-158.

Glattke, T.J., Pafitis, I.A., Cummiskey, C., and Herer, G.R. 1995. Identification of hearing loss in children and young adults using measures of transient otoacoustic emission reproducibility. *American Journal of Audiology* 4(3):71-86.

Gorga, M.P., Reiland, J.K., Beauchaine, K.L., Worthington, D.W., and Jesteadt, W. 1987. Auditory brainstem responses from graduates of an intensive care nursery: Normal patterns of response. *Journal of Speech and Hearing Research* 30:311-318.

Holte, L., Margolis, R.H., and Cavanaugh, R.M. 1991. Developmental changes in multifrequency tympanograms. *Audiology* 30:1-24.

Prieve, B.A. 1992. Otoacoustic emissions in infants and children: Basic characteristics and clinical application. *Seminars in Hearing* 13(1):37-52.

Salamy, A. 1984. Maturation of the auditory brainstem response from birth through early childhood. *Journal of Clinical Neurophysiology* 1:293-329.

Sininger, Y. 1995. Filtering and spectral characteristics of ABR and noise in infants. *Journal of the Acoustical Society of America* 98:2048-2055.

Stapells, D.R. 1989. Auditory brainstem response assessment of infants. *Seminars in Hearing* 10:229-251.

Tympanometric Detection of Middle Ear Effusion in Infants and Young Children

Jack L. Paradise, M.D., Clyde G. Smith, M.S., and Charles D. Bluestone, M.D.
From the Departments of Pediatrics, Community Medicine, and Otolaryngology, University of Pittsburgh School of Medicine, the Ambulatory Care Center, Children's Hospital of Pittsburgh, and the University of Pittsburgh Cleft Palate Center and the Department of Speech and Theatre Arts, Pittsburgh, Pennsylvania

Abstract

Tympanometry, a test of middle ear status new to clinical pediatrics, was carried out on 280 subjects, 10 days through 5 years of age. The tympanograms obtained were compared with otoscopic findings and, in 107 of the subjects, with findings at myringotomy. Seven distinct tympanometric curve types were identified and defined, based on their degree of correlation with the presence or absence of middle ear effusion.

In subjects 7 months of age and older, curves suggesting normal (high) tympanic membrane compliance in combination with atmospheric or near-atmospheric middle ear air pressure were rarely associated with effusion. Conversely, curves suggesting low tympanic membrane compliance were highly correlated with the presence of effusion. Curves suggesting intermediate compliance or reduced middle ear air pressure were also correlated with effusion, but the degree of correlation was dependent on the shape of the curve.

In infants less than 7 months of age, many of the ears with effusion had " normal" tympanograms, presumably because external auditory canal walls in such infants tend to be highly distensible.

Tympanometry is a simple, rapid, atraumatic, valid, and objective test, easily administered by paraprofessional personnel. Its use can result in improved detection of middle ear effusion and other middle ear abnormalities, and also appears to promote improvement in diagnostic acumen. *Pediatrics, 58:198-210, 1976, Ear, Tympanometry, Diagnosis.*

Middle ear disease is widely prevalent among infants and young children,[1-6] but readily escapes detection since (1) symptoms are often absent or inapparent; (2) otoscopic examination is often difficult to accomplish satisfactorily; and (3) tympanic membrane abnormalities are often subtle and difficult to appreciate. Therefore a method for detecting middle ear disease that does not depend on observation of the tympanic membrane would seem valuable. Pure-tone audiometry has traditionally been used for this purpose as a screening test, but in infants and young children it is impracticable, and in older children it may often fail to detect significant middle ear abnormalities, particularly effusion.[1,5,7-11]

Several studies[7-17] reported in otolaryngologic and audiologic journals suggest that tympanometry—a simple, objective test procedure—can detect middle ear effusion reliably in preschool and school-age children. When compared with pure-tone audiometry in this regard, tympanometry has been found appreciably superior.[8-11] However, the results of these studies have not been readily applicable to pediatric clinical practice because (1) systems for classifying tympanometric data have been imprecise; (2) detailed correlations of tympanometric and otoscopic data have not been presented; (3) data correlating tympanometric findings with findings at myringotomy are scant [7,8,16,17]; and (4) virtually no data have been reported for infants or children under 3 years of age.

In order to further assess the feasibility and validity of tympanometry in the clinical diagnosis of middle ear effusion during the first six years of life, we compared tympanometric findings with independent otoscopic findings in 280 infants and children. In 107 of these subjects, tympanometric and otoscopic findings were compared with middle ear findings at myringotomy.

Tympanometry

Tympanometry is a technique for indirectly characterizing tympanic membrane compliance and estimating middle ear air pressure by means of electroacoustic and

Reproduced with permission from *Pediatrics*, 58:198-210. Copyright 1976 by the AAP.

(Received August 8, 1975; revision accepted for publication March 18, 1976.) Read in part before the second annual meeting of the Society for Ear, Nose, and Throat Advances in Children, San Francisco, California, October 18, 1974.

A portion of this study was done in partial fulfillment of requirements for the degree of Master of Science at the University of Pittsburgh (C.G.S.).

Address for reprints: (J.L.P.) Children's Hospital of Pittsburgh, 125 De Soto Street, Pittsburgh, Pennsylvania 15213.

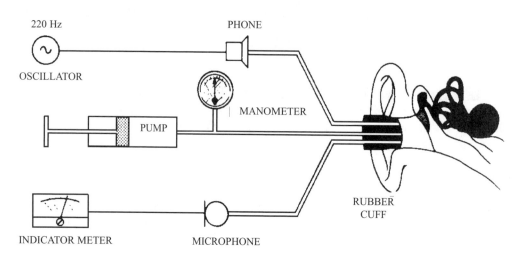

Figure 1. Simplified schematic diagram of the electroacoustic impedance bridge.

manometric measurements. These measurements are carried out in the external auditory canal by an instrument known as an *electroacoustic impedance bridge.* The instruments in current use derive from one described in 1934 by Schuster,[18] first applied clinically in 1946 by Metz,[19] and subsequently modified by Terkildsen and Nielsen[20] and Zwislocki.[21]

The design and function of the impedance bridge and the details of the test procedure have been reviewed previously.[7,12-14,22] Briefly stated, a probe tip is hermetically sealed in the external auditory canal by means of a tightly fitting rubber cuff, thus converting the external canal into a closed chamber (Fig. 1). The tip carries three tubes connected respectively to (1) an oscillator-receiver that delivers a fixed-frequency tone, (2) a microphone that monitors sound-pressure level, and (3) a pump-manometer that varies and measures air pressure. The tone is introduced at a given intensity, and the sound-pressure level in the external canal is monitored while air pressure is artificially varied from +200 mm to –400 mm H_2O. Under normal circumstances, as the tympanic membrane is stiffened by either positive or negative external-canal air pressure, its impedance is increased and its compliance reduced. Sound reflection by the tympanic membrane increases accordingly, and the sound-pressure level in the canal rises. Since the sound-pressure level is being continuously monitored, and since changes in the level are directly translatable into changes in tympanic membrane compliance, a continuous reading of tympanic membrane compliance is made available. A curve showing the changes in tympanic membrane compliance that occur in response to changes in external-canal air pressure is plotted; this curve is referred to as a *tympanogram* (Fig. 2,a).

As described by Brooks,[7] the tympanogram may be defined in terms of its three major characteristics: (1)

height of the peak; (2) location of the peak in relation to atmospheric pressure; and (3) rate of change in curve height in the vicinity of the peak, or gradient.

A variety of conditions may produce alterations in the shape of the tympanogram or the location of its peak. A flattened tympanogram, with low peak and gradual gradient (Fig. 2, b), suggests that tympanic membrane compliance is reduced and that its response to changes in external-canal air pressure is dampened. Tympanograms of this type are found when liquid has replaced much or all of the air in the middle ear cavity, or when the tympanic membrane or ossicular chain have been stiffened by scarring or other pathological change.

A tympanogram whose peak is shifted toward the negative (Fig. 2, c) is indicative of negative air pressure in the middle ear, a condition commonly attributed to eustachian tube dysfunction. The negative pressure causes retraction of the tympanic membrane, with resultant stretching and reduction in compliance. Peak compliance is restored only when, during the tympanometric procedure, air pressure in the external canal is artificially lowered to the point that the tympanic membrane is returned momentarily to the neutral position.≠

An "open" tympanogram (Fig. 2, d) results when tympanic membrane compliance exceeds the recording capacity of the instrument. Such curves are recorded from some ears that are normal, and from others with atrophic scarring of the tympanic membrane.

True tympanograms cannot be recorded from ears with perforated tympanic membranes or with tympanostomy tubes. Curves that resemble flattened tympanograms can sometimes be obtained from such ears, but they are almost always readily distinguishable on the basis of certain technical readings obtained in the course of carrying out the test procedure.

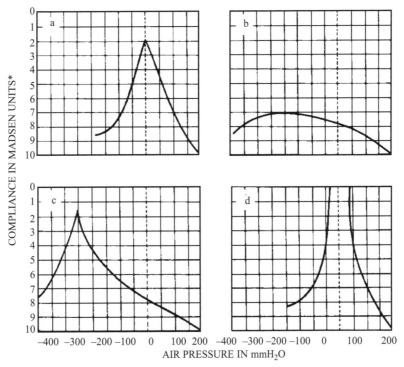

Figure 2. Some typical tympanograms: *a*, peaked (high peak and steep gradient), with peak located at or near atmospheric pressure; *b*, flattened or rounded (low peak and gradual gradient); *c*, peaked, with peak located in negative-pressure zone; *d*, open. *Madsen units are the arbitrarily designated units of compliance displayed by the Model ZO 70 instrument. Note that they are numbered paradoxically, so that 0 is the maximum and 10 is the minimum.

Tympanometry seems ideally suited as a test procedure for infants and young children because it (1) is entirely objective and does not depend on the subject's perception of, or response to sound; (2) can be carried out in practically any acoustic environment; (3) requires little, if any, immobilization of the subject; (4) is atraumatic; (5) can be administered quickly; and (6) is not affected by amounts of cerumen ordinarily present in the external auditory canal.

Subjects and Methods

Two groups of patients were studied during the period from May 25, 1972, through May 9, 1974. Group A consisted of 107 infants and children who had been scheduled by physicians other than the authors for

myringotomy and insertion of tympanostomy tubes because of recurrent acute otitis media or persistent middle ear effusion or both. Group B consisted of 173 infants and children not receiving myringotomy, but selected on the basis of availability and parental willingness from among those in various outpatient waiting areas of the Children's Hospital of Pittsburgh. Inquiry was not made as to the nature of their presenting complaints, but some were attending for well-child care, some had respiratory symptoms, some had miscellaneous medical or surgical problems, and some were siblings of patients. The study subjects ranged in age from 10 days through 5 years 11 months; 66 were black and 214 were white. Table I shows their distribution by age and sex.

Each subject received both tympanometry and otoscopic examination within a one-hour period. In group A subjects, both procedures were completed within the two-hour period preceding myringotomy. For each subject the findings of each procedure—tympanometry, otoscopy, and myringotomy if done—were recorded independently and without knowledge of other findings.

Children old enough to cooperate for the tympanometric procedure were usually seated (Fig. 3); younger children and infants either lay on an examining table or were held by parents. In order to maintain the degree of inactivity necessary for completing the test, some infants

≠Previous descriptions of tympanometry have failed to take cognizance of the fact, recently emphasized by Ingelstedt,[23] that negative middle ear air pressure is but one of various forces that may oppose outward movement of the tympanic membrane as external canal air pressure is lowered. Other such forces include elasticity and/or scarring of the membrane itself, or surface-tension effects attributable to the presence of small amounts of liquid in the middle ear. Thus, when the curve peak is shifted toward negative, its location does not necessarily, as commonly thought, provide an indirect measure of actual middle ear air pressure, but rather, indicates the amount of negative pressure in the external auditory canal necessary to exert an outward-pulling force on the tympanic membrane equal to the resultant of all countervailing forces within the middle ear or tympanic membrane itself.

Table I. Age and sex of 280 subjects receiving both tympanometric and otoscopic examination.

Age (mos)	Total in Age Group	Myringotomy (Group A)		No Myringotomy (Group B)	
		Male	Female	Male	Female
1 to 6	43	9	2	19	13
7 to 11	20	2	3	12	3
12 to 23	38	10	4	15	9
24 to 35	39	4	8	20	7
36 to 47	48	8	8	17	15
48 to 59	49	19	6	9	15
60 to 71	43	10	14	11	8
Total	280	62	45	103	70

were given a pacifier or fed from a bottle. All tympanometric procedures were carried out by an audiologist (C.G.S.), using a Madsen Electroacoustic Impedance Meter, Model Z0 70.† For subjects with external canals too small to admit the probe tip fitted with a standard rubber cuff, the tip was fitted instead with a short (one-half inch) sleeve of 8 ˘ Œ-inch rubber tubing, which was in turn inserted firmly into the canal in order to achieve an airtight seal. Tympanograms were plotted manually on the basis of readings obtained at intervals of 50 mm H_2O over a pressure range of +200 to –400 mm H_2O. The locations of tympanogram peaks were determined by monitoring the movement of the balance meter needle continuously. Peak locations that fell between the 50-mm demarcations were ascertained within 10 mm.‡ When minor oscillations of the meter needle occurred as a result of infants' sucking, readings were recorded at the midpoints of these oscillations. Crying sometimes affected meter readings, but consistent readings could usually be obtained during the short intervals between cries. The duration of the test procedure varied from about 5 to 15 minutes.

All otoscopic examinations were performed by a pediatrician (J.L.P.) using a standard, hermetically intact, pneumatic otoscope. When necessary, cerumen was removed from the external auditory canal with a blunt curette or cotton-tipped metal applicator. The following characteristics of each tympanic membrane were recorded: presence of either bulging or retraction, color, degree of translucency, presence of appreciable scarring, presence of air-fluid level, and degree of mobility on an arbitrary scale of 0 to +4. In diagnosing effusion all abnormalities of the tympanic membrane were taken into account, but

the minimum criterion for the diagnosis was impaired mobility, except in a few instances in which air-fluid levels were visible. For each ear, effusion was recorded as either "present," "absent," or "suspected."

Myringotomy was carried out under general anesthesia, and with an operating microscope, by or under the supervision of one of two otolaryngologists, who recorded the presence or absence of effusion in the middle ear after each operation.

Results

Correlations Between Otoscopic Diagnoses and Findings at Myringotomy

Table II shows that in 107 group A subjects receiving myringotomy, effusion was found in 139 of the 214 ears and not found in 75. Among the 139 ears with effusion at myringotomy, the otoscopic diagnosis had been "effusion" in 127 (91%) and "suspected effusion" in 9 (7%). Of the remaining three ears (2%), two had been considered effusion-free and one had not been examined. Among the 75 ears without effusion at myringotomy, 56 (75%) had been considered effusion-free, 6 (8%) had been considered suspect, and 13 (17%) had been thought to contain effusion.

Overall, in the 214 ears, there was agreement between otoscopic diagnoses and findings at myringotomy in 86% and disagreement in 7%, while in the remaining 7% otoscopic diagnoses had been indefinite. These correlations seemed sufficiently high to justify using the investigator's otoscopic diagnosis as the standard for validating the tympanometric curves recorded from group B subjects.

Feasibility of Tympanometric Testing

Tympanometric curves were recorded from 531 ears of the 280 subjects in groups A and B. Curves could not be obtained from one ear in each of 29 subjects: 19 had a tympanic membrane perforation or an indwelling tympanostomy tube; in 5 there was inadequate subject cooperation or excessive movement; and in 5 the external auditory canal could not be hermetically sealed.

---

†Madsen Electronics (Canada) Limited, 1074 South Service Road, Oakville, Ontario L6J5B4.

‡Linear X-Y plotters that record automatically are available, and in cooperative subjects offer somewhat greater ease of operation and less risk of error. However, in infants and young children who are crying or moving about, automatic plotting often results in artifact-filled curves that cannot be readily interpreted.

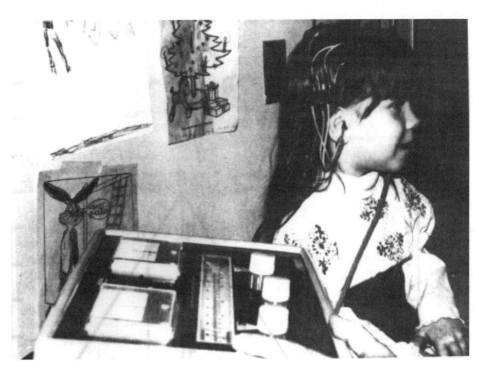

Figure 3. Four-year-old child receiving tympanometry.

Types of Tympanograms and Correlations with Middle Ear Effusion

For the most part, the tympanograms appeared to be of types similar to those described in studies of older children.[7,8,14] On the other hand—and also as noted in other series[12]—the three main characteristics of the tympanograms—peak height, peak location, and peak gradient—appeared each to vary so widely, and to occur in such a variety of combinations, as to constitute a virtual continuum. In order to arrive at a scheme for classifying tympanograms that would be practical clinically, we set out to group them according to their association with the

Table II. Otoscopic diagnoses and findings at myringotomy (214 ears of 107 subjects 2 months through 5 years of age).

Otoscopic Diagnoses	Findings at Myringotomy	
	No. of Ears With Effusion	No. of Ears Without Effusion
Effusion	127≠	13
Suspect	9	6
No effusion	2	56†
Not examined	1	0
Total	139	75

≠Two ears were discharging.
†Eleven ears had tympanostomy tubes or perforations.

presence or absence of effusion at myringotomy, or when myringotomy was not done, diagnoses at otoscopy.

Poor Correlation Below 7 Months of Age—Early in the study it became apparent that correlations between tympanometric curves and clinical findings were much less consistent in infants 6 months of age or younger than in older subjects. *Therefore, only curves from subjects 7 months of age and older were used in formulating the following classification scheme.*

Classification Criteria—All of the individual curve peaks were plotted on a matrix in which the X coordinate represented air pressure and the Y coordinate represented compliance units. Peaks of tympanograms of ears with effusion and of ears without effusion tended to cluster separately, but there were also transitional areas and areas of appreciable overlap. On inspection of the individual curves whose peaks were located within areas, it became apparent that the gradients of these curves (Fig. 4) influenced their correlations with the presence or absence of effusion. It therefore seemed logical to develop a classification scheme whose primary divisions were based on *air pressure-compliance relationships,* and whose secondary divisions were based on *gradient.* Numeric demarcations were chosen to create categories and subcategories most strongly correlated with the presence or absence of effusion.

Air Pressure Compliance Relationships—Five air pressure (in mm H_2O)-compliance (in Madsen units) zones defining curve peak locations were designated (Fig. 5):

(1) Normal (NL)—air pressure at or near atmospheric (−100 to +50), and compliance high (< 4.5).

(2) High-negative pressure (HN)—air pressure high-negative (< −100), and compliance high (< 5.0).

(3) Transitional (TR)—air pressure at or near atmospheric (−100 to +50), and compliance intermediate (4.5 through 5.5).

(4) Effusion (EFF)—air pressure covers a wide range (< +50), and compliance low, but to some extent pressure-related (> 5.5 if pressure > −100; < 5.0 if pressure < −100).

(5) High-positive pressure (HP)—air pressure high (∅ +50), and compliance high (0 through 4.4).

Gradient—Curve gradient proved *consistently* important in distinguishing effusion from noneffusion in only two of the zones: HN and TR. Gradients equal to or less than 0.15 were designated "gradual" (g); those greater than 0.15 were designated "steep" (s). Thus, a tympanogram whose peak was located in the transitional zone and whose gradient was gradual was designated TR-g; one whose peak was in the high-negative pressure zone and whose gradient was steep was designated HN-s.

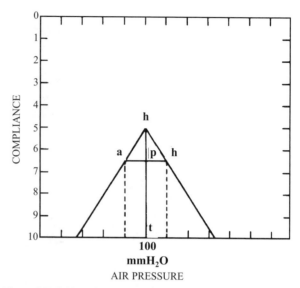

Figure 4. Definition of tympanometric gradient. Gradient is defined as the ratio hp/ht, where ht equals the overall height the overall height of the tympanogram, and hp equals the vertical distance from the peak of the tympanogram to a horizontal line intersecting the tympanogram so that its width between the points of intersection (a,b) is 100 mm H₂O. The higher the ratio hp/ht, the steeper the gradient. (Adapted from Brooks[12]).

Clinical Correlations in Subjects 7 Months Through 5 Years of Age

The correlations between tympanogram types and the presence or absence of effusion that emerged from this classification scheme are summarized in Table III (subjects receiving myringotomy—group A) and Table IV (subjects not receiving myringotomy—group B). The results in the two groups were quite similar even though the prevalence of effusion was relatively high in group A and relatively low in group B. Taken together, the tables show that type NL tympanograms were *rarely* associated with effusion, whereas types TR-g and EFF were *usually* associated with effusion. Between these extremes, and in increasing order of likelihood of being associated with effusion, lay types TR-s, HN-s, and HN-g.

Type HP curves were found in only seven ears; of these, four appeared normal and three had otoscopic findings indicating acute infection.

As the combined data indicate, tympanographic elements associated with effusion are (1) low curve peak, (2) displacement toward negative of the curve peak, and (3) gradual gradient. Review of the individual curves indicated further that *within* each of the zones shown in Figure 5, the curves that had one or more of these elements in extreme degree were the ones most consistently associated with effusion.

While the data from groups A and B are similar, those from group B are more appropriate for estimating the general probability of effusion in relation to specific types of tympanograms, since group B subjects were more representative of the population at large. These probabilities are shown in Figure 5. Probabilities in other populations might differ slightly depending on the prevalence of effusion.

Figure 6 shows commonly encountered variants of the tympanogram types defined above.

Age, Sex, and Race—Within the group of patients from 7 months through 5 years of age, further subdivision into narrower age categories identified no significant age-related differences in the correlations between tympanometric patterns and the presence or absence of effusion. Similarly, neither sex nor race appeared to be factors in these correlations.

Subjects Less Than Seven Months of Age

Of the 43 infants less than 7 months of age, 6 (10 ears studied) were aged 1 month or less; 22 (43 ears studied) were aged 2 or 3 months; and 15 (28 ears studied) were aged 4 through 6 months.

Among the 11 infants receiving myringotomy (group A), effusion was found in each of the 21 ears operated on. (Otoscopically the diagnosis of effusion had been considered certain in 19 and suspect in 2 of these ears.) Among

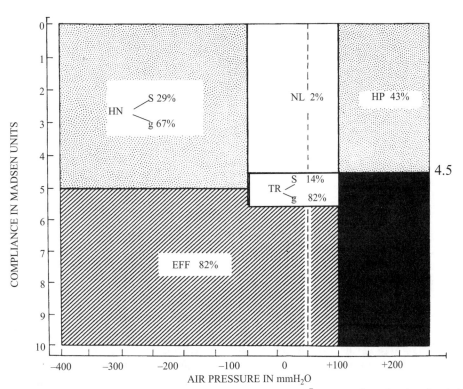

Figure 5. Probability of middle ear effusion in relation to tympanometric zones and gradients. See text for explanation of symbols. Percentages are derived from data summarized in Table IV.

the 32 infants who did not receive myringotomy (group B), otoscopic diagnoses were available for 60 ears. Thus, correlations between tympanometric findings on the one hand, and myringotomy or otoscopic findings on the other, were available for 81 ears. These correlations are shown in Table V.

As seen in Table V, 12 of the 13 "most abnormal" curves (each of the eight type EFF curves and four of the five type TR-g curves) were associated with definite or presumed middle ear effusion. Thus, the curve types that in subjects aged 7 months or older had been found to be associated with middle ear effusion were also associated with effusion in this age group. Conversely, however, curves that in the 7-months or over age group were almost invariably associated with normal ears were in this age group often associated with effusion: of the 64 "most normal" curve types (60 type NL and 4 type TR-s), 32 were associated with definite, presumed, or suspected effusion.

External-Auditory-Canal Wall Compliance as a Variable in Tympanometry

Previously reported analyses of tympanometric curves have been predicated on an assumption that during tympanometry, while external-auditory-canal air pressure is

being artificially altered, the wall of the canal remains essentially rigid. Yet, during pneumatic otoscopy in many infants and young children, the canal wall can easily be seen to distend. Surmising that this distensibility (compliance) might be an additional factor of consequence in determining the characteristics of the tympanogram, and might help explain the poor correlation between tympanometric findings and otologic status in infants less than 7

Table III. Tympanogram types and finding at myringotomy (177 ears of 96 subjects 7 months through 5 years of age).

Type of Tympanogram	Total		No. of Ears With Effusion		No. of Ears Without Effusion	
	No.	%	No.	%	No.	%
NL	38	100	2	5	36	95
HN-s	13	100	4	31	9	69
HN-g	28	100	24	86	4	14
TR-s	3	100	0	0	3	100
TR-g	6	100	5	83	1	17
EFF	89	100	79	89	10	11
HP	0	0	—	—	—	—
Total	177	100	114	64	63	36

Table IV. Tympanogram types and otoscopic diagnoses (273 ears of 141 selected outpatients and others 7 months through 5 years of age).

Type of Tympanogram	Total		No. of Ears With Effusion		No. of Ears With Suspect Effusion		No. of Ears Without Effusion	
	No.	%	No.	%	No.	%	No.	%
NL	129	100	2	2	0	0	127	98
HN-s	46	100	10	22	3	7	33	72
HN-g	15	100	9	60	1	7	5	33
TR-s	27	100	2	7	2	7	23	85
TR-g	11	100	9	82	0	0	2	18
EFF	38	100	31	82	0	0	7	18
HP	7	100	3	43	0	0	4	57
Total	273	100	66	24	6	2	201	74

months of age, we graded the canal wall distensibility of all study subjects on an arbitrary scale of 0 to +4. These data are summarized in Figure 7, and indicate that distensibility indeed appears to vary inversely with age, with the sharpest drop-off occuring just after 6 months of age.

Discussion

Correlations Between Tympanograms and Middle Ear Effusion and the Effects of Age

The present study provides new information concerning the validity of tympanometric testing in three pediatric age groups. In 4- and 5-year-old children it affords more precise correlations than heretofore available between specific tympanometric curve types and the presence or absence of middle ear effusion. In the 7-month through 3-year age group it indicates that tympanometric curve types and their correlations with the presence or absence of effusion are essentially the same as in 4- and 5-year-olds. And, in infants less than 7 months of age it demonstrates that while "abnormal" tympanograms appear to have the same significance as in older subjects, "normal" tympanograms are of no diagnostic value, since they may be associated in such infants with either effusion or the absence of effusion.

It appears reasonable to relate this latter finding to the hitherto unnoted fact that in infants less than 7 months of age, external auditory canal wall compliance is much greater than in older individuals. Given high compliance of the canal wall, it seems expected that electroacoustic-manometric measurements *within* the sealed canal might be unable to differentially identify reduced compliance of the tympanic membrane.

These presumably related structural and tympanometric features that distinguish very young infants would

appear to render untenable the assumption in certain recent studies[24-26] that, in newborns, "normal" tympanograms can be taken as evidence of mobile tympanic membranes and effusion-free middle ears.

It remains to be established whether the inability of tympanometry to identify effusion in infants less than 7 months of age can be overcome by using another instrument, the Grason-Stadler Otoadmittance Meter,§ which, among other differences from the Madsen bridge, is designed to measure components of impedance separately. In children 1 year of age and older, testing with this instrument has produced results[16,17] that appear comparable to those obtained in the present study, but studies of the

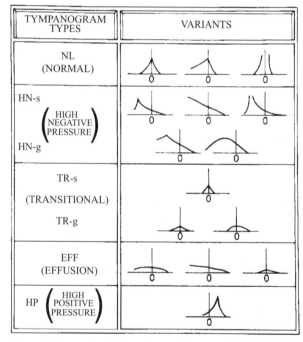

Figure 6. Commonly encountered examples of types of tympanograms.

Table V. Tympanogram types and middle ear status as determined by findings at myringotomy or otoscopic diagnoses (81 ears of 43 infants less than 7 months of age).

Type of Tympanogram	Total	Findings at Myringotomy or Otoscopic Diagnoses		
		No. of Ears With Effusion	No. of Ears With Suspected Effusion	No. of Ears Without Effusion
NL	60	24	6	30
HN-s	3	2	0	1
HN-g	1	0	0	1
TR-s	4	2	0	2
TR-g	5	4	0	1
EFF	8	8	0	0
HP	0	—	—	—
Total	81	40	6	35

validity of otoadmittance curves in younger infants have not been reported.

Why Detect Apparently Asymptomatic Effusions?

The value of any method of clinical detection depends first of all on the degree to which the condition to be identified threatens health, well-being, and present or future function. It is well known that middle ear effusion causes hearing impairment of varying degree in subjects old enough to test audiometrically, and it seems expected that the same relationship obtains in younger subjects as well. If in fact young children and infants with long-standing effusions (chronic serous otitis media) are hearing-deficient, to what extent are they thereby handicapped or at risk?

Persistent, severe impairment of hearing is obviously disabling, but the immediate and longterm effects of mild or moderate impairments that persist for long periods are unknown and difficult to assess. A few studies[27-29] suggest that such impairments, even if they are ultimately relieved, may have lasting adverse effects (inasmuch as they occurred during critically formative periods) on both cognitive development and skill in the use of language. In view of the high prevalence of chronic middle ear effusion, further study of these possible relationships is urgently needed.

Other possible effects or sequelae of chronic middle ear effusion include heightened susceptibility to middle ear infection,[30] adhesions and scarring,[31] and cholesteatoma.[32,33]

Although the clinical importance of chronic middle ear effusion remains insufficiently understood, and its natural history insufficiently elaborated, information now available points to the advisability of identifying persis-

tent effusion in apparently asymptomatic infants and children.

Tympanometry for Screening

Tympanometry appears promising at present as a screening test not only for school-age children, but also for infants and children in day-care and nursery-school settings, for whom no practicable screening test is now available. However, both the present study and most previous studies of tympanometry have dealt mainly with patients who had otologic or other clinical problems, whereas few studies of the validity of tympanometry as a screening test have been reported.[9-11,34] These, moreover, have been limited in both scope and detail. Further evaluation of its feasibility and validity is therefore needed in pediatric populations of various ages and backgrounds.

Tympanometry and Abnormalities Other Than Effusion

Middle ear effusion is the main but not the only significant otologic abnormality in infants and children that is detectable tympanometrically. Impacted cerumen is often associated with abnormal or bizarre curve patterns. Scarring of the type that limits compliance of the tympanic membrane or ossicles results in type TR-g or EFF tympanograms. Mild audiometric air-bone gaps, but without effusion, are often associated with type HN-s or HN-g tympanograms[35]; such tympanograms may also be forerunners of effusion.[7,8,35] If the identification of these various conditions were included among the goals of tympanometric testing its yield would be somewhat higher. Finally, it should be noted that the tympanometric procedure itself indirectly identifies the presence of tympanic membrane perforations or of patent tympanostomy tubes

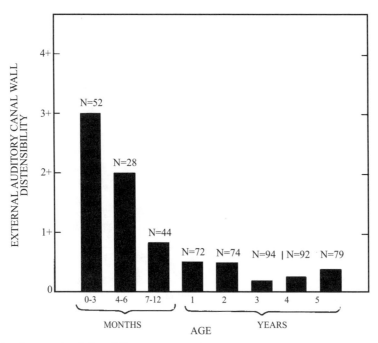

Figure 7. Average external auditory canal wall distensibility (0 to +4), as estimated otoscopically.

(and can therefore also be of diagnostic value when the patency of such tubes is in doubt).

Other Values of Tympanometry

Efficiency and Patient Comfort—Since middle ear disease in infants and young children is not only prevalent but often asymptomatic, many clinicians routinely carry out otoscopic examination in all pediatric patients, even those without symptoms. However, adequate visualization of the ear drum often requires that patients be forcibly restrained, and in addition, that cerumen be removed from the external auditory canal—procedures that may be time-consuming and that ordinarily result in some measure of anxiety and discomfort.

Tympanometry, on the other hand, is a simple, atraumatic procedure that can be carried out by paraprofessional aides after a few hours' training and is almost always readily accepted by infants and young children. Moreover, tympanometry appears so sensitive in detecting middle ear effusion in individuals 7 months of age or older that, in such subjects who are asymptomatic and who also have type NL tympanograms, otoscopy seems virtually unnecessary.

It would thus appear that instituting tympanometry as a routine diagnostic procedure would permit ready identification of a large number of individuals in whom otoscopy could safely be omitted. Much clinician time might thereby be saved, and appreciably patient anxiety and discomfort avoided.

Objectifying Follow-up Examinations—In following patients with known middle ear disease, difficulty frequently arises in deciding whether significant changes in clinical status have occurred, especially if the previous examinations had been carried out by other individuals. Serial tympanograms can help resolve such uncertainty, since they provide objective measurements as well as graphic records of middle ear status.

Teaching and Quality Control—Clinicians vary in the degree of their interest in and experience with middle ear disease in infants and young children, and they vary in their otoscopic diagnostic skills. Few studies of the validity of otoscopic diagnoses have been reported, but even among experienced observers disagreements about ear drum findings and their significance are commonplace. In our everyday practice in a busy pediatric teaching hospital, and in a study currently in progress, tympanometric findings have often led students and physicians at various levels of training and experience to call into question their otoscopic diagnoses and, after further consideration or reexamination, to revise them. In other instances, compatible tympanometric curves have reassured clinicians that their otoscopic diagnoses were in all probability correct. All in all, the use of tympanometry appears to have resulted in heightened interest in middle ear disease, better resolution of disagreements about middle ear status, more

§Grason-Stadler Co., Inc., Concord, Massachusetts 01742

critical self-appraisal with regard to otoscopic diagnosis, and improved diagnostic skills.

Summary and Conclusions

Tympanometry as a technique for detecting middle ear effusions was studied in 280 patients, 10 days through 5 years of age. Of these, 107 had been scheduled for myringotomy because of concurrent or recent middle ear effusion, and 173 were outpatients with miscellaneous complaints. Tympanometric curves were recorded using a Madsen ZO 70 Electroacoustic Impedance Meter, and were compared with independent otoscopic and myringotomy findings.

Five major categories of tympanograms comprising seven distinct curve types were identified, based on their degree of correlation with the presence or absence of middle ear effusion. This classification scheme differs somewhat from previously reported schemes and seems more useful clinically.

In subjects 7 months of age and older, curves suggesting normal (high) tympanic membrane compliance in combination with atmospheric or near-atmospheric middle ear air pressure were rarely associated with effusion. Conversely, curves suggesting reduced compliance of the tympanic membrane or of its attachments were highly correlated with the presence of effusion. Curves suggesting intermediate compliance or reduced middle ear air pressure or both were also correlated with effusion, but the degree of correlation was highly dependent on curve gradient. In general, the more these compliance, air-pressure, and gradient measurements departed from "normal," either singly or in combination, the greater was the likelihood of effusion.

In infants less than 7 months of age many of the ears with effusion had "normal" tympanograms, presumably because the external auditory canal walls of such infants tend to be highly distensible.

Tympanometry is a simple, rapid, atraumatic, valid, and objective test. It can be easily administered by trained paraprofessional personnel in almost any acoustic environment. Its incorporation into pediatric routines for subjects 7 months of age and older should result in improved and often more comfortable and efficient detection of middle ear effusion and certain other middle ear abnormalities. Tympanometric testing can also provide graphic records of middle ear status that are useful in following patients with known middle ear disease.

The use of tympanometry in conjunction with pneumatic otoscopy is helpful in teaching, and appears to promote both interest in middle ear disease and improvement in diagnostic acumen.

References

1. Lowe, J.F., Bamforth, J.S., Pracy, R.: Acute otitis media: One year in a general practice. *Lancet* 2:1129, 1963.
2. Reed, D., Struve, S., Maynard, J.E.: Otitis media and hearing deficiency among Eskimo children: A cohort study. *Am J Public Health* 57:1657, 1967.
3. Eagles, E.L., Wishik, S.M., Doerfler, L.G.: Hearing sensitivity and ear disease in children: A prospective study. *Laryngoscope*, suppl, pp 1-274, 1967.
4. Robinson, G.C., Anderson, D.O., Moghadam, H.K., *et al.*: A survey of hearing loss in Vancouver school children: I. Methodology and prevalence. *Can Med Assoc J* 97:1199, 1967.
5. Fay, T.H., Hochberg, I., Smith, C.R., *et al.*: Audiologic and otologic screening of disadvantaged children. *Arch Otolaryngol* 91:366, 1970.
6. Kessner, D.M., Snow, C.K., Singer, J.: Assessment of Medical Care for Children. Institute of Medicine, National Academy of Sciences, 1974, vol 3, pp 43-51.
7. Brooks, D.N.: An objective method of detecting fluid in the middle ear. *Int Audiol* 7:280, 1968.
8. Bluestone, C.D., Beery, Q.C., Paradise, J.L.: Audiometry and tympanometry in relation to middle ear effusions in children. *Laryngoscope* 83:594, 1973.
9. Brooks, D.N.: Hearing screening: A comparative study of an impedance method and puretone screening. *Scand Audiol* 2:67, 1973.
10. McCandless, G.A., Thomas, G.K.: Impedance audiometry as a screening procedure for middle ear disease. *Trans Am Acad Ophthalmol Otolaryngol* 78:98, 1974.
11. Cooper, J.C. Jr, Gates, G.A., Owen, J.H., Dickson, H.D.: An abbreviated impedance bridge for school screening. *J Speech Hear Dis* 40:260, 1975.
12. Brooks, D.: The use of the electroacoustic impedance bridge in the assessment of middle ear function. *Int Audiol* 8:563, 1969.
13. Alberti, P., Kristensen, A.: The clinical application of impedance audiometry. *Laryngoscope* 80:735, 1970.
14. Jerger, J.: Clinical experience with impedance audiometry. *Arch Otolaryngol* 92:311, 1970.
15. Jerger, S., Jerger, J., Mauldin, P.: Studies in impedance audiometry. *Arch Otolaryngol* 99:1, 1974.
16. Beery, Q.C., Bluestone, C.D., Andrus, W.S., Cantekin, E.I.: Tympanometric pattern classification in relation to middle ear effusion. *Ann Otol Rhinol Laryngol* 84:56, 1975.
17. Beery, Q.C., Bluestone, C.D., Cantekin, E.I., Gould, E.C.: A comparative study of tympanometric patterns in relation to middle ear effusion. Read before the 50th annual meeting of the American Speech and Hearing Association, Las Vagas, Nevada, November 6, 1974.

18. Schuster, K.: Eine Methode zum Vergleich akustischer Impedanzen. *Physikal Z*, 35:408, 1934.

19. Metz, O.: The acoustic impedance measured on normal and pathological ears. *Acta Otolaryngol* 63(suppl):2, 1946.

20. Terkildsen, K., Nielsen, S.: An electroacoustic impedance measuring bridge for clinical use. *Arch Otolaryngol* 72:339, 1960.

21. Zwislocki, J.: Acoustic measurement of the middle ear function. *Ann Otol Rhinol Laryngol* 70:599, 1961.

22. Ehrlich, M.A., Tait, C.A.: The application of acoustic impedance measurements to pediatric clinical practice. *Pediatrics* 55:666, 1975.

23. Ingelstedt, S.: Physiology of the eustachian tube. Read before the International Symposium on Recent Advances in Middle Ear Effusions, Columbus, Ohio, May 30, 1975.

24. Keith, R.W.: Impedance audiometry with neonates. *Arch Otolaryngol* 97:465, 1973.

25. Cannon, S.S., Smith, K.E., Reece, C.A., Thebo, J.L.: Middle ear measurements in neonates: A normative study. Read before the 50th annual meeting of the American Speech and Hearing Association, Las Vegas, Nevada, November 8, 1974.

26. Keith, R.W.: Middle ear function in neonates. *Arch Otolaryngol* 101:376, 1975.

27. Ling, D.: The education and general background of children with defective hearing, thesis Cambridge, Cambridge University Institute of Education, 1959.

28. Holm, V.A., Kunze, L.H.: Effect of chronic otitis media on language and speech development. *Pediatrics* 43:833, 1969.

29. Paradise, J.L., McWilliams, B.J., Bluestone, C.D.: Associations in cleft palate children between early otologic management and later mental, speech, and language development. Read before the 30th annual meeting of the American Cleft Palate Association, Phoenix, Arizona, April 14, 1972.

30. Jaffe, B.F., Hurtado, F., Hurtado, E.: Tympanic membrane mobility in the newborn (with seven months' follow-up). *Laryngoscope* 80:36, 1970.

31. Siirala, U.: Otitis media adhesiva. *Arch Otolaryngol* 80:287, 1964.

32. Jordan, R.E.: Secretory otitis media in etiology of cholesteatoma. *Arch Otolaryngol* 78:261, 1963.

33. Buckingham, R.A.: A. Kodachrome study of otitis media. In, Glorig, A., Gerwin, K.S. (eds): Otitis Media: Proceedings of the National Conference, Callier Hearing and Speech Center, Dallas, Texas. Springfield, Illinois, Charles C Thomas, 1972, pp 92-102.

34. Brooks, D.N.: Electroacoustic impedance bridge studies on normal ears of children. *J Speech Hear Res* 14:253, 1971.

35. Paradise, J.L., Smith, C.G., Bluestone, C.D.: Unpublished data.

Acknowledgments

The myringotomies were performed by or under the supervision of Herman Felder, M.D., and Edward S. Weisberg, M.D. The authors are grateful to Ernest J. Burgi, Ph.D., and Kenneth C. Stewart, M.S., for helpful technical suggestions concerning the study, and to Thomas K. Oliver, Jr., M.D., and Kenneth D. Rogers, M.D., for valuable suggestions concerning the manuscript.

Tympanometric Gradient Measured from Normal Preschool Children

Katherine A. Koebsell and Robert H. Margolis
Syracuse University, Communication Sciences and Disorders Program, Syracuse, N.Y., USA

Abstract

Tympanometric gradient is a quantitative expression of the shape of a tympanogram in the vicinity of the peak. Previous work suggests that gradient measures may be diagnostically and prognostically useful in the assessment and management of middle ear disease. However, since almost all previous work on the subject was performed on tympanograms recorded in 'arbitrary compliance units' which are not comparable to the physical admittance units provided by currently available instrumentation, at this point the tympanometric gradient can only be viewed to be a potentially-useful clinical measure. In this investigation, eight tympanometric gradient measures were calculated from tympanograms obtained from normal preschool age children. The measures were evaluated on the basis of distribution characteristics, relation to static admittance, and effect of pump speed. One of the measures—the pressure interval defined by a 50% reduction in peak eardrum admittance—appears to be the procedure of choice. Measurements obtained from abnormal ears are needed to evaluate the clinical utility of this measurement.

Key Words: Tympanometry • Tympanogram • Middle ear disease

Tympanometry is a widely used measurement technique which provides an indirect assessment of middle ear status. Two approaches have been used to separate tympanometric results into normal and abnormal groups: qualitative analysis (evaluation of tympanometric shape) and quantitative analysis (estimation of static admittance and tympanometric peak pressure). An additional measure, the tympanometric gradient, has been suggested as a means to combine qualitative and quantitative properties, by quantifying important aspects of the tympanometric shape.

The gradient is a measure of the shape of the tympanogram around the tympanometric peak. It has been quantified by various formulae by different investigators, whose measurements were obtained in different units. Brooks [1969] defined the gradient as the change in 'compliance' from the peak value to the value obtained at a pressure interval of 50 daPa on either side of the peak (fig.1). Brooks considered this gradient measure to represent 'the ratio between stress and strain' [Brooks, 1968 p. 281]. Margolis and Shanks [1985] suggested that a low gradient with normal static impedance may reflect an abnormally large resistive component. In a subsequent report, Brooks [1969] attempted to identify the boundary values between normal and abnormal middle ear function with respect to middle ear pressure, 'compliance' and gradient, from a total of 1053 children that he tested. He concluded that acoustic immittance measurements, including the tympanometric gradient, offer a simple and objective means of detecting middle ear disease in children at an early stage. His measurements were made with a Madsen Acoustic Impedance Meter (model number unspecified) [Brooks, 1968] or a 'Madsen ZO70 bridge coupled to an X-Y plotter' [Brooks, 1969]. In the 1968 paper, tympanograms are presented in cubic centimeters; in the 1969 paper no units are specified on the tympanograms, although tabulated gradient data are purportedly in cubic centimeters. It is not clear how the 'arbitrary compliance units' produced by the Madsen ZO70 instrument in the automatic recording mode were converted to cubic centimeters.

Paradise et al. [1976] attempted to correlate tympanometric peak pressure and the shape of the tympanogram with middle ear effusion. They employed a Madsen ZO70 Electroacoustic Impedance Meter which plotted tympanograms in 'compliance in Madsen Units'. A ratio method was used to calculate the gradient (fig.1). On the basis of their results, Paradise et al. [1976] concluded that the likelihood of effusion became greater 'the more these compliance, air pressure and gradient measurements departed from normal, either singly or in combination' [p. 209].

In a series of studies on tympanometry and secretory otitis media (SOM) in children, Fiellau-Nikolajsen [1983] recorded tympano-grams with Madsen ZO72 and ZO73 instruments in the automatic recording mode. Like the Madsen ZO70, these instruments record tympanograms in

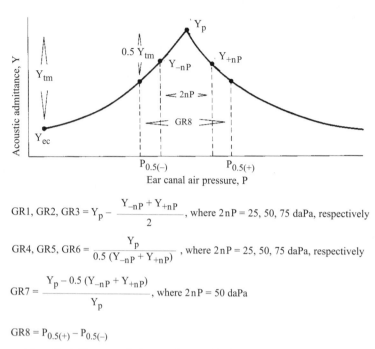

$$GR1, GR2, GR3 = Y_p - \frac{Y_{-nP} + Y_{+nP}}{2}, \text{ where } 2nP = 25, 50, 75 \text{ daPa, respectively}$$

$$GR4, GR5, GR6 = \frac{Y_p}{0.5\,(Y_{-nP} + Y_{+nP})}, \text{ where } 2nP = 25, 50, 75 \text{ daPa, respectively}$$

$$GR7 = \frac{Y_p - 0.5\,(Y_{-nP} + Y_{+nP})}{Y_p}, \text{ where } 2nP = 50 \text{ daPa}$$

$$GR8 = P_{0.5(+)} - P_{0.5(-)}$$

Figure 1. Calculation of tympanometric gradients. To correct admittance values used in the calculations to the plane of the tympanic membrane, the minimum tail admittance (Y_{ec}), which usually occurred at –400 daPa, was set to zero (MAX/MIN method). GR1, GR2, and GR3 are difference measures based on the method of Brooks [1969]. These measures represent the peak height over the pressure interval $2nP$ with $2nP = 25$, 50 and 75 daPa. GR4, GR5, and GR6 are ratio calculations modified from the method of Paradise et al. [1976]. These measures represent the ratio of the peak eardrum admittance Y_p to the mean admittance $\pm nP$ away from the peak. GR7 is the Paradise et al. method. It is the ratio of the height of the peak over the pressure interval $2nP$ to the peak eardrum admittance Y_p. GR8 is the pressure interval defined by a 50% reduction in peak eardrum admittance (Y_p), after de Jonge [1983].

'arbitrary compliance units'. He examined the relationship between the tympanometric gradient, calculated by the Brooks [1968] and Paradise et al. [1976] methods, the amount of middle ear effusion, and magnitude of hearing loss. He found that both the gradient and the magnitude of the hearing loss separately correlated with the amount but not the viscosity of the middle ear effusion. Moreover, the gradient of the tympanogram was more strongly correlated than hearing loss to presence of effusion. Fiellau-Nikolajsen [1983] concluded 'to the clinician the gradient is among the individual tympanogram components which affords the most information about SOM' [p. 50]. For this reason he argued that the gradient concept be incorporated into classification of tympanograms. In light of the high prevalence of otitis media in children [see Fiellau-Nikolajsen, 1983, for a review], tympanometric gradient may provide important diagnostic information in pediatric populations.

De Jonge [1983] reported normal gradient values obtained from adult tympanograms recorded in physical units of admittance. He calculated the gradient by the Brooks method and as the pressure interval defined by a 50% reduction in peak eardrum admittance (fig. 1). De Jonge studied the relationships between these gradient measures and static admittance. The Brooks gradient correlated very highly with static admittance, indicating that the two quantities reflect the same middle ear characteristics. De Jonge's pressure interval measure did not correlate highly with static admittance, suggesting that it reflects different middle ear characteristics. This gradient measure may complement static admittance in the evaluation of middle ear pathology.

Due to the differences in measurement units employed in these investigations, the results are not quantitatively comparable. Gradient data obtained from tympanograms recorded in 'arbitrary compliance units' are, at best, ordinal data, and are not amenable to parametric statistical analysis. The large differences in gradient measures that can result from different measurement procedures was demonstrated by Feldman [1975]. Most currently available acoustic-immittance instruments record in physical units, either acoustic admittance (acoustic mmhos) or equivalent volume (cm^3). Of the previous investigations of tympanometric gradient, only de Jonge's [1983] data, expressed in admittance magnitude, are comparable to values produced by currently produced instruments. In addition, the availability of faster pump speeds on these new instruments raises the question of the effect of rate of pressure change on tympanometric gradient.

This investigation was undertaken to evaluate eight gradient measures recorded from the population for whom the gradient measure may be most useful, children between the ages of 3 and 6 years. Each gradient measure was evaluated on the basis of the relation to static admittance, distribution characteristics, and effect of the rate of pressure change during tympanometric recording (pump speed).

Method

Subjects

Subjects in this study consisted of 88 ears of 46 children between the ages of 3.7 and 5.8 years (mean 4.54 years) who had participated in a hearing screening conducted at the Village Nursery School in Fayetteville, N.Y.

Parental consent and a brief medical history were obtained for each child prior to testing. Criteria for inclusion in the study were based on medical history, otoscopy, pure tone audiometry and acoustic immittance testing. The following criteria were used to determine subject eligibility: (1) positive behavioral responses to air conduction tones presented at 500, 1000, 2000 and 4000 Hz at a level of 20 dB HL [re: ANSI S3.6-1969 norms], missing no more than one frequency per ear; (2) single peaked tympanograms with a tympanometric peak pressure between –250 and +50 daPa; (3) presence of an ipsilateral acoustic reflex obtained in response to 1000 Hz, 105 dB SPL stimulus; (4) ear canals reasonably free of debris with no apparent signs of infection; (5) absence of recent history of otologic disease.

Procedure

Pure tone audiometric screening was conducted using a conventional pure tone audiometer (Maico MA-16) with TDH-39 headphones. A Madsen Electronics ZO174 Immittance Audio-meter monitor (VM 174), and printer (TP 174) were used to record all immittance test results.

The probe tone (226 Hz) and ipsilateral acoustic reflex stimuli of the Madsen ZO174 Immittance Audiometer were calibrated with a Brüel & Kjaer precision sound level meter (Type 2209) in a 2 cm^3 (HA-1) coupler. The immittance measurement portion of the Madsen ZO174 was calibrated against 2.0 and 0.5 cm^3 enclosed volumes of air. Tympanometric data were recorded in acoustic admittance magnitude with units of acoustic mmhos (i.e., 1 m^3 $\times$ 10^{-9}/Pa/s).

Tympanograms for all subjects (n = 88 ears) were recorded using a 50 daPa/s pump speed and for some subjects (n = 60 ears) tympanograms were recorded using a 200 daPa/s pump speed.[1] Each tympanometric recording was followed by two acoustic reflex recordings, employing a 1000-Hz, 105-dB SPL, ipsilateral stimulus.

For analysis, each tympanogram was projected by an opaque projector onto graph paper mounted on a wall. With this enhanced resolution, eleven different admittance and pressure values were determined. These values were recorded and later used in the calculation of various gradient values.

Calculation of the Gradient

The eight gradient measures that were calculated are described in figure 1. All admittance values used to calculate the gradient measures were corrected to the tympanic membrane by subtracting the minimum tail admittance Y_{ec}, which usually occurred at –400 daPa◊. In figure 1, then, Y_{ec} was set to zero. This is the MAX/MIN method of estimating the admittance at the tympanic membrane [see Margolis and Shanks, 1985, for a discussion]. The gradient measures fall into three categories: (1) GR1, GR2, and GR3: these measures represent the difference between two admittance values [after Brooks, 1969]; (2) GR4, GR5, GR6, and GR7: these measures express the ratio of two eardrum admittances [after Paradise et al., 1976]; (3) GR8: the pressure interval defined by a 50% reduction in peak eardrum admittance [after de Jonge, 1983].

GR1, GR2, and GR3 differ only in the pressure interval at which the admittance values were ob-tained from the tympanogram. Since the 50 daPa interval employed by Brooks [1969] was arbitrary, three different intervals were examined in this investigation. Note that since the measures are the difference between two admittance values, these gradient measures are in units of acoustic admittance (acoustic mmhos).

GR4, GR5, GR6, and GR7 are ratio measures adapted from the method of Paradise et al. [1976]. GR7 is exactly that employed by Paradise et al. The others were modified to allow a wider range of possible values. The Paradise et al. measure can vary between 0 and 1, where the others can assume values from 1.0 to infinity. The wider range of possible values was thought to allow greater deviation from normal in ears with middle ear disease. Since the measures are ratios of two admittance values, they are unitless quantities.

....

[1]For the slow pump speed Y_{ec} occurred at –400 daPa for 61 cases and at +400 daPa for 27 cases. For the fast speed Y_{ec} occurred at –400 daPa for 43 cases and at +400 daPa for 17 cases.

GR8, the method of de Jonge [1983], is the pressure interval (in daPa) over which peak eardrum admittance is reduced by 50%.

Results and Discussion

Static admittance results for the two pump speeds are presented in table I. The effect of pump speed was significant beyond the 0.001 level (Wilcoxon sign ranks test). The higher admittance obtained with the faster pump speed is consistent with observations of Creten and Van Camp [1974] and is thought to result from the nonlinear viscoelastic properties of the tympanic membrane. These results indicate that pump speed must be considered in the establishment of normative static admittance.

The following criteria were used to select the most clinically useful gradient measure: (1) A low correlation with static admittance was desired to identify a gradient measure which may contribute information that is supplemental to rather than redundant with static admittance. (2) A narrow distribution with values clustered closely about the mean was desired to facilitate the identification of abnormal values. (3) The optimal gradient measure would allow a large range of possible values outside the normal range. (4) Finally, invariance with respect to pump speed was desired as this would eliminate the need to establish separate norms for different recording speeds.

Table II presents descriptive and comparative statistics for the eight gradient measures obtained from tympanograms recorded in the slow and fast pump conditions. The Pearson product-moment correlation coefficients listed in this table indicate the strength of the association of each gradient measure with static admittance. The coefficient of variation [Daniels,1974, pp. 12-13] was computed to represent the relative variation in these data and thereby facilitate comparison between gradient measures. Additionally, a two-tailed Wilcoxon signed ranks test [Mendenhall and Ott, 1980, pp. 369-370] was used to test the effect of pump speed on each gradient measure and the significance levels are presented in table II.

Relation to Static Admittance

For both pump speeds, the strongest associations exist between static admittance and the gradient measures calculated using Brooks' method (GR1, GR2, and GR3) with GR3 exhibiting the highest correlation. This is not surprising as the formula used to calculate these gradient quantities closely resembles the calculation of static admittance. Since GR3 employs admittance values close to the tail of the tympanogram, it shows the closest relation to static admittance.

The ratio and pressure interval gradient measures (GR4, GR5, GR6, GR7, and GR8) display lower correlations with static admittance. The lower correlations suggest that these gradient measures convey information which is supplementary to the information contained in the static admittance measure, while GR1, GR2, and GR3 are redundant with static admittance.

Distribution Characteristics

The coefficient of variation statistic was selected for use as an index of the relative width of the distribution of each gradient measure. Expressed as a ratio of the mean to the standard deviation, this statistic is virtually independent of the unit of measurement or numeric inequalities between sets of data, provided that the data have interval or ratio properties. Note that the largest coefficients of variation were obtained for the gradient measures calculated by the Brooks method (GR1, GR2, and GR3). The smallest values were observed for the ratio measures (GR4, GR5, GR6, and GR7) with GR8 (pressure interval measure) producing an intermediate value. The gradients which exhibit the smaller coefficients of variation have narrow relative distributions around their means, and would potentially be more useful for detecting abnormalities.

Range of Possible Values

The relationship between the distribution of normal values and the range of possible values determines the ability to detect abnormalities. It is important to note that the effect of most high impedance middle ear abnormalities (e.g. secretory and acute otitis media) is to reduce the value of all gradient measures except GR8, which is increased by the presence of these pathologies. For detecting these abnormalities with all but GR8, we must examine the distance from the low end of the normal range to the lowest possible value. For GR8, we must examine the distance from the high end of the normal range to the highest possible value.

For all gradient measures except GR7 and GR8, the distance from the low end of the 90% range to the lowest possible value is about 1 sd, a range that is not adequate

Table I. Static acoustic admittance was calculated by subtracting the admittance at –400 daPa from the peak admittance. Means and standard deviations (sd) are in acoustic mmhos.

Pump speed, daPa/s					
50			200		
mean	n	sd	mean	n	sd
0.55	88	0.18	0.67	60	0.22

Table II. Descriptive and comparative statistics for eight gradient measures obtained from slow and fast speed tympanograms. Data for gradients GR1-GR3 are presented in units of acoustic mmhos, GR4-GR7 are unitless quantities and GR8 is in daPa.

Gradient	Possible values	Slow pump					Fast pump					Significance level‡
		0	sd	sd/0*	90% range	r†	0	sd	sd/0*	90% range	r†	
GR1	0-4	0.11	0.06	0.55	0.04-0.23	0.81	0.13	0.09	0.65	0.03-0.28	0.81	p ≤0.0002
GR2	0-4	0.23	0.11	0.47	0.10-0.44	0.85	0.28	0.16	0.57	0.11-0.56	0.87	p <0.0001
GR3	0-4	0.33	0.13	0.40	0.15-0.60	0.90	0.39	0.19	0.47	0.18-0.70	0.93	p <0.0001
GR4	1-4	1.23	0.10	0.08	1.10-1.38	0.45	1.24	0.12	0.09	1.07-1.50	0.51	p ≤0.2925
GR5	1-4	1.66	0.28	0.17	1.32-2.28	0.45	1.73	0.39	0.22	1.30-2.38	0.63	p ≤0.0011
GR6	1-4	2.35	0.62	0.26	1.63-3.50	0.38	2.45	0.69	0.28	1.65-3.90	0.63	p ≤0.0007
GR7	0-1	0.38	0.09	0.24	0.21-0.53	0.43	0.40	0.11	0.28	0.25-0.59	0.58	p ≤0.0022
GR8$_{n=60}$	0-4	0.31	0.30	-0.46\	81-180	-0.36	33.17		0.27	67.50-187	-0.60	p ≤0.0933
GR8$_{n=88}$			80-200									

*Coefficient of variation.

†Pearson product-moment correlation coefficient between static admittance and individual gradient measures.

‡Wilcoxon signed ranks test for same gradient measures, different pump speeds.

to detect abnormalities with statistical confidence. GR7 provides a range of about 2 sd between the lowest possible value and the low end of the 90% range.

Because there is no theoretical upper limit to GR8, and because GR8 increases with most high impedance abnormalities, there is a theoretically infinite range between the high end of the normal range and the highest possible value. Of course, GR8 is limited by the pressure interval over which the tympanogram is recorded. This measure, however, appears to provide the widest range for detection of abnormalities.

Effect of Pump Speed

The results of the Wilcoxon signed ranks test used to determine the effect of pump speed for each gradient measure are also listed in table II. The difference between each pair of means was significant at the 0.001 level or beyond, with two exceptions, gradients GR4 and GR8. The implication of these results is that separate norms would be needed for each gradient measure and both pump speeds with the exception of gradients GR4 and GR8. For these measures, results obtained using either a slow or fast pump speed may be considered roughly equivalent.

Selection of the Optimal Gradient Measure

Based on the information presented above, it appears that gradient measure GR8, de Jonge's pressure interval calculation, may be the most clinically useful gradient measure. It has a low association with static admittance, a comparatively small coefficient of variation, and it would not require separate norms for the two pump speeds employed in this investigation. In addition, there is a wide range of values between the normal range and the limits of possible values which will facilitate identification of pathologic ears. GR8 appears to be potentially useful for the detection of high impedance abnormalities which increase its value. In addition, the measure may be useful for detecting the narrow tympanometric peaks often associated with otosclerosis [Ivey, 1975].

As GR8 appears to be the preferred gradient measure, it is recommended that the results presented for the larger population (n = 88 ears), be used as tentative normative values for 3- to 6-year- old children. While this investigation provides normative gradient data for preschool age children, future research is needed to determine the behavior of gradient GR8 in pathologic populations. Additionally, the utility of this measure as a diagnostic tool would be enhanced by longitudinal studies of tympanometric gradient through various stages of disease or recovery processes. Only measures expressed in real physical units provide the capability to describe and analyze the data in a manner that provides insight into the selection of an optimal clinical measurement.

Mesure du gradient tympanométrique chez des enfants normaux en âge préscolaire

Le gradient tympanométrique est une expression quantitative de la forme du tympanogramme à proximité du pic. Des études antérieures suggèrent que les mesures de gradient peuvent être utiles sur le plan diagnostique et pronostique dans l'étude et le traitement des affections de l'oreille moyenne. Toutefois, la quasi-totalité de ces travaux a été effectuée avec des unités arbitraires de compliance, qui ne peuvent être comparées aux unités physiques d'admittance employées avec les appareils courants. Dans ces conditions, le gradient tympanométrique ne peut être que d'une utilité clinique potentielle. Dans cette étude, on a calculé 8 mesures de gradient tympanométrique à partir de tympanogrammes enregistrés sur des enfants normaux d'âge préscolaire. On a analysé les mesures en fonction des caractéristiques de distribution, de la relation avec l'admittance statique et de l'effet de la vitesse de la pompe. Une de ces mesures—l'intervalle de pression défini par une baisse de 50% du pic d'admittance tympanique—apparaît comme le procédé de choix. Des mesures sur des oreilles pathologiques sont nécessaires pour apprécier l'utilité clinique de cette méthode.

Acknowledgments

We are grateful for the support of Madsen Electronics who provided the instrument with which this research was executed. Without the capable assistance of the staff of the Village Nursery School, Fayetteville, N.Y., this project would not have been possible.

References

American National Standards Specification for Audiometers. ANSI S3.6 1969 (American National Standards Institute, New York 1970).

Brooks, D.: An objective method of determining fluid in the middle ear. *Int. Audiol.* 7:280-286 (1968).

Brooks, D.: The use of electro-acoustic bridge in the assessment of middle ear function. *Int. Audiol.* 8:563-565 (1969).

Creten, W.L.; Van Camp, K.J.: Transient and quasitransient tympanometry. *Scand. Audiol.* 3:39-42 (1974).

Daniel, W. W.: *Biostatistics: a foundation for analysis in the health sciences* (Wiley, New York 1974).

Feldman, A.S.: Acoustic impedance/admittance measurements; in Bradford, *Physiological measures of the audio-vestibular system* (Academic Press, New York 1975).

Fiellau-Nikolajsen, M.: Tympanometry and secretory otitis media. *Acta oto-lar.,* suppl. 394 (1983).

Ivey, R.G.: Tympanometric curves and otosclerosis. *J. Speech and Hearing Res.* 18:554-558 (1975).

Jonge, R.R. de: Normal tympanogram slope. *ASHA* 25:114 (1983).

Margolis, R.H.; Shanks, J.E.: Tympanometry; in Katz, *Handbook of clinical audiology*; 3rd ed., pp. 438-475 (Williams & Wilkins, Baltimore 1985).

Mendenhall, W.; Ott, L.: *Understanding statistics* (Duxbury Press, North Scituate 1980).

Paradise, J.L.; Smith, C.G.; Bluestone, C.D.: Tympanometric detection of middle ear effusion in infants and young children. *Pediatrics* 58:198-210 (1976).

Received October 8, 1985
Accepted February 10, 1986

Robert H. Margolis,
Syracuse University,
805 South Crouse Avenue,
Syracuse, NY 13244 (USA)

Identification of Middle Ear Dysfunction in Young Children: A Comparison of Tympanometric Screening Procedures

Jackson Roush, Ph.D; Amelia Drake, MD; and John E. Sexton, MS

Division of Speech and Hearing Sciences (J.R., J.E.S.), and Division of Otolaryngology—Head and Neck Surgery (A.D.), University of North Carolina, Chapel Hill, North Carolina

Abstract

Two acoustic immittance screening procedures were evaluated in conjunction with pneumatic otoscopy, performed by a pediatric otolaryngologist. The subjects were 204 3- and 4-yr-old children from a rural area in eastern North Carolina. Pass-fail criteria were examined using two middle ear screening procedures: (1) a "traditional" procedure based on measures of tympanometric peak pressure and acoustic reflexes, and (2) the tympanometric measures contained within the American Speech-Language-Hearing Association's (ASHA) revised Guidelines for Screening for Hearing Impairment and Middle Ear Disorders. The traditional procedure resulted in low specificity but high sensitivity, whereas ASHA's immittance procedure resulted in high specificity but only moderate sensitivity. The negative predictive value was very high for both procedures; however, positive predictive value was low, especially for the traditional procedure. Advantages and disadvantages of the two procedures and future research needs are discussed. (*Ear Hear* 13 2:63-69)

Middle ear disorders are among the most common diseases affecting young children. Teele, Klein, and Rosner (1983) reported that over one-third of all illness-related office visits for children under the age of 5 yr involve middle ear disease. Similar findings have been reported by other investigators, including Howie (1975), who reported that two-thirds of the children seen in their pediatric practice had experienced at least one episode of otitis media by their second birthday; nearly 15% had experienced more than six episodes.

Because of the high prevalence of middle ear disease in young children and the convenience of modern tympanometric instrumentation, many educational and health care institutions now routinely conduct acoustic immittance screening of children at the preschool and early elementary grade levels. Numerous studies have examined the efficacy of acoustic immittance screening (Brooks, 1973, 1977; Cooper, Gates, Owen, & Dickson, 1974; Lous, 1983; McCandless & Thomas, 1974; Orchik & Herdman, 1974) and it is generally agreed that these measures are easy to obtain and highly sensitive to middle ear dysfunction. Unfortunately, they are considerably less accurate in identifying children without disease. That is, several investigators have reported an excessively high rate of false positive medical referrals (e.g., Lucker, 1980; Paradise & Smith, 1978; Roeser & Northern, 1988; Roush & Tait, 1985; Schow, Pederson, Nerbonne, & Boe,

1981; Wachtendorf, Lopez, Cooper, Hearne, & Gates, 1984). Consequently, many authorities now advocate immittance screening only for those children considered to be at high risk for middle ear disease (Bluestone, Fria, Arjona, et al, 1986). As noted recently by Bluestone and Klein (1990), however, referral criteria based on acoustic immittance measurements are not well established even in high risk groups, and additional research in this area is needed.

Two sets of guidelines have been widely used in recent years for immittance screening: (1) the 1979 Guidelines of the American Speech-Language-Hearing Association (ASHA) for Acoustic Immittance Screening of Middle Ear Function (ASHA, 1979), and (2) the recommendations of the Nashville Task Force, which met at Vanderbilt University in 1977 (Harford, Bess, Bluestone, & Klein, 1978). ASHA's original protocol, variations of which are still in widespread use, recommended a combination of tympanometry and acoustic reflex measures, which resulted in three possible outcomes: pass (no additional follow-up), at-risk (schedule for rescreening), or fail (medical referral). An individual was passed if the tympanometric peak pressure was between +100 and −200 mm H$_2$O* and an acoustic reflex was present. If a peak was identifiable but outside this range, and the acoustic reflex was present, or, if peak pressure was within this range but the acoustic reflex absent, the individual was considered to be at risk and rescreening was performed in 3 to 5 weeks, at which time the result was reclassified as either a pass or fail. Immediate medical referral was recommended if tympanometric peak pressure was outside the +100 to −200 range and the acoustic reflex absent, or in the event of a flat (type B) configuration.

The Nashville Task Force recommendations included similar tympanometric and acoustic reflex criteria; however, they differed from the original ASHA guidelines with respect to referral criteria. In contrast to the original ASHA protocol, which, in some cases, recommended medical referral on the basis of initial immittance findings, the Nashville guidelines recommend rescreening all individuals with abnormal tympanometric results 4 to 6 weeks after the initial test was failed. Those children who were again classified as being at risk were to be scheduled for periodic monitoring rather than medical referral.

Several studies have sought to evaluate the efficacy of immittance screening and, in general, have reported moderately high sensitivity but low specificity (e.g., Lous, 1983; Lucker, 1980; Paradise & Smith, 1978; Roeser & Northern, 1988; Roush & Tait, 1985; Wachtendorf et al, 1984). In an effort to improve the specificity of its screening guidelines and to acknowledge a new American standard for acoustic immittance instruments (ANSI, 1988), ASHA recently adopted revisions to these guidelines. ASHA's revised protocol (ASHA, 1990), summarized in Table 1, consists of four components: history, visual inspection, identification audiometry, and tympanometry. Three individual acoustic immittance measurements are contained within the new set of guidelines: static admittance, equivalent ear canal volume, and tympanometric width (gradient). As noted in the guidelines, low static admittance (peak Y) is often seen in cases of active middle ear disease, whereas abnormally large ear canal volume estimates are often observed when tympanic membrane perforations exist in the presence of normal middle ear mucosa (ASHA, 1990). An abnormally wide tympanometric gradient is often indicative of middle ear effusion. Normative data, based on the work of Margolis and Heller (1987), are published as an appendix to the Guidelines, pending a larger scale normative study.

It is important to note that the new guidelines do not include measures of tympanometric peak pressure and acoustic reflex. The revised ASHA guidelines cite evidence that these measures contribute little to the sensitivity of immittance screening while substantially lowering specificity. It should also be noted that the revised guidelines never recommend immediate medical referral on the basis of initial immittance findings alone, except in cases of abnormally large ear canal volume estimates accompanied by low static admittance (i.e., when there is reason to

Table 1. Referral criteria for ASHA's revised Guidelines for Screening for Hearing Impairment and Middle Ear Disorders (ASHA, 1990). The present study examined only the acoustic immittance component of these guidelines.

History
  Otalgia
  Otorrhea
Visual inspection of the ear
  Structural defect of the ear, head, or neck
  Ear canal abnormalities
    Blood or effusion
    Occlusion
    Inflammation
    Excessive cerumen, tumor, foreign material
    Eardrum abnormalities
    Obvious perforation
    Obvious inflammation
    Severe retraction
Identification audiometry
  Fail air conduction screening at 20 dB HL at 1, 2, or 4 kHz in either ear
Tympanometry
  Flat tympanogram with equivalent ear canal volume outside normal range
  Low static admittance on two successive occurrences in a 4- to 6-week interval
  Abnormally wide tympanometric width on two successive occurrences in a 4- to 6-week interval

suspect a perforation of the tympanic membrane). When tympanometric results are abnormal, rescreening is done after 4 to 6 weeks. If results are again abnormal, an audiological/medical referral is made. In revising the screening guidelines, the ASHA Committee has attempted to address the problems associated with previous screening protocols, as well as the need to consider advances in acoustic immittance instrumentation and standards. The present study was designed to compare the acoustic immittance portion of the revised ASHA guidelines to a more traditional middle ear screening procedure consisting of tympanometric peak pressure and acoustic reflex measures.

Method

Subjects The subjects for this study were 204 3- and 4-yr-old children enrolled in Head Start preschool programs in a rural area located in eastern North Carolina. Males and females were equally represented. Approximately 95% of the children were black, and all were from low income families.

Instrumentation Acoustic immittance data were obtained using an automatic tympanometer (Micro Audiometrics Earscan). This device uses a 226 Hz probe tone with a positive to negative pressure sweep, at a rate of 150 daPa/sec. The static value is obtained by subtracting the amplitude at +200 daPa from the peak value. The immittance measures obtained for each subject were: (1) tympanometric peak pressure, expressed in daPa; (2) ipsilateral acoustic reflex, displayed graphically on a strip chart recording; (3) equivalent ear canal volume,

---

*ANSI S3.39-1987 recommends the use of the international units system (SI). For air pressure, the SI unit decapascal (daPa) replaces mm H_2O, previously used for tympanometry. For practical purposes, the two units can be considered equivalent (Margolis & Shanks, 1991).

expressed in millimhos; (4) static admittance, expressed in millimhos; and (5) tympanometric width, determined manually,† using a template constructed for this purpose (see ASHA, 1990).

Procedures   Initially, 242 subjects were seen in mid-January for acoustic immittance screening only. Six weeks later, acoustic immittance measures were repeated for all children present on the day of rescreening, including those who had normal immittance findings on the initial test. In addition, otoscopic examination, performed by a pediatric otolaryngologist, was conducted for each child.

Otoscopic Examination   Pneumatic otoscopy was performed on all children seen at the time of the second screening by the same physician, an otolaryngologist whose regular caseload consists primarily of pediatric patients, and whose otoscopic sensitivity and specificity (∅85%) have been established at surgery (Bluestone & Cantekin, 1979). Otoscopic findings were classified according to position, appearance, color, and any other remarkable characteristics. When fluid was thought to be present by otoscopy, a judgment was made regarding quantity and type. An otoscopic "failure" was judged to be an ear that required medical attention because of middle ear effusion, or because of abnormalities in color or appearance. The otoscopic examination was conducted immediately before, or just after the acoustic immittance measures. The examiner was unaware of the immittance findings.

Tympanometric Classification   The acoustic immittance results were analyzed according to the screening and classification procedures described in Table 2. The "traditional procedure"‡ is essentially the original ASHA procedure, but without immediate medical referral. That is, all ears with abnormal immittance results were rescreened before medical referral. Results obtained using this procedure were compared to those acquired using the tympanometric procedures contained within the revised ASHA Guidelines for Screening for Hearing Impairment and Middle Ear Disorders (ASHA, 1990).

Results

Table 3 compares the results obtained by applying the traditional and the revised ASHA immittance procedures to the 395 ears for which valid measurements could be obtained (13 ears were eliminated because of pressure equalization tubes or impacted cerumen). The traditional

Table 2. Referral criteria for the traditional and revised ASHA immittance screening procedures. According to the revised guidelines (ASHA, 1990), immittance findings must be abnormal on two successive occasions separated by a 4- to 6-week interval. The Guidelines also recommend that immittance be performed in conjunction with pure tone screening, visual inspection, and case history.

Referral criteria for "traditional" procedure	
Tympanometric peak pressure	< –200 daPa
Acoustic reflex	Absent
or	
Flat (type B) tympanogram	
Referral criteria for revised ASHA immittance measures	
Static acoustic admittance	< 0.2 mmho
Equivalent ear canal volume	> 1.0 cmΔ
Tympanometric width	> 150 daPa

screening procedure classified 122 ears as needing medical referral (31% of the total sample). Results for the same ears classified according to the revised ASHA immittance procedure resulted in a much larger number of ears being passed on the first screen (82%); however, for those requiring rescreening, the proportion of ears passed and referred was similar. The 43 ears needing medical attention according to the revised ASHA tympanometric procedure comprised 11% of the total sample.

A summary of results obtained using the two procedures is shown in Tables 4 and 5, based on the otoscopic findings at the second screening. It can be seen that both procedures were successful in identifying most of the ears needing medical referral based on otoscopic findings. As shown in Table 4, there were no false negatives using the traditional procedure. The two false negatives obtained using ASHA's middle ear screening procedure (Table 5) were characterized by markedly negative pressure, a measurement not included in that criteria. One of those ears was also characterized by significant abnormality of appearance (color).

Both immittance procedures were less accurate in the correct classification of nondiseased ears. As shown in Table 4, the traditional procedure correctly classified only 40% of the ears judged to be normal otoscopically (49 out of 122). Examination of data for the individual ears comprising this group revealed that nearly three-fourths failed because of absent acoustic reflexes, even though tympanometric peak pressure was less negative than –200 daPa. Most of the remainder failed because of tympanometric peak pressure more negative than –200 daPa (nearly all of these subjects had absent acoustic reflexes as well). Three

---

†The Earscan instrument now calculates tympanometric width automatically by determining the pressure interval associated with a 50% reduction in admittance on either side of the peak.

‡The term "traditional" is used here because the procedure is based on tympanometric peak pressure and acoustic reflexes, measures commonly used in screening for middle ear dysfunction. Although these measures have been widely used, procedures have varied considerably with respect to instrumentation, screening methods, and pass-fail criteria.

Table 3. Results of acoustic immittance screening applied to the traditional screening procedure and to the immittance measures contained within the revised ASHA protocol.

Screen 1 (n = 395 ears)		Screen 2 (n = 172 ears)	
Pass	Retest	Pass	Refer
Traditional screening procedure			
223 (56%)	172 (44%)	50 (29%)	122 (71%)
Percent of total sample referred: 31%			
Revised ASHA immittance procedure			
(n = 395 ears)		(n = 70 ears)	
324 (82%)	70 (18%)	27 (39%)	43 (61 %)
Percent of total sample referred: 11%			

ears categorized as false positives had flat tympanograms (i.e., static admittance <0.2 mmho).

The revised ASHA tympanometric procedure (Table 5) resulted in a much lower number of false positives, correctly classifying nearly three-fourths of the nondiseased ears. Examination of the 10 ears classified as false positive revealed that all failed because of abnormal tympanometric width and/or static admittance.

Comparison of the data shown in Tables 4 and 5 is complicated by the fact that different ears comprise each follow-up group. In an effort to accomplish a more direct comparison of the two immittance procedures at a single point in time, and to permit calculation of sensitivity, specificity, and predictive values, all 374 ears available for screening and otoscopic examination were classified according to the two procedures. As shown in Tables 6 and 7, comparison of sensitivity and specificity for the two procedures revealed that the traditional procedure, although highly sensitive (95%), achieved low specificity (65%). In contrast, the revised ASHA tympanometric procedure (Table 7) achieved high specificity (95%), but lower sensitivity (84%). Also of interest in Tables 6 and 7 are the predictive values calculated for the two screening procedures. For the traditional procedure (Table 6), it can be seen that a negative finding (i.e., normal tympanometric peak pressure and acoustic reflexes) was highly predictive of normal middle ear function as judged otoscopically (negative predictive value = 99%). In contrast, a positive finding predicted only about one-fourth of

Table 4. Screening results obtained when the traditional procedure was applied to the subgroup failing the initial screen (n = 158 ears). Only 158 of the 172 ears identified for referral in Table 3 are reported here because 14 ears could not be fully visualized otoscopically, even though valid acoustic immittance measures were obtained.

		Otoscopy	
		Fail	Pass
Immittance	Refer	36	73
	Pass	0	49

Table 5. Screening results obtained when ASHA's revised immittance procedures were applied to the subgroup failing the initial screen according to that procedure (n = 65 ears). Only 65 of the 70 ears identified for referral in Table 3 are reported here because 5 ears could not be fully visualized otoscopically, even though valid acoustic immittance measures were obtained.

		Otoscopy	
		Fail	Pass
Immittance	Refer	29	10
	Pass	2	24

the ears judged by otoscopy to need medical attention (positive predictive value = 27%). For the ASHA immittance measures (Table 7), the predictive value of a negative test was also very high (98%). The predictive value of a positive test (69%), although less than optimal, was considerably higher than that observed for the traditional procedure.

Examination of individual ear data for Table 6 revealed that for the two ears with normal immittance but abnormal otoscopic results, one was referred because of abnormal color/ appearance, the other because of retraction and abnormal appearance. For the revised ASHA tympanometric procedures (Table 7), examination of the seven ears with normal immittance but abnormal otoscopic findings, revealed that all were characterized by negative tympanometric peak pressure, a measurement not included in that protocol. Otoscopic findings for those ears revealed abnormal color/appearance for five of the seven, and severe retraction for the remainder.

Discussion

This study was designed to examine the practical application of two immittance screening procedures, based on otoscopic examination at the time of rescreening. As such, it attempted to stimulate the practical application of the two immittance procedures, but without the inevitable delays that normally occur between referral and medical examination. Also atypical was the benefit of pneumatic otoscopy performed by a validated pediatric otolaryngologist. Most children identified in a screening program are referred to a pediatrician or family practice physician, many of whom do not use pneumatic otoscopy.

Although considerable effort was undertaken to optimize the validation criteria used in this study, several important issues must be considered. First, as Bluestone and Klein (1990) have noted, actual verification of middle ear effusion, judged otoscopically, can only be achieved by performing a myringotomy immediately after examination. Because such a validation procedure is unfeasible in a study of this nature, there is undoubtedly some degree of error in using otoscopy as a "gold standard,"

Table 6. Screening results and calculation of sensitivity, specificity, and predictive values for the traditional procedure, based on data from 374 ears evaluated by immittance screening and otoscopy.

		Otoscopy	
		Fail	Pass
Immittance	Refer	42	115
	Pass	2	215

Sensitivity	=	95%
False negatives	=	5%
Specificity	=	65%
False positives	=	35%
Positive predictive value	=	27%
Negative predictive value	=	99%

Table 7. Screening results and calculation of sensitivity, specificity, and predictive values for the revised ASHA immittance procedures, based on data from 374 ears evaluated by immittance screening and otoscopy.

		Otoscopy	
		Fail	Pass
Immittance	Refer	37	17
	Pass	7	313

Sensitivity	=	84%
False negatives	=	16%
Specificity	=	95%
False positives	=	5%
Positive predictive value	=	69%
Negative predictive value	=	98%

even though otoscopic judgments were all made by the same validated otoscopist. It is also important to note that our findings are reported "by ear" rather than "by child." This distinction is important because, as Rockette and Casselbrant (1988) have shown, different levels of sensitivity and specificity may result depending on which methodological approach is taken.§ It is also important to emphasize that judgments regarding the acceptability of a given level of sensitivity or specificity can be made only in the context of disease prevalence. Although sensitivity and specificity are independent of prevalence, positive and negative predictive values (the frequency with which test results represent correct identification of individuals as affected or not affected) are highly influenced by prevalence. Thus, estimates of predictive values should be made only if there is knowledge of disease prevalence (Thorner, 1981). In the present study, 44 ears were classified as abnormal out of 395 examined, indicating a prevalence of approximately 11%. Our estimates of predictive value will undoubtedly differ from those obtained in a medical setting, where the prevalence of ear disease is much higher. This was shown in a recent study by Karzon (1991), who applied ASHA's revised immittance measures to a group of children seen in an otolaryngology setting. Fifty-five ears from a subset of 3- to 5-yr-olds yielded a negative predictive value of 81% for static acoustic admittance and 61% for tympanometric width (positive predictive value was not reported). Sensitivity and specificity were also lower than that observed in the present study for both static admittance and tympanometric width; however, the combined hit and false alarm rates for these measures was not computed.

Attempts to use acoustic immittance for identification of middle ear dysfunction have, in general, resulted in moderate sensitivity, but low specificity. That is, most screening protocols have been reasonably accurate in identifying ears with middle ear dysfunction, but less so in correctly classifying subjects not found to require medical intervention (see Bluestone & Klein, 1991). In gener-

al, our findings using the more traditional approach were similar to those of previous investigators. The over-referral problems associated with absent acoustic reflexes and/or negative tympanometric peak pressure have been demonstrated previously (e.g., Paradise & Smith,1978; Roush & Tait, 1985; Wachtendorf et al, 1984). The acoustic reflex, in particular, seems to contribute little to sensitivity while substantially lowering specificity.

When the two procedures are compared, the traditional immittance screening procedure, which included acoustic reflexes and measures of tympanometric peak pressure, was more successful in identifying ears needing medical attention than was the immittance procedure contained within ASHA's revised Guidelines, which is based on measures of static admittance, physical volume, and tympanometric width. Specifically, the revised ASHA tympanometric procedure classified as normal seven ears judged by the otolaryngologist as needing medical attention. In contrast, only two false negatives occurred when the traditional procedure was applied.

It is important to emphasize that the present study examined only the immittance component contained within the revised ASHA guidelines. Margolis and Heller (1987) suggest that specificity may be increased without lowering sensitivity by providing tympanometric rescreening and by including other components, such as otological history, visual inspection, and audiometric screening, in conjunction with acoustic immittance measures. This philosophy also guided the development of the revised ASHA procedures, and specific guidelines are recommended for each of these components (ASHA, 1990). In the present study, case history information was not included, and pure tone screening, although conducted previously for these children, was not done in conjunction with middle ear screening as recommended in the revised

§In this study, the prevalence calculated "by child" (24 referrals out of 204 subjects, or 12%), was similar to the prevalence calculated "by ear" (44 ears out of 395 examined, or 11%).

ASHA guidelines. Hence, the specificity achieved by applying ASHA's revised immittance measures, although significantly higher than that obtained with the more traditional approach, might have been even higher had the ASHA procedure been applied in its entirety (i.e., in conjunction with history, visual inspection, and pure tone audiometry). Likewise, the inclusion of case history information and pure tone screening would most likely improve the overall performance of the protocol. The effects of including visual inspection are less predictable. Because five of the seven ears missed by the ASHA immittance screening protocol had marked evidence of abnormal color and appearance as well as significant retraction, a skilled nonmedical otoscopist applying the revised ASHA protocol in its entirety might have identified those individuals as needing medical referral, even though they were not identified on the basis of tympanometric findings alone. On the other hand, specificity might have been lower if the inclusion of otoscopic inspection had resulted in an excessive number of false positive medical referrals. The ASHA committee debated the issue of visual inspection at length (R.H. Margolis, personal communication), but decided that the benefits of prompt medical attention for those who needed it justified the risk of additional false positive medical referrals. The visual inspection component will need careful evaluation, however, and programs electing to include it will need to evaluate the efficacy based on their screening personnel and the nature of their target populations (Roush, 1990). This seems particularly important in view of the relatively small proportion of subjects likely to need immittance follow-up under the revised ASHA protocol. It would be regrettable if the improvements in specificity brought about by the revised tympanometric criteria were negated by excessive over-referrals based on otoscopic inspection by nonmedical personnel.

Until the new ASHA guidelines are evaluated in their entirety, the overall validity and predictive value of that protocol will be unknown. In the meantime, audiologists responsible for middle ear screening programs, regardless of the protocol they select, should evaluate their procedures carefully to ensure that they are achieving an acceptable balance between sensitivity and specificity. It is well known that failure to achieve adequate sensitivity results in absence or delay of appropriate medical management, whereas low specificity results in wasted financial resources, strained interprofessional relations, and unnecessary concern on the part of parents and caretakers. Unfortunately, few programs engage in systematic monitoring of screening outcomes. Bluestone et al (1986), at the conclusion of a conference on screening for middle ear disease, noted that "existing screening programs appear to be functioning as massive case-finding mechanisms with-

out informed guidelines to govern their activities" (p. 68). It is imperative that audiologists and health care providers work cooperatively to ensure accurate, cost-effective identification procedures and appropriate medical referral criteria.

Conclusions

The implications of this study may be summarized as follows:

1. Those electing to apply ASHA's revised immittance measures to a population with characteristics similar to the one studied here should achieve a moderate level of sensitivity, but not as high as that achieved using a more traditional procedure based on measures of tympanometric peak pressure and acoustic reflex. Specificity, on the other hand, should be much higher using ASHA's revised immittance procedures. With regard to predictive values, assuming application of the procedures to an unselected group having a similar prevalence of middle ear dysfunction, negative findings would appear to have good predictive value for both procedures. That is, normal tympanometric results should be highly predictive of normal middle ear function. In contrast, the predictive value of a positive (abnormal) outcome would appear to be much lower for both procedures. The positive predictive value for the traditional procedure was 27%, meaning that only about one-fourth of the ears failing the screen were classified otologically as needing medical intervention. The positive predictive value of the revised ASHA immittance measures, although considerably higher (69%), would still be rejected by many practitioners as too low for routine screening purposes.

2. Those electing to continue the use of a more traditional approach to middle ear screening would be well advised to eliminate the acoustic reflex from the test procedure. The acoustic reflex, as routinely applied, appears to substantially lower the specificity, while contributing little to sensitivity.

3. Applied in its entirety, the revised ASHA protocol may achieve higher or lower sensitivity, specificity, and predictive values than those observed in the present study, depending on the time interval between assessment and medical examination and the combined effects of case history, visual inspection, audiometric screening, and acoustic immittance measures. Further research is needed to determine the relative contribution of each.

References

American National Standard Specifications for Instruments to Measure Aural Acoustic Impedance and Admittance (aural acoustic immittance), ANSI S3.39-1987. American National Standard Institute, New York, 1988.

American Speech-Language-Hearing Association. Guidelines for screening for hearing impairment and middle ear disorders. *Asha* 1990;32(Suppl 2):17-24.

American Speech-Language-Hearing Association. Guidelines for acoustic immittance screening of middle ear function. *Asha* 1979;21:550-558.

Bluestone, C., and Cantekin, E. Design factors in the characterization and identification of otitis media and certain related conditions. *Ann Otol Rhinol Laryngol* 1979;88:13-27.

Bluestone, C., Fria, T., Arjona, S., et al. Controversies in Screening for middle ear disease and hearing loss in children. *Pediatrics* 1986;77(1): 57-70.

Bluestone, C., and Klein, J. Otitis media, atelectasis, and eustachian tube dysfunction. In Bluestone, C.D., Stool, S.S., and Scheetz, M.L.S., Eds. *Pediatric Oto-laryngology*, 2nd ed, Philadelphia: WB Saunders Company, 1990:320-486.

Brooks, D.N. A comparative study of an impedance method and pure tone screening. *Scand Audiol* 1973;2:67.

Brooks, D.N. Mass screening with acoustic impedance. In Proceedings of the Third International Symposium on Impedance Audiometry. New York: American Electromedics Co, 1977.

Cooper, J.C., Gates, G., Owen, J., and Dickson, H. An abbreviated impedance bridge technique for school screening. *J Speech Hear Disord* 1974;40: 260.

Harford, E.R., Bess, F.H., Bluestone, C.D., and Klein, J.O., Eds. *Impedance Screening for Middle Ear Disease in Children*. New York: Grune & Stratton, 1978.

Holte, L., and Margolis, R. Screening tympanometry. *Sem Hear* 1987;8(4):329-337.

Howie, V.M. Natural history of otitis media. *Ann Otol Rhinol Laryngol* 1975;19(Suppl):67-72.

Karzon, R. Validity and reliability of tympanometric measures for pediatric patients. *J Speech Hear Res* 1991;34:386-390.

Lous, J. Three impedance screening programs on a cohort of seven-year-old children. *Scand Audiol* 1983; (Suppl 17):60-64.

Lucker, J.R. Application of pass-fail criteria to middle-ear screening results. *Asha* 1980;22:839-840.

Margolis, R.H., and Heller, J.W. Screening tympanometry: criteria for medical referral. *Audiology* 1987;26: 197-208.

Margolis, R., and Shanks, J. Tympanometry: Basic principles and clinical applications. In Rintelmann, W., Ed. *Hearing Assessment*. Austin: Pro-Ed, 1991:179-245.

McCandless, G.A., and Thomas, G.K. Impedance audiometry as a screening procedure for middle ear disease. *Trans Am Acad Opthalmol Otolaryngol* 1974; 78:98.

Orchik, D.J., and Herdman, S. Impedance audiometry as a screening device with school-age children. *J Audiol Res* 1974;14:283.

Paradise, J.L., and Smith, C.G. Impedance screening for preschool children-state of the art. In Harford, E.R., Bess, F.H., Bluestone, C.D., and Klein, J.O., Eds. *Impedance Screening for Middle Ear Disease in Children*. New York: Grune & Stratton, 1978:113-124.

Queen, S., Moses, F., and Wood, S. The use of immittance screening by the Kansas City, Missouri Public School District. *Semin Speech Lang Hear* 1981;2:119.

Rockette, H., and Casselbrant, M. Screening and diagnosis: methodologic issues in screening for otitis media. In Lim, D., Bluestone, C., Klein, J., and Nelson, J., Eds. *Recent Advances in Otitis Media with Effusion*. Toronto: BC Decker, 1988: 42-44.

Roeser, R.J., and Northern, J.L. Screening for hearing loss and middle ear disorders. In Roeser, R.J., and Downs, M.P., Eds. *Auditory Disorders in School Children*, 2nd ed. New York: Thieme-Stratton, 1988:53-82.

Roush, J. Identification of hearing loss and middle ear disease in preschool and school-age children. *Semin Hear* 1990;11:357-371.

Roush, J., and Tait, C. Pure tone and acoustic immittance screening of preschool-age children: An examination of referral criteria. *Ear Hear* 1985; 6(5):245- 249.

Schow, R.L., Pederson, J.K., Nerbonne, M.A., and Boe, R. Comparison of ASHA's immittance guidelines and standard medical diagnostic procedures. *Ear Hear* 1981;2(6):251-255.

Teele, D.W., Klein, J., and Rosner, B. Epidemiology of otitis media in children. *Ann Otol Rhinol Laryngol* 1980:89(Suppl 68):5-6.

Wachtendorf, C.A., Lopez, L.L., Cooper, J.C., Hearne, E., and Gates, G. The efficacy of school screening for otitis media. In Lim, D.J., Bluestone, C.D., Klein, J.O., and Nelson, J.D., Eds. *Recent Advances in Otitis Media*. Toronto: BC Decker, 1984:242-246.

Acknowledgments

The authors thank Robert Margolis and Joseph Hall for their comments and recommendations on an earlier draft of the manuscript. We are also grateful to reviewers Robert Nozza and Ross Roeser for their helpful suggestions on improving this report. Special thanks to the children and staff of the Headstart programs of Duplin County, North Carolina.

Address reprints requests to J. Roush, Campus Box 7190, Wing D-Medical School, University of North Carolina, Chapel Hill, NC 27599.

Received February 4, 1991
Accepted April 18, 1991

Identification of Middle Ear Effusion by Aural Acoustic Admittance and Otoscopy

Robert J. Nozza, Charles D. Bluestone, David Kardatzke, and Ruth Bachman

Children's Hospital of Pittsburgh [R.J.N., C.D.B., R.B.] and the Department of Otolaryngology, School of Medicine, University of Pittsburgh [R.J.N., C.D.B.], Biostatistics, Graduate School of Public Health, University of Pittsburgh [D.K.]

The ability of aural acoustic immittance measures and validated pneumatic otoscopy to identify middle ear effusion (MEE) was determined for a group of children with chronic or recurrent otitis media. The measures were made immediately prior to surgery for placement of tympanostomy tubes, with the validating diagnosis of MEE made by the surgeons. Aural acoustic admittance measures were made by a certified and licensed clinical audiologist using an instrument that meets current standards and otoscopic examinations were made by a nurse practitioner validated for use of otoscopy in the identification of MEE. Logistic regression analyses were done to determine the ability of admittance variables, otoscopy, and their combination to discriminate between ears with and ears without MEE. Of the individual admittance variables, tympanometric width had the best performance. Otoscopy alone had good sensitivity but only fair specificity. Combining acoustic admittance data with the otoscopist's findings did not improve sensitivity greatly, but improved the specificity relative to that of the otoscopist. The criterion tympanometric width >150 daPa or $Y_{tm} < 0.2$, a criterion commonly used based on interim norms published in an appendix of ASHA guidelines for screening, had good sensitivity but very poor specificity in the group of children scheduled for surgery. Also, a comparison was made for tympanometric width measures from the children undergoing surgery with those from a group of children more representative of the general population. Three distributions were found; one for ears with MEE, one for ears with no MEE of children scheduled for otologic surgery and one for ears with no MEE from the group of children from the general population. The data illustrate the importance of the population characteristics on the test measure used and have implications for choosing test criteria. In addition, group estimates of performance of acoustic admittance variables were approximately the same when otoscopy was used as the gold standard for identification of MEE as when findings at surgery were used. However, when comparing the two diagnostic methods on a case-by-case basis, it was determined that the otoscopist's diagnosis disagreed with the diagnosis of the surgeons in over 21% of the ears. (*Ear & Hearing* 1994;15;310-323)

In a previous report (Nozza, Bluestone, Kardatzke, & Bachman, 1992b), we discussed the need to develop standardized criteria for identification of middle-ear effusion (MEE). Standardization is particularly important when conducting clinical research on the diagnosis and/or natural history of otitis media (OM), on the efficacy of treatments for OM, and on screening for MEE. Aural acoustic admittance measures are often used for identifying ears with MEE and are incorporated often into the diagnostic decision making both in research studies and in the clinical setting. However, clinicians with skill in pneumatic otoscopy argue that clear visual evidence of MEE is found often in the presence of acoustic immittance findings that are negative or equivocal for MEE and that inclusion of validated pneumatic otoscopy could optimize decision rules for identification of MEE.

Data on the relation between aural acoustic admittance measures and the presence or absence of MEE in children were presented in our previous report (Nozza et al., 1992b). Acoustic admittance measures were analyzed with respect to the effusion status (MEE versus no MEE) of the ears of children who were undergoing myringotomy and tube (M&T) surgery, with the surgeon determining the presence or absence of MEE. It was shown that several different criteria based on various admittance measures, such as gradient and peak admittance (Y_{tm}), individually and in combination, had good sensitivity and specificity with respect to identification of MEE. In that study, the criterion that was the best at separating ears with MEE from those with no MEE was to call the test positive for MEE when the gradient was ≤ 0.1 or when the gradient was 0.2 or 0.3 and the acoustic reflex was absent. The sensitivity and specificity were 90% and 86%, respectively. We reported data that showed that the latter rule worked well with a group of children more representative of the general population as well. However, we pointed out also that admittance test characteristics are different in the population of children undergoing M&T surgery than they are in the group representing the general population. Consequently, it is important to remember that criteria developed on one

Reprinted by permission of authors and Williams & Wilkins. Copyright 1994. *Ear & Hearing*, 15, No. 4, pp. 310-323.

group or population may not be suitable for use with another group or population.

Validated otoscopists, trained and tested using surgical verification of MEE, can have high sensitivity and specificity, although there is considerable variability among them (Cantekin, Bluestone, Fria, Stool, Berry, & Sabo, 1980; Gates, Avery, Cooper, Hearne, & Holt, 1986; Toner & Mains, 1990). In previous studies, combining the otoscopist's diagnosis with acoustic immittance data has yielded diagnostic ability that is better than either otoscopy or immittance alone (Bluestone & Cantekin, 1979; Cantekin et al., 1980). The latter studies were based on measures using acoustic impedance meters that plotted "compliance" in arbitrary units. Today, acoustic immittance instruments must conform to a new ANSI standard (ANSI, 1987) that requires, among other things, that absolute physical quantities be used. More recent studies (Finitzo, Friel-Patti, Chinn, & Brown, 1992; Le, Daly, Margolis, Lindgren, & Giebink, 1992; Toner & Mains, 1990; Vaughan-Jones & Mills, 1992) have used immittance instruments that meet current standards and otoscopy to test diagnostic ability using findings of surgeons upon myringotomy as the gold standard. However, Toner and Mains (1990), Finitzo et al. (1992), and Vaughan-Jones and Mills (1992), rather than using the absolute physical quantities of aural acoustic immittance to categorize tympanograms, used a categorization scheme based on the "A, B, C" classifications that were originally described by Jerger (1970) and that were developed using impedance meters that used arbitrary compliance units. Le et al. (1992) used absolute physical quantities (admittance) rather than the pattern classifications after Jerger (1970). They defined normal and abnormal for tympanometric variables based on normative data from Margolis and Heller (1987) and included them in development of a clinical profile. None of the above studies reported an analysis of the data that was designed to determine what might be the best tympanometric or tympanometric/otoscopic criteria for identifying MEE with findings at surgery as the gold standard.

The purpose of the present investigation was to estimate the performance of acoustic admittance alone, validated otoscopy alone and the combination of acoustic admittance and otoscopy for determining the presence or absence of MEE in a group of children with history of chronic or recurrent middle ear (ME) disease. The need to standardize the diagnosis of MEE in clinical research studies as well as in ENT clinic has been strong motivation for this work. In addition, the characteristics of acoustic admittance alone with respect to ME status, as verified using myringotomy, will provide valuable information for the use of acoustic admittance measures in screening for ME disease. It should be noted that our current guidelines for screening for ME disease (ASHA, 1990) offer interim norms only. As pointed out in the guidelines, it is necessary that more data on ears with MEE be collected using currently available acoustic immittance instruments either to validate or to modify, based on data, our recommendations in the guidelines.

Because we were collecting otoscopic data, we added as a secondary aim the examination of the acoustic admittance data with the otoscopic diagnosis as the gold standard. Also, admittance values were compared for ears with and ears without MEE based on the diagnosis of the surgeon versus the diagnosis of the otoscopist.

Method

Subjects

One-hundred-seventy-one children between 1 and 12 yr of age (median age 3.8 yr), who were brought to the operating room at Children's Hospital of Pittsburgh for M&T surgery, served as subjects. Subjects were unselected, beyond the above criterion, except as demanded by the logistics of the testing situation. Of the 171 subjects, complete data were obtained on 249 ears. One-hundred-seventy-three (69.5%) of the ears tested were ears of children of ≤ 60 mo of age.

Instrumentation

A GSI-33 Version I Middle Ear Analyzer (Grason-Stadler, Inc.) was used for all acoustic admittance tests. The admittance tests were done by a clinically certified and licensed audiologist. A Welch-Allyn pneumatic otoscope was used by the validated otoscopist, who was a Pediatric Nurse Practitioner with many years' experience in pneumatic otoscopy in children and who had served as the otoscopist for the children in the outpatient group of our previous investigation (Nozza et al., 1992b). As discussed in the latter article, she had been validated by achieving a high level of performance using otoscopic diagnosis against findings of a surgeon at the time of myringotomy for the diagnosis of MEE.

Procedure

Each child was admitted to the Same-Day Surgery Unit of Children's Hospital of Pittsburgh. Unlike our previous study (Nozza et al., 1992b), in which patients were tested immediately outside of the operating room in a holding area, patients in the present study were tested in the Same-Day Surgery admission area. The admittance test and the otoscopic examination were done with the child sitting upright.

For admittance tests, the GSI-33 Middle Ear Analyzer was used in the "diagnostic" (as opposed to "screening") mode. Admittance tympanograms were recorded using a 226 Hz probe tone over a pressure range of +400 to –600 daPa with a positive to negative sweep. The rate of pressure change was 600/200 daPa, which means 600 daPa/s at first, slowing to 200 daPa/s in the region of change in admittance associated with the tympanogram peak, and then returning to the higher rate to complete the measure. The instrument was set also to "baseline" to provide compensated admittance changes as a function of the changing pressure. That is, the admittance of the volume of air in the external ear canal was estimated (at +400 daPa) and then subtracted from the dynamic admittance measure.

An attempt to elicit an acoustic reflex was made following tympanometry. A 1000 Hz tone was presented ipsilaterally at 100 dB HL a maximum of three times while the ear canal pressure was held at tympanometric peak pressure. In ears for which no peak could be determined, the stimulus was presented with ear canal pressure at 0 daPa.

The GSI-33 provides both a plot of the admittance change versus pressure (i.e., a tympanogram) and a table of the values for equivalent volume of the ear canal (V_{ec}), Y_{tm}, gradient and tympanometric peak pressure. Although gradient can be computed in several different ways (Brooks, 1969; de Jonge, 1986; Koebsell & Margolis, 1986), the GSI-33 that was used in this investigation computed gradient in a way similar to that recommended by Paradise, Smith, and Bluestone (1976). It is the ratio a/b, such that a is the difference between the Y_{tm} and the mean of the two admittance values at +50 and at –50 daPa from tympanometric peak pressure, and b is Y_{tm}. Tympanometric width (TW), another way of quantifying tympanometric shape or gradient, was measured after the fact. TW is the interval in daPa between the sides of the tympanogram at one half Y_{tm}. It was measured from the recorded tympanogram using a computerized optical digitization system that was designed for making measurements of anatomical structures in slide preparations. Acoustic reflex was recorded as present or absent based on a minimum 0.02 mmho change in admittance.

Following the acoustic admittance tests, the otoscopist examined the ear canal and tympanic membrane using the pneumatic otoscope. She characterized the ear as having effusion or no effusion while remaining unaware of the admittance findings. The time between our admittance and otoscopic tests and the time the patients entered the operating room was no longer than 60 minutes.

The surgeon was unaware of the admittance test and otoscopic exam results at the time of surgery. The surgeon was required to indicate only whether MEE was present or absent upon myringotomy. Several surgeons, experienced in research studies requiring verification of ME status during M&T surgery, participated in the study.

Surgery

All procedures were performed under general anesthesia using oxygen, nitrous oxide, and halothane by inhalation. A radial myringotomy incision was made in the anterosuperior quadrant of the tympanic membrane and the presence or absence of MEE was determined by aspirating the ME with a fine needle suction. The results were recorded by the surgeon on the standardized form. An Armstrong-type tympanostomy tube was then inserted into the myringotomy incision.

Results

Findings by Surgeon as the Gold Standard

Of the 249 ears for which complete data (myringotomy, otoscopy, and tympanometry) were obtained, 137 (55%) had MEE and 112 (45%) had no MEE as determined by the surgeon at the time of M&T. The primary analyses of acoustic admittance and otoscopy used the findings at surgery as the validating criterion (i.e., the gold standard). For comparison, the validated otoscopist diagnosed MEE in 148 (59%) ears and diagnosed no MEE in 101 (41%) ears.

The means and the 5th and 95th percentiles for tympanometric variables V_{ec}, Y_{tm}, tympanometric peak pressure, gradient, and TW are provided in Table 1. The values are displayed for ears with and without MEE as determined at surgery. Data on ears from a group of children unselected with respect to otologic history and otoscopically normal (Nozza et al., 1992b), as well as data from two other published studies of admittance in young children with normal hearing and no otoscopic evidence of ME dysfunction (Koebsell & Margolis, 1986; Margolis & Heller, 1987), are presented for comparison. The small differences in values across studies may be due to differences in ages of the subjects, differences in instrumentation settings and/or different means of compensating for ear canal volume across studies (see Table 1, footnotes a, b, and c).

A test of the acoustic reflex that was considered valid (i.e., free of artifact, reflex present or absent) was obtained for 218 (87.5%) of the 249 ears in the sample. Of those 218 ears, 124 (57%) had MEE and 94 (43%) had no MEE as determined at surgery. Thirty-one (12.5%) ears were recorded as "could not test" (CNT) due to crying, fussing, or movement.

Table 1. Myringotomy as gold standard. Group mean admittance values for ears with MEE and without MEE as determined by the surgeon from our group of children undergoing surgery (M&T group). Norms are taken from three recent studies.

| Variables | M&T Group Surgical diagnosis | | Norms Otoscopic diagnosis | | |
| | Current investigation | | Nozza et al.[a] | Koebsell/Margolis[b] | Margolis/Heller[c] |
	MEE	No MEE	No MEE	No MEE	No MEE
V_{ec} (cc)					
Mean	0.65	0.69	0.90	N/A[d]	0.74
SD	0.19	0.20	0.26		N/A
5-95% range	0.4 to 1.0	0.5 to 1.1	0.6 to 1.4	0.42 to 0.97	
N	137	112	130		92
Y_{tm} (mmho)					
Mean	0.28	0.58	0.78	0.67	0.50
SD	0.18	0.30	0.31	0.22	0.19
5-95% range	0 to 0.6	0.2 to 1.2	0.4 to 1.4	N/A	0.22 to 0.81
N	137	112	130	60	92
TPP (daPa)					
Mean	−174	−114	−34	N/A	−30
SD	123	115	58	N/A	
5-95% range	−415 to 0	−325 to 30	−207 to 15		−139 to 11
N[e]	122	110	130		92
Gradient					
Mean	0.14	0.30	0.45	0.40	N/A
SD	0.12	0.13	0.08	0.11	
5-95% range	0-0.4	0.1 to 0.5	0.3 to 0.6	0.25 to 0.59	
N	137	112	130	60	
TW[f] (daPa)					
Mean	373	216	104	124	100
SD	118	90	32	33	N/A
5-95% range	143 to 542	84 to 394	60 to 168	68 to 187	59 to 151
N	137	112	130	60	92

[a]Nozza et al. (1992b): +400 to −600 daPa; 3 to 16 years old.
[b]Koebsell and Margolis (1986): MAX/MIN Method, +400 to −400 daPa; 2.8- to 5.8-year-olds.
[c]Margolis and Heller (1987): +200 to −300 daPa; 3.7 to 5.8-year-olds.
[d]Not available from report.
[e]N for TPP is smaller than for other measures because "no peak" tympanograms were excluded.
[f]TW measures were not provided by the GSI-33 used in this investigation. Rather, a measurement was made with the help of an optical digitization and measurement system (see text). V_{ec}, equivalent ear canal volume; Y_{tm}, peak compensated admittance; TW, tympanometric width; TPP, tympanometric peak pressure; gradient (ratio of a/b, where a = difference in admittance between peak and a baseline drawn at point where width of tympanogram is 100 daPa and b = peak admittance).

Table 2 provides selected criteria for declaring a test positive for MEE and the associated sensitivity, specificity and predictive values based on our data. The validated otoscopist had sensitivity of 85% and specificity of 71% relative to the findings upon myringotomy. A logistic regression analysis was done to determine which variables alone and in combination best discriminated between ears with MEE and those with no MEE. The logistic regression, used for regression analyses in which one variable is binary (e.g., effusion present or absent), provides information on the relative ability of the different test measures, either alone or in combinations, to discriminate between the two groups (Agresti, 1984). After determining the relative ability of the various admittance variables to discriminate MEE from no MEE ears, specific cutoffs were evaluated to determine performance characteristics. The criteria in Table 2 represent those that had the best performance as determined using the logistic regression analysis or were chosen because they were suggested by data from previous research as potentially useful criteria.

TW was identified as the best single tympanometric variable for discriminating between ears with and ears without MEE. Following TW, in order of their ability to discriminate based on the logistic regression analysis, the other tympanometric variables were Y_{tm}, gradient, acoustic reflex, and tympanometric peak pressure. The best performance cutoff using TW alone was to call the test positive for MEE when TW was >275 daPa. Sensitivity and specificity were 81% and 82%, respectively (Table 2). Positive predictive value (PPV) is the percentage of those with a positive test outcome who truly have the disease and the negative predictive value (NPV) is the percentage of those with a negative test outcome who truly do not have the disease. To interpret test results properly, the sensitivity and specificity of the test, as well as a good estimate of the likelihood that disease will be present in the population tested (i.e., prevalence), must be known ahead of time. PPV and NPV, for a specific test criterion with known sensitivity and specificity, are the probabilities that the individual tested does or does not have the disease and, as such, relate directly to the question asked by the practitioner; namely, given this test outcome, what is the probability that the patient has the disease or condition in question (Griner, Mayewski, Mushlin, & Greenland, 1981)?

For the 218 ears on which there was a reliable test of the acoustic reflex, sensitivity and specificity of the acoustic reflex alone were 86% (106/124) and 65% (61/94), respectively. However, because 31 (12.5%) of the ears were recorded as CNT, or in other words, did not provide information sufficient to classify, the sensitivity and specificity values may be misleading.

Figure 1 presents some of the performance data in a receiver operating characteristic (ROC) space. In the ROC space, sensitivity and specificity data may be presented in a way that permits us to see easily which criteria perform best (Griner et al., 1981). With sensitivity on the y-axis and 1-specificity (false positive rate) on the x-axis, the closer to the upper left corner in the space the data point falls, the better is the overall performance. Points along the positive diagonal represent equal sensitivity and false positive rate; that is, chance performance. One can plot in the ROC space single points to represent performance of specific criteria for discriminating between MEE and no MEE or one can plot functions, or curves, that represent the effects on performance of different criteria (cutoffs) for a specific variable. For example, ROC curves for the variables Y_{tm} and TW are given in Figure 1, as are points representing selected other criteria. The difference in ROC curves for the two admittance variables are not substantial, although TW does achieve the greatest values. For example, for a specificity of around 80% (i.e., 1-specificity of 20% in Fig. 1), Y_{tm} (≤ 0.3) has a sensitivity of 70% while TW (>275) has sensitivity of over 80%. The other points in the ROC space represent the best performance that could be achieved using otoscopy alone and tympanometric variables combined with otoscopy. The specific cutoffs for the criteria that are given in Figure 1 can be obtained from Table 2. As is evident from Table 2 and Figure 1, combining otoscopy with TW did not improve the performance achieved by TW, but did improve the specificity of otoscopy. For example, if the test is called positive for MEE either when TW > 350, or when TW lies between 250 and 350 and otoscopy is positive, sensitivity is 80% and specificity is 81%.

Y_{tm} and TW are thought to have a low correlation, a relationship that might favor their use together in a diagnostic scheme (Koebsell & Margolis, 1986). For all ears, the Pearson product-moment correlation coefficient (r) between Y_{tm} and TW was –0.57, a measure close to that reported by Koebsell and Margolis (1986) for normal ears. However, in the present data set, the correlations between Y_{tm} and TW for ears with no MEE, $r = -0.41$, and for ears with MEE, $r = -0.37$, were lower than for all ears together. This finding is consistent with a data set with two subgroups, each with lower correlation than the overall group and separated with respect to the variables of interest. The lack of a strong relationship suggested that TW and Y_{tm} together might have better ability to discriminate between ears with MEE and ears with no MEE than either variable alone. However, a variety of combinations of TW with Y_{tm} were evaluated and none was better than TW alone. The best criterion, TW > 300 or Y_{tm} <0.1, produced sensitivity of 80% and specificity of 82%. Changes in the cutoff for either TW or Y_{tm} reduced one or both performance values.

Some criteria were such that the presence or absence of an acoustic reflex was included to disambiguate tympanometric findings. For example, the criterion of gradient ≤ 0.1, or gradient = 0.2 along with an absent acoustic reflex, provided sensitivity and specificity of 81% and 83%, respectively. However, criteria that required a valid test of the acoustic reflex to classify ears that were equivocal by tympanometry invariably left some ears unclassified. In the latter example, 10 ears could not be classified because they had gradient = 0.2 but the acoustic reflex was recorded as CNT. This typically occurred in cases of crying or extreme movements by the patients.

To summarize, there were a variety of criteria that produced a variety of different sensitivity and specificity values for the diagnosis of MEE. Many were similar in performance, with the best criteria producing sensitivity and specificity values in the low 80% range. Our otoscopist had good sensitivity and fair specificity. Table 2 provides information on the performance of specific criteria. However, it should be kept in mind that the performance of the tests used in this study are specific to the population tested; children with a history of chronic or recurrent MEE who were candidates for placement of tympanostomy tubes.

Findings of the Otoscopist as the Gold Standard

When surgery is not indicated, otoscopy is considered the standard against which to measure other test proce-

Table 2. Sensitivity, specificity, and predictive values of various criteria using acoustic admittance measures for the diagnosis of MEE as determined at myringotomy, in ears with a history of chronic or recurrent otitis media ($N = 249$).

Variables	Criterion	Sens (%)	Spec (%)	PPV (%)	NPV (%)
Otoscopy[a]		85	71	78	79
Gr + AR	Gr ≤ 0.1, OR Gr = 0.2 or 0.3 with AR absent (20 ears could not be classified)[b]	82	72	80	77
	Gr ≤ 0.1, OR Gr = 0.2 with AR absent (10 ears could not be classified)[b]	81	83	86	77
Y_{tm} + AR	Y_{tm} ≤ 0.2, OR Y_{tm} = 0.3 or 0.4 or 0.5 with AR absent (19 ears could not be classified)[b]	82	78	83	77
	Y_{tm} ≤ 0.2 OR Y_{tm} = 0.3 or 0.4 with AR absent (10 ears could not be classified)[b]	76	86	87	74
	Y_{tm} ≤ 0.3 OR Y_{tm} = 0.4 or 0.5 with AR absent (12 ears could not be classified)[b]	84	68	77	76
AR	AR absent (31 ears could not be classified)[b]	86	65	76	77
Gr					
	GR ≤ 0	23	98	94	51
	Gr ≤ 0.1	66	91	90	69
	Gr ≤ 0.2	85	62	73	78
	Gr ≤ 0.3	93	38	65	81
Y_{tm}[a]					
	Y_{tm} ≤ 0	11	98	88	47
	Y_{tm} ≤ 0.1	26	97	92	52
	Y_{tm} ≤ 0.2	46	92	88	58
	Y_{tm} ≤ 0.3	70	80	81	69
	Y_{tm} ≤ 0.4	83	69	76	77
Gr and Y_{tm}					
	Gr ≤ 0.1 OR Y_{tm} ≤ 0.2	72	87	87	71
	Gr ≤ 0.1 OR Y_{tm} ≤ 0.3	81	77	82	77
	Gr ≤ 0.1 OR Y_{tm} ≤ 0.4	87	67	76	81
TW[a]					
	TW > 150	94	26	61	78
	TW > 200	89	47	67	78
	TW > 250	85	68	76	78
	TW > 275	81	82	85	78
	TW > 300	77	85	86	75
	TW > 325	70	88	87	71
	TW > 350	61	89	88	65
	TW > 400	49	96	94	61
TW and Y_{tm}					
	TW > 150 OR Y_{tm} < 0.2	95	25	61	80
TW Plus Otoscopy (OTO)					
	TW > 350 or 250 ≤ TW ≤ 350 and OTO positive[a]	80	81	84	77
	TW > 300 or 250 ≤ TW ≤ 300 and OTO positive	82	79	82	78
	TW > 350 or 150 ≤ TW ≤ 350 and OTO positive[a]	85	75	81	87
	TW > 400 or 150 ≤ TW ≤ 400 and OTO positive	83	75	80	78
Y_{tm} Plus Otoscopy					
	Y_{tm} ≤ 0.1 or 0.1 < Y_{tm} ≤ 0.6 and OTO positive[a]	81	85	87	79
	Y_{tm} ≤ 0.1 or 0.1 < Y_{tm} ≤ 0.7 and OTO positive[a]	84	81	85	81

[a]See figure 1 for graphic representation in ROC space.
[b]Ears could not be classified because a valid test of the AR was not obtained, but was required to make the diagnosis based on the criterion.
AR, acoustic reflex; Gr, gradient; Y_{tm}, peak compensated admittance; OTO, otoscopy; Sens, sensitivity; Spec, specificity; PPV, positive predictive value; NPV, negative predictive value.

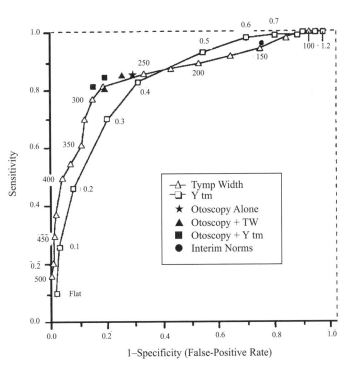

Figure 1. Sensitivity and specificity of selected criteria presented in ROC (receiver operating characteristic) space. Performance estimates of all single points in the ROC space are taken from Table 2. Criterion based on interim norms comes from Koebsell and Margolis (1986) as reported in ASHA guidelines (ASHA, 1990).

dures used in the identification of MEE. In the present study, we wanted to evaluate otoscopy as a diagnostic measure alone and in combination with admittance measures using surgery as the validating criterion. We did not do otoscopy with the intention of using it to validate the admittance data, but it is instructive to view the data in that context. In fact, one might argue that the otoscopist's view is the one that must be considered because, in most cases, surgical verification of MEE is not appropriate. Further, some of the data that have been reported on the relationship between acoustic admittance measures and MEE have used otoscopy as the standard (e.g., Karzon, 1991; Roush, Drake, & Sexton, 1992; Silman, Silverman, & Arick, 1992). Finally, and perhaps most importantly, when using tympanometry in a screening application, it is the physical exam (otoscopy) of a physician that is the outcome of a referral. Therefore, in practice, it is the otoscopy of the managing physician that will determine the "validity" of the screening test and/ or program. Table 3 presents descriptive statistics for admittance variables using otoscopic diagnosis to categorize the ears. Table 4 presents the performance characteristics of various acoustic admittance criteria using otoscopy as the standard. The group data using otoscopy (Tables 3 and 4) are very similar to the outcome using surgery as the standard (Tables 1 and 2).

Although the overall (group) performance of acoustic admittance does not change substantially when using otoscopy rather than surgery to confirm MEE, it is interesting to note that the group descriptive statistics obscure the outcome relative to individual ears. A closer look at the degree of disagreement between the two validating measures is necessary to fully appreciate the importance of the standard used. The otoscopist disagreed with the surgeon on 53 (21.3%) of the 249 ears in the study (Table 5). By otoscopy, 32 ears were false positives (negative by surgery but positive by otoscopy) and 21 ears were false negatives (positive by surgery but negative by otoscopy). That is, while there were similar proportions of the sample declared to have MEE by surgery (55%) and by otoscopy (59%), there was disagreement between the two diagnostic procedures in over 21% of the ears. Table 5 provides descriptive statistics for the tympanometric variables for ears for which there was diagnostic agreement between surgical findings and otoscopy, as well as for the group of ears for which there was disagreement. As one might predict, the group mean admittance measures for the ears for which there was agreement of MEE are quite different from the group mean tympanometric measures for the ears for which there was agreement of no MEE. The mean tympanometric values for ears for which there was disagreement lie between the two groups for which

Table 3. Otoscopy as gold standard. Group mean admittance values for ears with MEE and without MEE as determined by the otoscopist from our group of children undergoing surgery (M&T group). Norms are taken from three recent studies.

Variables	M&T Group Otoscopic diagnosis Current investigation		Norms Otoscopic diagnosis		
	MEE	No MEE	Nozza et al.[a] No MEE	Koebsell/Margolis[b] No MEE	Margolis/Heller[c] No MEE
V_{ec} (cc)					
Mean	0.68	0.65	0.90	N/A[d]	0.74
SD	0.22	0.15	0.26		N/A
5-95% range	0.4 to 1.1	0.5 to 1.0	0.6 to 1.4		0.42 to 0.97
N	148	101	130		92
Y_{tm} (mmho)					
Mean	0.31	0.56	0.78	0.67	0.50
SD	0.26	0.25	0.31	0.22	0.19
5-95% range	0 to 0.7	0.3 to 1.1	0.4 to 1.4	N/A	0.22 to 0.81
N	148	101	130	60	92
TPP (daPa)					
Mean	−189	−89	−34	N/A	−30
SD	127	91	58		N/A
5-95% range	−420 to 0	−245 to 25	−207 to 15		−139 to 11
N	131[e]	101	130		92
Gradient					
Mean	0.14	0.31	0.45	0.40	N/A
SD	0.12	0.13	0.08	0.11	
5-95% range	0 to 0.4	0.1 to 0.5	0.3 to 0.6	0.25 to 0.59	
N	148	101	130	60	
TW (daPa)					
Mean	370	204	104	124	100
SD	118	78	32	33	N/A
5-95% range	143 to 537	84 to 335	60 to 168	68 to 187	59 to 151
N	148	101	130	60	92

[a]Nozza et al. (1992b): +400 to −600 daPa; 3-16 yr old.
[b]Koebsell and Margolis (1986): MAX/MIN method, +400 to −400 daPa; 2.8- to 5.8-yr olds.
[c]Margolis and Heller (1987): +200 to −300 daPa; 3. 7 to 5.8-yr-olds.
[d]Not available from report.
[e]17 ears had NP (no peak) tympanograms.
V_{ec}, equivalent ear canal volume; Y_{tm}, peak compensated admittance; TW, tympanometric width; TPP, tympanometric peak pressure; gradient (ratio of a/b, where a = difference in admittance between peak and a baseline drawn at point where width of tympanogram is 100 daPa and b = peak admittance).

there was agreement. Table 6 presents the data for only the 53 ears for which there was disagreement between the findings at surgery and the otoscopic findings, this time separated by otoscopic false positives and false negatives relative to surgical diagnosis. There do not appear to be any easily derived tympanometric criteria that would help to discriminate these ears based on the group data.

Immittance Screening in the General Population

In our previous report (Nozza et al., 1992b), we presented acoustic admittance data from children who were visiting a hospital outpatient allergy clinic. However, we did not have TW measurements for the tympanograms in that study because the instrument that we used provided gradient as a ratio. For this report, we measured TW for the tympanograms from that group in the same way as

done for our surgery group so that we could investigate the performance of TW as it might apply to screening school-age children who were more representative of the general population. Although the subject sample is described in detail in our earlier article (Nozza et al., 1992b), a summary of the subjects is provided here. Seventy-seven children (ages 3-16, mean age 9 yr) were examined otoscopically and tympanometrically. Of the 77 children, tympanograms were obtained on 144 ears for which otoscopic diagnosis of ME condition was made; 135 ears had no MEE and nine ears had MEE. The mean, standard deviation, and 90% range for the 130 ears of children who were free of MEE bilaterally can be found in Table 1 or Table 3. Table 7 provides the sensitivity, specificity, and predictive values for TW and TW combined with Y_{tm} for ears from this group of children. Other admittance variables were presented in our earlier article

Table 4. Sensitivity, specificity, and predictive values of various criteria using acoustic admittance measures for the diagnosis of MEE as determined by otoscopy, in ears with a history of chronic or recurrent otitis media ($N = 249$).

Variables	Criterion	Sens (%)	Spec (%)	PPV (%)	NPV (%)
AR Alone	(31 ears not classified)	77	77	76	77
Gr					
	≤ 0	23	100	100	47
	≤ 0.1	64	94	94	64
	≤ 0.2	85	65	78	74
	≤ 0.3	93	32	67	76
Y_{tm}					
	≤ 011		100	100	44
	≤ 0.1	26	100	100	48
	≤ 0.2	47	97	96	55
	≤ 0.3	70	85	87	66
	≤ 0.4	77	66	77	66
TW					
	>150	95	29	66	78
	>200	89	51	72	75
	>225	86	62	77	75
	>250	85	73	82	76
	>275	79	86	89	74
	>300	75	89	91	71
	>325	70	94	95	68
	>350	62	95	95	63

AR, acoustic reflex; Gr, gradient; Y_{tm}, peak compensated admittance; TW, tympanometric width; Sens, sensitivity; Spec, specificity; PPV, positive predictive value; NPV, negative predictive value.

Table 5. Descriptive statistics for admittance variables for ears for which the diagnosis of No MEE (negative) or MEE (positive) by surgery and by otoscopy was in agreement and was in disagreement.

Variables	Both negative (No MEE)	Disagreement	Both positive (MEE)
V_{ec} (cc)			
Mean	0.67	0.68	0.66
SD	0.16	0.24	0.20
5-95% range	0.5 to 1.0	0.5 to 1.2	0.5 to 1.1
N	80	53	116
Y_{tm} (mmho)			
Mean	0.59	0.52	0.24
SD	0.27	0.30	0.16
5-95% range	0.3 to 1.2	0.1 to 1.0	0 to 0.5
N	80	53	116
TPP (daPa)			
Mean	−8	−171	−184
SD	88	122	126
5-95% range	−233 to 30	−375 to 25	−420 to 0
N^a	80	51	101
Gradient			
Mean	0.33	0.24	0.11
SD	0.12	0.13	0.10
5-95% range	0.2 to 0.5	0.1 to 0.5	0 to 0.3
N	80	53	116
TW (daPa)			
Mean	193	261	396
SD	69	107	106
5-95% range	83 to 300	103 to 408	186 to 546
N	80	53	116

[a]17 ears had no peak (NP) tympanograms and were not included in estimate of TPP. V_{ec}, equivalent ear canal volume; Y_{tm}, peak compensated admittance; TW, tympanometric width; TPP, tympanometric peak pressure; gradient (ratio of a/b, where a = difference in admittance between peak and a baseline drawn at point where width of tympanogram is 100 daPa and b = peak admittance).

(Nozza et al., 1992b). Because all ears in this group with $Y_{tm} < 0.2$ also had TW > 150, the performance of the criterion, TW > 150 or $Y_{tm} < 0.2$, is the same as using TW > 150 alone. For our data set, TW > 200 and TW > 250 had better performance than TW > 150 daPa.

In the context of screening, a more meaningful analysis for this outpatient group is one with the child, rather than the ear, as the unit of analysis (Fig. 2). Of the 77 children examined otoscopically, nine had at least one ear with ME disorder. According to the current ASHA guidelines (ASHA, 1990), a child reporting ear pain or with otoscopic evidence of drainage through the tympanic membrane should be immediately referred for medical examination. Based on those criteria, two children of the nine with ME disorders would have been immediate screening failures. Of the remaining seven, all but one would have been positive on the initial screening based on tympanometric findings in at least one ear, using any of the TW cutoffs considered above (TW > 150, TW > 200, or TW > 250). The child who didn't fail based on tympanometry had an otoscopic diagnosis of unilateral MEE with evidence of a fluid level or bubbles, $Y_{tm} = 2.3$ and TW = 100. This ear would not fail any reasonable tympanometric criterion designed to identify MEE.

Of the 68 children with no MEE bilaterally, tympanometric results were obtained for both ears for 63 children, for only one ear for four children, and for neither ear for one child. Rather than exclude the five children for whom incomplete tympanometric data were obtained, we have included them as screening positives on the initial test. This conservative approach gives a "worst-case" estimate of the number of children in our group who would have to be screened again according to the protocol in the ASHA guidelines (ASHA, 1990).

Unlike the group with MEE, the outcome for the group of 68 would change based on the tympanometric criterion (Fig. 2). That is, the specificity and PPV of the test vary with the tympanometric cutoff used. The criterion of history, visual inspection, and TW > 150 yielded 14 false positive identifications, whereas the change to TW > 200 produced 7 false positive identifications. With TW > 250, there were five false positives (consisting only of the five with incomplete data). Because for this data set the

Table 6. Descriptive statistics for admittance variables for ears for which the diagnosis by otoscopy (OTO) disagreed with that by surgery (MYR) ($N = 53$).

Variables	OTO : MEE MYR : No MEE	OTO : No MEE MYR : MEE
V_{ec} (cc)		
Mean	0.75	0.58
SD	0.28	0.11
5-95% range	0.5 to 1.4	0.5 to 0.7
N	32	21
Y_{tm} (mmho)		
Mean	0.55	0.48
SD	0.36	0.14
5-95% range	0 to 1.2	0.3 to 0.7
N	32	21
TPP[a] (daPa)		
Mean	−204	−124
SD	130	94
5-95% range	−390 to 50	−255 to 25
N	30	21
Gradient		
Mean	0.23	0.27
SD	0.12	0.14
5-95% range	0 to 0.4	0.1 to 0.5
N	32	21
TW (daPa)		
Mean	272	244
SD	112	99
5-95% range	103 to 443	127 to 387
N	32	21

[a]Two ears had no peak (NP) tympanogram. V_{ec}, equivalent ear canal volume; Y_{tm}, peak compensated admittance; TW, tympanometric width; TPP, tympanometric peak pressure.

sensitivity does not improve by adding any value of Y_{tm} to the criteria (i.e., the one false negative ear has $Y_{tm} = 2.3$, a value considered consistent with abnormally high admittance rather than low admittance), but specificity can decrease (Table 4 in Nozza et al., 1992b), there is no value to examining TW combined with Y_{tm}. It should be noted that the differences in ages of the subjects and the ear canal pressure at which V_{ec} was estimated between the interim norms provided in the ASHA guidelines (ASHA, 1990) and the data from our investigations (present study; Nozza et al., 1992b) may account for some of the differences in test performance. As the guidelines (ASHA, 1990) properly point out, if different age groups and/or different instrumentation settings are to be used, different normative standards may be called for. It should be noted also that for a first screening, in which disposition is a retest rather than a referral for medical examination in most cases, even a high false positive rate may be considered acceptable. Such judgments are made administratively based on a number of factors.

Discussion

The results of this investigation reveal the extent to which acoustic admittance, otoscopy, and their combination can be relied upon to discriminate between ears with and ears without MEE. The data have implications for several issues related to the identification and diagnosis of MEE in children.

Identification of MEE Using Acoustic Admittance and/or Otoscopy with Myringotomy as the Gold Standard

The admittance data from this investigation are consistent with data from our previous study (Nozza et al., 1992b). We have found that a variety of admittance criteria, with and without otoscopy, have good sensitivity and specificity for identification of MEE. Of the admittance variables taken singly, TW was best at discriminating between ears with MEE and ears with no MEE in the group with history of chronic or recurrent MEE (Fig. 1). The diagnostic performance of otoscopy alone varies widely among otoscopists, but as in the present investiga-

Table 7. Sensitivity, specificity, and predictive values for tympanometric width (TW) and TW combined with peak admittance (Y_{tm}) for ears of children representative of the general population (Nozza et al., 1992b). Diagnosis of middle ear effusion was done by otoscopy.

Variables	Criterion	Sens (%) ($N = 9$)	Spec (%) ($N = 135$)	PPV(%)	NPV(%)
TW	>150	89	93	44	99
	>200	78	99	78	99
	>250	78	100	100	99
TW or Y_{tm}	TW > 150 or Y_{tm} < 0.2[a]	89	93	44	99
	TW > 200 or Y_{tm} < 0.3	78	98	70	99
	TW > 250 or Y_{tm} < 0.3	78	99	88	99

[a]Interim norms (ASHA, 1990).
TW, tympanometric width; Sens, sensitivity; Spec, specificity; PPV, positive predictive value; NPV, negative predictive value.

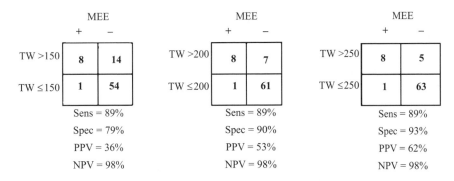

Figure 2. Two-by-two matrices representing outcome of three different screening criteria using tympanometric width (TW) and using the child, rather than the ear, as the unit of analysis. For all three matrices, children were positive outcomes if they failed the history, visual inspection or the criterion for TW. Also, children for whom tympanometry was completed on only one ear were considered positive on the screening. The children were described in detail in a previous article (Nozza et al., 1992b) and are considered to be representative of the general population. (Ages: 3-16, mean age, 9 yr) MEE = middle ear effusion; + = MEE present; – = MEE absent; Sens = sensitivity; Spec = specificity; PPV = positive predictive value; NPV = negative predictive value.

tion, specificity is typically lower than sensitivity. Some combinations of otoscopic diagnosis and tympanometric findings performed well also (Table 2).

Diagnosis of MEE

One problem that is inherent in the nature of studies of OM is the difficulty of defining the disease and deciding how to classify ears into a fixed, small number of categories (two to four) when the disease states lie on a virtual continuum. The typical way to handle the problem is to develop either a set of diagnostic rules that include an equivocal category (e.g., Finitzo et al., 1992; Toner & Mains, 1990) or a diagnostic scheme that attempts to break the disease continuum into more than the two categories of presence and absence of disease (e.g., Le et al., 1992).

From the standpoint of the practitioner attempting to interpret test data, equivocal categories are not very helpful. The approach of Finitzo et al. (1992) and Toner and Mains (1990) to disregard equivocal immittance data makes their sensitivity and specificity values appear quite high. However, as illustrated by the data from the present investigation, such maneuvers do not really provide useful information to the practitioner trying to decide in ambiguous cases.

In the present investigation, we have attempted to provide a number of different test criteria that are free of an equivocal category. By providing a variety of diagnostic criteria based on our various tests, we have given the practitioner the opportunity to see how the test performance varies and permits assessment of our data based on the needs of those who would apply the findings to their own situation. Things that must be taken into account by one who would use acoustic immittance and/or otoscopic information for diagnosis of ME disease include char-

acteristics of the population under study (general population, high-risk, chronic MEE, etc.), the ability of the practitioner to use pneumatic otoscopy to diagnose ME disease, and the definition of disease for which the test is being used (i.e., at what point on the continuum of disease the practitioner chooses to categorize).

Otoscopy as the Gold Standard

In other studies, specific acoustic admittance criteria were evaluated with respect to diagnosing MEE with otoscopy as the gold standard. Karzon (1991) found that criteria based on the interim norms provided in current ASHA guidelines (ASHA, 1990) had performance that was good but below 90% accuracy in a clinic setting. Roush et al. (1992) found better performance in a preschool screening. However, Silman et al. (1992) reported that there are acoustic immittance criteria that can achieve very high (> 90%) sensitivity and specificity. Silman et al. (1992) also used otoscopic diagnosis in a clinic setting to validate their admittance findings. Advocating the use of the acoustic reflex, they reported that adding the acoustic reflex to the protocol and interim norms provided in the ASHA guidelines (ASHA, 1990) could improve performance and that a criterion combining tympanometric peak pressure with acoustic reflex also could produce very high performance values. They were able to produce sensitivity and specificity values from their data set that were ∅ 90%. However, it should be noted that their sensitivity is based on ears diagnosed by the otolaryngologist/otoscopist as having MEE and the specificity is based on "normal hearing, normal ME" ears. Therefore, it is possible that there is a third group that consists of *neither normal hearing, normal ME ears, nor ears with MEE.* That is, there may be a group of ears with "*abnormal ME, but no MEE,*" that were not included in the sample. Such a group apparently was not included in the study by Silman et al. (1992), but probably represents a large proportion of ears in a pediatric otolaryngological practice. As pointed out in the present investigation, 45% of the ears referred for M&T surgery were *without MEE* at the time of surgery but were *abnormal* by most standards (e.g., Table 1). Silman et al. (1992) may have reduced the likelihood of dealing with equivocal data by eliminating a large source of the equivocal ears by their subject selection procedure. Our data may be used to illustrate such effects if such a sampling bias were to occur.

In Figure 3, the distributions for three groups of ears for the immittance variable TW are displayed. The distribution of TW for the ears *with MEE* from the present investigation, the ears *with no MEE* from the present investigation, and a group of ears *with no MEE* from children (outpatients) who were unselected with respect to otologic history and who were bilaterally effusion free by otoscopy at the time of testing. If we choose to pick a criterion that can discriminate between the ears with MEE and those with normal ME (i.e., between ears with MEE from children with a history of chronic or recurrent OM and ears with no MEE from an independent group with normal ME from the general population), we could find a cut point that will perform quite well. In fact, TW > 150 would produce sensitivity of 95% (Table 4) if we use the ears with MEE from the surgery group and specificity of 93% (Table 7) if we use the ears with no MEE from the outpatient group. However, with that maneuver, the *group with no MEE but abnormal ME* from the surgery group in the present study is excluded. Of course, that group should not be ignored and represents a part of the diagnostic dilemma. Failure to consider the group with abnormal ME but with no MEE in studies of diagnostic testing for MEE can misrepresent test performance and lead to selection of a test criterion with performance below that suggested by the data. Our premise is that the diagnosis of MEE is the important factor and that ears with MEE should be distinguished from ears with no MEE.

On the other hand, some might argue that a screening program should be designed to discriminate between those with normal ME (such as the no MEE ears of our children from the outpatient clinic) and those with abnormal ME (effusion present or absent). In that case, the group with abnormal ME with no MEE, rather than ignored, is included in the targeted group. If we can assume that all of the ears scheduled for M&T surgery, with or without MEE, are abnormal, and we screen for abnormal ME, then performance of our test criterion changes again. We already know that by using our normal ears from the general population our estimate of specificity is 93%. However, by using all ears going to surgery,

rather than just those with MEE, to estimate sensitivity, there is a drop in sensitivity from 95% to 84%. This illustrates the important point that the definition of the disease or condition targeted by the screening protocol and the nature of the population screened will influence performance of a given test criterion.

Agreement and Disagreement Between Otoscopic and Surgical Diagnosis of MEE

As we review data on the performance of acoustic immittance testing with respect to the identification of MEE, we see that some investigators have used surgical inspection of the ME as the gold standard while others have used otoscopy. Besides the differences in the population characteristics of those eligible for ME surgery and many of those who are examined by otoscopy, there is a sizable difference in how individual ears are categorized by the two methods. In our study, there was disagreement between otoscopy and the surgeons' findings in over 21% of the ears. The degree of discrepancy between the two methods may be affected by several factors, including the definition of the disease, the criteria used by the surgeon(s) in the study, the time delay between otoscopic examination and surgery, the possible effects of anesthesia on status of the ME during surgery, the skill and experience of the otoscopist and possibly others. Those attempting to apply acoustic immittance test results, with or without otoscopy as an adjunct, must be aware of how the data that are reported in the literature are obtained and must use all of that information in making decisions about how to apply the tests to their own situation in the clinic or the research laboratory.

ASHA Guidelines for Screening for Middle Ear Disorders

Current ASHA guidelines for screening for ME disorders (ASHA, 1990) recommend choosing criteria based on an estimate of the "normal range" (5th to 95th percentile) for Y_{tm} and TW. The interim norms accompanying the guidelines suggest $Y_{tm} < 0.2$ mmho or TW > 150 daPa as the criterion for a positive test result. The tympanometric criterion is designed to set the specificity (the percent of normal ears that are negative) at 95% for each measure. In our group undergoing M&T surgery, the criteria based on the interim norms yielded specificities of 26% and 97% for TW and Y_{tm}, respectively (See Table 2, TW > 150 and $Y_{tm} \leq 0.1$). The two combined, TW > 150 or $Y_{tm} \leq 0.1$, have a specificity of 25% (Table 2) because a positive outcome on either test causes the ear to be classified as positive. The ears with no MEE from our surgery group have TW distributed quite differently than the ears

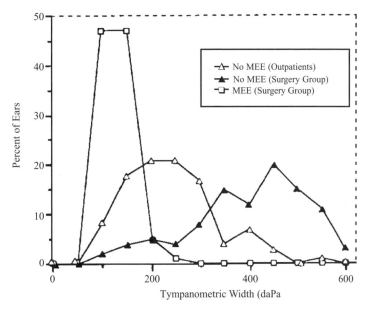

Figure 3. Distributions of tympanometric width (TW) for ears with MEE (surgery group) and two separate groups of ears with no MEE. Of ears with no MEE, one group is from the surgery group and one group is from a group representative of the general population which was tested previously as part of a different study (Nozza et al., 1992b).

with no MEE from a normal population. Consequently, the specificity estimates based on "normal" ears do not apply very well to the ears with no MEE from the surgery group.

The screening guidelines (ASHA, 1990) do point out clearly that the criteria used in a screening program should be representative of the population on which the test will be used. They suggest that if the population has different characteristics, then the prediction of 95% specificity might not be valid and different criteria might serve better. The guidelines mention also that the recommended protocol is based on estimating a normal range and screening for those outside that range. That is, the protocol is designed to have a high specificity (95% of normal ears should be negative on the test), but there is a lack of data on ears with MEE on which to get good estimates of sensitivity. In addition to specificity, the value of the screening test cannot be determined without an understanding of the sensitivity of the test and the predictive values for the population screened. As our data illustrate (Tables 2 and 4), maximizing specificity does not maximize sensitivity and does not assure good overall performance of the protocol. Setting cutoffs based on the specificity, without consideration of the sensitivity, could lead to poor test performance.

It is interesting to note that, with respect to tympanometric screening, the ASHA guidelines (ASHA, 1990) call for all those positive on one immittance screening test to be screened a second time prior to referral for medical evaluation. This is important for controlling the over-referral rate. However, because we know that the test may

perform differently with different populations, it is not clear that the same test criteria should be used for the second screening as were used for the first. By performing the initial screening, a smaller group with a higher prevalence of disease will be identified for rescreening. When the prevalence of disease changes, the predictive values of the test change. The consequences and costs of a positive outcome on a first screening are different than those on a second screening and should be taken into account in the screening protocol. Those positive on a first screening are simply rescreened at a later date while those positive on the second screening enter the health care system as referrals to physicians for medical evaluation, diagnosis and possibly treatment. A high overreferral rate may be easily tolerated in the first screening but may be problematic if associated with the second screening. By using different criteria for an initial screening than for a follow-up screening, Lous (1983) demonstrated better performance relative to both of the criteria that were being recommended at the time (ASHA, 1979; Harford, Bess, Bluestone, & Klein, 1978). Research into the effects of prevalence on initial and follow-up test performance in screening protocols must be done to address this important question.

Summary and Conclusions

We have presented data on acoustic admittance measures and validated pneumatic otoscopy for 249 ears of 171 children undergoing M&T surgery. One-hundred-thirty-seven ears were found to have MEE and 112 ears were found to have no MEE at the time of surgery. Rather than test specific admittance and/or admittance-otoscopic criteria that had been preselected, we submitted our data to a logistic regression analysis to determine which criteria, acoustic admittance and acoustic admittance combined with otoscopy, would best discriminate between ears with MEE and ears with no MEE. The best performance, which was achieved by several different criteria, was sensitivity and specificity around or slightly above 80% (Table 2; Fig. 1). TW had the best performance of any single acoustic admittance measure.

TW measurements were made also for tympanograms from a group of subjects from a previous study (Nozza et al., 1992b). The distribution of TW in the ears with no MEE from that group was different from the distributions of ears either with or without MEE from the group undergoing surgery that are reported in the present article (Fig. 3). Similar differences in distributions between the groups exist for Y_{tm} and for gradient (Nozza, Bluestone, & Kardatze, 1992a) as well. The data illustrate that, because the distribution of different acoustic admittance variables will differ depending not only on ME status but on the population being tested, different criteria for identifying MEE may be required for different populations. The criteria that work best for a high-risk population such as those scheduled for M&T surgery do not necessarily work best for the general population.

We examined also the difference between using findings by a surgeon during M&T surgery and the findings of a validated otoscopist as the "gold standard" for determining whether or not an ear had MEE. Although the performance of each admittance variable is similar whether using findings at surgery or the observations of the otoscopist as the validating criterion, for 21% of the ears there was disagreement between the surgeon and the otoscopist on the diagnosis.

The tympanometric screening criteria based on the interim norms reported in the ASHA guidelines (ASHA, 1990) perform reasonably well with a group representative of the general population; that is, low prevalence of MEE and unselected with regard to history of ME disease. Further, the tympanometric criterion based on the interim norms has a very high false positive rate and poor positive predictive value in the group with history of chronic or recurrent MEE. This illustrates the importance of knowing the population characteristics of those used to develop the criteria and knowing those of the group on whom the test will be used. As the ASHA guidelines suggest (ASHA, 1990), different criteria may be better than those recommended in the guidelines depending on the population being tested. Hopefully, the information in this report will help those using tympanometry for screening to see the need for developing criteria specific to the population tested and will provide information on performance of the various criteria that could be used with a high risk group or with those more representative of the general population (Nozza et al., 1992b). More research on performance of acoustic admittance measures in children with and without MEE of all ages is required so that our programs for identification and diagnosis of ME disorders can be optimized.

Acknowledgments

The help and cooperation of the following people is gratefully acknowledged: In Pittsburgh, Tamala Sobek, M.A., CCC-A, who performed the acoustic admittance tests; Doug Swarts, Ph.D., who performed the programming for digitization of tympanograms; Michele Chirdon, M.A., for digitizing the tympanograms; Herman Felder, M.D., who performed many of the surgeries; Carol Hatcher, R.N., operating room supervisor; D. Ryan Cook, M.D., chief of anesthesiology and the anesthesiologists who supported our project; and especially Howard Rockette, Ph.D., for many helpful discussions on issues related to analysis of audiologic data; and at The University of Georgia, Denise Ruggiere who assisted in the preparation of the manuscript and tables, and Virginia Calder for preparing the graphs.

Portions of the data from this project were reported at the International Symposium on Screening Children for Auditory Function, Nashville TN, June 27-29, 1991 and were presented as a poster at the annual convention of the American Speech-Language-Hearing Association, Seattle, WA, November 16-19, 1990.

Current affiliation of Dr. Nozza: Department of Communication Sciences and Disorders, University of Georgia.

Address for correspondence: Robert J. Nozza, Ph.D., Department of Communication Sciences and Disorders, 570 Aderhold Hall, University of Georgia, Athens, GA 30602-7152.

Received October 13, 1993; Accepted March 21, 1994

References

Agresti, A. (1984). *Analysis of ordinal categorical data.* New York: Wiley.

American National Standards Institute. (1987). American national standard specifications for instruments to measure aural acoustic impedance and admittance (aural acoustic immittance). *ANSI S3.39,* New York.

American Speech-Language-Hearing Association. (1979). Guidelines for acoustic immittance screening of middle ear function. *ASHA, 21,* 283-288.

American Speech-Language-Hearing Association. (1990). Guidelines for screening for hearing impairment and middle ear disorders. *ASHA, 32,* 17-24.

Bluestone, C.D., & Cantekin, E.I. (1979). Design factors in the characterization and identification of otitis media and certain related conditions. *Annals of Otology, Rhinology and Laryngology, 88,* 13-28.

Brooks, D.N. (1969). The use of the electro-acoustic impedance bridge in the assessment of middle ear function. *International Audiology, 8,* 563-569.

Cantekin, E.I., Bluestone, C.D., Fria, T.J., Stool, S.E., Beery, Q.C., & Sabo, D.L. (1980). Identification of otitis media with effusion in children. *Annals of Otology, Rhinology and Laryngology, 89,* 190-195.

de Jonge, R. (1986). Normal tympanometric gradient: a comparison of three methods. *Audiology, 25,* 299-308.

Finitzo, T., Friel-Patti, S., Chinn, K., & Brown, O. (1992). Tympanometry and otoscopy prior to myringotomy: issues in diagnosis of otitis media. *International Journal of Pediatric Otorhinolaryngology*, 24, 101-110.

Gates, G.A., Avery, C.A., Cooper, J.C., Hearne, E.M., & Holt, G.R. (1986). Predictive value of tympanometry in middle ear effusion. *Annals of Otology, Rhinology and Laryngology*, 95, 46-56.

Griner, P.F., Mayewski, R.J., Mushlin, A.I., & Greenland, P. (1981). Selection and interpretation of diagnostic tests and procedures. *Annals of Internal Medicine,* 94, 553-570.

Harford, E.R., Bess, F.H., Bluestone, C.D., & Klein, J.O., (1978). *Impedance screening for middle ear disease in children.* New York: Grune & Stratton.

Jerger, J. (1970). Clinical experience with impedance audiometry. *Archives of Otolaryngology*, 92, 311-324.

Karzon, R.G. (1991). Validity and reliability of tympanometric measures for pediatric patients. *Journal of Speech and Hearing Research*, 34, 386-390.

Koebsell, K.A., & Margolis, R.H. (1986). Tympanometric gradient measured from normal preschool children. *Audiology*, 25, 149-157.

Le, C.T., Daly, K.A., Margolis, R.H., Lindgren, B.R., & Giebink, G.S. (1992). A clinical profile of otitis media. *Archives of Otolaryngology Head and Neck Surgery*, 118, 1225-1228.

Lous, J. (1983). Three impedance screening programs on a cohort of seven-year-old children. *Scandanavian Audiology*, 17, 60-64.

Margolis, R.H., & Heller, J.W. (1987). Screening tympanometry: criteria for medical referral. *Audiology*, 26, 197-208.

Nozza, R.J., Bluestone, C.D., & Kardatze, D. (1992a). Sensitivity, specificity, and predictive values of immittance measures in the identification of middle-ear effusion. In F.H. Bess & J.W. Hall (Eds.), *Screening children for auditory function* (pp. 315-329). Nashville: Bill Wilkerson Press.

Nozza, R.J., Bluestone, C.D., Kardatzke, D., & Bachman, R.N. (1992b). Towards the validation of aural acoustic immittance measures for diagnosis of middle ear effusion in children. *Ear and Hearing*, 13, 442-453.

Paradise, J.L., Smith, C.G., & Bluestone, C.D. (1976). Tympanometric detection of middle ear effusion in infants and young children. *Pediatrics*, 58, 198-210.

Roush, J., Drake, A., & Sexton, J.E. (1992). Identification of middle ear dysfunction in young children: A comparison of tympanometric screening procedures. *Ear and Hearing*, 13, 63-69.

Silman, S., Silverman, C.A., & Arick, D.S. (1992). Acoustic-immittance screening for detection of middle-ear effusion in children. *Journal of the American Academy of Audiology*, 3, 262-268.

Toner, J.G., & Mains, B. (1990). Pneumatic otoscopy and tympanometry in the detection of middle ear effusion. *Clinical Otolaryngology*, 15, 121-123.

Vaughan-Jones, R., & Mills, R.P. (1992). The Welch Allyn Audioscope and Microtymp: Their accuracy and that of pneumatic otoscopy, tympanometry and pure tone audiometry as predictors of otitis media with effusion. *The Journal of Laryngology and Otology*, 106, 600-602.

Developmental Changes in Static Admittance and Tympanometric Width of Infants and Toddlers

Jackson Roush, Kristin Bryant, Martha Mundy, Susan Zeisel, Joanne Roberts

Division of Speech and Hearing Sciences, University of North Carolina [J.R.] Capitol ENT, Raleigh, North Carolina [K.B.], Carolina Otits Media Project, Frank Porter Graham Child Development Center, University of North Carolina at Chapel Hill [M.M., S.Z.]

Longitudinal measures of peak-compensated static acoustic admittance and tympanometric width are reported for infants and toddlers from 6 months to 30 months of age, based on over 1600 assessments of 88 children during a 24-month period. The subjects wee all African American children in full-time day care. Significant age effects were observed, with younger children displaying lower static admittance values and wider tympanograms. The results of this investigation underscore the importance of age- and population-specific norms when using acoustic immittance measures to evaluate middle ear status in children.

Aural acoustic immittance measures are used routinely in the audiologic assessment of middle ear function. A battery of immittance measures often includes peak-compensated static acoustic admittance (static admittance) and calculation of tympanometric gradient or width. Static admittance is an estimate of the acoustic immittance at the lateral surface of the tympanic membrane. It is calculated by subtracting the admittance obtained with the ear canal pressurized from the admittance measured at the peak value. Although static admittance has considerable variability in normal subjects, low static admittance measured with a low-frequency probe tone is often associated with middle ear effusion. Measures of static admittance can also enhance the classification of tympanometric shape, since most classification procedures are based on the height of the admittance peak (Margolis and Heller, 1987).

Methods of calculating the shape of a tympanogram have varied substantially, but several investigators have noted that measures of tympanometric gradient or width are potentially more sensitive to middle ear effusion than static admittance or tympanometric peak pressure (Brooks, 1968; Paradise et al, 1976; Haughton, 1977; Fiellau-Nikolajsen, 1983; Nozza et al, 1994).

Most commercially available immittance instruments now report tympanometric width according to the pressure interval defined by a 50 percent reduction in peak admittance, expressed in dekaPascals (daPa) (see Fig. 1). Support for this method, first proposed by Liden et al (1970), comes from the work of Koebsell and Margolis (1986) and deJonge (1986), who compared various methods of calculating tympanometric gradient.

In an effort to collect normative data using contemporary instrumentation and standardized recording measures, Margolis and Heller (1987) reported admittance, tympanometric width, equivalent ear canal volume, and tympanometric peak pressure in adults and preschool subjects. The children in their study ranged in age from 2.8 years to 5.8 years, with a mean age of 4.7 years. The resulting data were subsequently reported in ASHA's *Guidelines for Screening for Hearing Impairment and Middle Ear Disorders* (ASHA, 1990) as "interim norms," which appear in an appendix to the revised guidelines.

The present study was undertaken to acquire normative data for static admittance and tympanometric width in children under 3 years of age. In particular, we were interested in determining if there are developmental changes that need to be considered when applying these measures to the evaluation of middle ear function in young children.

METHOD

Subjects

The 88 subjects in this investigation were part of an onging prospective study designed to explore the relationship between otitis media in early childhood and the development of language and learning (Roberts et al, 1995). There were 40 males and 48 females. All subjects were low- and middle-income African-American children attending full-time day care in one of nine child care centers in the central Piedmont region of North Carolina. Their average age at entry to day care was 5.2 months (SD=3.0 months).

Otoscopic Examination

The children were seen biweekly for pneumatic otoscopy performed by an experienced pediatric nurse practitioner (PNP). Their ears were examined an average of 9.2 times between the ages of 6 and 30 months. During the 24-month observation period, the children experienced bilateral otitis media with effusion (OME) in 51 percent of the cases, unilateral OME in 12 percent of the cases, and no OME in 37 percent of the cases. Diagnosis of OME was based on otoscopic observation; tympanometry was used to corroborate the OME diagnosis. When otoscopic examination was not successful, tympanometry was used as the primary diagnostic tool. OME was classified as purulent (acute) when the fluid in the middle ear was opaque and yellowish/white. OME was classified as serous when the fluid in the middle ear was clear or straw-colored in appearance. Fluid was presumed to be present when the tympanic membrane was immoble and/or fluid levels were observed in the middle ear.

Agreement between judgment of mobility on pneumatic otoscopy and tympanometry was evaluated throughout the investigation. Interobserver agreement between the PNP and the pediatrician was 90 percent (kappa+.65) for mobility and 91 percent (kappa=.68) for diagnosis. Interobserver agreement between the

Table 1 Means, SDs, and 90% Ranges for Static Admittance Measures, Grouped by Age and for All Observations

Age (mo)	*Static Admittance (mmhos) (N = 1827 Ears)*			
	Ears	Mean	SD	90% Range
6-12	286	.39	.15	.20 to .50
12-18	546	.41	.16	.20 to .60
18-24	590	.48	.18	.30 to .70
24-30	405	.52	.24	.30 to .80
All Ages	1827	.45	.19	.20 to .70

Table 2 Means, SDs, and 90% Ranges Tympanometric Width, Grouped by Age and for All Observations

Age (mo)	*Tympanometric Width (daPa) (N = 1636 Ears*)*			
	Ears	Mean	SD	90% Range
6-12	248	160	54	102-234
12-18	477	148	42	102-204
18-24	543	149	43	102-204
24-30	368	142	44	96-192
All Ages	1636	148	40	102-204

(*Peak Y $\geq$ 0.3 mmho).

PNP and a pediatric otolaryngologist, whose otoscopy skills have been validated against myringomtomy, was 89 percent (kappa=.65) for mobility and 89 percent (kappa=.64) for diagnosis, based on 76 ear observation.

Data from ear examinations used in the present analysis were limited to those in which the diagnosis was normal based on otoscopic examination and for which immittance measures were judged to be accurate and complete. In general, the otoscopic examiner was blind to the tympanometric results; however, in some cases, practical considerations required tympanometry to precede otoscopy. Thus, the examiner was sometimes aware of the tympanometric findings prior to otoscopy.

Instrumentation

Acoustic immittance data were obtained using an automatic tympanometer (Micro Audiometrics Earscan), which was calibrated according to ANSI standards. This device uses a 226-Hz probe tone at 85 dB SPL with a positive to negative air pressure sweep, at a rate of 150 daPa/sec. Acoustic admittance magnitude was measured in acoustic mmhos (1 acoustic mmho=$1m^3$ x 10^{-9}/Pa/sec) over an ear canal pressur range of +200 to -300 daPa. The static value was obtained by subtracting the admittance at +200 daPa from the peak value.

Tympanometric width was calculated automatically by the tympanometer according to the pressure interval corresponding to a 50 percent reduction in static admittance (see Fig. 1). The instrument did not attempt to calculate tympanometric width unless the static admittance value was greater than or equal to 0.3 mmhos.[1] Daily calibration measurements were made in the hard-walled calibration cavity supplied by the manufacturer.

RESULTS

Tympanograms displayed peak pressure that was similar for all ages ranging from -174 daPa to + 18 daPa,

with a mean value of -64 daPa (SD=75 daPa). The means, standard deviations, and 90 percent ranges for static admittance and tympanometric width are shown in Tables 1 and 2. For static admittance, the mean for all ages combined was 0.45 mmhos (SD=0.19), with a 90 percent range of 0.2 mmhos to 0.7 mmhos. Tympanometric width for all ages combined was 148 daPa (SD=40), with a 90 percent range of 102 daPa to 204 daPa.

Age and gender effects were studied using general linear mixed models (Laird and Ware, 1982; McLean et al, 1991). These methods can be viewed as a generalizaation of repeated measures analysis of variance in which systematic individuals effects on the repeated assessments are represented in the analysis model by random effects. Accordingly, these methods take into account the fact that multiple assessments on the same individual are likely to be correlated. Specifically, the static admittance and tympanometric width were analyzed with a model that included age as a continuous variable, gender and age x gender as fixed effects, and the individual as a random effect. Results indicated that age differences were reliably detected for both static admittance (F=27.7) and tympanometric width (F=44.0). There were no significant gender differences.

DISCUSSION

Direct comparison of these data to previous studies is complicated by technical and procedural differences. Many of the earlier studies of acoustic immittance were based on measurements performed using tympanograms expressed in "arbitrary compliance units" and thus are not amenable to comparison. For contemporary instruments, the most important variables are (1) the method of compensating for ear canal volume; (2) the method of calculating tympanometric width from the peak-compensated static admittance value; (3) pump speed; and (4) probe-tone frequency. Regarding correction for ear canal volume, Margolis and Shanks (1991) note that

---

[1]The Earscan, like most tympanometric screening instruments, does not compute tympanometric width on tympanograms having a static admittance less than 0.3 mmhos due to the loss of accuracy that occurs when calculations must be made at or near the "noise floor."

compensation at +200 daPa is slightly less accurate than "maximum/minimum" calculations or compensation at extreme negative values (e.g., -400 daPa); however, this method has been used successfully in several studies (e.g., Shanks and Wilson, 1986); Margolis and Heller, 1987). Regarding calculatin of tympanometric width, Margolis and Heller (1987) note that tympanometric gradient based on the pressure interval corresponding to a 50 percent reduction in static admittance, expressed in daPa, appears to have several advantages over other methods. Advantages include (1) relative invariance to pump speed; (2) a wide range of values between normal and abnormal values, thus facilitating identification of diseased ears; and (3) low correlation with static admittance, thus supplementing rather than duplicating other immittance measures. Pump speed is likely to have a significant effect only on peak admittance, with faster pump speeds (e.g., 400 daPa/sec) producing higher values of peak Y than slower speeds. Regarding probe tone, a low-frequency probe (e.g., 226) has been generally considered well suited for detecting middle ear effusion in all but neonatal populations, although some have challenged this assumption (Keefe et al, 1993).

The study by Margolis and Heller (1987), whose 50 pediatric subjects (92 ears) ranged in age from 2.8 years to 5.8 years and whose results are reported as "interim norms" in an appendix to the 1990 ASHA guidelines, was procedurally similar to the present investigation and therefore amenable to comparison. Using a screening instrument that measured acoustic admittance magnitude in acoustic mmhos over an ear canal pressure range of +200 to -300 daPa (90% range = 59-151 daPa). Although data were not reported for specific age groups, significant age effects were observed.

There is no obvious explanation for the lower static admittance and wider tympanograms observed in younger children although the differences may be related to changes in the anatomy and physiology of the external and middle ear known to continue throughout childhood (Anson and Donaldson, 1981). It is also possible that younger subjects, known to exhibit a higher prevalence of middle are effusion, may experience subtle and presumably temporary changes in the mechanical properties of the tympanic membrane, in the absence of otoscopic abnormalities. Although our measures were limited to single component (Y) tympanograms, these changes would most likely have their primary influence on the resistive components of middle ear impedance (Margolis and Shanks, 1985), the effects of which would be seen in a "broadening" and "flattening" of the admittance tympanogram. All of the subjects in the present investigation were in full-time day care, a factor often associated with higher prevalence of OME. Indded, the prevalence of

OME was very high in this sample. Although ears were judged to be free of OME at the time these tympanograms were obtained, the recurrent OME history characterizing many of these subjects most likely had residual effects on middle ear function. This might account for the relatively wide tympanograms we observed even in our oldest subjects (mean =144 daPa for the 24- to 30-month age group), compared to those of Margolis and Heller (1987). That is, the subjects in the present investigation most likely had a higher incidence of OME than the subjects studied by Margolis and Heller (1987).

Normative data for static admittance, tympanometric width, and other immittance variables has also been reported by Nozza et al (1992), who studied subjects ranging in age from 3 to 16 years. The children were unselected with regard to OME history and thus were characteristic of the general population. Not surprisingly, means for peak admittance (0.78 mmho) and tympanometric width (104 daPa) differed from those of the present investigation. Nozza and colleagues have also reported immittance findings in children with recurrent OME histories who were tested just prior to undergoing surgery for myringotomy and tube placement (Nozza el al, 1994). In general, acoustic immittance measures revealed substantially lower peak admittance (0.28 mmho) and wider tympanograms (373 dPa), even when the children were free of middle ear effusion at the time of testing. These findings are consistent with those of the present investigation in demonstrating that middle ear status is likely to differ for children with and without OME histories, even when middle ear effusion is not present.

In summary, our findings suggest that infants and young toddlers with normal middle ear status, as judged otoscopically, are likely to exhibit lower static admittance values and wider tympanograms than those of older preschoolaged children drawn from the same population. The results of this study underscore the need for age- and population-specific norms, especially if the data are to be used in screening for middle ear dysfunction. The values reported here, however, should be applied only to the age groups included in our sample (6 months to 30 months), since younger infants are likely to show a variety of tympanometric findings that differ from older children and adults (e.g., Holte et al, 1991), and the mechanisms underlying these observations appear to be affected by the complex interaction of ear canal growth, resonance, and vibration (Keefe et al, 1993). Application of these norms also assumes that the acoustic immittance measures are obtained using instrumentation having similar technical specifications, that is, a low-frequency probe tone (e.g., 226 Hz), automatic compensation for ear canal volume by subtracting the admittance at +200 daPa from the peak value, and calculation of tympanometric width based on the pres-

---

[2]Margolis and Heller (1987) also reported norms for a pump speed of 400 daPa/second.

sure interval corresponding to a 50 percent reduction in static admittance. Finally, these norms will be most applicable to populations having a similar prevalence of OME, since children with a high rate of recurrence may exhibit residual changes in middle ear function, even during periods when OME has resolved.

The broad normative range of tympanometric widths observed for this age group and population may reduce the utility of this measure as a screening tool; however, further research is needed to determine the optimal immittance screening battery and cut-off values for each measure in the battery, for diseased as well as nondiseased ears.

ACKNOWLEDGMENTS

This research was supported by grant MCJ-370599 and MCJ-370649, Maternal and Child Health Bureau, Health Resources and Services Administration, U.S. Department of Health and Human Services. The authors are grateful to Dr. Margaret Burchinal for statistical consultation and Ms. Elizabeth Gunn for assistance with data analysis. Dr. Robert Margolis, Dr. Donald Schum, and two anonymous reviewers provided helpful comments on an earlier version of this manuscript. Portions of this paper were presented at the Annual Convention of the American Speech-Language-Hearing Association, Anaheim, CA, November, 1993.

REFERENCES

American Speech-Language-Hearing Association. (1990). Guidelines for screening for hearing impairment and middle ear disorders. *ASHA* 32 (Suppl 2), 17-24.

Anson, B., Donaldson, J. (1981). *Surgical Anatomy of the Temporal Bone and Ear*. Philadelphia: W.B. Saunders.

Brooks, D.N. (1968). An objective method of determining fluid in the middle ear. *Int Audiol* 7, 280-286.

deJonge, R. (1986). Normal tympanometric gradient: a comparison of three methods. *Audiology* 25, 299-308.

Fiellau-Nickolajsen, M. (1983). Tympanometry and secretory otitis media. *Acta Otolaryngol Suppl* 394, 1-73.

Haughton, P.M. (1977). Validity of tympanometry for middle ear effusions. *Arch Otolaryngol* 103, 505-513.

Holte, L., Margolis, R., Cavanaugh, R. (1991). Developmental changes in multifrequency tympanograms. *Audiology* 30, 1-24.

Keefe, D., Bulen, J., Arehart, K., Burns, E. (1993). Ear-canal impedance and reflection coefficient in human infants and adults. *J Acoust Soc Am* 94(5), 2617-2638.

Koebsell, K.A., Margolis, R.H. (1986). Tympanometric gradient measured from normal preschool children. *Audiology* 25, 149-157.

Laird, N.M., Ware, J.H. (1982). Random effects models for longitudinal data. *Biometrics* 38, 963-974.

Liden, G., Peterson, J., Bjorkman, G. (1970). Tympanometry. *Arch Otolaryngol* 92, 248-257.

Margolis, R.H., Shanks, J.E. (1985). Tympanometry. In: Katz J. (ed.) *Handbook of Clinical Audiology*. Baltimore: Williams and Wilkins, 438-475.

Margolis, R.H., Heller, J.W. (1987). Screening tympanometry: criteria for medical referral. *Audiology* 26, 197-208.

Margolis, R.H., Shanks, J.E. (1991). Tympanometry: basic principles and clinical applications. In: Rintelmann W. (ed.) *Hearing Assessment*. Austin, TX: Pro-Ed, 179-245.

McLean, R.A., Sanders, W.L., Stroup, W.W. (1991). A unified approach of mixed linear models. *The American Statistician* 45, 54-64.

Nozza, R.J., Bluestone, C.D., Kardatzke, D. (1992). Sensitivity, specificity, and predictive values of immittance measures in the identification of middle-ear effusion. In: Bess F.H., Hall J.W. (eds.) *Screening Children for Auditory Function*. Nashville: Bill Wilkerson Press, 315-329.

Nozza, R.J., Bluestone, C.D., Kardatzke, D., Bachman, R. (1994). Identification of middle ear effusion by aural acoustic admittance and otoscopy. *Ear and Hearing* 15, 310-323.

Paradise, J.L., Smith, C.G., Bluestone, C.D. (1976). Tympanometric detection of middle ear effusion in infants and young children. *Pediatrics* 58, 198-210.

Roberts, J.E., Burchinal, M., Medley, L., Zeisel, S., Mundy, M., Roush, J., Hooper, S., Bryant, D., Henderson, F. (1995). Otitis media, hearing sensitivity, and maternal responsiveness in relation to language during infancy.

Shanks, J.E., Wilson, R.H. (1986). Effects of direction and rate of ear-canal pressure changes on tympanometric measures. *Journal of Speech and Hearing Research* 29, 11-19.

Identification of Neonatal Hearing Impairment: Ear-Canal Measurements of Acoustic Admittance and Reflectance in Neonates

Douglas H. Keefe, Richard C. Folsom, Michael P. Gorga, Betty R. Vohr, Jay C. Bulen, and Susan J. Norton

Multicenter Consortium on Identification of Neonatal Hearing Impairment, Seattle, Washington; Boys Town National Research Hospital (D.H.K., M.P.G.), Omaha Nebraska; Children's Hospital and Regional Medical Center (S.J.N.), Seattle, Washington; University of Washington Medical Center (R.C.F.), Seattle, Washington; Women's and Infant's Hospital (B.R.V.), Providence, Rhode Island; Truman State University (J.C.B.), Kirksville, Missouri

Objectives: 1) To describe broad bandwidth measurements of acoustic admittance (Y) and energy reflectance (R) in the ear canals of neonates. 2) To describe a means for evaluating when a YR response is valid. 3) To describe the relations between these YR measurements and age, gender, left/right ear, and selected risk factors.

Design: YR responses were obtained at four test sites in well babies without risk indicators, well babies with at least one risk indicator, and graduates of neonatal intensive care units. YR responses were measured using a chirp stimulus at moderate levels over a frequency range from 250 to 8000 Hz. The system was calibrated based on measurements in a set of cylindrical tubes. The probe assembly was inserted in the ear canal of the neonate, and customized software was used for data acquisition.

Results: YR responses were measured in over 4000 ears, and half of the responses were used in exploratory data analyses. The particular YR variables chosen for analysis were energy reflectance, equivalent volume and acoustic conductance. Based on the view that unduly large negative equivalent volumes at low frequencies were physically impossible, it was concluded that approximately 13% of the YR responses showed evidence of improper probe seal in the ear canal. To test how these outliers influenced the overall pattern of YR responses, analyses were conducted both on the full data set ($N = 2081$) and the data set excluding outliers ($N = 1825$). The YR responses averaged over frequency varied with conceptional age (conception to date of test), gender, left/right ear, and selected risk factors; in all cases, significant effects were observed more frequently in the data set excluding outliers. After excluding outliers and controlling for conceptional age effects, the dichotomous risk factors accounting for the greatest variance in the YR responses were, in rank order, cleft lip and palate, aminoglycoside therapy, low birth weight, history of ventilation, and low APGAR scores. In separate analyses, YR responses varied in the first few days after birth. An analysis showed that the use of a YR test criterion to assess the quality of probe seal may help control the false-positive rate in evoked otoacoustic emission testing.

Conclusions: This is the first report of wideband YR responses in neonates. Data were acquired in a few seconds, but the responses are highly sensitive to whether the probe is fully sealed in the ear canal. A real-time acoustic test of probe fit is proposed to better address the probe seal problem. The YR responses provide information on middle-ear status that varies over the neonatal age range and that is sensitive to the presence or absence of risk factors, ear, and gender differences. Thus, a YR test may have potential for use in neonatal screeening test for hearing loss.

Multicenter Consortium on Identification of Neonatal Hearing Impairment, Seattle, Washington; Boys Town National Research Hospital (D.H.K., M.P.G.), Omaha, Nebraska; Children's Hospital and Regional Medical Center (S.J.N.), Seattle, Washington; University of Washington Medical Center (R.C.F.), Seattle, Washington; Women's and Infant's Hospital (B.R.V.), Providence, Rhode Island; Truman State University (J.C.B.), Kirksville, Missouri.

Work Supported by the NIDCD (DC01958).

A central goal of any neonatal screening test is to correctly identify ears with normal hearing. Current interest centers on tests such as evoked otoacoustic emissions (EOAEs), which are sensitive to middle-ear and cochlear status, and auditory brain stem responses (ABRs), which are sensitive to middle-ear, cochlear and neural status. A difficulty in interpreting such tests is that the acoustic response of the middle ear is not independently assessed in the absence of the influence of other levels of the auditory system. The response of the middle ear is mechanical in nature, with a direct acoustic correlate in the ear canal. For EOAEs and, under some conditions, for ABRs, a resonse may be absent either due to the presence of a cochlear or a conductive hearing loss. Because transient middle-ear dysfunction may be more prevalent in neonatal ears than cochlear or sensorineural hearing losses, there is a critical need for a better understanding of middle-ear functioning in neonates. The scope of this report is to describe results obtained from an acoustical test of middle-ear function in a large population of neonatal ears, and to examine the relationship of the acoustic resonses to subject age, gender, left/right ear, and selected risk factors.

There does not currently exist a clinically accepted acoustic test of middle-ear status applicable to a neonatal population. A problem with tympanometry is that static pressurization of the ear canal produces large changes in ear canal volume due to changes in ear canal diameter. For example, in most ears tested in a population of infants of age 1 to 5 day old, the ear canal diameter changed up to 70% in response to positive and negative pressure transients of magnitude 250 to 300 daPa (Holte, Margolis, & Cavanaugh, 1991). The more fundamental ear-canal dimension from the standpoint of acoustical measurements is area, which scales inversely with the characteristic impedance of the ear canal (Keefe, Bulen, Arehart, & Burns, 1993), and a nominal 70% change in diameter would produce an area change of 290%. Holte et al. (1991) recommended a tympanometric frequency of 226 Hz for infants less than 4 mo old, as the tympanometric shapes are more easily interpreted than those obtained at higher frequencies. Other investigators have recommended higher test frequencies in measuring neonatal tympanograms. McKinley, Grose, and Roush (1997) compared the use of tympanometric probe frequencies of 226, 678, and 1000 Hz in neonates, and found no clear association between tympanometric patterns and pass/fail rates in a transient evoked otoacoustic emission (TEOAE) test.

In older children and adults, tympanometry is the clinical standard for acoustic testing of middle-ear status. A microphone, inserted in a leak-free manner in the ear canal, records the response to a sinusoidal tone generaged by a sound source while static pressure is varied within the ear canal. Tympanometry is effective in identifying various forms of middle-ear dysfunction, and can thus be used to help interpret EOAE and ABR measurements in the same ear. However, tympanometric measurements in neonatal ears may be unreliable because the use of static pressure distorts the ear canal shape in the more compliant ear-canal walls of neonates. As reviewed by McKinley et al. (1997), some other factors complicating the interpretation of middle-ear measurements in neonates include the presence of vernix in the ear canal, and the presence of residual amniotic fluid or mesenchyme in the middle ear.

An alternative line of research on the functioning of the middle ear in adults and children has focused on the use of acoustic immittance measurements at ambient static pressure, but across a wide frequncy bandwidth. These are termed admittance-reflectance (YR) tests. Keefe et al. (1993) measured acoustic impedance, acoustic admittance and (pressure) reflectance responses from 125 to 10,700 Hz in adults and in full-term infants of age 1 to 24 mo, and found systematic developmental changes. They hypothesized that the 2 to 4 Hz range might be useful for clinical tests of middle-ear status because it is the frequency range over which the normal-functioning middle ear, terminated by a normal-functioning cochlea, is most efficient at absorbing sound energy delivered into the ear canal. This hypothesis suggests an approach that is a significant departure from standard clinical practice, in which low-frequency tympanometry is used. Another large effect was that the low-frequency reflectance increased with increasing age. A hypothesis for the younger subjects in the current study is that their measured reflectances are predicted to be lower in magnitude at these lower frequencies.

This report describes YR measurements in neonates, identifies the presence and cause of artifact in the YR data set, and examines the YR responses as a function of test site, ear (left or right), ethnicity, age, and selected risk factors. These YR responses are of interest because they have been shown to be useful in predicting the preseence of conductive loss in a population of children from 2 to 11 yr old (Piskorski, Keefe, Simmons, & Gorga, 1999). Because the YR responses are indicative of middle-ear status, and because the presence of middle-ear status, and because the presence of middle-ear pathology may increase the likelihood that the evoked OAE or ABR responses are weak or absent, it is of interest to examine the characteristics of YR responses in a neonatal population within a hearing screening protocol.

METHODS

SUBJECTS

The test group of subjects was a subset of those described in Vohr et al. (2000). The admittance-reflectance (YR) measurements were performed on neonates at four of the test sites: Boys Town National Research Hospital, Children's Hospital and Regional Medical Center, University of Washington Medical Center, and Women's and Infant's Hospital.

ADMITTANCE-REFLECTANCE (YR) MEASUREMENT PROCEDURES

An admittance-reflectance (YR) measurement procedure comprised two steps, a calibration procedure followed by data collection in the ear canal. The calibration phase took approximately 5 minutes, and was usually performed once a day before the first ear-canal measurement. Small in accuracies in the calibration procedure, such as the presence of a tiny leak between probe and calibration tube, generally caused the calibration to fail. When this occurred, the calibration procedure was repeated after obtaining a leak-free fit. In contrast, data collection in the neonate was rapid and straightforward. A desired requirement was that a seal between the probe and ear canal be present, and that the baby be relatively quiet for the measurements. The duration of data acquisition was 0.7 sec.

The methodology for measuring input admittance (Y) and energy reflectance (R) has been described in detail previously (Keefe, Ling, & Bulen, 1992). The probe assembly consisted of a customized version of a probe used in a commercial otoacoustic emission measurement system (Otodynamics, ILO92) along with non-commericial hardware and software. The probe has two miniature loudspeakers and one microphone. The YR measurement used one of the loudspeakers, driven by a digital-to-analog converter, and the microphone signal, output from the microphone preamplifier and connected to an analog-to-digital converter. Data were collected at a 25 kHz sample rate using an Ariel DSP 16+ data acquisition system with 16-bit digital-to-analog converter and analog-to-digital converter, and stored and analyzed in a computer running customized software.

The system was calibrated using a broadband chirp of 82 msec duration applied to the probe loudspeaker. The probe was inserted into each of six calibration tubes of different lengths, each closed at its opposite end. The acoustic pressure in each tube was transduced and digitized in response to the chirp.

The diameter of each calibration tube was 4.85 mm, which was chosen sufficiently small so as to approximate the ear-canal diameter of older neonates, yet sufficiently large that the probe could be conveniently affixed to the open end of each tube. The nominal lengths of the tubes were chosen to ensure the robustness and accuracy of the calibration procedure. The set included tubes of length 268.3, 324.5, 431.6, 415.9, 346.5, and 684.4 mm. The calibration procedure calculated the Thevenin pressure and impedance associated with the probe and measurement system by fitting the measured pressure responses to modeled impedance functions based on a cylindrical-tube geometry including an ideal closed end.

After calibration, the probe was inserted into the ear to be tested and data were acquired using the same broadband chirp stimulus. At each frequency f, the acoustic admittance $Y(f)$, and impedance $Z(f) = 1/Y(f)$, at the tip of the probe assembly were calculated. The complex acoustic admittance is expressed in terms of its real part, the conductance $G(f)$, and its imaginary part, the susceptance $B(f)$, by:

$$Y(f) = G(f) + jB(f), \qquad (1)$$

where j is the unit imaginary number corresponding to a time dependence t on all variables of e^{j2pft} at frequency f. The equivalent volume $V(f)$ is defined by:

$$V(f) = pc^2 B(f)/(2\pi f) \qquad (2)$$

where p is the density of air, and c is the phase velocity of sound. The (energy) reflectance is defined in terms of the admittance $Y(f)$. The complex acoustic impedance may be expressed in terms of its resistance and reactance.

The conductive and equivalent volume, or the resistance and reactance, describe the acoustic response of each ear. Although the reflectance can be expressed in terms of either pair of variables, it is informative to study its frequency response along side that of the admittance or impedance variables, because it is an alternative representation that is less sensitive to the location of the probe within the ear canal.

DATA INTERPRETATION

Data interpretation involved as a first step the decision on whether the data were valid. A number of conditions can make these measurements inaccurate. These include leaky seals, environmental noise, breathing noise and vocalization, debris in the probe, improper insertion, and inappropriateness of the calibration to the system being measured. Additionally, responses can be changed by the insertion, because the act of inserting the tube can artificially distend the enonatal ear canal, which is much more flaccid than that of an older child or adult.

For adult ears, a good seal is indicated by relatively high reflectance at frequencies of 500 Hz and below. This is not true in neonates. Indicators of leaks are the following:

· R (Energy Reflectance). Figure 1 shows energy reflectance (top), resistance (middle), and reactance (bottom) of the same neonatal ear, first with a good seal (left), and then with the probe loosened somewhat (right). Energy reflectance is high at low frequencies because the resistance and reactance are close to zero,

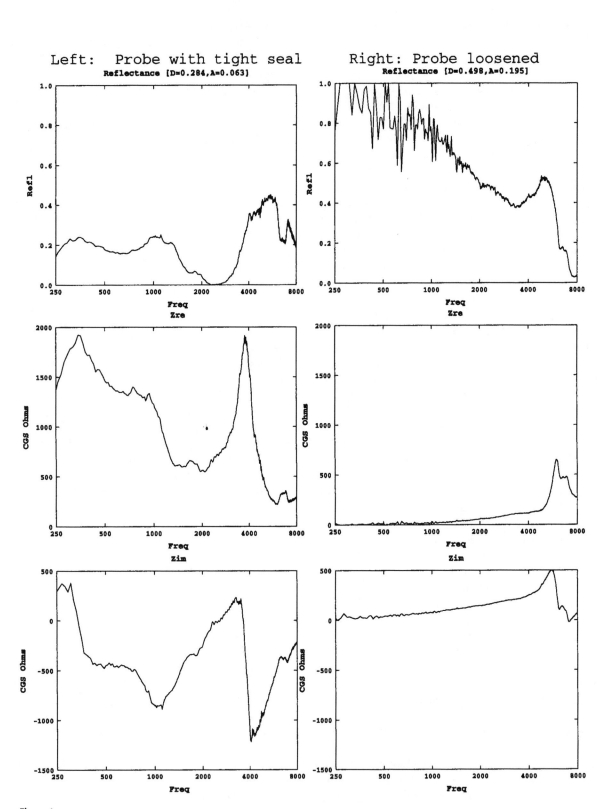

Figure 1.

indicative of a large acoustic discontinuity associated with a leak.

The resistance and reactance tend toward very low values when there is a leak present, from which it follows that the equivalent volume associated with a leak tends towards a large negative value. These tendencies are more noticeable in neonates than adults, because the resistance in adults is already low at low frequencies.

Once a trained observer recognized a leak, it could be remedied by reinserting the probe, changing its orientation, or using a larger probe tip. Converting the data in Figure 1 to equivalent volume, the presence of a leak produced equivalent volumes at 500 to 1000 Hz in the rang eof -5 cm^3. Such values can be regarded as evidence of artifact. The reactance $X(f)$ for the leaky fit rises approximately lineaarly with frequency (Fig. 1), and can therefore be expressed as $X(f) = 2\pi fm$, in which the frequency is f, and the acoustic inertance ("mass") is m. Neglecting the resistance for simplicity, the equivalent volume $V(f)$ for such a reactance is inversely proposal to the product of the acoustic ineertance and the square of the frequency. This equivalent volume is strongly negative when the acoustic inertance is small (as is the case for a leaky fit) and the frequency is low.

The probe tip could sometimes be inserted in such a way that it was blocked against the wall of the ear canal. Depending on how the probe tip was occluded and to what degree, this produced a variety of results. It could behave like a blocked probe, with low levels and attendant low reflectances. If the tip was pushed close to a wall or if the ear canal were collapsed, high reflectances were produced. Reflectance values exceeding 1.0 are unphysical in a passive system and unlikely to occur in the ear at these stimulus levels. These results are not representative of a normally functioning middle ear. The testers were trained to detect a blocked probe (or collapsed ear canal), and adjust the probe fit until a satisfactory response was obtained.

GENERAL NEONATAL SCREENING
PROTOCOL PROCEDURES

Data collection consisted of the standard neonatal screening protocol (Harrison et al., 2000) augmented by the YR test. The standard protocol included tests of ABR (Sininger et al., 2000), TEOAEs (Norton et al., 2000), and distortion product otoacoustic emissions (DPOAE) (Gorga et al., 2000). The order of these three tests was randomized across subjects. When the YR test was added, the single alteration in this protocol was that the YR test always preceded the TEOAE test. YR data were obtained for both ears of each subject whenever possible.

RESULTS

The YR variables used in subsequent analyses were equivalent volume, acoustic conductance and energy reflectance. The database included the repsonses from 4163 ears. This population was split into two halves and exploratory data analyses were conducted on the first-half data set, which included $N = 2081$ responses. The overall number of subjects in the INHI study was dictated by the need to achieve a sufficiently large number of subjects with sensorineural hearing loss. However, for the purposes of this report, which is not concerned with sensorineural hearing loss, the availability of more than 2000 responses was more than enough to characterize the acoustical transmission properties of the neonatal external and middle ears.

IDENTIFY INVALID YR RESPONSES

The equivalent volume (or susceptance in the ears of 1-mo-olds may be slightly negative at low frequencies. A model has been proposed to account for such negative values at low frequencies based on a resonant motion of the external ear-canal wall, or resonant motion in a shunt pathway of the middle ear (Keefe et al., 1993). This behavior exemplifies the need to refer to this admittance variable as an equivalent volume rather than a volume, because volume is always a positive quantity. In contrast, equivalent volume is a dynamical variable that may be positive or negative.

As discussed in Methods, however, a leaky probe fit results in large negative values of the equivalent volume in the lower frequencies. Therefore, a criterion to determine the validity of the data was based on the presence of large, negative values of equivalent volume that would not reasonably be expected to occur when an adequate probe seal was attained.

Preliminary studies were conducted on a subset of the subjects tested at one of the sites, and it was found that the distribution of equivalent volumes had a pronounced tail extending out to large negative values. Therefore, an analysis of outliers was conducted on the first-half population.

The average equivalent volume was calculated in the frequency range from 250 to 1000 Hz, and the resulting outlier analysis is represented in the two box-and-whiskers plots in Figure 2. This 2.5 octave range was chosen as the low-frequency end of the measured response, in which the qualify of probe fit can most easily be assessed. The data are plotted over different ranges of equivalent volumes, from -2 to 2 cm^3 (left), and over the complete range from -48 to +3.5 cm^3 (right). The lower, middle and upper horizontal lines of the box show the 25th, median (50th), and 75th per-

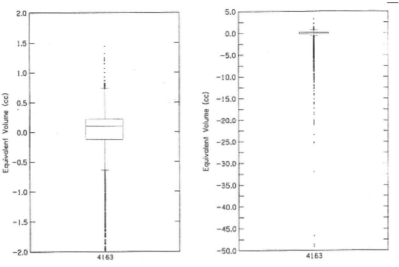

Figure 2. Box-and-whiskers plots of average equivalent volume (cm³) from 250 to 1000 Hz for the first-half sample population over a narrow (left plot) and wide (right plot) range of values.

centiles of the distribution. That is, 50% of the responses had an average equivalent volume in the range from -0.10 to 0.24 cm³, so that the inter-quartile range (IQR) was 0.34 cm³. The upper whisker (i.e., a short horizontal line connected to the box by a vertical line), is drawn at a distance of 1.5 IQRs above the top line of the box, and the lower whisker is drawn at a distance of -.15 IQRs below the bottom line of the box. Individual responses that were larger than the upper whisker, or smaller than the lower whisker, were defined as outliers. There are many more negative than positive outliers; the full-range plot on the right shows the negative outliers extend down to -48 cm³, which is well beyond any credible range of physiologic variation.

A common approach in statistics (e.g., Kleinbaum, Kupper & Muller, 1988) is to define as outliers any observations that extend more than 3.0 IQRs from the box, and to exclude such outliers from further analyses. Because a leak produced a negative equivalent volume at low frequencies, only the negative detached outliers were excluded from the sample population, corresponding to observations with equivalent volumes less than -1.15 cm³. This criterion identified approximately 13% of the responses to be outliers. After exclusion, the distribution of averaged, low-frequency equivalent volumes showed a central peak near 0.2 cm³, and a slight tail towards negative values (see Fig. 3). Across all 4163 ears, there were far fewer responses (13 responses) identified as positive outliers, defined as those ears with equivalent volumes exceeding 0.91 cm³. The largest such outlier exceeded 1000 cm³, clearly an invalid measurement, and the next largest outlier was slightly larger than 3 cm³. This largest (positive) outlier occurred in the second-half population that is not included in the detailed analyses that follow.

It is reasonable to hypothesize that were a leak to be present in some probe fittings (operationally defined as a YR response with a large negative equivalent vol-

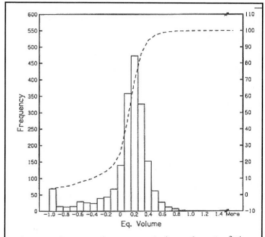

Figure 3. Histogram of average equivalent volume (cm³) from 250 to 1000 Hz for the first-half sample population after excluding outliers.

ume), its tendency to appear might vary with the tester, and, therefore, might vary with test site. Figure 4 illustrates the equivalent volume distributions at each of the test sites for the first-half data set including outliers. The five curves within each panel range from low to high equivalent volumes, corresponding to the 10th, 25th, 50th, 75th, and 90th percentiles of the distribution. Large numbers of negative outliers occurred more frequently in some test sites than in others. The large negative equivalent volumes at low frequencies are physiologically implausible. Thus, the large differences observed between test sites are concluded to be evidence for differences in test technique.

We conclude that a significant number of ears had responses with artifact, consistent with a leaky probe fit. The largest differences across test sites occurred at the 10th and 25th percentiles of the distributions, whereas the median and larger percentiles had much smaller differences between sites.

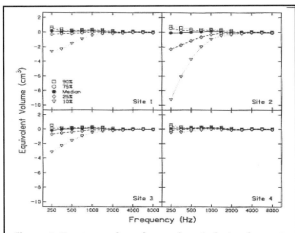

Figure 4. Frequency dependence of equivalent volume at each of four test sites, showing the 10%, 25%, 50%, 75%, and 90% of the distribution at each frequency.

REFLECTANCE, EQUIVALENT VOLUME, AND CONDUCTANCE SPECTRA

The YR responses chosen for detailed analyses were the (energy) reflectance, equivalent volume and (acoustic) conductance. These variables are plotted versus frequency in Figure 5 for the first-half population with outliers excluded. Each plot shows the median response (solid line) as well as responses at the 10th, 25th, 75th, and 90th percentiles.

The median reflectance remained near 0.2, which means that 20% of the energy incident on the neonatal ear was reflected, and 80% was absorbed within the middle ear and cochlea. However, 10% of the responses had a reflectance exceeding approximately 0.50. The middle 50% of the responses had reflectances in the range from 0.1 to 0.3 with only a modest variation with frequency.

The median equivalent volume varied between approximately +0.1 cm^3 down to slightly below 0 cm^3 at high frequencies. The 10th and 90th percentiles of the distribution had more pronounced differences at frequencies up to approximately 707 Hz, relative to their differences at higher frequencies. The middle 50% of the responses were within approximately ±0.15 cm^3 of the median equivalent volume for all frequencies above 250 Hz.

The median conductance varied over a range from 0.6 mmho at low frequencies up to 1.7 mmho at 5657 Hz. The shape of the conductance plot across frequency was similar in all the percentiles, with a relative maximum at the 2000 Hz and 5657 Hz half-octaves. The middle 50% of the responses typically varied across frequency by ±0.4 mmho relative to the median conductance, with increased variability above 5657 Hz.

These median responses form the baseline against which the magnitude of shifts in these YR variables

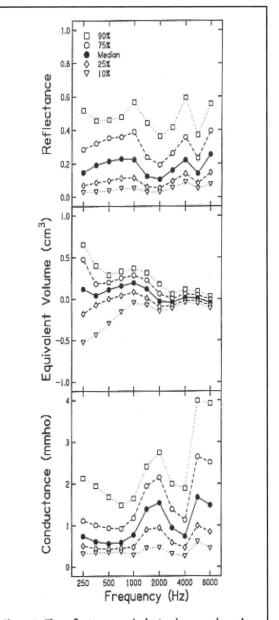

Figure 5. The reflectance, equivalent volume, and conductance of the population across all ages, but with outliers excluded, are plotted as a function of frequency in the top, middle, and bottom panels, respectively.

produced by gender, ear, risk and age effects can be compared.

GENDER AND EAR EFFECTS

Comparisons of YR responses across different variables were conducted both on all the ears in the first population (Table 1) and on those ears after excluding negative outliers (Table 2). Each element in this table is blank if significance was not achieved, based on a 2-way, paired *t*-test using a *p*-value of 0.05. Each non-blank element contains a numerical value equal to the

Table 1. All Subjects.

	Ear (L-R)	Gender (M-F)	Family Hist? Diff	Dysmorphic? Diff	Low Weight? Diff	Pinna Abno.? Diff	Craniofac..? Diff	Other Malf.? Diff	Bilrubin? Diff	Low Apgar? Diff	Meningitis? Diff	Aminogly? Diff	Ventilation? Diff	Syndromes? Diff	Infections? Diff
R250			-0.059				-0.118			0.030					
R353	0.016		-0.038				-0.090			0.027					
R500	0.023		-0.030				-0.077			0.022					
R707	0.017		-0.038				-0.125			0.019					
R1000			-0.044		-0.049		-0.216					-0.032	-0.089		
R1414			-0.042		-0.082		-0.350					-0.025	-0.090		
R2000	-0.021				-0.084		-0.431						-0.057		
R2828	-0.025				-0.027		-0.396					0.029			
R4000	-0.033				-0.028		-0.316	0.069	0.075	0.031		0.056	0.069		
R5657	-0.022						-0.264					0.028			
R8000			0.026		0.032	-0.071	-0.245			0.040			0.050		
V250															
V353															
V500															
V707			0.201												
V1000	0.089	0.109											-0.065		
V1414	0.071	0.083													
V2000							-0.066								
V2828					0.035		-0.135			0.033		0.033			
V4000							-0.253								
V5657															
V8000															
G250															
G353	-0.209														
G500	-0.159														
G707	-0.127														
G1000				0.243	0.168		0.839	0.254		0.088	0.187	0.081	0.213		
G1414	0.143			0.369	0.235			0.269			0.198		0.293		
G2000				0.684			1.167								
G2828				0.625			0.779								
G4000															
G5657							-4.669								
G8000															

Table 2. Outlier subjects excluded.

	Ear (L-R) Diff	Gender (M-F)	Family Hist? Diff	Dysmorphic? Diff	Low Weight? Diff	Pinna Abno.? Diff	Craniofac.? Diff	Cleft Diff	Other Malf.? Diff	Bilrubin? Diff	Low Apgar? Diff	Meningitis? Diff	Aminogly? Diff	Ventilation? Diff	Syndromes? Diff	Infections? Diff
R250			-0.059				-0.060	-0.124			0.032					
R353	0.024	0.024	-0.036				-0.042	-0.093			0.030					
R500	0.031	0.022					-0.037	-0.079			0.022					
R707	0.022	0.018	-0.033				-0.057	-0.130								
R1000			-0.041		-0.065		-0.108	-0.232					-0.040	-0.103		
R1414			-0.042		-0.108		-0.135	-0.379					-0.030	-0.103		
R2000	-0.023				-0.100		-0.165	-0.481						-0.065		
R2828	-0.026						-0.160	-0.440					0.039			
R4000	-0.036				0.042		-0.118	-0.326			0.042		0.069	0.081		
R5657	-0.026						-0.092	-0.269					0.036			
R8000		0.026				-0.073	-0.111	-0.258					0.048			
V250	-0.087		-0.189		0.230				-0.249		0.117		0.101	0.179		
V353		0.039	-0.144		0.111						0.060		0.061	0.094		
V500	0.052	0.040	-0.087		0.082						0.045			0.057		
V707	0.057	0.032	-0.062		0.079		0.050	0.086			0.037			0.044		
V1000	0.049	0.027	-0.047		0.058		0.060	0.116			0.027			0.037		
V1414	0.030	0.016	-0.053				-0.033	-0.076		-0.087	0.021		-0.031	-0.036		
V2000			-0.028				-0.052	-0.135			0.030		-0.015	-0.055		
V2828	-0.011				0.024								0.022			
V4000		0.010	-0.027		0.059		-0.058	-0.160		0.046	0.035	0.061	0.033	0.051		
V5657	-0.015				0.023								0.013	0.024	0.022	
V8000	-0.015		0.011		-0.013			0.046								
G250	-0.087		0.167													
G353	-0.071															
G500	-0.079															
G707																
G1000	0.142				0.196		0.229	0.370	0.221				0.090	0.199		
G1414					0.269		0.427	0.887						0.261	0.260	
G2000	0.182		-0.185	0.461	-0.244		0.466	1.074		-0.706			-0.234	-0.178		
G2828	0.097			0.436			0.324	0.726					-0.245	-0.476		
G4000	0.106	0.090	-0.187								0.199			-0.177		
G5657		0.199	-0.561		0.931		-0.744	-2.609			0.504		0.320	0.560		
G8000	-0.192	0.171		0.826			0.337						0.193	0.416	0.658	

difference in the corresponding reflectance, equivalent volume, and conductance variables at the indicated half-octave frequency. These variable names are listed in column 1 with the first letter R, V., and G denoting reflectance, equivalent volume and conductance, respectively, and the succeeding number denoting frequency in Hz, e.g., R500 is reflectance in the half-octave centered at 500 Hz. The magnitude of all the significant differences can be compared in absolute terms to the median responses plotted in Figure 5 to assess the extent of the relative difference.

A comparison of the distribution of significant differences in the two tables shows that significant differences were more often found in the subject populaton after excluding outliers. In nearly every case in which a significant difference was observed in the entire population, a corresponding significant difference was also observed in the population with outliers excluded, and the differences nearly always had the same polarity. A reasonable explanation is that the responses from ears in the outlier group were contaminated by noise, thereby making it more unlikely to observe a significant effect. For this reason, further discussion of results is restricted to the subject population with outliers excluded (Table 2).

At frequencies below 1414 Hz, the left-ear response had larger reflectance and equivalent volume, and smaller conductance than the right-ear response in the same subject; at frequencies above 1414 Hz, the left-ear response had smaller reflectance and equivalent volume, and larger conductance than the right-ear response. Males tended to have larger reflectance and larger equivalent volumes than females at low frequencies, and higher conductance at frequencies at and above 4000 Hz. The absolute values of reflectance shifts for effects of ear and gender were in the range 0.02 to 0.03, whereas the median reflectances are approximately 0.2. The absolute values of equivalent volume shifts were in the range 0.01 to 0.06 cm^3, which is only slightly smaller than median equivalent volume and in the same range as the middle 50% of observations. The absolute values of conductance shifts were in the range of 0.07 to 0.2 mmho, whereas the median conductance varied across frequency from 0.7 to 1.8 mmho. The reflectance and conductance shifts are typically 10% or larger than the corresponding median values, and the relative shifts in equivalent volume were somewhat larger. The shifts between ears across all YR variables tended to be slightly larger than the shifts due to gender.

RISK FACTOR EFFECTS

The risk factors that were investigated in regards to the YR responses were selected from those discussed by

Vohr et al. (2000). Each risk factor is a dichotomous variable indicating presence or absence of the condition in the particular subject, and are as follows: cleft lip or palate (CLEFT LIP/PAL.), dysmorphic characteristics (DYSMORPH), pinna abnormalities (PINNA), other malformations (OTHER MALFORM.), low birthweight (WEIGHT), family history of hearing loss (FAMILY HISTORY), aminoglycosides (AMINOGLY.), whether the neonate was placed on a ventilator (VENTILATION), low APGAR scores (APGAR), meningitis (MENINGITIS), other syndromes (SYNDROMES), infections (INFECTIONS), and bilirubin exchange levels (BILIRUBIN). The additional risk factor of craniofacial anomolies is the union of the first four risk factors.

The possible presence of various risk factors accounted for significant changes in the YR variables. The risk factors in Table 2 (and Table 1) were defined as the difference in the mean YR response for the group without the risk factor relative to the mean YR response for the group with the risk factor.

Responses from neonates with a cleft lip or palate had higher reflectance at all frequencies, which means that less energy was absorbed by the middle ears of neonates with cleft lip or palate than in the middle ears of neonates without cleft lip or palate. The associated change in energy reflectance was as large as 0.48 at 2000 Hz, on a scale that varies only between zero and one. By comparison, the median value of reflectance at 2000 Hz was only 0.1. The cleft-lip subjects had the largest shifts in equivalent volume and conductance as well, which exceeded the absolute values of the corresponding median values.

The subjects with cranial-facial anomalies, which includes the cleft lip or palate subjects as a subgroup, also showed large shifts in the YR variables, for example, a shift in reflectance of at least 0.16 at 2000 and 2828 Hz. It turns out that the cleft lip or palate subjects were largely responsible for the significant differences in the subjects with cranial-facial anomalies. The risk factors for low weight at birth and whether the neonate was placed on a ventilator showed moderate shifts in YR responses. For example, the largest reflectance shifts were on the order of 0.1, relative to the nominal absolute reflectance of 0.2. It is possible that covariations in age-related differences (discussed below) may account for some of the differences listed, but it is unlikely because the age-related differences across age are relatively modest for frequencies above 250 Hz and conceptional ages (CAs) less than 46 wk or so.

The shifts in YR responses with variables with three or more values are listed for the group of ears after excluding outliers (Table 3). Significant differences for RISK TYPE were observed depending on

Table 3. Outlier subjects excluded

YR	RISKTYPE (1,2,3 = Hi wRF, woRF)		SITENUM (1,2,3,4 denote sites)			ETHNIC	GA	CA	Chronological Age (days) re: YR score in < 1-day-olds						
	1 vs.3	2 vs.3	1 vs.4	2 vs.4	3 vs.4				1-1.5	1.5-2	2-2.5	2.5-3	3-4	4-14	15-28
R250	-0.035	0.039	0.047	0.057	0.030	0.0027	0.0000	0.0000	-0.076	-0.078	0.092	0.119	-0.048	-0.055	-0.058
R353	-0.023	0.056	0.024	-0.053	0.034		0.0045	0.0000	-0.072	-0.104	0.081	-0.107	0.053	-0.043	-0.049
R500	-0.023	0.072	0.031	-0.097	0.057	0.0088	0.0000	0.0000	0.020	-0.091	0.030	-0.094	-0.158	-0.077	-0.121
R707	-0.040	0.059	0.145	-0.123	0.037	0.0077	0.0000	0.0000		-0.089		-0.082	0.020	-0.123	-0.156
R1000	-0.093	0.040	0.077	0.212	0.215	0.0194	0.0000	0.0000		-0.324		0.070		-0.141	-0.087
R1414	-0.049	0.063	0.030	0.146	0.167	0.0023	0.0000	0.0000		-0.123		0.338		-0.102	-0.142
R2000	-0.068	0.104	0.043	0.079	0.127	0.0162	0.0000	0.0001		0.047		0.541		-0.150	-0.266
R2828	-0.165	0.020	0.036	0.065	0.101	0.0187	0.0000	0.0253		-0.038				-0.207	-0.115
R4000	-0.081	0.027	0.258	0.074	0.068	0.0029	0.0000	0.0000		-0.027				-0.088	-0.068
R5657	-0.042	-0.021	0.150	0.096	0.039	0.0198	0.0000	0.0000		-0.027				0.054	0.083
R8000	-0.032	-0.139	0.085	0.079	0.023	0.0031	0.0000	0.0000		0.336				0.064	-0.038
V250	0.024	0.200	0.080	0.018	0.017	0.0000	0.0000	0.0000		0.507				-0.047	-0.033
V353	-0.018	0.641	0.068	0.039	0.024	0.0017	0.0042	0.0000		-0.652				-0.033	-0.033
V500	-0.045		0.070	0.234	0.019	0.0441	0.0001	0.0000						-0.024	0.306
V707	-0.046		0.075	0.311	-0.310	0.0096	0.0002	0.0000						0.199	0.252
V1000	-0.020		0.047	0.284	-0.267	0.0378	0.0488	0.0000						0.169	0.265
V1414	0.108		0.062	0.265	-0.288	0.0014	0.0000	0.0000						0.152	0.199
V2000	0.350		0.020	0.195	-0.212	0.0011	0.0000	0.0000						0.475	0.302
V2828	0.171		-0.175	0.295	-0.151	<0.0005	0.0000	0.0000						0.721	0.797
V4000	-0.563		0.123	0.682	-0.105		0.0000	0.0000						0.361	0.573
V5657	-0.412		0.286	0.562	-0.146		0.0000	0.0000						-0.439	0.369
V8000			0.787	0.824	0.202		0.0015	0.0000							-0.588
G250			0.297	0.924	0.416		0.0000	0.0000							
G353							0.0000	0.0000							
G500							0.0000	0.0000							
G707							0.0006	0.0000							
G1000							0.0000	0.0000							
G1414							0.0000	0.0000							
G2000							0.0000	0.0000							
G2828							0.0000	0.0000							
G4000							0.0000	0.0000							
G5657							0.0000	0.0000							
G8000							0.0000	0.0000							
N									138	72	35	29	239	517	249

(baseline group 0-1 day-old N = 96)

RISKTYPE, SITENUM and Chronological Age are not significant if blank, else any significant contrasts are given.
ETHNIC, GestAge and CurrGrp show significant p values, and 0 means <0.0005.

whether the neonates were in a normal nursery with no risk factors ($N = 697$, group 1), normal nursery with one or more risk factors ($N = 196$, group 2), or in an intensive care unit (high-risk) ($N = 1188$, group 3). Table 3 shows significant differences between the mean responses in the high-risk group relative to those in the well-baby group without risk factors, and between the mean responses from the well-baby group with risk factors versus those from the well-baby group without risk factors. These differences were observed in at least five half-octaves of each of the reflectance equivalent volume and conductance responses. The high-risk neonates had smaller reflectance and equivalent volumes than low-risk neonates across the frequency range. The magnitude of the reflectance, equivalent volume and conductance shifts fro RISK TYPE were approximately twices as large or more than the corresponding reflectance, equivalent volume and conductance shifts due to EAR and GENDER (Table 2). Relative to the median values of these YR variables plotted in Figure 5, the magnitude of relative shifts for RISK TYPE were typically 20 to 30%.

Also shown in Table 3 are the significant differences in the YR variables for three of the test-site pairs, 1 versus 4, 2 versus 4, and 3 versus 4 (SITE-NUM). The shifts in YR responses tended to be larger than those associated with RISK TYPE (and EAR and GENDER). The underlying data have already been discussed, but it is interesting to note that the means were more often significantly different in the population with outliers excluded than in the entire population (the YR differences are not tabulated), even though the 10th and 25th percentiles were so markedly different across site in the entire population (e.g., Fig. 4).

Results were obtained for ethnicity, gestational age (GA), and CA categories, which, because of the number of categories for each variable, are listed differently in Table 3 from the preceding variables discussed. Each element is blank if the corresponding variable did not account for a significant amount of the variance of the YR resonse; otherwise, the element is the p-value that was significant (at the 0.05 level). Significant differences due to ethnicity may have underlying covariate relationships that remain unexamined. GA and CA were significant for nearly every YR variable. Because these age variables are highly correlated, attention was restricted to CA.

The YR responses varied with CA from <33 wk through 48 wk. The half-octave-averaged reflectance, equivalent volume and conductance responses (outliers excluded) are plotted for each octave frequency in Figures 6 through 8 as a funciton of CA. Trends at the intermediate half-octaves were similar, but were not plotted. The medians of reflectance and equivalent vol-

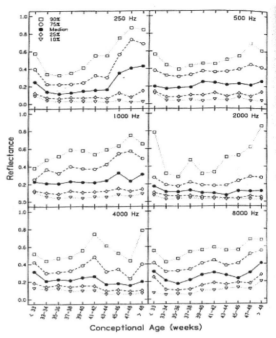

Figure 6. Plots of energy reflectance versus conceptional age at each octave from 250 to 8000 Hz.

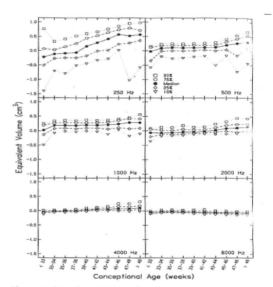

Figure 7. Plots of equivalent volume versus conceptional age at each octave from 250 to 8000 Hz.

ume slightly increased at low- and mid-frequencies with increasing CAs, except for the youngest age group (<33 wk CA), which had higher reflectance at most frequencies. The medians of conductance at 2000 and 4000 Hz increased with CA above 41 wk. The reflectance and conductance distributions are skewed in the sense that the 75th and 90th percentiles increased more mardedly with CA age, whereas the 25th and 10th percentiles showed little or no variability with age. These different trends may be due to underlying covariates, i.e., the group of neonates in the 90th percentile of a YR

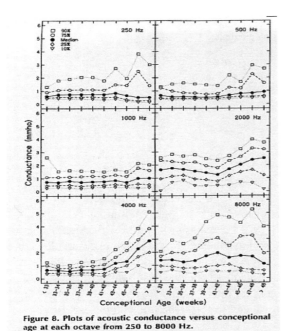

Figure 8. Plots of acoustic conductance versus conceptional age at each octave from 250 to 8000 Hz.

response may be different from the group of neonates in the 10th percentile. The CA variable encapsulated both the normal development of the middle ear as well as a shift in the risk-type characteristics of the distribution of infants, because older CA neonates in this study tended to be those who had been placed in a neonatal intensive care unit (NICU).

One hypothesis of interest is whether the YR responses changed in the first couple of days after birth, due to the influences of material including vernix present in the ear canal and middle ear. Table 3 shows the differences in YR responses at various chronologic ages (in days up to 28 days old) relative to the YR responses in the youngest chronologic age group (up to 1 day old). Any nonblank value is indicative of a difference in the YR responses of older infants to those infants tested within the first 24 hr after birth. A qualitative shift in the YR responses was observed in infants of age 1.5 to 2 days relative to the baseline younger group. These older infants have reduced reflectance at and above 2828 Hz, reduced equivalent volumes below 500 Hz and between 2828 and 5657 Hz, increased equivalent volume at 1414 Hz, and increased conductance from 1414 to 2000 Hz. Essentially all of the subjects less than 4 days old were from the normal nursery. There were only sparse changes in YR responses for subjects of chronologic ages from 2 to 4 days relative to the baseline younger group. A reduction in equivalent volume at low frequencies was observed in subjects of age up to 15 to 28 days old, even though the more typical developmental pattern is that equivalent volume increases with age. This suggests that the middle ears in

1-day-olds are different from the middle ears of somewhat older neonates and perinates.

Alternatively, it might be supposed that this result is due to sampling bias. Infants with craniofacial anomalies often were seen between 10 and 28 days of age, and might be expected to produce shifts in accordance with Table 2. However, the observed group shifts in Table 3 in the 15 to 28 days old group were in the opposite direction from the shifts due to the craniofacial anomaly risk factor. Thus, this aspect of sampling bias does not account for the observed shift in this older age group relative to the 1-day-old group.

This question was examined from a different perspective by evaluating the cumulative distributions of energy reflectance for subjects (excluding outliers) with chronologic age up to 3 days old. After averaging energy reflectance across the entire frequency range (250 to 8000 Hz), Table 4 shows the relative distribution of ears with average energy reflectance exceeding 0.6 (defining the High -R group) as a function of chronologic age. During the first 24 hr after birth, 5.2% of ears had high reflectance, and the relative proportion of high-reflectance ears decreased over the next few days. For example, in the chronologic age range of 1 to 3 days, 1.5% of ears had high reflectance. These trends are in the direction of the prior analysis, namely, that some ears just after birth have high reflectance, corresponding to low absorption of energy in the middle ear.

DISCUSSION

The equivalent volume in the neonatal ear can be negative at low frequencies, which means that the impedance at the probe tip is mass-dominated rather than stiffness-dominated as in the ears of adults and older children. This is consistent with Holte et al. (1991), who have reported mass-like values for the static admittance phase angle near 450 Hz. Keefe et al. (1993) reported a low-frequency resonance in full-term infants of age 1 and 3 mo, which includes a region of mass-like response. Holte et al. (1991) suggested that "material other than air in the middle ear cavity may add mass to the ossicular chain." Keefe et al. (1993) modeled the low-frequency admittance and reflectance responses at the youngest ages tested using an oscillator model, which has its resonance at low frequencies and which acts in parallel with the eardrum admittance. Although their data do not exclude the possibility that this shunt admittance might be due to some change within the middle ear, the most parsimonious explanation is that the oscillator model represents a resonanat ear-canal wall motion. This explanation is consistent with the low-frequency YR responses observed in this study. It is not apparent how adding mass to the ossicu-

Table 4. High reflectance neonates (R > 0.6) as function of chronological age.

Chronological Age (Days)	Total N	High-R N	High-R %
0-1	96	5	5.2
1-1.5	126	2	1.6
1.5-2	67	1	1.5
2-2.5	35	0	0.0
2.5-3	29	1	3.4
1-3 (all except 0-1 days)	267	4	1.5

lar chain would change the low-frequency eardrum impedance to a mass-dominated response. It would seem that such a change would produce a larger, rather than smaller, energy reflectance, in contrast to the results of this study (with the important exception that infants tested in the first day after birth have higher-reflectance, which may be due to the presence of vernix or material within the middle ear).

The YR variables showed significant ear differences, with the largest relative shifts for equivalent volume. At frequencies below 1414 Hz, the equivalent volume and reflectance in the left ear were larger than those in the right ear, and the conductance in the left ear was smaller than that in the right ear. The directions of these shifts were all reversed above 1414 Hz (with the single exception of the shift in conductance at 8000 Hz).

Adopting a simple stiffness, mass and resistance model of the acoustic response of the ear as used in related investigations (Feeney & Keefe, 1999; Johansen, 1948; Marfolis, Saly, & Keefe, 1999), shifts in reflectance, equivalent volume, and conductance can be predicted due to individual shifts in the stiffness, mass and resistance coefficients. Such a model can be useful in interpreting the patterns of shifts in YR variables across frequency, even though it is not intended to realistically model the response of the neonatal ear. The result of such an analysis is that the pattern of reflectance and conductance shifts across frequency for the ear effect is consistent with an increased stiffness in the left-ear response.

However, the predicted equivalent volume shift is in the opposite direction from that observed. Although reflectance and conductance were positive for all ears tested, it is clear from Figure 5 that the median equivalent volume was fairly close to zero, that is, there were many observations of both positive and negative equivalent volumes. This is perhaps the best explanation for why the relative shifts in equivalent volume were larger than the relative shifts in reflectance and conductance: it is because the median equivalent volume was close to zero. Given the separation at low frequencies between

the 25th and 75th percentiles of the distribution of equivalent volumes in Figure 5, it is apparent that the relative shift is not as meaningful as the absolute shift. This is in marked contrast to the equivalent volume in the adult ear, which is always positive. When the shift in equivalent volume due to stiffening is calculated for a simple ear model with a negative equivalent volume, the predicted shift is in accord with the experimental data.

The preponderance of evidence suggests that the difference across YR variables measured in left and right ears is related to a relative (acoustic) stiffening of the left ear, with a resonance frequency in the neighborhood of 1000 to 1414 Hz. That said, it is unclear how to assign the stiffness, mass, and resistance elements in the model to external- and middle-ear functioning. In part, this is because both the middle ear and the ear-canal walls may have resonant characteristics, and the dynamical response at the walls may be very different in neonatal ears than in the ears of older children and adults (Keefe et al., 1993).

The YR variables showed significant gender effects, with the largest relative shifts for equivalent volume. At frequencies below 2000 Hz, the equivalent volume and reflectance in the male ear were larger than those in the female ear, and there was no shift in conductance. At frequencies above 2000 Hz, the means of reflectance and equivalent volume showed no gender effect in three of four frequency bins, whereas the mean conductance of the males was higher than that of the females in three of four frequency bins (4000 to 8000 Hz). Adopting a simple stiffness, mass and resistance model of the acoustic response of the ear, the qualitative pattern of shifts up to 2000 Hz may be accounted for by psiting that the male ear is less stiff than the female ear. To account for the equivalent volume shifts, it is again necessary to assume that the baseline equivalent volume is negative at low frequencies. The data above 2000 Hz are not well accounted for by this model.

The significant differences in Table 2 do appear to have an underlying relatively simple form across frequency, i.e., the signs of the differences tend to shift slowly with respect to frequency. The simple-oscillator model of the ear is only partially successful at accounting for the qualitative pattern of the effects. An improved model of the neonatal ear is needed to understand the patterns of ear and gender effects on the YR responses.

The YR responses varied with CA, but the magnitude of the changes were modest (Figures 6 through 8) compared with postnatal development over the first 2 yr (Keefe et al., 1993). An interesting aspect of the neonatal development changes was the occasionally nonmonotonic behavior, e.g., the reflectance in the youngest CA group (<33 wk) as contrasted with older ages. The reflectances from the present study, although lower than previously reported (compare 43 to 44 and 45 to 46 wk CA responses in Figure 6 to the data for 1-mo-olds in Figure 4 of Keefe et al., 1993), follow similar patterns across frequency. Furthermore, there is qualitative similarity of the changes that occur with age. It should be noted that the reflectance measurements in the 1993 study were based on tests in healthy, full-term infants, whereas the older CA neonates in the present study included infants with health complications. The equivalent volume at low frequencies (250 to 1000 Hz) was also much smaller in the <33 wk group than in older age groups. The reduction in the low-frequency reflectance in the younger ages may be associated with a resonance, possibly related to the more compliant ear-canal walls.

The slight increase in the low-frequency reflectance in the much younger CAs tested in the present study is apparently inconsistent wit this model, although the corresponding reduction in the low-frequency equivalent volume is consistent with the model. This suggests the possibility of some additional dynamical factor in the <33 wk age group. One candidate is the presence of vernix in the ear just after birth, which may increase reflectance. This possibility is supported by the result that the incidence of ears with abnormally high reflectance was higher in enonates within 24 hr after birth (Table 4). Subjects tested at young conceptional and chronologic ages in this study included those subjects exiting the health care facility due to the absence of significant health complications. Thus, it is likely that the younger CA groups had a disproportional number of subjects tested at young chronologic age, in whom the presence of vernix is more likely. This may account for the increase in reflectance in the <33 wk age group.

These exploratory analyses demonstrated that several risk factors accounted for a significant amount of the variance in many of the YR responses, but did not determine the extent to which such relationships existed due to age interactions. That is, if the distribution of risk factors varied across age, an age effect in the YR responses may have appeared as a risk-factor effect (this possibility was not a concern in the analyses of ear and gender effects, because these effects were balanced with respect to age). Thus, the risk factor effects on the YR responses were assessed using an analysis of variance (ANOVA) that also took account of CA.

An ANOVA was performed for each risk factor to explain its YR response based on the risk factor (denoted by V, which should not be confused with equivalent volume V), CA, and the interaction of risk factor and CA (VxCA). Thus, each ANOVA answered the question whether any significant variation in the YR response was accounted for by the risk factor, CA, or by their interaction. The results are shown in Table 5A and B, which indicate whether or not each factor V was significant after controlling for CA and whether or not the interaction VxCA was significant for 27 to 33 of the YR responses (11 frequencies and three variables total 33 responses).

The first two columns in Table 5A show the pattern of significances for site (SITENUM), based on the YR responses in the four sites, and for group (RISK GROUP), based on membership in the well-baby group with no risk factors, the well-baby group with one or more risk factors, or the NICU group. The remaining columns in Table 5A, and continuing in Table 5B, list the pattern of significances for the individual dichotomous risk factors. The dichotomous variables in each column are sorted in decreasing order across Table 5A and B according to the number of significant results. Thus, the cleft lip or palate risk factor was most often significant as either a main effect or an interaction in explaining the YR responses, followed by the aminoglycoside risk factor, etc., Each risk factor in Table 5A had 16 or more significant tests across all YR variables, whereas each risk factor in Table 5B had 10 or fewer significant tests across all YR variables.

After accounting for the main effect of CA on the YR responses, those dichotomous risk factors that were most important in their effects on the YR responses include cleft lip or palate, aminoglycoside, low weight, use of ventilation, and low APGAR scores. The cleft lip or palate group is a special category of infants in whom middle-ear dysfunction is expected, so it was not surprising that their YR responses were so different. The risk factors of low weight, use of ventilation and low APGAR scores are risk factors that may be associated with hearing loss. These findings support the theory that such at-risk neonates had a different middle-ear status than a baseline group of otherwise healthy neonates. The importance of aminoglycosides was unexpected, as no obvious prior hypothesis existed to explain why this

Table 5. A. Significant coefficients from ANOVA on first-half population excluding outliers.

	SITENUM		Risk Group		Cleft Lip/Pal.?		Aminoglycoside?		Low Weight?		Ventilation?		Low Apgar?	
	V	CAxV	V	CAxV	V	CAxV	V	CAxV	V	CAxV	V	CAxV	V	CAxV
R250	s	s	s	s	s	s	s	s	s	s	s	s	s	s
R353	s	s	s	s	s	s	s	s	s	s	s	s	s	s
R500	s	s	s	s	s	s	s	s	s	s	s	s	s	s
R707	s	s	s	s	s	s	s	s	s	s	s	s	s	s
R1000	s	s	s	s	s	s	s	s	s	s	s	s	s	s
R1414	s	s	s	s	s	s	s	s	s	s	s	s	s	s
R2000	s	s	s	s	s	s		s	s	s	s	s	s	s
R2828	s	s	s	s	s	s		s	s	s	s	s	s	s
R4000	s	s	s	s	s	s		s	s	s	s			
R5657	s	s	s	s	s	s		s	s					
R8000	s	s	s	s	s	s		s						
V250	s	s	s	s	s	s		s						
V353	s	s	s	s	s	s		s						
V500	s	s	s	s	s			s						
V707	s	s	s	s	s			s						
V1000	s	s	s	s	s			s						
V1414	s	s	s	s	s			s						
V2000	s	s	s	s	s									
V2828	s	s	s		s									
V4000	s	s			s									
V5657	s	s			s									
V8000	s	s			s									
G250	s	s			s									
G353	s	s			s									
G500	s	s			s									
G707	s	s												
G1000	s	s												
G1414														
G2000														
G2828														
G4000														
G5657														
G8000														

CA = coverage; V = variable (listed in top row); CAxV = interaction.
"s" in cell denotes a significant factor <0.05.

risk factor might be related to middle-ear status. Its emergence may be due to the high correlation of the aminoglycoside risk group with the low birthweight risk group.

The fact that risk group was important in its effect on the YR responses (Table 5A) is not surprising given the preceding discussion. For example, membership in the NICU group was positively correlated with an increased likelihood for the risk factors of ventilation, low birthweight and low APGAR scores. The importance of the site variation, even after excluding outliers and accounting for CA effects, is consistent with either of two hypotheses. The first hypothesis is that testers at some sites may have used slightly different testing procedures than testers at other sites. For example, it may be that the criterion for excluding detached outliers was too conservative, and that responses from some sites were more often contaminated by probe-fit artifact than responses at other sites. The second hypothesis is that the distributions of neonates at the various sites were not identical in regards to covariates such as risk group, presence of specific risk factors, weight, GA, ethnicity, etc. These underlying covariates may account for the significant differences across sites. Most likely, both of these effects contributed to these differences.

Measurements of wideband admittance and reflectance may have utility in neonatal hearing screening programs. The YR responses take only seconds to acquire, and should be much less susceptible than EOAE and ABR measurements to environmental and patient noise because the inherent signal to noise ratio is larger. This is because the acoustical response to be

Table 5. Continued B. Additional significant coefficients from ANOVA on first-half population excluding outliers.

	Family History?		Dysmorphic?		Pinna Abnormal?		Meningitis?		Other Malform?		Syndromes?		Infections?		Bilirubin?	
	V	CAxV	V	CAxV	V	CAxV	V	CAxV	V	CAxV	V	CAxV	V	CAxV	V	CAxV
R250	s	s	s	s	s	s	s	s	s	s	s	s	s	s		
R353	s	s	s	s	s	s	s	s	s	s	s	s	s	s		
R500	s	s	s	s	s	s	s	s	s	s	s	s	s	s		
R707	s	s		s	s	s	s	s	s	s	s	s	s	s		
R1000	s	s		s	s	s	s	s	s	s	s	s	s	s		
R1414				s	s	s	s	s	s	s	s	s	s	s		
R2000					s	s	s		s	s	s	s	s	s		
R2828					s	s	s		s	s	s	s	s	s		
R4000					s	s	s		s	s	s	s				
R5657					s	s	s		s							
R8000					s	s	s									
V250					s	s	s									
V353					s	s	s									
V500					s		s									
V707					s		s									
V1000					s		s									
V1414					s		s									
V2000					s											
V2828					s											
V4000					s											
V5657					s											
V8000					s											
G250					s											
G353					s											
G500					s											
G707																
G1000																
G1414																
G2000																
G2828																
G4000																
G5657																
G8000																

CA = coverage; V = variable (listed in top row); CAxV = interaction.
"s" in cell denotes a significant factor <0.05.

measured is at the same moderate sound pressure level as the evoking ear-canal stimulus, unlike the much smaller acoustical response comprising an EOAE signal in the ear canal.

The YR responses varied with risk factors that are thought to be related to middle-ear-status, and the structure of YR responses in the first day after birth is consistent with the hypothesis that the presence of material in the ear canal and middle ear reduced the transmission of energy into the middle ear and, thus, into the cochlea. The YR responses provide frequency-specific information on middle-ear status across a broad frequency range. It is evident from prior work on older children that there is not a simple mapping from a YR response at a particular frequency to the prediction of a conductive hearing loss at that frequency. It turns out that a multivariate approach utilizing information from all frequencies is needed to accurately predict the presence or absence of a conductive hearing loss at a particular frequency (Piskorski et al., 1999). This is because the YR responses at some frequencies may be controlled by middle-ear factors that are directly related to transfer of energy to the cochlea, and at othe frequencies may be controlled by middle-ear factors that have little relationship to the cochlear termination. Thus, the use of admittance-reflectance responses in a neonatal hearing screening program, in conjuction with EOAE and/or ABR measurements, may require a sophisticated analytical approach to unravel the subjects with conductive, cochlear and mixed hearing losses.

Nevertheless, the detection of an unusually high reflectance (for example, the high-reflectance condition for the analysis in Table 4 was that the reflectance exceeded 0.6, corresponding to a pressure reflectance magnitude of 0.77) means that there exists a corresponding reduction in the forward transfer of stimulus energy into the middle ear and thence to the cochlea, and a concomitant reduction in the retrograde transfer of energy in any EOAE. Thus, it is predicted that unusually high reflectances will be associated with unusually low or absent EOAE responses, elevated thresholds, and perhaps prolonged ABR latencies.

An issue in EOAE and ABR testing is ensuring a leak-free probe fit. The YR response is extremely sensitive to quality of probe fit, and, to the extent that some neonates in a hearing screening program have poor probe fit, the additional measurement of the YR response may help identify these ears. One approach would be to provide real-time feedback during the YR test when the low-frequency-averaged equivalent volume is less than some criterion value. The tester might be requested to adjust probe fit and measure a new response. In the present study, this criterion value was -1.15 cm^3. An experiment needs to be conducted in which such a criterion, or some generalization thereof, is implemented in real-time, and then compared with the results obtained by an independent "gold standard" as to whether or not a leak is present.

In the absence of such an experiment, an analysis addresses the issue whether the presence of a leak, as deduced from the YR response, may help account for the presence of low-amplitude or absent EOAEs. If such were found to be the case, a YR test in conjunction with an EOAE test could help reduce the number of "false positives," i.e., ears for which a sufficiently low-level EOAE would predict cochlear hearing loss in a subject with hearing in the normal range. This analysis used a relatively crude technique to classify each EOAE response as "present" (above a threshold stopping criterion) or "absent" (below a threshold stopping criterion). These stopping crieria are described in Norton et al. (2000).

A subset of 1301 subjects were available for this analysis, in which a single ear per subject was included. Because the YR test always preceded the TEOAE test in the test protocol, the analysis was confined to interpreting the TEOAE responses delivered at a level of 86 dB pSPL, as it is likely that the status of the probe seal was similar in the two tests.

Of the 1301 ears, 86 ears or 6.6% of the population had an "absent" TEOAE response. Of the (negative) outlier population of 170 ears as classified by the YR test, 21 ears or 12.4% had an "absent" TEOAE response. Of the population of 1131 ears that were not

outliers according to the YR test, the rate of "absent" TEOAE responses was 5.8%. This more than 2-fold increase in the proportion of ears in which the TEOAE response was "absent" suggests that an acoustic leak was present in these ear canals, because, for a leaky probe fit, the stimulus level delivered through the middle ear to the cochlea is decreased, and, probably, the level of the TEOAE was decreased. Hence, the ear tested with a leaky probe seal is more likely to fail the TEOAE test. This failure is due to insufficient energy transmitted to the cochlea as well as poor coupling of the resulting TEOAE signal to the probe microphone. Even though TEOAEs were measurable in most ears with leaky probe fits, a reduction in the fail rate on an TEOAE test by nearly a factor of two would have significance in controlling the fails rates in typical screening populations.

Although this analysis did not utilize the more carefully constructed definition of classifying a TEOAE response as present or absent, which was used in studying all the TEOAE responses in the database, nevertheless the large difference in TEOAE test performance in the outlier and nonoutlier populations should not be strongly influenced by differing definitions of TEOAE test performance. In addition, the ability to place a probe in the ear canal in a leak-free manner should be independent of whether there exists a cochlear hearing loss in the ear. Thus, the results of this analysis support the view that a contributor to the false-positive rate of TEOAEs was improper probe seal, and may account for roughly half the false positives in the sample population. It is possible that an improper probe seal may degrade DPOAE test performance as well. A YR test with a real-time indicator of probe seal might be beneficial for subsequent EOAE testing, but additional research is needed to validate that confirmed tester errors in fitting the probe lead to equivalent volume responses that are highly negative and that EOAE levels are correspondingly reduced.

In the much more typical cases in which an adequate probe seal is achieved, it may be that combining the results of the acoustic YR response will assist in interpreting the results of EOAE and ABR tests. This is because the YR response assesses middle-ear status, and variations in middle-ear status can influence test outcomes based on EOAE and ABR. Although this hypothesis is plausible, the magnitude of the expected influence needs to be assessed both in terms of basic research and clinical efficacy. The CA variations in the YR responses were significant but modest. In the 1000 to 4000 Hz frequency range at which EOAEs are often tested in neonates, as CA increased, reflectance was relatively constant, equivalent volume increased slightly, and conductance increased markedly (at least for 2000 and 4000 Hz) for CAs exceeding 43 wk. This latter increase indicates either greater power loss within the external ear (in particular, in the lossy ear-canal walls) and middle ear, or greater power transferred to the cochlea. It remains to be determined the extent to which YR responses in neonatal ears, which are indicative of forward transfer of power into the middle ear, account for the characteristics of EOAE and ABR responses, both in comparisons across ears in normal-hearing subjects, hearing-impaired populations.

CONCLUSIONS

Admittance-reflectance responses were acquired in a clinical setting at four sites in 4031 neonatal ears. The evidence suggests that the left ear was acoustically stiffer than the righ ear, and that the female ear was acoustically stiffer than the male ear. The YR technique requires a leak-proof insertion into the ear canal, which was achieved in approximately 87% of ears tested. An analysis showed that the false positive rate associated with TEOAE testing may be significantly reduced when a leak-proof insertion is obtained, as assessed by a criterion of seal provided by the YR test. Systematic changes occurred in YR responses 24 hr after birth, which suggests that the YR test may be sensitive to the presence of vernix and other material in the external and middle ears that clears up within the first couple of days after birth. The YR responses in the youngest CA group (<33 wk) tested showed some departures from the otherwise monotonic relationship of YR variables across CA. Such departures may be due to vernix-induced effects on the acoustical ear-canal response. The variation in YR responses with age from 33 to 48 wk CA is consistent with data in older infants, with lower energy reflectance (near 0.25). The YR responses differed on neonates across risk type, and varied based on such dichotomous risk factors as cleft lip or palate, aminoglycosides, low weight, use of ventilation, and low APGAR scores. the admittance-reflectance test shows promise in providing information on the middle-ear status of neonates, which may be useful in interpreting neonatal tests for screening hearing loss.

ACKNOWLEDGMENTS

We are grateful to Robert Ling for his expertise in developing the YR measurement software, Kelly Mascher and Pawel Piskorski for technical support, Laurie Winney for document preparation, and Kristin A. Fletcher for her central role in statistical analyses of data. This work was primarily supported by NIDCD grant #R10 DC10958. Software engineering was supported by NIDCD #P01-00520.

REFERENCES

Feeney, M.P., & Keefe, D.H. (1999). Acoustic reflex detection using wide-band acoustic reflectance, admittance, and power measurements, *Journal of Speech Language and Hearing Research*, 42, 1029-1041.

Gorga, M.P., Norton, S.J., Sininger, Y.S., Cone-Wesson, B., Folsom, R.C., Vohr, B.R., & Widen, J.E. (2000). Identification of neonatal hearing impairment: Distortion product otoacoustic emissions during the perinatal period. *Ear and Hearing*, 21, 400-424.

Harrison, W.A., Dunnell, J.J., Vohr, B.R., Gorga, M.P., Widen, J.E., Cone-Wesson, B., Folsom, R.C., Sininger, Y.S., & Norton, S.J. (2000). Identification of neonatal hearing impairment: Implementation of neonatal test protocol. *Ear and Hearing*, 21, 357-372.

Holte, L., Margolis, R.H., & Cavanaugh, Jr., R.M. (1991). Developmental changes in multifrequency tympanograms. *Audiology*, 30, 1-24.

Johansen, H. (1948). Relation of audiograms to the impedance formula. *Acta Oto-Laryngologica (Stockholm)*, 74, 66-75.

Keefe, D.H., Bulen, J.C., Arehart, K.H. & Burns, E.M. (1993). Ear-canal impedance and reflection coefficient in human infants and adults. *Journal of the Acoustical Society of America*, 94, 2617-2638.

Keefe, D.H., Ling, R., & Bulen, J.C. (1992). Method to measure acoustic impedance and reflection coefficient. *Journal of the Acoustical Society of America*, 91, 470-485.

Kleinbaum, D.G., Kupper, L.L., & Muller, K.E. (1988). *Applied Regression Analysis and Other Multivariable Methods* (pp. 189-192). Boston: PWS-Kent.

Margolis, R.H. Saley, G.L., & Keefe, D.H. (1999). Wideband reflectance tympanometry in normal adults. *Journal of the Acoustical Society of America*, 106, 265-280.

McKinley, A.M., Grose, J.H., Roush, J. (1997). Multifrequency tympanometry and evoked otoacoustic emissions in neonates during the first 24 hours of life. *Journal of the American Academy of Audiology*, 8, 218-223.

Norton, S.J., Gorga, M.P., Widen, J.E., Vohr, B.R., Folsom, R.C., Sininger, Y.S., Cone-Wesson, B., & Fletcher, K.A. (2000). Identification of neonatal hearing impairment: Transient otoacoustic emissions during the perinatal period. *Ear and Hearing*, 21, 425-442.

Piskorski, P., Keefe, D.H., Simmons, J., & Gorga, M.P. (1999). Prediction of conductive hearing loss based on acoustic ear-canal response using multivariate clinical decision theory. *Journal of the Acoustical Society of America*, 105, 1749-1764.

Sininger, Y.S., Cone-Wesson, B., Folsom, R.C., Gorga, M.P., Vohr, B.R., Widen, J.E., Ekelid, M., & Norton, S.J. (2000). Identification of neonatal hearing impairment:

Auditory brainstem response in the perinatal period. *Ear and Hearing*, 21, 383-399.

Vohr, B.R., Cone-Wesson, B., Widen, J.E., Sininger, Y.S., Gorga, M.P., Folsom, R.C., & Norton, S.J. (2000). Identification of neonatal hearing impairment: Characteristics of infants in the neonatal intensive care unit (NICU) and well baby nursery. *Ear and Hearing*, 21, 373-382.

Development of Auditory Function in Newborn Infants Revealed by Auditory Brainstem Potentials

Arnold Starr, M.D., Ragnar N. Amlie, M.D., William Hal Martin, and Stephen J. Sanders

Departments of Neurology, Pediatrics, and Psychobiology, University of California, Irvine

Abstract

Auditory brainstem potentials were recorded from scalp electrodes in 42 infants ranging in gestational age from 25 to 44 weeks. The latencies of the various potential components decreased with maturation. Wave V, evoked by 65-dB sensation level clicks, changed in latency from 9.9 msec at 26 weeks of gestation to 6.9 msec at 40 weeks of gestation. Central conduction times in the auditory pathway also decreased with maturation from 7.2 msec at 26 weeks to 5.2 msec at 40 weeks. The effects of brainstem and cochlear disorders on auditory brainstem potentials were noted in several abnormal infants. The application of all of these techniques could permit an objective definition of both normal and abnormal sensory processes in newborn infants. *Pediatrics* 60:831-839, 1977, Auditory Development, Brainstem Potentials, Newborn Infants.

The clinical assessment of neurological and sensory functions of the newborn infant requires considerable experience and the results are usually described in qualitative terms. Recently, scalp-derived cortical brain potentials evoked by auditory,[1-4] visual,[5] and somatosensory stimuli[6] have been used to provide quantitative measures of changes in sensory function in the newborn. These techniques primarily sample cortical activity and the evoked potentials' amplitude and latency can vary with the infant's level of arousal. Procedures have now been developed for measuring sensory function in subcortical portions of one of the sensory systems, the auditory brainstem pathway, where arousal asserts relatively little effect.[7]

Auditory brainstem potentials are the far-field reflection of electrical events generated within the auditory pathway in its course through the brain. These potentials can be recorded from scalp electrodes in humans, using computer averaging techniques, and consist of seven deflections of submicrovolt amplitudes in the initial 10 ms following a click signal.[8] The components, designated by Roman numerals, are thought to derive from the sequential activation of the nuclei and pathways comprising the auditory system. Studies in both animals[9,10] and humans[11] suggest that wave I represents activity of the VIII nerve, wave II represents activity of the cochlear nuclei, wave III represents activity of the superior olive, and waves IV and V represent activity of the inferior colliculus. The origins of waves VI and VII have not yet been established. The latencies of the brainstem potentials change in an orderly manner with signal intensity and are not influenced by level of arousal. The technique has been used to assess hearing in newborn infants,[12] to measure maturation of newborn infants,[13] and to evaluate brainstem function in neurological disorders in adults.[14-17]

The present study utilized measures of auditory brainstem potentials in newborn and preterm infants to define the maturation of both peripheral (i.e., the cochlea) and central portions of the auditory pathway. In the course of study, we have encountered instances in which abnormalities of these potentials could be related to the infants clinical condition.

Methods

The infants were patients in the neonatal intensive care unit, the term nursery, or the intermediate nursery of the University of California Irvine Medical Center. Informed consent for the evoked potential study was obtained from the parent. Assessment of gestational age was based on (1) the date of the first day of the mother's last normal menstrual cycle and (2) a detailed physical examination performed shortly after birth using a composite scoring system.[18] The results from 42 infants ranging in original conceptional age from 25 to 44 weeks provide the data for this report.

The infants were tested in their bassinets or incubators. The equipment was on a small cart that was wheeled close to the patient. Three tin disc electrodes, 5 mm in diameter, were attached at the vertex (Cz) and mastoids, using a standard conducting medium (Grass electrode paste) and adhesive tape to hold the electrodes in place. The electrical potentials were recorded between the vertex electrode and mastoid electrode ipsilateral to the ear

Reproduced with permission from *Pediatrics*, 60:831-839. Copyright 1977 by the AAP.

Received January 4; revision accepted for publication April 25, 1977. Supported by U.S. Public Health Service grant NS11876-03.

Address for reprints: (R.N.A.) Department of Pediatrics, University of California, Irvine, CA 92717.

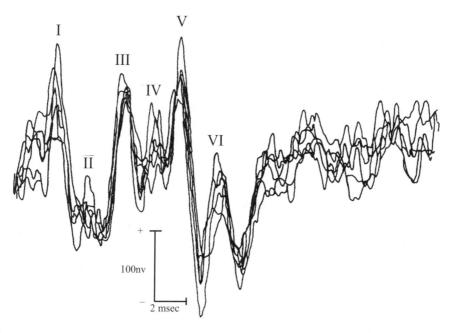

Figure 1. Auditory brainstem potentials from normal term infant at 40 weeks' gestation, measured six separate times over two-hour period. Six distinct components designated I through VI can be identified. Click rate was 10/sec; click intensity, 65 dB SL. Positivity at vertex electrode in this and all subsequent illustrations is represented by upward deflection.

receiving the click signal. The other mastoid electrode served as the patient ground. The responses were amplified by a factor of 10^5, filtered between 100 Hz and 3 kHz (3 dB down points) and averaged by a small digital computer. A 20-msec time base with a resolving capacity of 20 to 80 μsec per point for 1,024 points was used. A total of 2,048 stimulus trials was averaged and a duplicate average was made at each signal intensity to assess reproducibility of results. The average auditory brainstem potentials were plotted by an X-Y plotter for measurements of the latency and amplitude of the various components.

The acoustic signals were clicks generated by passing alternating-polarity, 0.5-msec square waves through an attenuator and power amplifier before actuating a TDH 39 earphone housed in an MX-41 coupler. The earphone was held in place over the ear taking care that the pinna was not compressed. Only one ear was tested in each infant. The intensity of the signals was calibrated in decibels of sensation level (dB SL) referred to the mean hearing threshold of six normal hearing adults measured in the nursery environment.

Auditory brainstem potentials were measured with a click rate of 10/sec in response to signal intensities of 65, 45, and 25 dB SL. In some of the infants born before 28 weeks of gestation, additional tests were carried out at 75 dB SL. The potentials were measured within four days of birth in all infants. The evoked potentials in 24 of the 42 infants were reexamined at a later date.

Figure 1 shows averaged auditory brainstem potentials derived from a normal term infant (40 weeks' gestation) measured six separate times over a two-hour period. The components were remarkably consistent in both form and amplitude except for waves II and IV. The latencies of the most reproducible and easily defined components (waves I, III, the IV-V complex, or V) were defined at their peak. Waves II, VI, and VII were too variable in appearance to allow systematic study. In those instances where a peak was flattened, lines were extended from the rising and falling slopes of the component in question and the peak defined by the intersection. The recording accuracy on repeated measures of the same waves was ±0.1 msec. Waves IV and V were often fused into a single component designated as the "IV-V complex." Data on the latency of the complex have been included with wave V, based on studies in five sets of twins in whom one member of each set had distinct waves IV and V while the other member had a IV-V complex. The difference in latency between the measurements in each member of the twin set was within the error of the measuring technique.

A listing of the infants studied arranged according to gestational age; latency of the components I, III, IV-V at three signal intensities; birth weight; and clinical diagnosis is available on request from the National Auxiliary Publications Service.

Slow cortical evoked potentials to clicks were also studied in the four infants who were born before the 28th week of gestation. The same recording electrodes were used. The amplifier band pass was changed to 1 to 100 Hz. The click intensity was 65 dB SL and the click rate was 1/sec. A total of 256 clicks comprised the averaged response recorded on a 512-msec time base. The infants were quiet and appeared asleep at the time of testing. The EEG was not recorded simultaneously, preventing staging of the sleep cycle.

Results

The latencies of the most prominent components (I, III, IV-V) of the brainstem potential from each infant to 65-dB SL clicks are plotted in Figure 2 as a function of gestational age. The latencies of all of the components decrease as gestational age at birth increases, with the maximal shift occurring before 34 weeks.

For instance, a two-week difference in gestational age between 32 and 34 weeks was associated with a 0.8-msec decrease in the latency of the IV-V component. A comparable two-week difference between the 38th and 40th weeks of gestation was accompanied by only a 0.1-msec latency change.

The first infant tested in the most immature group (less than 28 weeks of gestation) did not have auditory brainstem potentials to the 65-dB SL click but they subsequently appeared when the infant was retested several weeks after birth. Absence of auditory brainstem potentials at this early age was confirmed in two of the next three infants in this group. The possibility that these results indicated the presence of a critical period for the appearance of auditory function in human infants around the 28th week of gestation was rejected by additional studies. First, an increase in the intensity of the click signal by 10 dB SL to 75 dB SL resulted in the appearance of brainstem potentials in the two infants (Fig. 3). The IV-V complex occurred at latencies of 10.5 and 15 msec, respectively. Second, an examination of slow cortical evoked potentials to the same 65-dB click signals that were ineffective in eliciting brainstem potentials revealed a negative-going deflection between 100 and 200 msec in these infants (Fig. 3). Thus, auditory brainstem potentials can be recorded from preterm infants even as young as 25 weeks of gestation, if the signal is sufficiently intense. However, at this early age the click intensity necessary to elicit cortical potentials is lower than that needed for evoking brainstem potentials.

Retesting preterm infants after birth revealed that maturation of auditory function proceeded at about the same rate in both extrauterine and intrauterine environments. Figure 4 contains the mean latency of auditory brainstem potentials to 65-dB SL clicks of the initial test in all of the infants as well as the later tests in some of the infants. The age of retest in designated as the conceptional

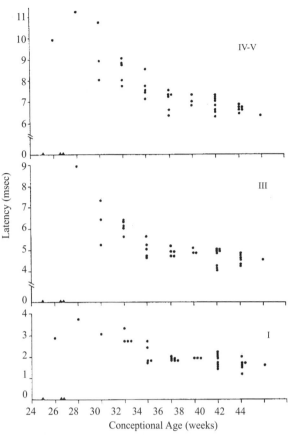

Figure 2. Auditory brainstem potentials from 42 newborn infants tested within four days of birth to clicks at 65 dB. Latencies of most prominent components, waves I, III, and IV-V complex, are plotted as a function of conceptional age. Triangles refer to tests in which no potential components could be identified.

age for this comparison. For instance, an infant born at 30 weeks' gestation and tested on the fourth week of life is included in the 34- to 35-week conceptional age group and can be compared with the results of the initial test at birth obtained from our preterm population born at the 34th to 35th week of gestation.

The relative contribution of peripheral (cochlea and middle ear) and central auditory pathway processes to the maturational changes can be derived from measures of auditory brainstem potentials. Wave I is assumed to represent activity of the VIII nerve while the other components (II to VII) represent activity arising from auditory pathway structures within the brainstem.[9,11,19] The long latency of wave I in the most preterm infants and the subsequent shortening of latency with increases in gestational age are evidence of changes in peripheral processing during this period. Since cochlear microphonic potentials were not recorded, we are unable to establish the proportion of the latency change of wave I that can be attributed to modifications of middle ear and cochlear receptors during devel-

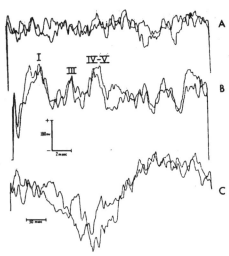

Figure 3. Effects of stimulus intensity of auditory brainstem potentials prior to 28 weeks' conceptional age. (A) No clear potential components are evoked by 65-dB SL clicks. (B) Potentials evoked by 75-dB SL clicks have definite components. (C) Slow cortical evoked potential to the same 65-dB SL clicks msec in A, showing clear negativity at 150 msec.

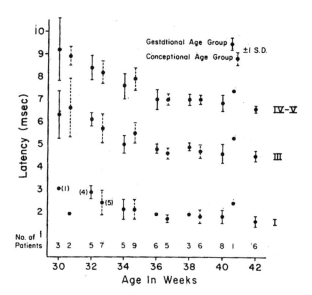

Figure 4. Comparison of mean latencies at 65 dB SL of major waves between gestational age group tested at birth and conceptional age group tested several weeks after birth at comparable ages. One SD of the mean is indicated by bars; numbers in parentheses indicate number of infants with clearly defined components of total group tested, indicated at lower part of graph.

opment and the proportion that represents changes in the transduction of receptor potentials into VIII nerve activity.

The time difference between the various components (i.e., waves III minus wave I, wave IV-V minus wave III, or wave IV-V minus wave I) can be used as a measure of maturation of the central auditory pathway. Figure 5 contains a plot of the time difference between waves IV-V and I as a function of gestational age. It is apparent that central conduction time as measured by the difference between the IV-V complex and wave I decreases with gestational age. The scatter in the measures of central conduction times between adjacent waves (waves III and I or waves IV-V and III) is too large to allow an estimate as to the site of maximal change along the central pathway.

Signal intensity had significant effects on the latency of auditory brainstem potentials. A decrease in signal intensity was accompanied by a lengthening of latency of brainstem potentials for all infants that varied with gestational age. The latency change of the IV-V complex in preterm infants for a 20-dB decrease of signal intensity (65 to 45 dB) varied from 0.2 to 2.0 msec, whereas the same intensity change in adults results in a latency shift of less than 0.9 msec. The effect of signal intensity on the latency of auditory brainstem potentials in preterm infants is most likely due to immaturity of peripheral auditory mechanisms, since central conduction times in the auditory pathway (wave IV-V minus wave I) were unaffected by the same 20-dB change in signal intensity.

The amplitude of the brainstem potentials varies considerably in both adults and newborn infants. However, measurements of the IV-V complex suggest that there is an increase in amplitude during maturation.

Disorders of Auditory Brainstem Potentials in Newborn Infants

There were several newborn infants whose auditory brainstem potentials deviated significantly from the normal patterns. These infants were neurologically or audiologically impaired and were not included in the core population.

Their auditory brainstem potentials were either delayed in latency or altered in amplitude. The components' designation as wave I, II, etc., could be uncertain

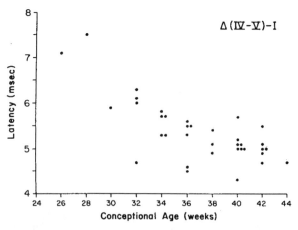

Figure 5. Time difference in milliseconds between various auditory brainstem potential components for each infant evoked by 65-dB SL click signal.

from inspection of the averaged potentials to just one click intensity. Several strategies were used to help delineate the components. First, waves I, II, and III are attenuated as click rates increase above 25/sec, whereas the amplitude of wave V is little affected.[12] Second, all of the components shift in latency as click intensity is reduced, whereas the time difference between each of the components remains unchanged. Thus, there is an orderly relationship between the components independent of click intensity.[6] Finally, the amplitude of certain of the components (waves I and III) can be profoundly modified by moving the mastoid electrode to the ear contralateral to the click stimulation, whereas the other components are little affected.[14] Nevertheless, the identity of some of the components of an abnormal auditory brainstem potential may still be imprecise even after all of these techniques have been utilized. An example of one such case that has come to postmortem examination was associated with multiple diffuse lesions of the brainstem (case 6 in reference 11).

Results from representative infants in the present study suggest some clinical applications of this procedure in the newborn nursery.

Patient 1. This infant was born at term and was normal except for a petechial rash localized to the face. She was admitted at 6 weeks with failure to thrive, abnormal head lag, seizures, and lack of clear behavioral response to sounds. Audiometric testing with a 3,000-Hz tone at 100 dB evoked "a marked startle and ocular reflex." In contrast, at 2 months and 4 months of age, auditory brainstem potentials were absent to click signals presented to either ear at 75 dB SL. At 5 months a definitive diagnosis of congenital cytomegalovirus disease was established. The child is now 8 months of age and both the parents and the pediatrician feel the child is deaf. Her psychomotor development is otherwise normal.

Comment. The recording of auditory brainstem potentials provides an objective means for defining auditory function in difficult-to-test newborn and developing infants and particularly infants suspected of hearing loss.

Patient 2. This term infant was noted to bleed from the left external ear canal at birth. Measurement of auditory brainstem potentials revealed a marked disparity between latencies of the IV-V complex evoked by stimulation of the two ears (Fig. 6). The potentials were of normal latency for the infant's age for the right ear but delayed 1.0 msec in the left ear. The potentials were absent in response to 45-dB SL clicks in the affected ear. No other hearing tests were carried out and follow-up has been unsuccessful.

Comment. Auditory brainstem potentials provide sufficiently precise measures to distinguish differences in auditory sensitivity between the ears due to trauma of the cochlea or middle ear at birth.

Patient 3. The patient was a normal full-term infant who was febrile on the second day of life. The diagnosis of *Escherichia coli* meningitis was established and the infant was treated. The meningitis resolved and auditory brainstem potentials were requested to assess hearing function at 3 weeks of age. The IV-V component was of normal latency when evoked by stimulation of one ear but considerably delayed on stimulation of the opposite ear at both 65 and 75 dB SL (Fig. 6). The latency difference was comparable to a 40-dB hearing loss. Repeated auditory brainstem potential measurement at 11 weeks of age showed marked improvement in the affected ear with the components returning to normal latency. There were no other tests of auditory brainstem performed. It is likely that the child experienced ischemia of one of the cochlea secondary to meningitis with almost complete recovery.

Comment. Auditory brainstem potentials provide early evidence of the presence of a temporary hearing loss (in this patient, a unilateral deficit) that followed meningitis.

Patient 4. The patient had a gestational age of 32 weeks and weighted 1,360 g. She had severe respiratory distress syndrome and required assisted ventilation. There was a sudden deterioration of the clinical condition on the second day of life compatible with an intracranial hemorrhage. Her condition stabilized for a week but then she gradually developed signs of hydrocephalus. A ventri-

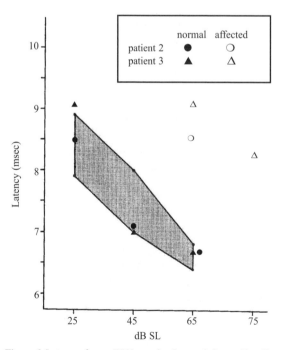

Figure 6. Latency of wave IV-V complex for two infants with unilateral hearing losses. Shaded region represents range of values for normals in this age group.

culostomy was performed but the baby developed sepsis and died on the 22nd day of life.

Auditory brainstem potentials were recorded on the day before death while she required complete respiratory assistance. She had intermittent generalized seizures with hypotonia in the periods between seizures. The pupils were 4 mm in diameter and did not react to light. Auditory brainstem potentials consisted of an abnormally high-amplitude wave I of normal latency and a IV-V complex appearing at a delayed latency of 20 msec. The central conduction time (wave V minus wave I) was considerably prolonged to 17 msec (upper limit of normal in our core population at this age was 6 msec). The brain was covered by a gray exudate, most severe around the brainstem. There was a massive intracerebral hemorrhage, extensive necrosis, and advanced encephalomalacia of both hemispheres and the brainstem. *Citrobacter diversus* was identified on tissue sections and culture.

Comment. Measures of auditory brainstem potentials revealed severe impairment within the CNS manifested by markedly prolonged central conduction times. These potentials provide an objective method for assessing the integrity of the brainstem in neurologically impaired infants.

Patient 5. The infant was born after 38 weeks' gestation. The neurological examination revealed marked hypotonia. All of the components of the auditory brainstem potentials were present, but the central conduction time (wave V minus wave I) was prolonged (7.0 msec). At 19 months of age the brainstem potentials still showed a prolonged central conduction time of 6.6 msec (normal, 4.3 msec) (Fig. 7). The patient was severely retarded and could not sit without support. She could not crawl, had poor coordination of the upper extremities, and made sounds that were not intelligible. Horizontal nystagmus was noted in addition to the severe hypotonia.

Comment. This infant's hypotonia is probably due to a disorder of the CNS. The detection of prolonged central conduction times in the auditory brainstem potentials is evidence of such a brainstem abnormality. The basis for the abnormality has not yet been defined.

Discussion

Far-field recording of auditory brainstem potentials in newborn infants provides information as to the integrity of function of both peripheral and central portions of the auditory pathway. The test requires technical skills for electrode application and electrophysiological data acquisition, but both are within the area of expertise of the electrodiagnostic technician.

There is evidence that the various components of the brainstem potential represent the sequential activation of neural structures comprising the auditory pathway in its course from the cochlea to the cortex.[9-11] We have demonstrated that measurement of the various components of the auditory brainstem potential can provide the clinician with objective evidence of (1) the status of auditory function in newborn infants in whom the question of altered hearing has been raised and (2) the integrity of brainstem structures in infants with neurological dysfunction.

The results from the present study of auditory brainstem potentials in newborn infants show that reliable components to a 65-dB SL click signal first appear at about the 28th week of gestation. The latencies of the components then decrease as gestation proceeds, with the rate of change being maximal between the 28th and 34th weeks. Auditory maturation is still not complete at birth, as Salamy and McKean[20] have shown that brainstem potentials continue to decrease in latency throughout the first year of life and are not at adult values even at that age.

The failure to detect auditory brainstem potentials prior to the 28th week of gestation is not due to an absence of auditory function at this stage of development, as a slight increase in the intensity of the click signal evokes the brainstem potentials. Furthermore, in both the present study and those of Weitzman and Graziani,[1] the initial negative component of the slow cortical evoked

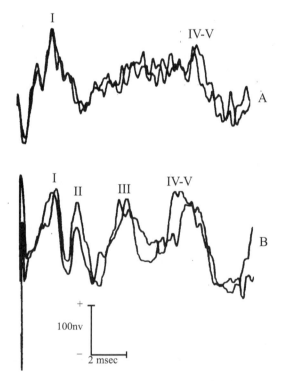

Figure 7. Patient 5 tested at birth (A) and at 19 months of age (B). Central conduction time (wave IV-V minus wave I) is prolonged on both tests. Value at birth is 7.0 msec (upper limit of normal is 5.5 msec) and 6.6 msec at 19 months of age (upper limit of normal is 4.4 msec).

potential could also be recorded in preterm infants as early as the 25th week of gestation. The basis for the threshold difference between the brainstem and cortical potentials is unclear but three possibilities will be considered.

First, the relative difference in amplitude between the cortical potentials (1 to 10 µV) and the far-field brainstem potentials (less than 0.50 µV) may be a technical factor favoring the detection of the cortical potentials. This possibility is not supported by experimental studies in cats,[21] in which auditory brainstem potentials abruptly appear postpartum on the 13th day, whereas other authors have reported that cortical evoked potentials to acoustic signals appear earlier, at about the tenth postpartum day.[22,23]

The discrepancy between the detection of far-field auditory brainstem and cortical potentials may depend on different requirements for neural synchrony of these two events. Auditory brainstem potentials are best elicited by transient acoustic signals with rapid rise times. These signals evoke synchronous discharges in VIII nerve fibers followed by the sequential activation of synchronous events at each higher level of the auditory system. The detection of these sequential sets of synchronous neural events probably accounts for the distinct components of the auditory brainstem potentials. Acoustic signals that have gradual rise times are less effective in evoking neural synchrony and do not evoke brainstem potentials. In contrast, temporal dispersion of neuronal events has considerably less effect on cortical evoked potentials. Acoustic signals with rather slow onset (up to 50 msec) can still evoke cortical potentials, and the long time period employed in recording the cortical potentials (256 msec) favors temporal integration.[24] An experimental study of neural synchrony during development in cats[25] reveals that the immature auditory system is impaired. If there were a corresponding alteration of neural synchrony in the immature infant, auditory brainstem potentials would also be altered.

A change in cochlear responsiveness during maturation could account for the differences in detecting cortical and brainstem potentials. In adults with normal hearing, cortical potentials can be evoked by a wide range of signal frequencies within the acoustic spectrum, whereas auditory brainstem potentials are evoked predominantly by signals containing acoustic energy above 2 kHz.[24] The *click* signals used in this and most evoked potential studies will not select for either type of potential, as the energy is widely distributed across the acoustic spectrum though peaks occur at the resonant frequency of the particular transducer employed. There is experimental evidence that low-frequency sensitivity is selectively enhanced during cochlear maturation. Electrophysiological experiments in animals[26,27] reveal that

cochlear function is initially restricted to the low acoustic frequencies and that the extension of sensitivity to both the higher and lower frequency ranges appears only later with maturation. It may be that the difficulty in detecting brainstem potentials before the 28th week of gestation in the infants in this study due in part to such a delayed maturation of high-frequency sensitivity.

In the present experiment, there is evidence that auditory maturation involves both peripheral and central auditory sides. The peripheral changes are manifest by the decrease in latency of wave I (representing VIII nerve activity) to a constant click intensity as gestation progresses. The central changes are evident by the decrease in conduction time between wave I and other brainstem components. The mechanisms accounting for the change in central conduction time could involve changes in nerve conduction velocity associated with myelination and/or changes in synaptic efficiency at the various nuclei of the auditory pathway. The mechanisms accounting for the peripheral change could include impedance changes in the middle ear, the maturation of high-frequency sensitivity of the cochlea, or changes in transduction between hair cells and the dendrites of VIII nerve.

Auditory brainstem potentials provide an objective means for quantifying auditory development in the human infant with implication of assessing the effects of environmental and congenital factors during the critical period after birth. The technique allows the clinician to obtain a precise measure of the function of one of the sensory pathways independent of factors of arousal or attention. It is possible that similar studies of subcortical visual and somatosensory function will be developed in the near future.

A table containing all clinical data with data of the latencies of the various components at 65, 45, and 25 dB SL is available from the National Auxiliary Publication Service, American Society for Info Science, 1440 Connecticut Avenue, N.W., Washington, D.C. 20036.

References

1. Weitzman, E.D., Graziani, L.J.: Maturation and topography of the auditory evoked response of the prematurely born infant. *Dev Psychol* 1:79, 1968.
2. Barnet, A.B., Goodwin, R.S.: Averaged evoked electroencephalographic responses to clicks in the human newborn. *Electroencephalogr Clin Neurophysiol* 18:441, 1965.
3. Akiyama, Y., Schulte, F.J., Schultz, M.A., Parmelee, A.H. Jr: Acoustically evoked responses in premature and full term newborn infants. *Electroencephalogr Clin Neurophysiol* 26:371, 1969.
4. Rapin, I., Graziani, L.J.: Auditory evoked responses in normal, brain-damaged and deaf infants. *Neurology* 17:881, 1967.

5. Umazaki, H., Morrell, F.: Developmental study of photic evoked responses in premature infants. *Electroencephalogr Clin Neurophysiol* 28:55, 1970.

6. Desmedt, J.A., Brunko, E., Debecker, J.: Maturation of the somatosensory evoked potentials in normal infants and children, with special reference to the early N_1 component. *Electroencephalogr Clin Neurophysiol* 40:43, 1976.

7. Picton, R.W., Hillyard, S.A.: Human auditory evoked potentials: II. Effects of attention. *Electroencephalogr Clin Neurophysiol* 36:179, 1974.

8. Jewett, D.L., Williston, J.S.: Auditory-evoked far fields averaged from the scalp of humans. *Brain* 94: 681, 1971.

9. Jewett, D.L.: Volume-conducted potentials in response to auditory stimuli as detected by averaging in the cat. *Electroencephalogr Clin Neurophysiol* 28:609, 1970.

10. Buchwald, J.S., Huang, C.M.: Far-field acoustic response: Origins in the cat. *Science* 189:382, 1975.

11. Starr, A., Hamilton, A.: Correlation between confirmed sites of neurological lesions of far-field auditory brainstem responses. *Electroencephalogr Clin Neurophysiol* 41:595, 1976.

12. Hecox, K., Galambos, R.: Brain stem auditory evoked responses in human infants and adults. *Arch Otolaryngol* 99:30, 1974.

13. Schulman-Galambos, C., Galambos, R.: Brain stem auditory-evoked responses in premature infants. *J Speech Hear Res* 18:456, 1975.

14. Starr, A., Achor, L.J.: Auditory brainstem responses in neurological disease. *Arch Neurol* 32:761, 1975.

15. Starr, A.: Clinical relevance of auditory brainstem responses, in Desmedt, J.E. (ed): Evoked Responses. Basel, Switzerland, S Karger & Co, 1976.

16. Starr, A.: Auditory brainstem responses in brain death. *Brain* 99:543, 1976.

17. Stockard, J.J., Rossiter, U.S.: Clinical and pathologic correlates of brainstem auditory response abnormalities. *Neurology* 27:316, 1977.

18. Dubowitz, L.N.S., Dubowitz, V., Goldberg, C.: Clinical assessment of gestational age. *J Pediatr* 77:1, 1970.

19. Sohmer, H., Feinmesser, M., Szabo, G.: Sources of electro-cochleographic responses as studied in patients with brain damage. *Electroencephalogr Clin Neurophysiol* 37:663, 1974.

20. Salamy, A., McKean, C.M.: Postnatal development of human brainstem potentials during the first year of life. *Electroencephalogr Clin Neurophysiol* 40:418, 1976.

21. Jewett, D.L., Romano, M.N.: Neonatal development of auditory system potentials averaged from the scalp of rat and cat. *Brain Res* 36:101, 1972.

22. Ellingson, R.J., Wilcott, R.C.: Development of evoked responses in visual and auditory cortices of kittens. *J Neurophysiol* 23:363, 1960.

23. Rose, J.E., Adrain, J., Santibanez, G.: Electrical signs of maturation in the auditory system of the kitten. *Acta Neurol Lat Am* 3:133, 1957.

24. Davis, H.: Brain stem and other responses in electric response audiometry. *Ann Otol* 85:3, 1976.

25. Javel, E., Brugge, J.F., Kitzes, L.M.: Response properties of single neurons in anterior ventral cochlear nucleus (AVCN) of the newborn cat: Frequency selectivity and temporal ordering of discharges. *J Acoust Soc Am*, 90th meeting, San Francisco, November 1975, 58:S64(A), 1975.

26. Aitkin, L.N., Moore, D.R.: Inferior colliculus: II. Development of tuning characteristics and tonotopic organization in central nucleus of the neonatal cat. *J Neurophysiol* 38:1208, 1975.

27. Konishi, M.: Development of auditory neuronal responses in avian embryos. *Proc Natl Acad Sci USA* 70:1795, 1970.

Auditory Brainstem Responses from Children Three Months to Three Years of Age: Normal Patterns of Response II

Michael P. Gorga, Jan R. Kaminski, Kathryn L. Beauchaine, Walt Jesteadt, and Stephen T. Neely

The Boys Town National Institute for Communication Disorders in Children

Auditory brainstem responses (ABR) were measured in 535 children from 3 months to 3 years of age. The latencies reported in this paper should be unaffected by peripheral hearing loss because each child had bilateral wave V responses at 20 dB HL_n. Wave V latencies decreased as age increased, at least to 18 months of age, while little or no change was noted in wave I latencies over the same age range. Thus, interpeak latency differences followed the same developmental time course as wave V. The shapes of wave V latency-level functions were comparable across age groups. These results suggest that changes in wave V latency with age are due to central (neural) factors and that age-appropriate norms should be used in evaluations of ABR latencies in children. Interaural differences in absolute wave V latencies and interpeak latency differences were similar to those observed in infants and adults, indicating that response symmetry is independent of age. Statistical analyses suggested that the distributions of absolute and relative latency measurements are normal, making it possible to describe norms in terms of means and standard deviations. A simple model is described that accounts accurately for changes in mean wave V latencies as function of age from preterm through the first three years of life.

This paper represents a continuation of our work describing developmental changes in auditory brainstem responses (ABR). Previous papers described ABRs from graduates of an intensive care nursery (ICN), ranging in age from 33 to 44 weeks conceptional age (Gorga, Kaminski, & Beauchaine, 1988; Gorga, Reiland, Beauchaine, Worthington, & Jesteadt, 1987). We viewed these data as normative ICN references because of the large sample size, the threshold criteria for inclusion in the database, the status of the babies at the time of testing, the range of stimulus conditions examined, and the sound-isolated conditions under which these measurements were made. The present paper extends the approach we used with infants to develop a similar normative ABR reference for children from 3 months to 3 years of age.

A number of studies, discussed below, have described developmental changes in ABRs over the first three years of life. In general, these studies report little or no change in wave I latency whereas the latencies of all response components after wave I decrease with age. The largest changes occur for wave V latency and for the interwave latency difference between waves I and V. It may be difficult, however, to use these data to develop normative references for children.

Some of the studies reporting developmental changes through early childhood were based on data from relatively small groups of subjects (Cox, Hack, & Metz, 1981; Hecox & Galambos, 1974; Mokotoff, Shulman-Galambos, & Galambos, 1977; Rotteveel et al., 1986). In some cases, the sample size was unspecified (e.g., Cox, 1985). In one study, it appears that the data from each ear of the same subject were treated as independent samples (Beiser, Himelfarb, Gold, & Shanon, 1985), which may not be valid, given the high correlation between ears (Gorga et al., 1987; Salamy, 1984).

In some cases, changes in ABR latencies were studied for only the first few months of life although developmental changes in ABR latencies appear to continue through at least the first year of life. For example, Zimmerman, Morgan and Dubno (1987) followed 22 full-term infants from birth to 26 weeks of age. Similarly, Hyde, Matsumoto, and Alberti (1987) studied ABRs only up to 4 months of age.

Despland (1985) described changes in ABRs for subjects whose ages ranged from preterm (30 weeks conceptional age) through 10 years. Unfortunately, criteria for subject inclusion were not explicitly stated, other than to report that "all infants were normal at birth." Also absent was any description of the variance in the data, which is necessary if they are to be used to develop normative references.

Fria and Doyle (1984) reported ABR latencies from 466 subjects ranging in age from 32 weeks postconcep-

Reprinted by permission of authors and American Speech-Language-Hearing Association. Copyright 1989. *Journal of Speech and Hearing Research*, 32, pp. 218-288.

tion to adulthood and having wave V responses at 20 dB HL_n. However, only 64 subjects ranged in age from 3 months to 3 years, these subjects were divided among five widely spaced age intervals, and the number of subjects per age group ranged from 3 (36 months of age) to 24 (6 months of age). Estimates of the variance in the data also were not provided.

Finally, a series of reports exist that describe developmental changes in ABR latencies through adulthood based on large sample sizes (Salamy, 1984; Salamy & McKean, 1976; Salamy, McKean, Pettett & Mendelson, 1978). In these studies, however, the ABR evaluation apparently did not include an examination of peripheral auditory sensitivity at the time of testing, the reported latencies were in response to binaural stimuli, and only one high-level stimulus was studied.

In the present paper, we describe ABR results from a large group of children ranging in age from 3 months to 3 years. Data are included only from those children for whom the ABR indicated that hearing sensitivity was within normal limits bilaterally. In addition to describing the distributions of absolute wave V latencies for a wide range of stimulus levels, interwave latency differences and interaural symmetry in ABR latencies also are evaluated. We know of no other paper describing interaural symmetry in ABR latencies for this age range.

Methods

The stimuli and recording procedures used here were virtually identical to those used in our previous work (Gorga et al., 1987). They are briefly reviewed below.

Stimuli

In all cases, responses were elicited by 100-μs rarefaction clicks, presented at a rate of 13/ second. These stimuli were transduced by a Beyer DT48 circumaural earphone. The time waveform and amplitude spectrum of these stimuli have been described elsewhere (Gorga, Abbas, & Worthington, 1985). Stimulus level ranged from 20 dB HL_n to 80 dB HL_n. Zero dB HL_n, which was determined by measuring the behavioral threshold for the click in a group of normal hearing adult subjects, was equivalent to a peak sound pressure of 30 dB (re: 20 μPa).

Recording Technique

Brain electrical activity (EEG) was measured between chlorided silver-silver disc electrodes placed at the vertex and at the ipsilateral mastoid process. An electrode placed at the forehead served as the ground electrode. Interelectrode impedances did not exceed 3000 ohms. The ongoing EEG activity was amplified (10^5), filtered (100-3000 Hz, 6 dB/octave), and digitized (either 10 μs or 15 μs dwell time, for a total of either 10.24 ms or 15.36 ms, respectively) prior to input to an averager (Nicolet, 1170). Responses to 1,024 stimulus presentations were averaged and each averaged response was replicated once. Averaged responses were transferred from the Nicolet to a laboratory computer for storage and analysis.

Subjects

The principal set of ABR data reported here was obtained from 535 children who ranged in age from 3 months to 3 years. Each child had wave V responses at 20 dB HL_n bilaterally. Thus, the latencies reported here should not be affected by peripheral hearing loss because any child with a wave V response at 20 dB HL_n in all likelihood would have normal peripheral auditory sensitivity, at least for the mid-to-high frequencies (Gorga, Worthington, Reiland, Beauchaine, & Goldgar, 1985; Jerger & Mauldin, 1978). No other criteria were used in the selection of subjects. For example, no effort was made to exclude children who may have had middle ear dysfunction. Additionally, the neurological status of these children typically was unknown. As a consequence, we did not include neurological status in the subject-selection criteria. However, many children with severe neurological involvement have completely normal ABRs as long as the auditory brainstem pathways are not involved (e.g., Weber, 1985). Furthermore, we have assumed that subjects are not likely to have wave V responses to 20 dB HL_n bilaterally if there is significant neurological involvement at the level of the auditory brainstem pathways. Few studies, however, include measurements for low-level stimuli in otoneurologic evaluations. Stein and Kraus (1985) provide a brief review of cases when neurological status might alter the agreement between ABR and behavioral thresholds.

For comparison purposes, we will review previously reported data from 585 graduates of an ICN. These infants ranged in age from 33 weeks to 44 weeks conceptual age and had bilateral wave V responses down to at least 30 dB HL_n (Gorga et al., 1987). They were tested under identical conditions to those used for the present group of older children, with the exception that infants were evaluated during periods of natural sleep (i.e., without sedation).

Finally, data are presented from 20 adult subjects who had pure-tone audiometric thresholds of 10 dB HL or less for the octave frequencies from 250 to 8000 Hz. These subjects had no history of middle ear or neurological dysfunction and were tested during periods of natural sleep.

Procedures

All ABR tests were performed in a double-walled sound-isolated chamber (IAC). Measurements were taken only when the child was either in a state of natural sleep or was sedated, typically with chloral hydrate (40-60 mg/kg). For each ear, the initial stimulus typically was a click at 80 dB HL_n, which always resulted in a clear response. Stimulus level was then decreased in 20-dB steps down to a level of 20 dB HL_n. Lower levels were not assessed. Even though every child had wave V responses at 20 dB HL_n for each ear, occasionally we were unable to obtain data at all four test levels or to start the evaluation with the high level stimulus because of limitations imposed by subject state. This problem was unrelated to subject age.

Data Analysis

Previous work indicated that the data from two ears of the same subject were highly correlated (Gorga et al., 1987). As a result, only the data from the left ear of each subject will be used in descriptions of both absolute latencies and interpeak latency differences. Data were divided further according to the chronological age of the child, which is defined as the age (in months) from birth. No effort was made to adjust ages to account for prematurity at birth. Eleven groups were formed, ranging from 3-6 months to 33-36 months of age (with interval midpoints ranging from 4.5 and 34.5 months). Within each age group, means and standard deviations were calculated for absolute and relative latencies and for interaural latency differences. These analyses resulted in 110 pairs of means and standard deviations.

Cumulative distributions were formed for each response component latency, interpeak latency difference, and interaural latency difference from each of the eleven age groups. To test the assumption that the underlying distributions were normal, each cumulative distribution was compared to a normal ogive that was computed from the mean and standard deviation of the latencies in that distribution, using the Kolmogorov-Smirnov D-statistic (Guilford, 1965). This statistical procedure can identify distributions that differ significantly from normal, but it cannot describe the extent to which the calculated ogive accounts for the actual data. To obtain this information, the correlation was computed between the actual distribution of latencies and corresponding points on the normal ogive. Correlations are reported in terms of r^2, the proportion of the variance in the cumulative distribution that is accounted for by the normal ogive.

Results and Discussion

Wave I Latency

Table 1 reports mean wave I latencies and standard deviations as a function of age. These data were obtained in response to a click at 80 dB HL_n. A significant Kolmogorov-Smirnov D-statistic ($p < .05$) was observed only for the distribution of scores in the 9 to 12-month age group. In all other cases, the D-statistic was not significant, suggesting that these distributions did not differ from normal. This outcome is not unexpected, given the total number of distributions (110) to which the Kolmogorov-Smirnov test was applied and the significance level (.05) at which this test was performed. Thus, we have used means and standard deviations to describe the distributions in all cases. Furthermore, the r^2 values that were obtained when the actual data were compared to the calculated ogives suggest that the means and standard deviations provide accurate descriptions of each distribution.

There was little or no change in wave I latency over this age range and no significant differences across age groups in a one-way analysis of variance. The standard deviations also varied little with age. If wave I latency can be viewed as a measure of peripheral response maturity, then it appears that the peripheral response to click stimuli is mature early in life. At the least, its latency does not change from three months to three years of life.

Wave V Latency

Table 2 reports mean wave V latencies and standard deviations for each age group at each of four click levels. There was a tendency for the standard deviations to

Table 1. Means (M) and standard deviations (SD) of wave I latency at 80 dB HL_n for each of eleven chronological age categories. The number of cases for each age group also is reported along with the proportion of variance accounted for by a normal ogive approximation to the observed cumulative distributions.

Age group (months)	Number	M (ms)	SD	r^2
3-6	78	1.594	0.171	0.93
6-9	65	1.592	0.161	0.94
9-12*	91	1.592	0.177	0.91
12 15	48	1.593	0.169	0.89
15-18	72	1.578	0.145	0.96
18-21	27	1.551	0.116	0.99
21-24	28	1.572	0.169	0.86
24-27	17	1.532	0.139	0.93
27-30	17	1.588	0.194	0.94
30-33	58	1.558	0.157	0.98
33-36	25	1.557	0.152	0.94

*Kolmogorov-Smirnov D-statistic significant at the 0.05 level.

decrease as the level increased. This results in part from the fact that response waveforms are better defined for high level stimuli, resulting in a more precise identification of the wave V peak. Once again, the standard deviations are independent of age. Finally, the high values of r^2 indicate that the means and standard deviations are sufficient to describe each distribution of scores.

Latencies are approximately 0.6 ms shorter for the children 33 to 36 months of age compared to children in the 3 to 6 month age category. Latencies are also 0.6 ms shorter for children 3 to 6 months of age when compared to the data from infants 39 to 40 weeks conceptional age (CA) (Gorga et al., 1987), which would be the age equivalent of a full-term baby. Our normative adult latencies for the same stimuli, on the other hand, are approximately 0.1 ms shorter than those found in children 33 to 36 months of age.

Some insight into the cause of the small difference between wave V latencies for adults and for children three years of age may be gained from Figure 1, in which mean latencies at 80 dB HL_n are plotted as a function of age. Wave V latencies are represented by circles, whereas wave I latencies are represented by triangles. In addition to plotting data from the children in the present study, we also included data from adults and from infants who were 39 to 40 weeks CA at the time of the ABR test. Note that the differences between latencies for adults and for children 33 to 36 months of age are the same for wave I as they are for wave V, suggesting that this 0.1 ms effect is due to factors peripheral to the generation of wave I. It is possible that some of the children had subclinical middle-ear dysfunction that was undetected by air-conduction ABRs, even with a threshold criteria of 20 dB HL_n. Standard deviations in both wave I and wave V latencies were larger for children, which could occur if some of the children had middle ear dysfunction at the time of the ABR test. Ear canal collapse, which can result in high frequency conductive hearing loss, also is more likely to occur in young children. Although unlikely, an alternative explanation might be that there are small developmental changes that occur in the peripheral auditory system after 3 years of age.

The mean wave V latencies from Table 2 are plotted in Figure 2 as a function of level, with age as the parameter. For comparison purposes, we have included data from adult subjects and from graduates of our ICN. There is a very orderly progression in wave V latency as either level or age increases. The largest changes occur early in life, with progressively smaller changes occurring in the second and third years. The fact that these systematic changes continue for approximately the first two years of life indicates that age-dependent norms should be used in evaluations of wave V latencies in children.

Table 2. Means (M) and standard deviations (SD) of wave V latencies at each of four levels in each of 11 age groups. The number of children in each group is also reported along with the proportion of variance accounted for by a normal ogive approximation to the observed cumulative distributions.

Level (dB HL_n)	Age group (months)	Number	M (ms)	SD	r^2
20	3-6	79	8.717	0.526	0.99
	6-9	68	8.591	0.612	0.99
	9-12	91	8.310	0.537	0.98
	12-15	48	8.280	0.601	0.98
	15-18	74	8.329	0.609	0.96
	18-21	28	8.219	0.624	0.88
	21-24	28	8.052	0.582	0.91
	24-27	18	8.301	0.457	0.95
	27-30	18	7.981	0.417	0.85
	30-33	58	8.115	0.528	0.99
	33-36	25	8.103	0.684	0.93
40	3-6	78	7.426	0.358	0.99
	6-9	68	7.276	0.375	0.99
	9-12	88	7.049	0.366	0.97
	12-15	48	7.009	0.454	0.98
	15-18	72	6.999	0.381	0.98
	18-21	28	6.949	0.356	0.93
	21-24	28	6.794	0.334	0.91
	24-27	18	6.888	0.291	0.95
	27-30	18	6.753	0.333	0.96
	30-33	53	6.789	0.323	0.99
	33-36	24	6.815	0.378	0.93
60	3-6	62	6.734	0.331	0.99
	6-9	56	6.563	0.286	0.99
	9-12	87	6.310	0.290	0.96
	12-15	44	6.295	0.333	0.96
	15-18	62	6.242	0.245	0.99
	18-21	23	6.190	0.180	0.97
	21-24	23	6.138	0.287	0.93
	24-27	15	6.088	0.224	0.90
	27-30	13	6.082	0.283	0.95
	30-33	45	6.073	0.310	0.98
	33-36	21	6.062	0.307	0.95
80	3-6	79	6.253	0.321	0.98
	6-9	67	6.101	0.265	0.99
	9-12	91	5.899	0.268	0.99
	12-15	48	5.913	0.273	0.98
	15-18	73	5.845	0.267	0.99
	18-21	28	5.736	0.194	0.99
	21-24	28	5.712	0.262	0.94
	24-27	18	5.711	0.187	0.97
	27-30	17	5.602	0.223	0.97
	30-33	58	5.675	0.267	0.99
	33-36	25	5.678	0.273	0.94

A two-way analysis of variance of the data in Table 2 is summarized in Table 3. In an effort to simplify the analysis, data were included only from those children on whom it was possible to measure responses at all four test

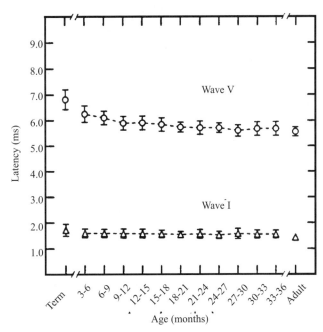

Figure 1. Mean wave I (open triangles) and wave V (open circles) latencies as a function of age in months. Error bars represent ± 1 standard deviation. Data from graduates of an ICN who were 39 to 40 weeks conceptional age at the time of the ABR tests are represented as "term." These data were taken from a previous paper, describing ABR latencies in graduates of an ICN (Gorga et al., 1987). Also shown are data from 20 adult subjects.

levels. Highly significant effects of both age and level were observed, but the interaction between age and level was insignificant.

The mean wave V latencies at 60 and 80 dB HL_n (see Table 2) are plotted in separate panels in Figure 3 in an effort to compare the present results to data from other studies. These two levels were selected for comparison because there are few previous data available at levels below 60 dB HL_n. In fact, the conditions of measurement were not identical even for those studies reporting results at similar levels to the ones used here. These differences in measurement notwithstanding, there is general agreement in wave V latencies across studies. Latencies in the present study tend to be either comparable to (80 dB HL_n) or slightly longer than (60 dB HL_n) previously reported values. In some of the previous studies, binaural stimuli were used (Salamy, 1984; Salamy & McKean, 1976; Salamy et al., 1978) which could account for their observation of slightly shorter wave V latencies.

Interpeak Latency Differences

Table 4 reports mean interpeak latency differences and standard deviations for each of the 11 age categories in this study. These data were obtained in response to clicks at 80 dB HL_n. As expected from the data in Tables 1 and 2, and in Figure 1, there was a systematic decrease in interpeak latency differences with increasing age. Adult values were achieved at approximately 18 to 24 months

of age for both the I-III interval and the III-V interval. Therefore, the I-V interval follows the same developmental time course. The standard deviations for all interpeak latency differences appear to be independent of age.

Figure 4 plots the mean I-V interpeak latency difference from Table 4 as a function of age. Error bars represent ± 1 standard deviation. For purposes of illustration, we have again included data from adults and from infants who were 39 to 40 weeks postconception at the time of the ABR test. There was approximately a 0.5-ms decrease in this interval from the full-term equivalent age of 39 to 40 weeks CA to 3 to 6 months of age and an additional decrease of about 0.5 ms from 3 to 6 months of age until the adult value of 4.12 ms is reached at about 2 years of age. This suggests that the neural pathways between the generator sites of waves I and wave V are mature at 2 years. This conclusion is consistent with our earlier observation that small differences between adult wave V latencies and those observed in children 33 to 36 months of age are due to factors peripheral to the generator site of wave I.

Interaural Symmetry

Interaural symmetries in wave V latencies and in the I-V interpeak latency differences were evaluated by subtracting the value for the left ear from the same measurement in the right ear. Table 5 reports mean interaural differences and standard deviations for wave V. Compara-

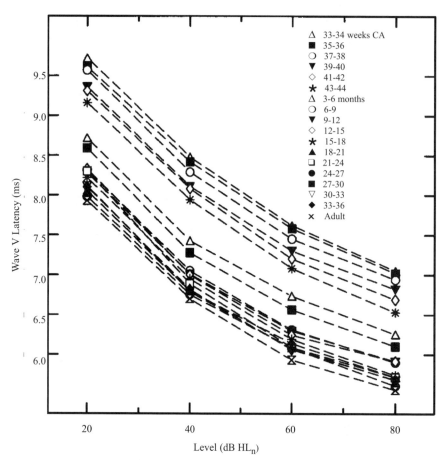

Figure 2. Mean wave V latencies as a function of level. The parameter in this figure is age at the time of the ABR test. Data for infants 33 to 34 through 43 to 44 weeks conceptional age (CA) were taken from Gorga et al. (1987). Also shown are data from 20 adult subjects.

ble data for the I-V interval are given in Table 6. The differences between ears in any age group were quite small, ranging from –0.031 ms to 0.078 ms, and these differences did not depend on age in any systematic way. The overall mean difference in wave V latencies was 0.006 ms ($SD = 0.167$), while the overall interaural difference in the I-V interval was 0.007 ms ($SD = 0.161$). This means that 95% of the interaural differences are less than about 0.35 ms. This value is virtually identical to the value reported for graduates of our ICN (Gorga et al., 1987) and is simi-

lar to the reported estimates for adults (Clemis & McGee, 1979; Feblot & Uziel, 1982). These data also offer further support for the premise that the data from the two ears of an individual are highly correlated. Although absolute latencies decrease as age increases, the correlation between ears appears to be independent of age.

Developmental Changes from Birth to 3 Years

The data reported here were obtained under conditions identical to those used to obtain similar data from graduates of our ICN (Gorga et al., 1987). These two sets of data can now be combined, forming a total sample of 1,120 infants and children on whom to base a description of developmental changes occurring from several weeks preterm through the first three years of life. Figure 5 plots mean wave V latencies as a function of conceptional age with stimulus level as the parameter. The vertical dashed line is drawn at the full-term CA of 40 weeks. The most rapid changes occur during the perinatal period, but slower changes continue through early childhood.

Table 3. Summary of two-way analysis of variance of wave V latencies as a function of age category and level. Data are included only from those children on whom latencies were measured for all four test levels. This restriction reduced the sample to 447 children.

Source	df	Mean square	F	Probability
Age	10	8.18	18.05	<0.001
Error	436	0.45		
Level	3	364.52	5954.71	<0.001
Level × Age	30	0.04	0.73	0.861
Error	1308	0.06		

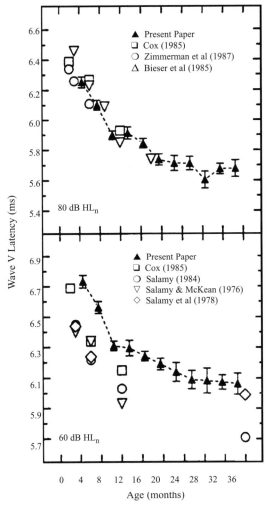

Figure 3. Filled triangles represent the present mean wave V latencies (± 1 *standard error of the mean*) as a function of age for clicks at 80 dB HL$_n$ (top panel) and at 60 dB HL$_n$ (bottom panel). Comparable data from other studies are represented according to the symbol legend within each panel.

Table 4. Means (M) and standard deviations (SD) of interpeak latency differences for each of 11 age groups. The number of subjects in each group also is given along with the proportion of variance accounted for by a normal ogive approximation to the observed cumulative distributions.

Interpeak latency difference	Age group (months)	Number	M (ms)	SD	r²
I-III	3-6	78	2.523	0.215	0.99
	6-9	65	2.416	0.225	0.99
	9-12	89	2.313	0.235	0.95
	12-15	47	2.313	0.149	0.99
	15-18	70	2.258	0.157	0.99
	18-21	27	2.259	0.238	0.96
	21-24	27	2.168	0.206	0.97
	24-27	17	2.278	0.172	0.87
	27-30	17	2.099	0.137	0.94
	30-33	58	2.210	0.157	0.99
	33-36	24	2.171	0.197	0.95
III-V	3-6	79	2.128	0.215	0.99
	6-9	67	2.082	0.215	0.99
	9-12	89	1.992	0.199	0.99
	12-15	47	2.006	0.219	0.98
	15-18	71	1.999	0.163	0.99
	18-21	28	1.992	0.189	0.98
	21-24	27	1.959	0.195	0.98
	24-27	18	1.912	0.182	0.91
	27-30	17	1.915	0.155	0.88
	30-33	58	1.904	0.180	0.99
	33-36	24	1.937	0.174	0.98
I-V	3-6	78	4.653	0.287	0.98
	6-9	65	4.502	0.270	0.99
	9-12	89	4.306	0.285	0.99
	12-15	48	4.320	0.240	0.99
	15-18	71	4.252	0.224	0.99
	18-21	27	4.182	0.227	0.98
	21-24	28	4.140	0.248	0.95
	24-27	17	4.197	0.171	0.94
	27-30	17	4.015	0.215	0.96
	30-33	58	4.117	0.226	0.97
	33-36	25	4.121	0.251	0.93

The data in Figure 5 were fitted with an exponential function of the form

$$\text{wave V latency} = 4.89 + 4.46e^{-0.0318a} + 5.31e^{-0.0251i}$$

where:

a = conceptional age in weeks, and
i = level in dB HL$_n$

Solutions of this equation are plotted as solid lines in Figure 5. This model assumes that age and level are independent variables, in agreement with the results of the two-way analysis of variance summarized in Table 3. Overall, this model accounts for 99.6% of the variance in mean wave V latencies. If the term related to age is removed, the equation predicts adult wave V latencies.

Fria and Doyle (1984) concluded that two exponential models were needed to describe chances in wave V latencies with age, in contrast the present findings that suggest that a single exponential model provides an accurate description to our data. Eggermont and Salamy (1988) have fitted human ABR latencies with both a single exponential and with the sum of two exponential functions. They report that mean latencies from children who were born after full term gestation are better described with a single exponential model, although data from children born prematurely are better fitted with the sum of two exponential functions. However, we were unable to separate children according to their gestational age at birth, at least for children over 3 months of age. As a consequence, we could not determine whether the sum of two

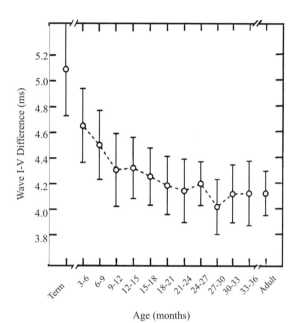

Figure 4. Mean wave I—wave V intervals (±1 SD) as a function of age. Data also are represented for adults and for infants tested at the equivalent term age of 39 to 40 weeks CA ("term").

exponentials would have resulted in a better fit for a subgroup of subjects. As might be expected, we were unable to account for additional variance beyond 99.6% by fitting the present mean data with two exponential functions.

Recently, we proposed a scheme for separating the peripheral and central contributions to wave V latencies (Neely, Norton, Gorga, & Jesteadt, 1988). The peripheral or mechanical (cochlear) component was assumed to depend upon both frequency and level although the central or neural component was assumed to be independent of frequency and level. If this model is correct, it can be used to evaluate the relative contributions of peripheral

and central development to changes in wave V latencies in early childhood. We would conclude that peripheral or cochlear factors are important, for example, if the changes in latency with age were dependent on level. This is clearly not the case. Although the asymptotic values in Figure 5 depend on level, the shapes of these functions are identical. Thus, these data support the premise that maturational changes in human wave V latencies are due to neural or central factors (such as myelinization) and are not dependent on mechanical (peripheral) factors. Of course, this conclusion is only valid for humans who are at least 33 weeks CA at the time of test. If measurements were possible on infants much younger than 33 weeks CA, then indications of peripheral immaturity also might be evident.

In contrast to the present conclusions, Folsom and Wynne (1987) reported data that suggest that the cochleae of children are not adultlike at 3 months of age. They noted that, for frequencies of 4000 and 8000 Hz, wave V tuning curves in infants were broader than those observed in adults. Assuming that frequency selectivity is determined at the periphery, their data suggest that the cochleae of infants are immature. The discrepancies between our data and theirs may be due to the spectral differences between stimuli. It is possible that responses to a broad spectrum stimulus, such as a click, will not demonstrate the same age dependence as the ABR to frequency specific stimuli.

Summary

There is a very orderly decrease in wave V latency and in interpeak latency differences as age increases from 3 months to at least 18 or 24 months of age. This finding

Table 5. Mean differences (D) between left and right ears in wave V latencies at 80 dB HL_n. Standard deviations (SD) and the number of children in each age group also are listed, along with the proportion of variance accounted for by a normal ogive approximation to the observed cumulative distributions.

Age group (months)	Number	D (ms)	SD	r^2
3-6	79	−0.013	0.196	0.99
6-9	67	0.002	0.143	0.97
9-12	91	0.011	0.157	0.99
12-15	48	0.038	0.194	0.96
15-18	73	0.036	0.172	0.98
18-21	28	−0.026	0.129	0.97
21-24	27	−0.026	0.197	0.94
24 27	18	0.074	0.102	0.98
27-30	17	−0.011	0.102	0.89
30-33	58	−0.009	0.164	0.98
33-36	25	−0.020	0.142	0.97

Table 6. Mean differences (D) between left and right ears in wave I-wave V interval at 80 dB HL_n. Also shown are the number of children and the standard deviations (SD) in each age group, along with the proportion of variance accounted for by a normal ogive approximation to the observed cumulative distributions.

Age group (months)	Number	D (ms)	SD	r^2
3-6	75	−0.005	0.200	0.98
6-9	65	0.009	0.138	0.98
9-12	89	0.001	0.174	0.99
12-15	47	0.030	0.186	0.96
15-18	70	0.019	0.151	0.99
18-21	27	0.012	0.155	0.93
21-24	27	0.003	0.112	0.95
24-27	17	0.078	0.173	0.93
27-30	17	−0.031	0.070	0.93
30-33	58	0.001	0.146	0.98
33-36	25	−0.030	0.114	0.99

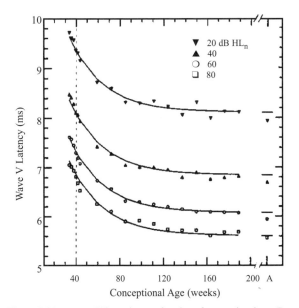

Figure 5. Mean wave V latencies as a function of conceptional age. Data from graduates of an ICN (Gorga et al., 1987) are represented as the first six points on each function. Data also are shown for adults. The ages of the children in the present study were converted to weeks and 40 was added to these numbers in order to convert chronological age to conceptional age. The parameter is click level. The vertical dashed line is drawn at the equivalent full-term age of 40 weeks CA. The solid lines drawn through the data represent the solution of the exponential model described in the text.

suggests that age appropriate norms are needed if ABR latencies are to be used in the assessment of children. The overall pattern of development from early infancy to 3 years of age is well described by a decaying exponential equation. The fact that age-dependent changes in wave V latencies are independent of stimulus level suggests that central (neural) factors are responsible for these developmental changes in ABRs. Interaural differences in either absolute wave V latency or in the I-V interval do not appear to depend on age and are within the range of values observed for adults on similar measures.

Acknowledgments

This work was supported in part by NIH. We would like to thank Theresa Langer, Margaret Cox, and Jo Peters for their help in data analyses and in figure preparation. Eric Javel and Donna Neff provided helpful suggestions as part of our internal review process. We also thank Aaron Thorton and two anonymous reviewers for helpful suggestions on an earlier version of this paper.

References

Beiser, M., Himelfarb, M.Z., Gold, S., & Shanon, E. (1985). Maturation of auditory brainstem potentials in neonates and infants. *International Journal of Pediatric Otorhinolaryngolgy,* 9, 69-76.

Clemis, J.D., & McGee, T. (1979). Brainstem electric response audiometry in the differential diagnosis of acoustic tumors. *Laryngoscope,* 89, 31-42.

Cox, L.C. (1985). Infant Assessment: Developmental and age-related considerations. In J.T. Jacobson (Ed.), *The auditory brainstem response* (pp. 297-316). San Diego, CA: College-Hill Press.

Cox, C., Hack, M., & Metz, D. (1981). Brainstem evoked response audiometry: Normative data from the preterm infant. *Audiology,* 20, 53-64.

Despland, P.A. (1985). Maturational changes in the auditory system as reflected in human brainstem evoked responses. *Developmental Neuroscience,* 7, 73-80.

Eggermont, J.J., & Salamy, A. (1988). Maturational time course for the ABR in preterm and full term infants. *Hearing Research,* 33, 35-47.

Feblot, P., & Uziel, A. (1982). Detection of acoustic neuromas with brainstem auditory evoked potentials: Comparison between cochlear and retrocochlear abnormalities. In J. Courjon, F. Mauguiere, & M. Revol (Eds.), *Advances in neurology: Clinical applications of evoked potentials in neurology* (pp. 169-176). New York: Raven Press.

Folsom, R.C., & Wynne, M.K. (1987). Auditory brain stem responses from human adults and infants: Wave V tuning curves, *Journal of the Acoustical Society of America,* 81, 412-417.

Fria, T.J., & Doyle, W.J. (1984). Maturation of the auditory brain stem response (ABR): Additional perspectives. *Ear and Hearing,* 5, 361-365.

Gorga, M.P., Abbas, P.J., & Worthington, D.W. (1985). Stimulus calibration in ABR measurements. In J.T. Jacobson (Ed.), *The auditory brainstem response* (pp. 49-62). San Diego, CA: College-Hill Press.

Gorga, M.P., Kaminski, J.R., & Beauchaine, K.A. (1988). Auditory brainstem responses from graduates of an intensive care nursery using an insert earphone, *Ear and Hearing,* 9, 144-147.

Gorga, M.P., Reiland, J.K, Beauchaine, K.A., Worthington, D.W., & Jesteadt, W. (1987). Auditory brainstem responses from graduates of an intensive care nursery: Normal patterns of response. *Journal of Speech and Hearing Research,* 30, 311-318.

Gorga, M.P., Worthington, D.W., Reiland, J.K., Beauchaine, K.A., & Goldgar, D.E. (1985). Some comparisons between auditory brainstem response thresholds, latencies, and the pure-tone audiogram. *Ear and Hearing,* 6, 105-112.

Guilford, J.P. (1965). *Fundamental statistics in psychology and education* (4th ed.). New York: McGraw Hill.

Hecox, K. & Galambos, R. (1974). Brainstem auditory evoked response in human infants and adults. *Archives of Otololaryngology,* 99, 30-33.

Hyde, M.L., Matsumoto, N., & Alberti, P.W. (1987). The normative basis for click and frequency specific BERA in high-risk infants. *Acta Oto-laryngologica (Stock.)*, 103, 602-611.

Jerger, J., & Mauldin, L. (1978). Prediction of sensorineural level from the brainstem evoked response. *Archives of Otololaryngology*, 104, 456-461.

Mokotoff, B., Schulman-Galambos, C., & Galambos, R. (1977). Brain stem auditory evoked responses in children. *Archives of Otolaryngology*, 103, 38-43.

Neely, S.T., Norton, S.J., Gorga, M.P., & Jesteadt, W. (1988). Latency of auditory brainstem responses and otoacoustic emissions using tone-burst stimuli. *Journal of the Acoustical Society of America*, 83, 652-656.

Rotteveel, J.J., Colon, E.J., Notermans, S.L.H., Stoel-Inga, G.B.A., Visco, Y., & Graaf, R. (1986). The central auditory conduction at term date and three months after birth. *Scandinavian Audiology*, 15, 11-19.

Salamy, A. (1984). Maturation of the auditory brainstem response from birth through early childhood. *Journal of Clinical Neurophysiology*, 1, 293-329.

Salamy, A., & McKean, C.M. (1976). Postnatal development of human brainstem potentials during the first year of life. *Electroencepalography and Clinical Neurophysiology*, 40, 418-426.

Salamy, A., McKean, C.M., Pettett, G., & Mendelson, T. (1978). Auditory brainstem recovery processes from birth to adulthood. *Psychophysiology*, 15, 214-220.

Stein, L., & Kraus, N. (1985). Auditory brainstem response measures with multiply handicapped children and adults. In J.T. Jacobson (Ed.), *The auditory brainstem response* (pp. 337-348). San Diego, CA: College-Hill Press.

Weber, B.A. (1985). Interpretation: Problems and pitfalls. In J.T. Jacobson (Ed.), *The auditory brainstem response* (pp. 99-112). San Diego, CA: College-Hill Press.

Zimmerman, M.C., Morgan, D.E., & Dubno, J.R. (1987). Auditory brain stem evoked response characteristics in developing infants. *Annals of Otology, Rhinology, and Laryngology*, 96, 291-299.

Received February 16, 1988
Accepted September 9, 1988

Requests for reprints should be sent to Michael Gorga, Boys Town National Institute for Communication Disorders in Children, 555 North 30th Street, Omaha, NE 68131.

Audiometric Accuracy of the Click ABR in Infants at Risk for Hearing Loss

Martyn L. Hyde, Krista Riko, and Kathy Malizia
*Otologic Function Unit, Mount Sinai and Toronto General Hospitals, University of Toronto,
Toronto, Ontario, Canada*

Abstract

The auditory brainstem response (ABR) to clicks is widely used for early detection of hearing loss in the child at risk for hearing dysfunction, but there is a lack of direct, large-sample estimates of test accuracy.

In this report, results and preliminary analyses are presented that relate click ABR thresholds obtained at 3 to 12 months corrected age to detailed follow-up behavioral puretone audiometry at 3 to 8 years of age, for 1,367 ears in 713 children at risk for hearing loss.

The data are analyzed in terms of conventional 2˜2 decision matrices and associated parameters, using dichotomous (binary) measures of hearing loss and ABR test outcome. The accuracy of the ABR appears to depend strongly on the precise criteria that are chosen to define both hearing loss and ABR outcome.

ABR accuracy is excellent for detecting average sensorineural hearing loss at 2 and 4 kHz in excess of 30 dB, and the overall results for a wide range of hearing loss and ABR abnormality criteria can be conveniently summarized in terms of relative operating characteristics (ROCs).

Key Words: Auditory brainstem response (ABR), accuracy, validity, infant hearing screening, relative operating characteristic

It is widely believed that early detection and management of hearing loss in the infant will improve the development of communicative skills. There is a lack of formal, direct scientific evidence that this is indeed so, but such evidence will be difficult to obtain. The hypothesis has much face validity, and it seems evident that accurate information about hearing must at least facilitate the early management of the multiply-handicapped child.

In 1982, the U.S. Joint Committee on Infant Hearing recommended that infants at risk for hearing loss should be screened by 3 months of age and that intervention should be started by 6 months of age, wherever possible. The Joint Committee did not specify any particular method of testing hearing, but a consensus is now emerging that behavioral observation audiometry and, more generally, any methods based on scoring of reflex responses to loud sounds are not sufficiently accurate, especially if it is desired to detect mild or moderate hearing losses. In 1987, the U.S. Committee on Hearing, Bioacoustics and Biomechanics (CHABA) concluded that the auditory

brainstem response (ABR) was the most objective available tool. In 1989, the ASHA Committee on Infant Hearing recommended audiometric screening using the ABR.

During the last decade, there have been many primary reports concerning the use of the ABR in infant hearing testing (Alberti et al, 1985; Swigonski et al, 1987), and there has been a proliferation of clinical programs for early detection of hearing loss, based on ABR techniques. Most commonly, a click stimulus is used to elicit the ABR. Thus, the click ABR has emerged as a commonly used tool for screening or for threshold estimation in infants.

Despite the popularity of the ABR, there is a need for more data concerning the audiometric accuracy of this tool in the high-risk infant population. While there have been several reports that address follow-up audiometry in ABR screening failures, a comprehensive review by Murray et al (1985) emphasized the need to verify ABR test outcomes not only in those who fail an ABR screening test, but also in those who pass. This was endorsed by CHABA in 1987, noting a need for statistically adequate studies of ABR test accuracy. This need continues to exist. The practice of validating neonatal or infant ABR data using a subsequent ABR test as the "gold standard" addresses the reproducibility of ABR results, but not their accuracy

Reprinted by permission of authors and Decker Periodicals Inc. Copyright 1990.
Journal of the American Academy of Audiology, 1, pp. 56-66.

Reprint requests: Martyn L. Hyde, Silverman Audiology Laboratory, Suite 200, 600 University Avenue, Toronto, Ontario M5G 1X5, Canada as estimators of true hearing thresholds. At present, it is probably necessary to use reliable behavioral audiometric results as the gold standard, despite the problems that arise from the time interval between the ABR testing and the point at which behavioral testing becomes sufficiently reliable to serve as a standard. To the present authors' knowledge, there have been only two relevant large-sample ABR accuracy studies to date (Durieux-Smith et al, 1987; Swigonski et al, 1987).

There are many variables that may influence the results of an ABR validation study. The most obvious include the test method itself, when and where the testing was performed, and the characteristics of the population to be tested. One of the most interesting variables is the age at test. To accommodate the Joint Committee guidelines it is necessary to test below 6 months of age, but is testing best done in the neonate prior to discharge, or as late as possible, consistent with the guidelines? Perhaps the most important factor is access to the patient, which is potentially guaranteed if testing is performed prior to discharge, whereas the parents may not comply with instructions to return for postdischarge testing. A question here is whether parents who will not bring the child back for later evaluation would comply in any useful way with management strategies based on a predischarge test. Clearly, this is not a straightforward question, and local conditions may dictate local solutions.

The practice at Mount Sinai Hospital, Toronto, since 1984 has been to test at-risk infants as outpatients at about 4 months corrected age, that is, at about 56 weeks postconception. One of the reasons for this was a finding from an earlier research study (Hyde et al,1984) that ABR results differed considerably in the neonatal period and at about 4 months of age. The later results are certainly more relevant to any subsequent intervention, and this view has been supported by Swigonski et al (1987). Thus, ABR results at 3 to 6 months of age are of particular importance; the ABR testing to be evaluated in this report was conducted in the first year of life, but never at less than 3 months corrected age.

Material and Methods

Subjects

Subjects were drawn from Mount Sinai Hospital (MSH) and the Hospital for Sick Children (HSC), which are adjacent teaching hospitals in the Toronto downtown core. MSH is a general hospital with a program for early detection of hearing loss that is based on ABR and a risk register similar to that recommended by the Joint Committee. The prevalence of ABR screening failure at 30 dB nHL is typically 8 percent. HSC, in contrast, is a tertiary center with a much higher prevalence of ABR abnormality, typically 60 percent.

The study sample comprised 1,065 at-risk infants from MSH, a complete at-risk sample over a 3-year period, targeted without regard to whether or not an ABR had been performed. To this was added a random sample of 135 children from HSC who had had an ABR test in the first year of life. Thus, a total of 1,200 children were targeted for follow-up audiometric evaluation.

ABR Protocol

At MSH, all ABR testing was carried out in an audiometric soundroom, using a Nicolet MED-80 system. Silver chloride disk electrodes were attached at the high midline forehead and on both mastoids. Recording bandwidth was 150 to 3000 Hz (Butterworth, 12 dB/octave), with a 25.6 ms window. Two averages of at least 2000 stimuli each were accumulated, per stimulus condition. Stimuli were monaural 100-μs clicks of alternating polarity; these were delivered at about 35 per second for threshold determination, and at 21 per second for otoneurologic assessment at 70 dB nHL or greater, via a hand-held TDH-49 earphone in an MX/41AR cushion. The lowest click level used was 30 dB nHL, and threshold was bracketed with steps of 10 dB. Thresholds were also obtained for 2-1-2 ms trapezoidal notch masked tonepips at 500 Hz and 4000 Hz, but this report deals exclusively with click results.

At HSC, the equipment and protocol were similar, except that general anesthesia was applied where necessary in order to obtain satisfactory EEG conditions, and only clicks were used.

The criterion for abnormality of an ABR record was presence or absence of wave V or its ensuing negative wave. All ABR thresholds were estimated by an experienced observer (MLH). ABR threshold was defined as the lowest click level at which a clear and reproducible waveform was judged to be present. Ears for which the level of spontaneous electromyogenic artifact was high were rejected from the analysis.

Follow-Up Protocol

Targeted subjects were recalled at age 3 to 8 years. All testing was carried out by two experienced audiologists in an audiometric soundroom. The testers had no knowledge of the ABR results in infancy. The protocol included conventional pure-tone air and bone conduction thresholds, speech recognition testing, acoustic impedance and reflex tests, and a language screening test, the TACL-R (Carrow-Woolfolk, 1985). Also, a questionnaire covering demographic factors and pertinent history was administered to parents. This report deals exclusively with the pure-tone audiometric data.

Data Management

All data from the risk assessment and ABR testing in infancy, and the follow-up results, were recorded in a relational database management system (Oracle RDBMS). Analysis was via Oracle SQL or SPSS-X (DEC Microvax II, VMS).

Results

Of the targeted group of 1200 children, reliable behavioral pure-tone audiometry under earphones was subsequently obtained in 865 children (72 percent); of these, 713 (82 percent) had had an ABR test in the first year. The results to be presented here are based on 1,367 ears that yielded reliable click ABR thresholds and follow-up pure-tone thresholds. Of these 713 children, 397 were male and 316 were female. The mean age at follow-up was 3.9 years, with an SD of 0.9 and range of 3.0 to 8.0; 99 percent were tested at 6 years or less.

Figure 1 shows a scatterplot of the click ABR threshold obtained in infancy, on the ordinate, versus the average pure-tone threshold at 2 and 4 kHz, on the abscissa. While there are many possible audiometric measures that might be chosen to summarize hearing loss severity, this measure was noted by Gorga et al (1985) to be one of the best correlates of the click ABR threshold, when obtained concurrently. It can be argued that the performance of the click ABR should be assessed in relation to audiometric measures that reflect appropriately the acoustic and electrophysiologic attributes of the click.

The use of ears, as opposed to individuals, as data points can lead to incorrect confidence interval width for estimates of means, because the two ears of any given individual rarely yield statistically independent data. However, the use of exclusively right ear or left ear data is excessively conservative for many purposes, and discards information. No confidence intervals are given here, but they may be estimated conservatively by halving the sample size. There were no statistically significant differences between ears, as reflected in chi-square tests at the 0.05 level of significance.

The scatterplot in Figure 1 is presented in a manner that permits direct comparison with the standard 2˜2 decision matrix or contingency table (Jerger, 1983; Sackett et al, 1985); the four cells of the table correspond directly to the four quadrants of the scatterplot delineated by the lines denoted as "disease criterion" and "test criterion." Here, the target disease is hearing loss, with subjects denoted as disease-positive if they exceed the disease criterion, and disease-negative otherwise. This is based on the follow-up audiometry and is considered to represent the "true" disease status. The subject tests positive for disease on the infant ABR test if the ABR threshold exceeds the test criterion. Any pair of disease and test criteria will generate a corresponding decision matrix. In principle, any disease and test criteria may be chosen, and the two criteria need not have the same numerical value. Indeed, because of the number of variables that affect the statistical relationship between the ABR threshold and the hearing loss measure (e.g., audiometric profile, EEG noise levels, ABR recognition criteria), there is no reason to assume that the two measures should intrinsically be the same.

The dichotomization of essentially continuous measures such as the ABR threshold or the average hearing level certainly results in a formal loss of information, but it permits the use of many powerful analysis techniques and is well suited to estimation of screening test performance. An alternative analytic approach is regression analysis, treating the ABR threshold as the independent variable (abscissa) that predicts the follow-up audiometric status; performance would be expressed in terms of bias and variability of the prediction. Here, the approach based on the decision matrix will be used.

In Figure 1, there is an obvious tendency for the ABR and behavioral thresholds to covary, clustering around the dotted diagonal that denotes equality. Furthermore, the audiologists' determination of the type of hearing loss at follow-up is also indicated by the symbol type. The term 'normal' denotes the fact that no behavioral threshold was greater than 20 dB, from 250 Hz to 8 kHz, which is a clinical criterion quite distinct from the outcome of applying a numerical criterion to the two-frequency average used in the figure. Thus, it is possible to have patients with clinical dysfunction at any point on the scatterplot.

When the criterion lines are overlaid on the scatterplot, it is immediately obvious that the criteria used to define the presence or absence of disease and pass or failure on the test under investigation (in this case, the infant ABR) will have a profound effect on the number of data points in the various quadrants of the

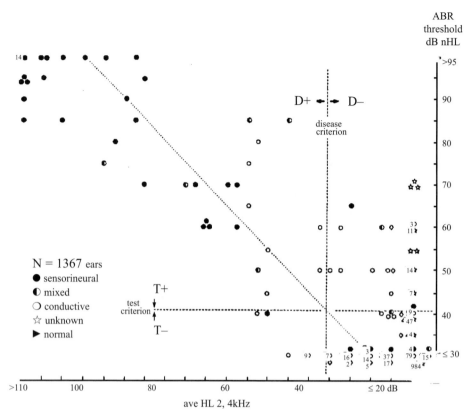

Figure 1. A scatterplot of average behavioral pure-tone hearing threshold at 3 to 8 years (ordinate) versus the click ABR threshold in the first year, for 1,367 ears in 713 children at risk for hearing loss. The axes are such that overlaying disease (hearing loss) and test (ABR) abnormality criteria upon the scatterplot will generate directly the four cells of the standard 2 × 2 decision matrix. See text for explanation of "abnormal" cases, eg., with "normal" abscissa values.

scattergram. It follows that the decision matrix and its attendant parameters of test performance, such as the sensitivity (the conditional probability that the ABR test is positive for disease, given that disease is present), specificity (the conditional probability that the test is negative, given that disease is absent), and the likelihood ratios for the two test outcomes (for each outcome, the ratio of its conditional probabilities when disease is present and absent) will depend on the disease and test criteria. Thus, some means of expressing the effect of criterion variation is required. One of the most elegant approaches is the Relative Operating Characteristic (ROC), known earlier as the receiver operating characteristic. Recently, Swets (1988) has emphasized the power and generality of the ROC approach to the analysis of test performance.

First, consider the generation of a single decision matrix. Suppose it is decided that average hearing losses greater than 40 dB, regardless of type of hearing loss, are the target disease, and it is required to evaluate a click ABR screening criterion level of 40 dB nHL (the equality is coincidental). The criteria would then have the positions shown in Figure 1. The 12 ears in

the false-negative (lower left) quadrant, for example, are obvious on the scatterplot. The associated 2˜2 table is shown in Table 1a; the sensitivity and specificity are 0.81 and 0.96, respectively, which is good performance.

To improve the sensitivity, the ABR abnormality criterion could be lowered, perhaps to 30 dB, and this would give the results shown in Table 1b. The sensitivity and specificity are now 0.84 and 0.91. Thus, lowering the ABR criterion reduces the false-negative rate from 0.19 to 0.16, but more than doubles the false-positive rate, from 0.04 to 0.09.

When defining the target hearing loss characteristics, there is more to consider than the nature of the hearing loss measure and the value of the abnormality criterion. For example, suppose it is desired to focus on sensorineural impairment. In terms of the scatterplot, this means that all unfilled circles in the two disease-positive quadrants are moved into the disease-negative column, becoming either false positives or true negatives. The revised scatterplot would yield the matrices shown in Table 1c and 1d, for 40 dB disease and 40 and 30 dB test criteria, respectively. Note

Table 1. Examples of 2~2 Contingency Tables (Decision Matrices) Derivable from Figure 1.

(a)		All Hearing Loss	
		Yes(D+)	No(D−)
ABR 40 dB nHL	Fail(T+)	51	50
	Pass(T−)	12	1254
		Sensitivity 0.81	
		Specificity 0.96	
		LR + 21.1 LR − 0.20	

(b)		All Hearing Loss	
		Yes(D+)	No(D−)
ABR 30 dB nHL	Fail(T+)	53	117
	Pass(T−)	10	1187
		Sensitivity: 0.84	
		Specificity: 0.91	
		LR + 9.4 LR − 0.17	

(c)		SN Hearing Loss	
		Yes(D+)	No(D−)
ABR 40 dB nHL	Fail(T+)	44	57
	Pass(T−)	1	1265
		Sensitivity 0.98	
		Specificity 0.96	
		LR + 22.7 LR − 0.02	

(d)		SN Hearing Loss	
		Yes(D+)	No(D−)
ABR 30 dB nHL	Fail(T+)	45	125
	Pass(T−)	0	1197
		Sensitivity 1.0	
		Specificity 0.91	
		LR + infinite LR − 0.0	

The hearing loss criterion used here is that the average pure-tone threshold at 2 and 4 kHz is over 40 dB HL.
The ABR criteria are a click ABR threshold of over 40 dB nHL or over 30 dB nHL.
The sensitivity, specificity, and likelihood ratios for positive (fail) and negative (pass) ABR outcomes are also shown.
LR+ = sensitivity/(1−specificity) and LR− = (1−sensitivity)/specificity.
Post-test odds for disease = pretest odds ~ LR(test outcome).

that the focus on sensorineural hearing loss changes the decision matrices radically, particularly improving the sensitivity of the test.

A more complete picture of the way in which ABR test accuracy depends on the various criteria is shown in Figure 2. Here, the ordinate is the true-positive rate, or sensitivity, and the abscissa is the false-positive rate, namely the complement of the specificity. In this so-called 'binormal plane,' the axes are linear in terms of standard deviations of the normal (Gaussian) distribution, but are thereby nonlinear in terms of probability. Relative to the linear probability axes of the classic ROC plane, this transformation expands the interesting regions with sensitivity close to 100 percent and false-positive rate close to 0 percent. Also, it transforms ROC curves that reflect an underlying binormal model into straight lines (Swets, 1988), that is, if the distributions of the test variable, namely the ABR threshold, were normal with the same variance for both the disease-positive and the disease-negative populations, then the ROC would be linear with unit slope (45 degrees). If the slope is less than unity, the usual cause is that the disease-positive distribution has larger variance. The dotted lines in the background of Figure 2 represent binormal ROCs at various integer values of the parameter d'. This parameter is essentially the distance between the means of the disease-negative and disease-positive distributions, expressed in terms of a number of standard deviations, and is a useful summary measure of test accuracy. A useless (random) test has a d' of zero, whereas an excellent test might achieve a value of about 3.0 or more. See Swets (1988) for a more detailed discussion of ROC techniques and test accuracy measures.

In Figure 2 are plotted six ROCs, three for a disease definition that includes all types of hearing loss and three for a definition restricted to sensorineural hearing loss. In each case, the hearing loss severity criterion takes values of 20, 30, and 40 dB as indicated. For every ROC, the four points correspond to four values of the ABR abnormality criterion, namely 60, 50, 40, and 30 dB nHL, reading from left to right.

For every ROC in Figure 2, the trading relationship between sensitivity and specificity as the test criterion is changed is apparent. Test accuracy improves as the hearing loss criterion increases, and the accuracy is generally higher for sensorineural hearing loss. All the ROCs show good linearity, and those for sensorineural loss tend to follow the normal, equal variance model most closely. For sensorineural loss of over 30 dB, averaged at 2 and 4 kHz, the ROC slope is close to unity and the d' is about 3.5, which means that the infant ABR is an excellent test for hearing loss thus defined. Note that changing the ABR abnormality cri

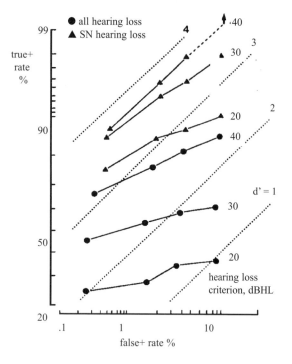

Figure 2. Relative operating characteristics (ROCs) for the click ABR test as a predictor of hearing loss. The axes are linear in standard deviations of the normal (Gaussian) distribution. A positive test means that the test is positive for disease, i.e., it indicates that hearing loss is present. Each data point is the result of applying one pair of dichotomous disease and test criteria to the data of Figure 1. The parameter is the value of the hearing loss criterion, and each criterion is applied either to all hearing loss or to exclusively sensorineural hearing loss. The four data points for each ROC arise from ABR abnormality criteria of 60, 50, 40, and 30 dB nHL, from left to right.

terion alters the sensitivity and specificity according to the bilinear normal ROC rule, but this does not alter the global accuracy of the test, as expressed by the approximately constant d' value of about 3.5.

For all hearing loss criteria other than those just noted, the ROC slope is very different from unity, so there is no unique value of d' that globally summarizes the test performance over a range of test criterion values. Here, it is necessary to resort to other global measures of test accuracy, such as the area under the ROC curve, usually denoted as A (Swets, 1988), or to deal with particular sensitivity-specificity pairs, in discussions of test accuracy.

Discussion

The results and analyses presented in this report are preliminary, but may be of interest to those who are about to establish, or are already engaged in, clinical programs for detection of hearing loss using ABR techniques. Insight into the relationships between sensitivity and specificity as a function of the test and disease

criteria is an essential prerequisite for meaningful cost benefit analysis and resource allocation.

The data outlined here suggest that as a detector of sensorineural hearing loss with an average value of greater than 30 dB at 2 and 4 kHz, the click ABR test performed at between 3 months and 1 year of age is an excellent tool. By varying the ABR test failure criterion from 30 dB through 60 dB, the sensitivity can be adjusted from over 98 percent down to about 85 percent, with concomitant change in the falsepositive rate from about 10 percent down to less than 1 percent. The choice of ABR criterion should depend on factors such as the prevalence of hearing loss in the tested population and the quantitative costs associated with test overhead and outcome error (Sackett et al, 1985).

In this study, the hearing status as determined at follow-up is used as a proxy for the true hearing status in the first year of life because there is no behavioral technique that has sufficient accuracy to constitute a gold standard at the time of the ABR test. The problem with a delay of several years is that the true hearing status may change. First, consider sensorineural hearing loss. In infants and young children, this will rarely fluctuate or remit, but certainly may be initiated or may progress in the period between the ABR and the follow-up audiometry. This will cause apparent false-negative ABR outcomes. From a regression standpoint, there will be negative bias in the ABR as a predictor of the true hearing level. In the scatterplot of Figure 1, there is one sensorineural loss point (at 55, 40) that is likely to be counted as false-negative. This arose from a child who was born at 1260 g after 30 weeks, with severe asphyxia and intraventricular hemorrhage. Also, at higher ABR thresholds there are several points for which the hearing loss is 20 dB or more greater than the ABR threshold. Because ABR thresholds are typically greater than concurrent behavioral thresholds, progression of hearing loss could be suspected for several of these points.

If sensorineural hearing loss rarely remits, resolving conductive impairment is by far the most probable cause of false-positive ABR findings.

If conductive hearing loss were to be encompassed in the disease definition, which is not unreasonable clinically, then there are much more serious difficulties inherent in the follow-up validation because of the greater probability of change in hearing. For example, even if the conductive hearing loss components in infancy and at follow-up were statistically unrelated, there would by chance be a certain proportion of test outcomes that are apparently, but not actually, correct. A more detailed analysis might take account of such factors, but the simplest approach, adopted here, is to focus on the data for sensorineural loss; in that regard, conductive pathology is a source of variation that can only degrade the apparent performance of the ABR test.

There are several techniques that might be used to improve the performance of the ABR. For example, it may be possible to identify conductive hearing loss on the basis of ABR wave latency increase, e.g., for wave I. If such a classifier performed well, then many of the false positives that limit the observed ABR performance might move to the true-negative region. It remains to be seen whether a latency rule can be derived that will produce a net performance enhancement.

In the bottom right-hand corner of the scatterplot of Figure 1, there are several points indicating the presence of sensorineural hearing loss. For example, hearing losses at low or high frequencies could and did occur, yet were not reflected in the behavioral outcome measure selected here, namely the 2 and 4 kHz average pure-tone hearing level. Because a hearing loss component in infancy at 8 kHz might indicate a progressive sensorineural disorder that should at least be flagged for monitoring, the 2 and 4 kHz average is imperfect as a clinical outcome measure. Indeed, there are many other measures that merit consideration in a more detailed analysis.

Furthermore, features of the audiometric contour may contribute in other ways to discrepancies between ABR and behavioral measures. For example, underestimation of average hearing loss by the ABR threshold may result from better hearing at frequencies outside the domain of the average but within the wide excitation bandwidth of the click (Kileny and Magathan, 1987).

When the ABR test is normal but there is sensorineural hearing loss at follow-up, progressive or adventitious dysfunction is one cause of apparent error, but the fault lies in the deferred gold standard. On the other hand, it is possible to see such a result even though the hearing loss was present throughout, if the dysfunction is more rostral than the site of generation of ABR wave V (probably subcollicular). This is a genuine error and limitation on the part of the ABR test. It is not yet clear if cortical dysfunction, for example, might have contributed to any of the data reported here.

False-positive ABR findings, in the sense of false-positive detection of disease, could arise due to poor recording conditions or techniques, but records that showed poor reproducibility were excluded from this dataset. A more subtle possible cause is poor ABR development due to inadequate neural synchronization; this is of concern in those at risk for neurodevelopmental disorders, such as the graduates of an intensive care nursery.

In conclusion, the results presented here are encouraging for advocates of the ABR as a tool for early detection of hearing loss, but much further analysis of this dataset is required, and is in progress. This analysis includes examination of the contribution that tonepip ABR thresholds and ABR wave latency measurements can make to test accuracy, introduction of the risk factors as covariates and sample stratifiers, and exploration of relationships among risk factors, ABR findings, and language screening outcomes. Further studies in this area are required to delineate fully the confidence that should be placed in infant ABR outcomes, either as bases for intervention or as secondary standards by which newer techniques such as evoked otoacoustic emission measurement may be evaluated.

Acknowledgments

This work was supported by the Ontario Ministry of Health, the Medical Research Council of Canada and the Saul A. Silverman Family Foundation.

The collaborative support of Peter Alberti, Marilyn Boyden, and Bill Crysdale is gratefully acknowledged. Special thanks are due to Gayle Chown, Naneve Hawke, Kris Madsen, and Susan Peberdy, who gathered the bulk of the data.

Presented in part at the meeting of the American Academy of Audiology, Kiawah Island, SC, April 1989.

References

Alberti, P., Hyde, M., Riko, K., Corbin, H., Fitzhardinge P. (1985). Issues in early identification of hearing loss. *Laryngoscope* 95:373-381.

ASHA Committee on Infant Hearing. (1989). Audiologic screening of newborn infants who are at risk for hearing impairment. *Asha* 32:89-92.

Carrow-Woolfolk, E. (1985). Test for auditory comprehension of language-revised edition. *TACL-R Examiner's Manual*. Allen, TX: DLM Teaching Resources.

Committee on Hearing, Bioacoustics, and Biomechanics. (1987). Brainstem audiometry of infants. *Asha* 29:47-55.

Durieux-Smith, A., Picton, T., Edwards, C., Goodman, J., MacMurray, T. (1987). Brainstem electric response audiometry in infants of a neonatal intensive care unit. *Audiology* 26:284-297.

Galambos, R., Hicks, G., Wilson, M. (1984). The auditory brainstem response reliably predicts hearing loss in graduates of a tertiary intensive care nursery. *Ear Hear* 5:254-260.

Gorga, M., Worthington, D., Reiland, J., Beauchaine, K., Goldgar, D. (1985). Some comparisons between auditory brain stem response thresholds, latencies, and the pure-tone audiogram. *Ear Hear* 6:105-112.

Hyde, M., Riko, K., Corbin, H., Moroso, M., Alberti, P. (1984). A neonatal hearing screening research program using brainstem electric response audiometry. *J Otolaryngol* 13:49-54.

Jacobson, J.T., Morehouse, C. (1984). A comparison of auditory brainstem response and behavioral screening in high risk and normal newborn infants. *Ear Hear* 5:247-253.

Jerger, S. (1983). Decision matrix and information theory analyses in the evaluation of neuroaudiologic tests. In: Jerger, J., Jerger, S., Neely, J., eds. The neuroaudiological evaluation. *Semin Hear* 4:121-133.

Joint Committee on Infant Hearing. (1982). Position statement. *Pediatrics* 70:496-497.

Kileny, P., Magathan, M. (1987). Predictive value of ABR in infants and children with moderate to profound hearing impairment. *Ear Hear* 8:217-221.

Murray, A., Javel, E., Watson, C. (1985). Prognostic validity of auditory brainstem evoked response screening in newborn infants. *Am J Otolaryngol* 6:120-131.

Sackett, D., Haynes, R., Tugwell, P. (1985). Clinical epidemiology—a basic science for clinical medicine. Boston: Little, Brown & Co.

Stein, L., Clark, S., Kraus N. (1983). The hearing impaired infant: patterns of identification and habilitation. *Ear Hear* 4:232-236.

Swets, J. (1988). Measuring the accuracy of diagnostic systems. *Science* 140:1285-1293.

Swigonski, N., Shallop, J., Bull, M., Lemons, J. (1987). Hearing screening of high risk newborns. *Ear Hear* 8:26-30.

Thresholds for Auditory Brain Stem Responses to Tones in Notched Noise from Infants and Young Children with Normal Hearing or Sensorineural Hearing Loss

David R. Stapells, Judith S. Gravel, and Brett A. Martin

Department of Otolaryngology, Albert Einstein College of Medicine, Bronx, New York

Objective: To assess the accuracy of threshold estimates determined using the auditory brain stem responses (ABRs) to brief tones presented in notched noise in a group of infants and young children with normal hearing or sensorineural hearing loss (SNHL).

Design: The thresholds for ABRs to brief duration 500, 2000, and 4000 Hz tones presented in notched-noise masking were evaluated in infants and young children with normal hearing ($N = 34$) or SNHL ($N = 54$). Tone-evoked ABR thresholds were compared with behavioral thresholds obtained at follow-up audiologic assessments, for a total of 220 comparisons.

Results: ABR thresholds for the infants with bilateral normal hearing were 23.6, 12.9, and 12.6 dB nHL for 500, 2000 and 4000 Hz, respectively. Most (92 to 100%) infants with normal hearing showed ABRs to 30 dB nHL tones. Across all subjects (i.e., those with normal hearing and those with impaired hearing), high ($\varnothing\,0.94$) correlations were found between the ABR and behavioral thresholds. The mean differences between ABR (dB nHL) and behavioral (dB HL) thresholds across all subjects were 8.6, –0.4, and –4.3 dB for 500, 2000, and 4000 Hz, respectively. Overall, 98% of the ABR thresholds were within 30 dB of the behavioral thresholds, 93% were within 20 dB, and 80% were within 15 dB.

Conclusions: These threshold results for the ABR to brief tones in notched noise obtained for infants and young children are similar to those obtained in similar studies of adults. The technique may be used clinically with reasonable accuracy to estimate pure-tone behavioral thresholds in infants and young children who are referred for diagnostic threshold ABR testing. (*Ear & Hearing* 1995;16;361-371)

The click-evoked auditory brain stem response (ABR) is the most widely employed procedure for the electrophysiological evaluation of auditory threshold in infants and young children when their behavioral audiometric results are unobtainable or unreliable. The ABR to clicks alone, however, cannot provide information concerning sensitivity for specific frequencies. Furthermore, hearing loss restricted to particular frequency regions may be underestimated or missed entirely by the click-ABR threshold (e.g., Picton, 1978; Picton & Durieux-Smith, 1988; Picton, Ouellette, Hamel, & Durieux-Smith, 1979; Stapells, 1989; Yamada, Yagi, Yamane & Suzuki, 1975). An alternative and more frequency-specific approach to obtain electrophysiologic thresholds is to record the ABRs to brief-duration tonal stimuli.

Numerous studies have investigated the ABRs to tonal stimuli (for a review, see Stapells, Picton, & Durieux-Smith, 1994). In terms of estimating behavioral thresholds in hearing-impaired subjects, most studies have indicated reasonably accurate and reliable results for frequencies from 500 to at least 4000 Hz (e.g., Hayes & Jerger, 1982; Kileny & Magathan, 1987; Kodera, Yamane, Yamada & Suzuki, 1977; McGee & Clemis, 1980; Munnerley, Greville, Purdy, & Keith, 1991; Picton et al, 1979; Stapells, Picton, Durieux-Smith, Edwards, & Moran, 1990; Suzuki, Kodera & Yamada, 1984; Suzuki & Yamane, 1982), although a small number have indicated inaccuracies and difficulties occurring for 500 Hz (Davis & Hirsh, 1976; Gorga, Kaminski, Beauchaine & Jesteadt, 1988; Hayes & Jerger, 1982; Laukli, 1983; Laukli, Fjermedal & Mair, 1988; Sohmer & Kinarti, 1984). Some of these difficulties may be attributed to various problems, including high-pass EEG filter set too high, use of EEG recording channel contralateral to the ear-stimulated, high levels of ipsilateral masking noise, high levels of acoustic ambient noise and/or electrically noisy environment (e.g., operating room), stimuli which were either too brief or too long, too few trials per average, and/or waveform interpretation issues.

Several studies have investigated the tone-evoked ABRs in infants and young children (Hyde, 1985;

Reprinted by permission of authors and Williams & Wilkins. Copyright 1995. *Ear & Hearing*, 16, No. 4, pp. 361-371.

Stapells, 1989; Stapells et al, 1994; Stockard, Stockard & Coen, 1983; Suzuki et al, 1984), and most indicate the responses are detectable at intensities similar to those in adult subjects. Our recent studies have indicated normal "screening" intensities for infants aged 2 weeks or older are 30-40 dB nHL at 500 Hz, and 20-30 dB nHL at 2000 and 4000 Hz (Stapells, 1989; Stapells et al, 1994). Studies of the tone ABR in infants and young children with hearing impairments are few but have indicated reasonable estimates of their behavioral audiograms (e.g., Kileny & Magathan, 1987; Suzuki et al, 1984). Generally, these studies have been in relatively small groups of children with hearing impairments or in children from whom behavioral audiometric information has been questionable.

The brief tones required to elicit synchronous ABRs contain significant acoustic splatter in frequencies above and below the tones' nominal frequencies. Studies in subjects with normal hearing have indicated that responses to brief tones presented at intensities greater than 40-50 dB nHL, or about 70 dB peak-to-peak equivalent SPL, contain contributions from this acoustic splatter and hence have reduced frequency specificity (for a review, see Stapells et al, 1994). This is true whether the tones be 500, 1000, 2000, or 4000 Hz. Furthermore, regardless of how "pure" a tonal stimulus may be (e.g., a tone of several seconds duration and thus containing essentially no acoustic splatter), above about 70 dB SPL upward spread of excitation occurring as a result of cochlear physiology rather than acoustic splatter will result in contributions arising from frequencies above the tones' nominal frequencies (Pickles, 1986). These issues have led to the suggestion of the use of simultaneous ipsilateral noise masking to improve the frequency specificity of the ABRs to these brief tones (Picton, 1978; Picton et al, 1979).

High-pass filtered noise may be employed to mask upward spread of excitation as well as the acoustic splatter to frequencies above the tone frequency (e.g., Kileny & Magathan, 1987); however, it does not mask splatter to frequencies lower than the tone frequency. This is particularly significant in the case of steeply sloping high frequency impairments where sensitivity at a lower frequency is much better than that at a higher frequency (Picton, 1978; Picton et al, 1979; Purdy & Abbas, 1989; Stapells, 1984; Stapells et al, 1990; Stapells et al, 1994). Mixing "notched" (band reject) masking noise with the brief tones has been suggested as a solution (Picton et al, 1979).The effects of the notched-noise masking on the ABRs to brief tones have been reviewed (Stapells et al, 1990, 1994). Results of two different centers' recent studies of adults with normal hearing (Purdy et al, 1989; Stapells et al, 1990) and impaired hearing (Stapells et al, 1990;

Munnerley et al, 1991) have indicated reasonably accurate ABR estimates of pure tone behavioral threshold using the technique of recording the ABR to brief tones in notched noise. No studies of this technique in groups of infants or young children with hearing impairments have been published.

The purpose of the present study was to assess the accuracy of threshold estimates determined using the ABR to brief tones presented in notched noise in a group of infants and young children with sensorineural hearing loss referred for clinical testing, as well as in a group of infants and young children with normal hearing. The ABR thresholds were compared with pure tone behavioral audiometric thresholds obtained at follow-up, usually at a later age.

Methods

A total of 88 infants and young children, aged 1 week to 8 yr (mean age at ABR = 31 mo; median age = 21 mo; 77% of subjects aged less than 48 mo) participated in this study. Thirty-four subjects had normal hearing, whereas 54 subjects had sensorineural hearing loss (SNHL). Six of the subjects had unilateral sensorineural impairments with normal hearing in the other ear. Subjects with bilateral normal hearing were recruited as part of their participation in a multivisit longitudinal research program.

Subjects with hearing loss were specifically referred for clinical ABR testing by our Auditory Behavioral Laboratory, by other clinical facilities associated with the Albert Einstein College of Medicine/Montefiore Medical Center (AECOM/MMC), as well as by outside agencies. Owing to the clinical nature of this study, the specific audiometric test equipment used to obtain behavioral audiograms and acoustic immittance measures varied by facility. All ABR testing (and same-day acoustic immittance measures) was completed in the AECOM Auditory Evoked Potential Laboratories.

Behavioral audiograms were obtained independently of the ABR assessment: approximately 90% of the behavioral tests were completed by our related AECOM/MMC laboratories and clinics (all of the normal-hearing group and the majority of the subjects in the SNHL group); 10% were obtained by other clinical facilities (SNHL group). The average age for behavioral audiometric testing was 33.9 ± 25.4 mo (median age = 28.1 mo). On average, these audiograms were obtained within 2.2 ± 18.0 mo of the ABR testing, with some audiograms for the older children being obtained before the ABR.

All audiograms considered in this investigation were deemed reliable by the audiologist completing the behavioral audiogram. This was based on the subjective judgment of the audiologist or an actual quantification of false-positive responding (percentage of responses to control trial intervals). If the reliability of the behavioral audiogram was questionable, the result was not considered. If more than one audiogram was available for a child, the one deemed most reliable was used in the analyses.

Only audiometric threshold data were considered. Behavioral test results that were obtained using behavioral observation audiometry or that were considered "minimal response levels" rather than threshold values were excluded from this study. Consequently, audiograms obtained using only visual reinforcement audiometry, play audiometry, or in a few cases, conventional audiometric test procedures, were included in the analyses. Air conduction thresholds were obtained using conventional supra-aural earphones (i.e., TDH-39, TDH-49, etc., with MX41/AR cushions). No thresholds obtained in sound field were considered. If masking was not used in cases of threshold asymmetry, the audiogram was excluded from the study.

Inclusion in this study required evidence of no conductive component at the time of the ABR and behavioral tests. This was determined by either the absence of an air-bone gap (when bone conduction thresholds were available) and/or by normal acoustic immittance results. Following the qualitative classification scheme suggested by Jerger (1970), a tympanogram with normal compliance and peak pressure between +50 and −150 daPa was considered as evidence of the absence of significant middle ear pathology. The presence of the acoustic reflex (when available and with consideration of the degree of the loss) provided further evidence of normal middle ear function. In the few cases with tympanometric pressure peaks less than −150 daPa (type C), present acoustic reflexes were required in order for the data to be included. In no case were threshold data included when a noncompliant (flat, type B) tympanogram was recorded on the day of testing. A 220 Hz probe frequency was used in the majority of cases.

Inclusion in the group with normal hearing required behavioral thresholds at or better than 25 dB HL for 500 to 4000 Hz. Inclusion in the group with sensorineural hearing loss required behavioral thresholds for one or more of 500, 2000, and 4000 Hz to be greater than 25 dB HL. Mean (and standard deviation) pure-tone behavioral thresholds are given for each group in Table 1.

Stimuli for ABR testing were 500, 2000, and 4000 Hz short duration tones presented in notched noise.

The tones had linear rise times equaling two cycles, plateau times of one cycle, and linear fall times of two cycles. The normal behavioral thresholds (0 dB nHL) for these stimuli are 24.6, 26.1, and 29 dB peak-to-peak equivalent (pe) SPL for the 500, 2000, and 4000 Hz tones, respectively (Stapells et al, 1990). The tones were presented monaurally at a rate of 39.1/sec using a Telephonics TDH-49 earphone (MX41/AR cushion). This rate was the fastest rate allowed by our equipment when using a 25-msec analysis time. The notched noise was produced by passing broadband noise through a band-reject filter (one octave-wide notch centered on the nominal frequency of the tone) with high-pass and low-pass rejection slopes of 48 dB per octave. The noise intensity (in dB SPL) before filtering was set 20 dB below the pe SPL of the tone. This tone-to-noise ratio was maintained for all tone intensities. These stimuli and noise maskers are the same as those used in an earlier study carried out in adults (Stapells et al, 1990). The ear contralateral to that being assessed was masked using white noise set 30 dB below the level required to mask ipsilaterally (Stapells, 1984). Stimuli and noise maskers were calibrated using a Brüel and Kjaer 2209 sound level meter and NBS 9-A earphone coupler (Brüel & Kjaer type 4152 with a 1-inch microphone type 4144).

Single-channel recordings of the brain stem responses were obtained using gold-plated cup electrodes placed at the vertex (noninverting) and mastoid (inverting) ipsilateral to the stimulated ear. A similar electrode placed on the forehead served as a ground. Interelectrode impedances were less than 3000 Ohms. The EEG filter was set to a band pass of 30 to 3000 Hz (12 dB/octave slope) and averaged using a poststimu-

Table 1. Pure-tone behavioral thresholds (dB HL) for normal-hearing and sensorineural-impaired (SNHL) ears.

	Frequency (Hz)		
	500	2000	4000
Normal-hearing ears:			
Mean	15.9	13.2	13.8
SD	7.9	6.8	6.1
N[a]	39	39	41
SNHL ears:			
Mean	64.6	74.2	79.2
SD	33.8	34.1	33.1
N[b]	77	78	70

[a]N, number of ears with normal thresholds contributing data to study. Includes results for six normal ears from subjects with unilateral SNHL.
[b]N, number of ears with SNHL contributing data to the study.

lus analysis time of 25 msec. Trials containing amplitudes exceeding ±25 μV were automatically rejected. At least two replications of 2000 trials each were obtained in each intensity/frequency condition.

All subjects were tested while asleep for ABR testing. Most slept in a crib, but some were seated in a reclining chair or in their parent's arms. Subjects in the group with normal hearing were tested in natural sleep. Subjects in the group with sensorineural hearing loss aged 6 mo or more were sedated by their physician (using chloral hydrate) as part of their clinical assessment; subjects in this group aged under 6 mo were tested in natural sleep. All testing was carried out in a double-walled, sound-attenuating room. Subjects were continuously monitored by intercom, direct visual observation, and by monitoring of their EEG on an oscilloscope. Testing proceeded only when this monitoring indicated the child was asleep and was interrupted during periods of waking or questionable sleep.

Tympanograms (age >5 mo: 220 Hz probe frequency; age ≤4 mo: 660 Hz probe frequency; Marchant, McMillan, Shurin, Johnson, Turczyk, Feinstein & Panek, 1986) were obtained during the same sleep session as the ABR test. Ipsilateral acoustic reflexes were also attempted. ABR testing was usually carried out after the acoustic immittance testing.

ABR stimulus/intensity/ear test order was different between the groups with bilateral normal hearing and SNHL. In the group with normal hearing, an ear was randomly chosen, and testing concentrated on that ear. One of the stimulus frequencies was randomly chosen, and threshold was obtained using 10-20 dB steps down to as low as 0 dB nHL. Thresholds for the remaining stimulus frequencies were then obtained for the same ear in random order. When sleep time permitted, thresholds for the other ear were obtained but are not included in this study. This protocol was part of these subjects' participation in a longitudinal study of children with and without otitis media.

ABR testing for the group with SNHL was dictated by clinical concerns. Typically, ABR testing began using 2000 Hz 30 dB nHL tones. If a response was present at 30 dB nHL, then the intensity was dropped to 20 dB nHL and recordings obtained. Recordings at lower intensities were not obtained. If a response was not observed in the 30 dB recording, testing was switched to the other ear, and a similar procedure was carried out. If no response was present to the 30 dB nHL 2000 Hz tones, then a decision regarding what to test next was made based upon the acoustic immittance findings: if immittance findings indicated normal middle ear function then we proceeded to obtain the ABR threshold for the 2000 Hz tones. If the immittance

results had not, to this point, been obtained they were then obtained. Ears with abnormal or noninterpretable immittance results were excluded from this study and generally would have received bone conduction ABR testing (Foxe & Stapells, 1993; Stapells & Ruben, 1989). After obtaining thresholds for 2000 Hz in each ear, recordings were then obtained to high-intensity clicks in order to assess VIIIth nerve and brain stem auditory pathway integrity bilaterally (Stapells, 1989). Subjects with abnormal wave V/wave I amplitude ratios (i.e., less than 0.6) were excluded from this study. Thresholds for 500 Hz tones were next obtained bilaterally, with 30 dB nHL being the lowest intensity tested. Finally, sleep time permitting, thresholds for 4000 Hz tones were obtained bilaterally, with 20 dB nHL being the lowest intensity tested. The minima of 20 dB nHL for 2000 and 4000 Hz and 30 dB nHL for 500 Hz were chosen based on normative results (Stapells, 1989; Stapells et al, 1990, 1994) and on clinical efficiency. The number of ABR/behavioral threshold combinations are shown in Table 2, broken down by normal hearing or SNHL, stimulus frequency, and by three age ranges (0 to 6 mo, 7 to 48 mo, >49 mo). These age ranges and their numbers are typical of the patient population seen for diagnostic threshold ABR evaluations.

Response presence required the agreement of two judges familiar with tone-evoked ABRs. The presence of an ABR in each condition was based primarily upon the replicability of the ABR V-V′ slow wave (Stapells & Picton, 1981; Takagi, Suzuki, & Kobayashi, 1985). Changes in latency and amplitude with stimulus intensity and frequency were also available and helpful to the judges. To rule out contamination by stimulus artifact, only the portion of tracings following the offset of the tonal stimuli (500 Hz: 10 to 25 msec; 2000 Hz: 2.5 to 25 msec; 4000 Hz: 1.25 to 25 msec) were considered by the judges. The judges were not aware of a subject's pure-tone behavioral thresholds. As indicated above, in the majority of cases in both groups, pure-tone behavioral thresholds were available only on follow-up.

Owing to equipment limits, maximum stimulus intensities for ABR testing were limited to 100 dB nHL for 500 Hz, 95 dB nHL for 2000 Hz, and 90 dB nHL for 4000 Hz. Maximum intensities for behavioral testing were 110 dB HL for the three frequencies. In cases where "no response" was obtained at the maximum equipment intensity, a threshold was arbitrarily assigned as being 10 dB above the maximum.

Threshold difference measurements were calculated by subtracting the pure-tone behavioral thresholds (in dB HL) from the ABR thresholds (in dB nHL).

Threshold results were analyzed using descriptive statistics, frequency distributions, linear regressions, and Student's t-tests. Results were considered significant if $p < 0.01$. Owing to incomplete repeated measures (and therefore missing data, see Table 2), the statistical significance of differences between means involving different stimulus frequencies, as well as data combined across frequencies, were not assessed.

Results

Overall, 220 ABR/behavioral threshold assessments were obtained from the 88 infants and young children. Seventy-three of these assessments were obtained for 500 Hz, 96 for 2000 Hz, and 51 for 4000 Hz. Most of these ABR thresholds were obtained for children aged under 4 yr (see Table 2).

Figure l shows the ABRs to 500, 2000, and 4000 Hz tones in notched noise recorded from a 2l-mo-old subject with normal hearing whose results are typical of her group. Vertex-positive waves V followed by vertex-negative waves V′ are clearly present to the three tones presented at 60, 40, and 20 dB nHL. The locations of the waves V (and the judges' rating of "present response") are indicated by the arrows. The ABR thresholds (20 dB nHL) are within 5 dB of her behavioral pure-tone thresholds (indicated at the top of the figure, obtained at age 24 mo).

Mean thresholds (in dB nHL) and response detectability statistics for the ABRs from the normal-hearing ears are presented in Table 3. The mean ABR thresholds for these infants and young children are similar to and slightly better (lower) than those previ-

ously presented for adult subjects (Stapells et al, 1990). The response detectability results are also similar between the adult and infant/child groups, suggesting no differences in ABR detectability for infants, young children, and adults. Over 90% of the normal-hearing group showed ABRs to 30 dB nHL 500 Hz tones and to 20 dB nHL 2000 and 4000 Hz tones. The mean ABR threshold for 500 Hz is about 10 dB higher than for 2000 and 4000 Hz. Owing to incomplete repeated measures and therefore missing data, the statistical significance of this and other frequency-related differences were not assessed.

Brain stem response waveforms obtained for the left ear of a 15-mo-old subject with a bilateral sensorineural hearing loss are shown in Figure 2. Location of waves V (and the judges' rating of "present response") are indicated by the arrows. The ABR thresholds (60, 40, and 60 dB nHL for 500, 2000, and 4000 Hz, respectively) are within 5 dB of his pure-tone behavioral thresholds (reliably obtained at age 30 mo) of 55, 35, and 60 dB HL for 500, 2000, and 4000 Hz.

The relationship of the pure-tone behavioral thresholds to the ABR thresholds obtained using the tones in notched-noise technique is illustrated for all ears in the graphs shown in Figure 3. Data points in these scatterplots are identified as to their hearing group (normal or sensorineural loss) and age (at time of ABR) group. With only a few exceptions, the ABR to tones in notched-noise technique provided reasonably accurate estimates of pure-tone behavioral sensitivity for all frequencies. The average (±1 SD) ABR minus behavioral threshold difference is 1.7 ± 13.1 dB (average across both hearing groups and all three frequencies), with a median difference of 0 dB. Results for normal and SNHL ears are similar, with overall threshold differences (average across three frequencies) of 1.5 ± 12.1 dB for the normal-hearing ears and 1.8 ± 13.7 dB for the SNHL ears. If the direction of the ABR minus behavioral threshold difference is not considered (i.e., if we take the absolute value of the difference score), the ABR estimated, on average, within 10.3 ± 8.2 dB of behavioral threshold. Table 4 compares the mean threshold difference scores for the normal-hearing and SNHL ears and for the three frequencies.

In total, 98% of the ABR thresholds were within 30 dB of the behavioral thresholds, 93% were within 20 dB, 80% were within 15 dB, and 66% were within 10 dB. Of the 43 cases where ABR/behavioral thresholds differed by greater than 15 dB, 26 were ABR overestimations (i.e., 12% of cases showed ABR 15 dB or greater overestimations of behavioral threshold). In only four threshold estimations (of a total of 220), all

Table 2. Number of ABR/behavioral threshold combinations[a] by subject group, stimulus frequency, and age.

	Frequency (Hz)		
	500	2000	4000
Normal-hearing ears (40 subjects[b]):			
All ages total	25	28	23
0-6 mo	3	6	3
7-48 mo	22	18	20
>49 mo	0	4	0
SNHL ears (54 Subjects):			
All ages total	48	68	28
0-6 mo	2	5	5
7-48 mo	35	42	15
>49 mo	11	21	8

[a]Number of ears contributing data.
[b]Includes six subjects with unilateral SNHL.

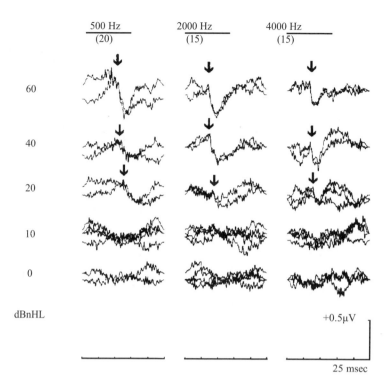

Figure 1. ABRs to brief tones in notched noise recorded from a 21-mo-old subject with normal hearing. Pure-tone behavioral thresholds, obtained at age 24 mo, are shown in parentheses. Traces judged to contain a replicable response are identified by the arrows, which also indicate the approximate location of ABR wave V or the V-to-V′ transition. ABR thresholds were judged to be 20 dB nHL for each of the three frequencies. Waveforms are plotted with positivity at the vertex represented as an upward deflection.

for 500 Hz, the ABR threshold to tones in notched noise overestimated the pure-tone behavioral threshold by greater than 30 dB. One of these >30 dB overestimations was due to the 30 dB nHL minimum intensity for 500 Hz (the 500 Hz pure-tone behavioral threshold was –5 dB HL; the 500 Hz ABR "threshold" was 30 dB nHL or better). If results are excluded where no-response was recorded for either ABR or behavioral measures, the above detectability rates improved such that 74% of the ABR thresholds are now within 10 dB of the behavioral thresholds, and only one difference score is greater than 30 dB.

The ABR threshold estimates appear to be equally accurate across the ages (at time of ABR) spanned by the subjects participating in this study. No significant relationship was found between the ABR minus behavioral threshold difference and the age at ABR evaluation (500 Hz: $r = 0.05$, df = 71, $p > 0.1$; 2000 Hz: $r = 0.18$, df = 94, $p > 0.05$; 4000 Hz: $r = 0.07$, df = 49, $p > 0.1$).

Table 5 (top) presents the results of the linear regression analyses performed on the data for all ears (normal and SNHL) for the ABR (Y) versus pure-tone behavioral (X) thresholds. These results show the same pattern as the threshold difference scores shown in Table 4. The high (>0.94) correlation coefficients at each fre-

quency indicate the good correspondence between the two thresholds, whereas the near unity (0.88-0.92 dB/dB) slopes indicate similar changes in both measures over a wide range of hearing loss. On the bottom of Table 5 are shown the results of the linear regression analyses when all no-response values have been removed. The primary change is to bring the slopes closer to unity and decrease the Y intercept. That is, the

Table 3. Tone-ABR thresholds and detectability for normal-hearing group[a].

	Frequency (Hz)		
	500	2000	4000
Mean threshold (dB nHL)	23.6	12.9	12.6
SD (dB)	9.9	9.0	8.1
N	25	28	23
Detectability (in percent):			
≤10 dB nHL	12	50	52
≤20 dB nHL	52	96	100
≤30 dB nHL	92	100	100
≤40 dB nHL	100	100	100

[a]Results from group with bilateral normal hearing, with data from only one ear per subject included.

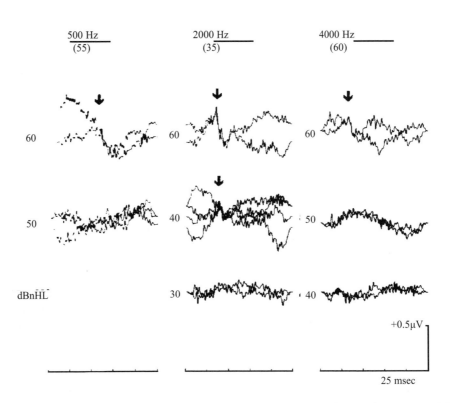

Figure 2. ABRs to brief tones in notched noise recorded from a 15-mo-old subject with a sensorineural hearing loss. Pure-tone behavioral thresholds, obtained at age 30 mo, are shown in parentheses. ABR thresholds were judged to be 60 dB nHL at 500 Hz, 40 dB nHL at 2000 Hz, and 60 dB nHL at 4000 Hz, all within 5 dB of the pure-tone behavioral thresholds. Stimulus intensities, in dB nHL, are plotted to the left of each waveform.

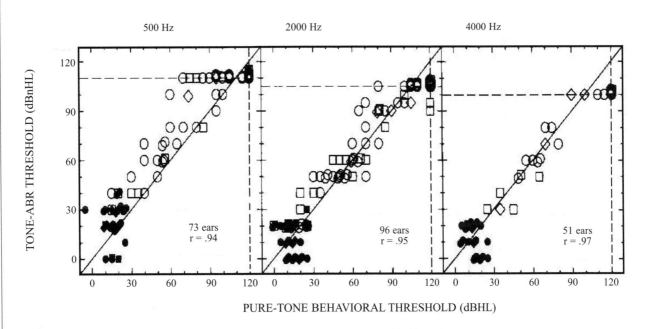

Figure 3. Threshold estimation using the ABR to 500 Hz (left), 2000 Hz (middle), and 4000 Hz (right) tones presented in notched noise. Results for normal-hearing (filled symbols) and sensorineural-impaired (open symbols) ears are plotted with three age ranges (at time of ABR) identified: 0-6 mo, diamonds; 7-48 mo, circles; 49 mo or greater squares. Shown also are the correlation coefficients for each frequency across all subjects and the number of ears involved. Dashed lines (-----) indicate the no-response range for each frequency and test, equivalent to the equipment maximum output plus 10 dB. Points plotted ∅ the dashed line indicate no-response for the measure. Points with multiple subjects have symbols offset (±1 dB per subject) to show clearly the overlapping data. Diagonals (solid lines) represent perfect ABR/behavioral threshold correspondence and are not regression lines.

Table 4. Difference scores (dB): tone-ABR threshold (dB nHL) minus pure-tone behavioral threshold (dB HL).

	Frequency (Hz)		
	500	2000	4000
Normal-hearing ears:			
Mean (dB)	6.8	−0.9	−1.3
SD	11.5	11.8	11.7
SNH ears:			
Mean (dB)	9.6	−0.2	−6.8
SD	13.4	12.0	11.0
All ears (normal and SNHL):			
Mean (dB)	8.6	−0.4	−4.3
SD	12.8	11.5	12.1

inclusion of the higher no-response levels for behavioral (120 dB HL) compared with ABR (100-110 dB nHL) results had distorted the slopes of the functions shown on the top of Table 5, making them less than unity.

The effect of "flat" versus "sloping" audiometric configuration was investigated next by dividing the ears with into three groups: (i) reverse slope SNHL (low-frequency behavioral thresholds at least 21 dB worse than high-frequency thresholds), $N = 4$; (ii) flat configuration (500 to 4000 Hz behavioral thresholds all within 20 dB of each other, including normal ears), $N = 96$; and (iii) high-frequency (HF) sloping SNHL (high-frequency behavioral thresholds at least 21 dB worse than low-frequency thresholds), $N = 44$. Across all three frequencies, high correlations remained between the ABR and behavioral thresholds (flat: $r = 0.91$; HF sloping: $r = 0.88$; reverse slope: too few data) and with no-response data excluded, slopes remained near unity. Differences between the ABR minus behavioral threshold difference scores for the three audiometric configurations were small and clinically insignificant (reverse slope: 8.8 ± 2.5 dB; flat: 0.7 ± 13.4 dB; HF sloping: 3.6 ± 14.5 dB), with these differences even smaller when no-response results were removed (reverse slope: 8.8 ± 2.5 dB; flat: 6.8 ± 10.4 dB; HF sloping: 2.1 ± 11.2 dB). Results separated for the three frequencies showed similar patterns, with no clear or statistically significant differences in the ABR minus behavioral threshold difference scores (no-response results excluded) between the flat and HF sloping configurations for 500 Hz (flat: 11.6 ± 11.9 dB; HF sloping: 10.7 ± 10.2 dB; $t = 0.17$, df = 24, $p > 0.1$), 2000 Hz (flat: 5.2 ± 9.2 dB; HF sloping: 1.8 ± 10.5 dB; $t = 1.17$, df = 45, $p > 0.1$), or 4000 Hz (flat: 0.6 ± 4.2 dB; HF sloping: $−6.7 \pm 8.2$ dB; $t = 2.00$, unequal variances adjusted df = 7.7, $p > 0.1$).

In clinical practice, ABR threshold(s) are used to estimate pure-tone behavioral thresholds. Presented below are equations for each frequency that provide these predictions from tone-ABR thresholds. The equations are derived from linear regression analyses of this study's data for all subjects (normal and impaired hearing), with no-response results excluded:

Discussion

The results of this study indicate that reasonably accurate estimates of 500, 2000, and 4000 Hz pure-tone behavioral thresholds in infants and young children can be obtained by recording the auditory brain stem response to brief tones presented in notched masking noise. In this study, the majority (66-74%) of the tone-ABR thresholds were within 10 dB of the subjects' pure-tone behavioral thresholds, and 93% were within 20 dB. These results are similar to results previously reported for this technique in adults with normal hearing (Picton et al, 1979; Purdy et al, 1989; Stapells et al, 1990) and adults with hearing loss (Picton et al, 1979; Stapells et al, 1990; Munnerley et al, 1991).

No differences were seen in the ABR minus behavioral threshold difference scores between the ears with normal hearing and those with SNHL. This is in contrast to previous studies in adults which have indicated that differences between brief-tone ABR and pure-tone behavioral thresholds are reduced in subjects

Table 5. Results of linear regression analyses[a] for each frequency: All ears (normal-hearing and SNHL).

	Frequency (Hz)		
	500	2000	4000
All data:			
Y intercept, dB nHL	13.11	6.27	3.22
Slope	0.92	0.88	0.85
Standard error of regression (dB)	12.50	10.95	9.75
Correlation coefficient (r)	0.94*	0.95*	0.97*
Number of ears	73	96	51
Excluding ABR or behavioral "No response":			
Y intercept, dB nHL	11.02	3.61	1.30
Slope	0.95	0.96	0.92
Standard error of regression (dB)	11.40	10.76	10.11
Correlation coefficient (r)	0.91*	0.93*	0.91*
Number of ears	52	76	39

[a] X = pure-tone behavioral threshold (dB HL); Y = tone-ABR threshold (dB nHL).
*$p < 0.001$ (one-tailed).

with SNHL compared to subjects with normal hearing (e.g., Picton et al, 1979; Stapells et al, 1990). This has been suggested to be due primarily to the influence (i.e., reduction of threshold) of temporal integration on pure-tone behavioral thresholds of subjects with normal hearing and the lack of such an influence for subjects with SNHL (Stapells et al, 1990). This lack of difference between pediatric subjects with normal hearing and SNHL may suggest poorer temporal integration in the pediatric population or may reflect attentional and motivational effects and the less reliable behavioral results seen in these young subjects (for reviews, see Werner & Rubel, 1992; Wilson & Thompson, 1984).

More generally, the results of this study complement and confirm the results of the large number of studies which have indicated that the ABRs to 500 to 4000 Hz brief tones (masked or nonmasked) are recordable down to acceptably low intensities and provide reasonable estimates of behavioral thresholds (e.g., Beattie & Boyd, 1985; Davis & Hirsh, 1979; Davis et al, 1985; Foxe & Stapells, 1993; Gorga et al, 1988; Gorga, Kaminski, Beauchaine, & Bergman, 1993; Hayes & Jerger, 1982; Hyde et al, 1987; Kileny & Magathan, 1987; Klein, 1983, 1984; Kodera et al, 1977; Kramer, 1992; McGee & Clemis, 1980; Munnerley et al, 1991; Picton et al, 1979; Purdy et al, 1989; Purdy & Abbas, 1989; Stapells & Picton, 1981; Stapells et al, 1990, 1994; Stapells & Ruben, 1989; Suzuki & Yamane, 1982; Suzuki et al, 1984; Suzuki et al, 1977). They are in contrast to a small number of studies that have indicated unsatisfactory results with tone-evoked ABRs, particularly at 500 Hz.

The results of the present study in infants and young children should lay to rest concerns about the applicability of previous adult tone ABR studies' results to the pediatric population. Many of the adult studies employed a near-40/sec stimulus rate (e.g., Picton et al, 1979; Purdy et al, 1989; Stapells et al, 1990; Munnerley et al, 1991) and must have contained both ABR wave V and the 40 Hz steady-state response (Galambos et al, 1981; Stapells, Linden, Suffield, Hamel, & Picton, 1984). Because infants and young children do not show the response amplitude enhancements seen in adults when stimuli are presented at about 40/sec (Stapells, Galambos, Costello & Makeig, 1988; Suzuki & Kobayashi, 1984), the possibility that the adult tone-ABR studies, especially for 500 Hz stimuli, would not be applicable to infants has recently been suggested (Picton, 1991; Picton, Champagne & Kellett, 1992; Stapells et al, 1990). In contrast to this concern, however, the majority (92 to 100%) of the infants and young children with normal hearing in the

500 Hz: Behavioral threshold (dB HL) = −3.25 + (0.87 * ABR threshold, dB nHL) ± 10.96 (SE, dB)
2000 Hz: Behavioral threshold (dB HL) = + 1.82 + (0.91 * ABR threshold, dB nHL) ±10.46 (SE, dB)
4000 Hz: Behavioral threshold (dB HL) = +4.12 + (0.90 * ABR threshold, dB nHL)± 10.00 (SE, dB)

present study produced clear ABRs to the tones at acceptably low stimulus intensities (≤30 dB nHL), and the ABR thresholds to tones in notched noise accurately estimated the pure-tone behavioral thresholds of the infants and children with SNHL. This was true for 500 Hz as well as for 2000 and 4000 Hz. The ABR to tones in notched-noise technique is thus applicable to pediatric clinical populations.

ABR thresholds to 500 Hz brief tones are elevated by about 10 dB compared to the thresholds for higher frequency stimuli. A −10 dB correction factor might therefore be appropriate when evaluating this frequency. Alternatively, the regression equations provided at the end of the "Results" section may be used to predict behavioral thresholds. In this study, the normal-hearing infants' mean 500 Hz ABR threshold was 23.6 dB nHL (48 dB pe SPL), compared with 12.9 dB nHL (39.0 dB pe SPL) for 2000 Hz and 12.6 dB nHL (41.6 dB pe SPL) for 4000 Hz. The 2000 and 4000 Hz normative results are similar to ours (Stapells et al, 1990) and others' previous studies (e.g., Purdy et al, 1989; Suzuki et al, 1984). The 500 Hz ABR normal thresholds are similar to our previous study in adults (Stapells et al, 1990), but are about 10 dB worse than others have reported (Purdy et al, 1989; Suzuki et al, 1984). We are currently compiling normative brief-tone ABR results in a larger sample of infants.

In general, brain stem responses to 500 Hz brief tones require more experience to recognize than do ABRs to higher frequency stimuli. These responses to low-frequency stimuli usually do not demonstrate the sharper peaks seen in response to 2000 or 4000 Hz brief tones. Because of this, they are also more susceptible to background electrical noise, whether of patient or environmental origin. This may be the reason for the one 500 Hz ABR overestimation of greater than 30 dB seen in this study (excluding data involving maximum or minimum stimulus intensities). In order to adequately assess 500 Hz thresholds using the ABR, patients must be sleeping quietly, clinicians must be experienced with these responses, and a sufficient number of trials and replications must be averaged to ensure low residual electrical noise levels in the waveforms.

Objective signal-to-noise measures (e.g., Elberling & Don, 1984; Picton et al, 1983) may help in this regard, although no studies of their application to tone-evoked ABRs have been published.

The clinical origin of the present study's infants and children with hearing loss likely added some variability to results as well as placing limitations on the number of thresholds and the minimum intensities tested. Further, the follow-up required for this and any study involving infants adds variability and inaccuracies often associated with the time lag between the ABR and behavioral measures.

One set of limitations is related to the behavioral audiometry. Because many of the behavioral audiograms were obtained at a later age, occasionally as much as 1 to 2 yr after the ABR assessment, there is the possibility that hearing thresholds worsened during this time. Other possible problems related to the different times for behavioral audiometry include: (i) variable procedures and criteria for behavioral audiometry (related to differing developmental levels), and (ii) differing middle ear status not revealed by acoustic immittance results or history (i.e., subclinical). Finally, it is likely that some of the infants' follow-up behavioral thresholds were still higher than adult levels due to their immaturity (i.e., in the 6- to 24-mo age range) (Wilson & Thompson, 1984). Keeping in mind these issues, the mean ABR behavioral time difference was 2.2 mo. Thus, for most subjects, results for both measures were obtained relatively close to each other. Further, we often had more than one set of behavioral results to confirm the reliability and stability of the behavioral results. Finally, infants with questionable or unobtainable acoustic immittance results were excluded.

Another set of limitations related to the clinical origin of the group with SNHL were the procedures necessitated by the need for specific clinical information. Because 2000 Hz thresholds were deemed most relevant, they were almost always obtained first, to the detriment of 500 and 4000 Hz. Thus, there are fewer data for these latter frequencies. We were careful, however, to ensure only data from quiet and sleeping subjects were included. Thus, some 500 and 4000 Hz data were excluded because the subject awoke during testing of these frequencies. Another limitation of these clinically obtained data concern our minimum intensities. Because of time constraints and need for clinical efficiency, we did not assess below 30 dB nHL for 500 Hz or below 20 dB nHL for 2000 and 4000 Hz in the group with SNHL. This affected results for a total of only nine data points (500 Hz: $N = 1$; 2000 Hz: $N = 7$; 4000 Hz: $N = 1$), but could have contributed to

the slightly less-than-unity slopes of the regression lines. Finally, there is an advantage to these clinical results: the subjects with SNHL probably slept quieter and longer because of their chloral hydrate-induced sleep and/or because of their being sleep deprived by parents anxious to obtain necessary clinical information. The infant and young children in the group with normal hearing were required to sleep naturally. They did not receive chloral hydrate and their parents did not always sleep deprive them for the study.

Considering the limitations outlined above, the results of the present study are very encouraging: the ABR to tones in notched-noise technique provided reasonably accurate estimations of these children and infants' pure-tone behavioral thresholds. Although this study did not compare these results to those obtained without notched-noise masking, previous studies have indicated the masking to be particularly useful for assessing hearing loss with rising or sloping configurations (Picton, 1978; Picton et al, 1979; Stapells et al, 1994). Because one does not know in advance the slope of an infant's audiometric configuration, notched-noise masking would be used for all cases.

There are likely to be improvements in techniques to obtain frequency-specific evoked potential thresholds in infants and young children. Nonlinear gating functions (e.g., Blackman window) improve the frequency specificity of the brief tones and may, therefore, improve the frequency specificity of the ABR elicited by these brief tones (Gorga & Thornton, 1989). ABR data supporting this suggestion, however, are currently lacking, and a recent paper by Purdy and Abbas (1989) reported no differences for linear versus Blackman tones. The use of such stimuli and the current availability of filters with very steep rejection slopes may allow for improvements in the notched-noise masker (e.g., notch width, noise intensity). Although not widely implemented on commercial equipment, notched-noise masking could be easily incorporated by equipment manufacturers if clinicians demanded this feature. Additionally, objective response measures are now available on commercial clinical equipment and should help in making decisions concerning response presence/absence, although research is required for their use with tone-evoked ABRs. Finally, although not reliably present in infants using 40/sec rates (Stapells et al, 1988; Suzuki & Kobayashi, 1984), brain stem steady-state responses to amplitude-modulated tones can be recorded in infants if very rapid (80 to 100/sec) modulation rates are used, allowing the use of rapid and objective, frequency-based, response measures (Aoyagi, Kiren, Kim, Suzuki, Fuse & Koike, 1993; Levi, Folsom, & Dobie, 1993).

In summary, the present study suggests that, using the ABR to brief tones in notched noise, reasonably accurate estimates of 500, 2000, and 4000 Hz pure-tone behavioral thresholds may be obtained in infants and young children with either normal hearing or sensorineural hearing loss. In the present study, 93% of the ABR thresholds were within 20 dB of the behavioral thresholds, and 80% were within 15 dB. No differences were seen as a result of age at ABR (1 week post-term to 8 yr) or as a result of audiometric configuration (rising, flat, sloping). Provided clinicians use appropriate protocols and have reasonable experience with tone-evoked ABRs, the technique is ready for clinical use, and should provide results that are more accurate than click-evoked ABR threshold results. Click ABR/ behavioral threshold regression equations, in addition to their lack of frequency specificity, show lower correlations, larger standard errors, and lower slopes (i.e., less than unity) compared with results for tone-evoked ABRs (Stapells et al, 1994). After several years of using both tone- and click-evoked ABR techniques in our clinic, we no longer use the click-evoked ABR for threshold estimations. Instead, we rely on ABR threshold\s for brief tones in notched noise to estimate hearing sensitivity in infants and young children.

Acknowledgments

This work was supported by United States Public Health Service, National Institute for Deafness and Other Communication Diseases (NIDCD) Clinical Center Grant 8 P50 DC00223, and by NICHD Mental Retardation Research Center Grant HD01799. Brett Martin was supported by a Graduate Research Assistantship from the City University of New York (CUNY).

Presented at the annual convention of the American Speech Language-Hearing Association, San Antonio, TX, November 22 1992, and at the 16th midwinter research meeting of the Association for Research in Otolaryngology, St. Petersburg Beach, FL, February 8, 1993.

Address correspondence to: David R. Stapells, Ph.D., Auditory Evoked Potential Laboratories, Albert Einstein College of Medicine, R.F. Kennedy Center Room 817, 1410 Pelham Parkway, Bronx, NY 10461.

Received May 5, 1994; accepted January 11, 1995

References

Aoyagi, M., Kiren, T., Kim, Y., Suzuki, Y., Fuse, T., & Koike, Y. (1993). Optimal modulation frequency for amplitude-modulation following response in young children during sleep. *Hearing Research,* 65, 253-261.

Beattie, R.C., & Boyd, R.L. (1985). Early/middle evoked potentials to tone bursts in quiet white noise, & notched noise. *Audiology,* 24, 406-419.

Davis, H., & Hirsh, S.K. (1976). The audiometric utility of the brain stem response to low-frequency sounds. *Audiology,* 15, 181-195.

Davis, H., & Hirsh, S.K. (1979). A slow brain stem response for low-frequency audiometry. *Audiology,* 18, 445-461.

Davis, H., Hirsh, S.K, Turpin, L.L., & Peacock, M.E. (1985). Threshold sensitivity, and frequency specificity in auditory brainstem response audiometry. *Audiology,* 24, 54-70.

Elberling, C., & Don, M. (1984). Quality estimation of averaged auditory brainstem responses. *Scandinavian Audiology*, 13, 187-197.

Foxe, J.J., & Stapells, D.R. (1993). Normal infant and adult auditory brainstem responses to bone-conducted tones. *Audiology,* 32, 95-109.

Galambos, R., Makeig, S., & Talmachoff, P.J. (1981). A 40-Hz auditory potential recorded from the human scalp. *Proceedings of the National Academy of Sciences U.S.A,* 78, 2643-2647.

Gorga, M.P., & Thornton, A.R. (1989). The choice of stimuli for ABR measurements. *Ear and Hearing,* 10, 217-230.

Gorga, M.P., Kaminski, J.R., Beauchaine, K.A., & Jesteadt, W. (1988). Auditory brainstem responses to tone bursts in normally hearing subjects. *Journal of Speech and Hearing Research,* 31, 87-97.

Gorga, M.P., Kaminski, J.R., Beauchaine, K.L., & Bergman, B.M. (1993). A comparison of auditory brain stem response thresholds, & latencies elicited by air-, & bone-conducted stimuli. *Ear and Hearing,* 14, 85-94.

Hayes, D., & Jerger, J. (1982). Auditory brainstem response (ABR) to tone pips: Results in normal and hearing-impaired subjects. *Scandinavian Audiology,* 11, 133-142.

Hyde, M.L. (1985). Frequency-specific BERA in infants. *Journal of Otolaryngology Supplement,* 14, 19-27.

Hyde, M.L., Matsumoto, N., & Alberti, P.W. (1987). The normative basis for click and frequency-specific BERA in high-risk infants. *Acta Oto-Laryngologica (Stockholm),* 103, 602-611.

Jerger, J. (1970). Clinical experience with impedance audiometry. *Archives of Otolaryngology, 92,* 311-324.

Kileny, P.R., & Magathan, M.G. (1987). Predictive value of ABR in infants and children with moderate to profound hearing impairments. *Ear and Hearing,* 8, 217-221.

Klein, A.J. (1983). Properties of the brain-stem response slow-wave component. I. Latency, amplitude, and threshold sensitivity. *Archives of Otolaryngology,* 109, 6-12.

Klein, A.J. (1984). Frequency and age-dependent auditory evoked potential thresholds in infants. *Hearing Research,* 16, 291-297.

Kodera, K., Yamane, H., Yamada, O., & Suzuki, J-I. (1977). Brain stem response audiometry at speech frequencies. *Audiology,* 16, 469-479.

Kramer, S.J. (1992). Frequency specific auditory brainstem responses to bone-conducted stimuli. *Audiology, 31,* 61-71.

Laukli, E. (1983) High-pass and notch noise masking in suprathreshold brainstem response audiometry. *Scandinavian Audiology, 12,* 109-115.

Laukli, E., Fjermedal, I., & Mair, I.W.S. (1988). Low-frequency auditory brainstem response threshold. *Scandinavian Audiology, 17,* 171-178.

Levi, E.C., Folsom, R.C., & Dobie, R.A. (1993). Amplitude-modulation following response (AMFR): Effects of modulation rate, carrier frequency, age, and state. *Hearing Research, 68,* 42-52.

Marchant, C.D., McMillan, P.M., Shurin, P.A., Turczyk, V.A., Feinstein, J.C., & Panek, D.M. (1986). Objective diagnosis of otitis media in early infancy by tympanometry and ipsilateral acoustic reflex thresholds. *Journal of Pediatrics, 109,* 590-595.

McGee, T.J., & Clemis, J.D. (1980). The approximation of audiometric thresholds by auditory brainstem responses. *Otolaryngology, Head and Neck Surgery, 88,* 295-303.

Munnerley, G.M., Greville, K.A., Purdy, S.C., & Keith, W.J. (1991). Frequency-specific auditory brainstem responses relationship to behavioral thresholds in cochlear-impaired adults. *Audiology, 30,* 25-32.

Pickles, J.O. (1986). *An introduction to the physiology of hearing* (2nd ed). London: Academic Press.

Picton, T.W. (1978). The strategy of evoked potential audiometry. In S.E. Gerber, & G.T. Mencher (Eds.), *Early diagnosis of hearing loss* (pp. 297-307). New York: Grune & Stratton.

Picton, T.W. (1991). Clinical usefulness of auditory evoked potentials: A critical evaluation. *Journal of Speech-Language Pathology and Audiology, 15,* 3-29.

Picton, T.W., & Durieux-Smith, A. (1988). Auditory evoked potentials in the assessment of hearing. *Neurologic Clinics, 6,* 791-808.

Picton, T.W., Ouellette, J., Hamel, G., & Smith, A.D. (1979). Brainstem evoked potentials to tone pips in notched noise. *Journal of Otolaryngology, 8,* 289-314.

Picton, T.W., Linden, R.D., Hamel, G., & Maru, J.T. (1983). Aspects of averaging. *Seminars in Hearing, 4,* 327-340.

Picton, T.W., Champagne, S.C., & Kellett, A.J.C. (1992). Human auditory evoked potentials recorded using maximum length sequences. *Electroencephalography and Clinical Neurophysiology, 84,* 90-100.

Purdy, S.C., & Abbas, P.J. (1989). Auditory brainstem response audiometry using linearly and Blackman-gated tone bursts. *ASHA, 31,* 115-116.

Purdy, S.C., Houghton, J.M., Keith, W.J., & Greville, K.A. (1989). Frequency-specific auditory brainstem responses. Effective masking levels and relationship to behavioural thresholds in normal hearing adults. *Audiology, 28,* 82-91.

Sohmer, H., & Kinarti, R. (1984). Survey of attempts to use auditory evoked potentials to obtain an audiogram. *British Journal of Audiology, 18,* 237-244.

Stapells, D.R. (1984). *Studies in evoked potential audiometry.* Unpublished doctoral dissertation, University of Ottawa, Ottawa, Ontario, Canada.

Stapells, D.R. (1989). Auditory brainstem response assessment of infants and children. *Seminars in Hearing, 10,* 229-251.

Stapells, D.R., & Picton, T.W. (1981). Technical aspects of brainstem evoked potential audiometry using tones. *Ear and Hearing, 2,* 20-29.

Stapells, D.R., & Ruben, R.J. (1989). Auditory brainstem responses to bone-conducted tones in infants. *Annals of Otology, Rhinology and Laryngology, 98,* 941-949.

Stapells, D.R., Linden, D., Suffield, J.B., Hamel, G., & Picton, T.W. (1984). Human auditory steady state potentials. *Ear and Hearing, 5,* 105-113.

Stapells, D.R., Galambos, R., Costello, J.A., & Makeig, S. (1988). Inconsistency of auditory middle latency and steady-state responses in infants. *Electroencephalography and Clinical Neurophysiology, 71,* 289-295.

Stapells, D.R., Picton, T.W., Durieux-Smith, A., Edwards, C.G., & Moran, L.M. (1990). Thresholds for short-latency auditory-evoked potentials to tones in notched noise in normal-hearing and hearing-impaired subjects. *Audiology, 29,* 262-274.

Stapells, D.R., Picton, T.W., & Durieux-Smith, A. (1994). Electrophysiologic measures of frequency-specific auditory function. In J.T. Jacobson (Ed.), *Principles and applications in auditory evoked potentials* (pp. 251-283). Needham Heights, MA: Allyn & Bacon.

Stockard, J.E., Stockard, J.J., & Coen, R.W. (1983). Auditory brain stem response variability in infants. *Ear and Hearing, 4,* 11-23.

Suzuki, J-I., & Yamane, H. (1982). The choice of stimulus in the auditory brainstem response test for neurological and audiological examinations. *Annals of the New York Academy of Sciences, 82,* 731-736.

Suzuki, J-I., Kodera, K., & Yamada, O. (1984). Brainstem response audiometry in newborns and hearing-impaired infants. In A. Starr, C. Rosenberg, M. Don, & H. Davis (Eds.), *Sensory evoked potentials. 1. An international conference on standards for auditory brainstem response (ABR) testing* (pp. 86-93). Milan, Italy: CRS Amplifon.

Suzuki, T., & Kobayashi, K (1984). An evaluation of 40-Hz event-related potentials in young children. *Audiology, 23,* 599-604.

Suzuki, T., Hirai, Y., & Horiuchi, K. (1977). Auditory brainstem responses to pure tone stimuli. *Scandinavian Audiology, 6,* 51-56.

Takagi, N., Suzuki, T., & Kobayashi, K. (1985). Effect of tone-burst frequency on fast and slow components of auditory brain-stem response. *Scandinavian Audiology, 14,* 75-79.

Werner, L.A., & Rubel, E.W. (Eds.) (1992). *Developmental psychoacoustics.* Washington, DC: American Psychological Association.

Wilson, W.R., & Thompson, G. (1984). Behavioral audiometry. In J. Jerger (Ed.) *Pediatric audiology* (pp. 1-44). San Diego: College-Hill Press.

Yamada, O., Yagi, T., Yamane, H., & Suzuki, J-I. (1975). Clinical evaluation of the auditory evoked brain stem response. *Auris-Nasus-Larynx,* 2, 97-105.

Auditory Brain Stem Responses to Air- and Bone-Conducted Clicks in the Audiological Assessment of At-Risk Infants

Edward Y. Yang, Andrew Stuart, George T. Mencher, Lenore S. Mencher, and Michael J. Vincer

School of Human Communication Disorders (E.Y.Y.) and Department of Psychology (A.S.), Dalhousie University, Halifax, NS, Canada; Nova Scotia Hearing and Speech Clinic (G.T.M., L.S.M.), Halifax, NS, Canada; and Grace Maternity Hospital and Department of Pediatrics (M.J.V.), Dalhousie University, Halifax, NS, Canada

Abstract

Auditory brain stem responses (ABRs) to air- and bone-conducted clicks were used to assess the auditory status of 170 at-risk neonates. During the perinatal period, 20.6% (35/170 cases) of the at-risk infants failed ABRs to air-conducted clicks at 30 dB nHL in at least one ear. Ear-specific results indicated an initial failure rate of 15.0% (51/340 ears). Approximately two-thirds (32/51 ears) of these initial failures showed purely conductive deficits, whereas the remaining one-third (19/51 ears) involved suspected sensorineural components. Follow-up audiological evaluations were performed for 87.1% (148 cases) of these at-risk infants at 4 mo and/or 1 yr corrected age. Based on the initial tests and follow-up assessments, the tentative operating characteristics of ABRs to both air- and bone-conducted clicks for identification of sensorineural deficits in at-risk neonates were calculated. It was found that the ABR to bone-conducted clicks yielded better specificity, predictive value of positive results, and overall efficiency. It is suggested that the ABR to bone-conducted stimuli should be viewed as a valuable addition in the assessment of cochlear reserve in infants who fail a newborn auditory screening to air-conducted stimuli.

The early identification of hearing loss in newborn infants has been advocated during the past four decades. Among several techniques studied for newborn auditory assessment during the past 15 yr, the ABR has emerged as the most consistent and reliable tool. The ABR provides an objective evaluation of the peripheral auditory status of infants (Hecox & Galambos, 1974). Currently, two methods are available for stimulus delivery: air conduction and bone conduction. The ABR using air-conducted stimuli has been widely used in testing pediatric populations, especially in audiological screening for at-risk infants (Alberti, Hyde, Riko, Corbin, & Abramovich, 1983; Durieux-Smith, Picton, Edwards, Goodman, & MacMurray, 1985; Galambos, Hicks, & Wilson, 1984; Jacobson & Morehouse, 1984; Schulman-Galambos & Galambos, 1979; Stein, Özdamar, Kraus, & Paton, 1983).

The incidence of severe to profound sensorineural hearing loss among at-risk infants has been reported to be approximately 2 to 4% compared to an incidence of 0.15% in an unselected population of newborn infants (Cox, Hack, & Metz, 1981). ABR abnormalities have

been found in 11 to 41% of initial testing in at-risk neonates (see Hall, Kripal, & Hepp, 1988, for a review). On follow-up evaluations at 3 to 12 mo of age, however, ABR abnormalities persist in only 2 to 5% of infants initially tested. The discrepancy between the confirmed sensorineural hearing loss at follow-up evaluation and that of initial ABR abnormalities during the perinatal period has raised notable clinical concerns regarding the effectiveness of ABR as a screening tool.

A number of factors have been speculated to account for the wide range in reported incidence of ABR abnormalities at initial screenings during the perinatal period (Hall et al, 1988). Of these factors, transient middle ear disorders have received considerable attention. The high incidence of middle ear effusion among neonatal intensive care unit infants (Balkany, Berman, Simmons, & Jafek, 1978; Derkay, Bluestone, Thompson, Stephenson, & Kardtzke, 1988; McLellan, Strong, Johnson, & Dent, 1962; Paradise, 1981; Proctor & Kennedy, 1990; Stockard & Curran, 1990) and the presence of residual substance and fluid in the middle ear cavity of newborn infants (Buch & Jorgensen, 1964; Proctor, 1964) have been suggested as potential contributors to the so called "inaccuracy" in ABR newborn auditory screening. Unfortunately, the

Reprinted by permission of authors and Williams & Wilkins. Copyright 1993.
Ear & Hearing, 14, No. 3, pp. 175-182.

conventional indices for detecting middle ear pathology such as otoscopic examination and tympanometry have proven to be difficult in the case of the former (Berman, Balkany, & Simmons, 1978; Groothius, 1982; Schreiner & Kiesling, 1981) and unreliable in the latter (Paradise, Smith, & Bluestone, 1979; Schwartz & Schwartz, 1978) with newborn infants. What remains, therefore, is the continuing challenge of distinguishing between ABR abnormalities due to conductive versus sensorineural losses in neonates.

In an effort to differentiate sensorineural from conductive hearing impairments and thereby improving the efficiency of ABR screening methods, the use of ABR to bone-conducted stimuli has been suggested (Hall, 1992; Hooks & Weber, 1984; Nousak & Stapells, 1992; Stapells, 1989; Stapells & Ruben, 1989; Stuart, Yang, & Stenstrom, 1990; Stuart, Yang, Stenstrom, & Reindorp, 1993; Weber, 1983; Yang, Rupert, & Moushegian, 1987; Yang & Stuart, 1990; Yang, Stuart, Stenstrom, & Green, 1993; Yang, Stuart, Stenstrom, & Hollett, 1991). To date, the contribution of ABR to bone-conducted stimuli in auditory screening of at-risk neonates has not been reported. Accordingly, the purpose of the present study was to investigate the use of ABRs to air- and bone-conducted clicks in the audiological assessment of at-risk infants.

Method

Subjects

One hundred and forty normal full-term newborn infants served as the control group. These infants presented the following criteria: (1) gestational age between 38 and 42 weeks, (2) no risk for hearing loss (Joint Committee on Infant Hearing, 1982), (3) Apgar scores of 8 or higher at l and 5 min, (4) birth weight no less than 2500 g, and (5) physically and neurologically normal as judged by pediatric house staff. Thirty-four of these subjects were followed at 4 mo (±2 weeks) of age and 29 at l yr (±l mo) of age. One hundred and seventy newborn infants at risk for hearing loss (Joint Committee on Infant Hearing, 1982) were tested in the Grace Maternity Hospital and Izaak Walton Killam Hospital for Children, Halifax, Nova Scotia. Among these at-risk newborn infants, 76 were selected from the Special Neonatal Care Unit (SNCU) and 94 were recruited from the well baby nursery (WBN). These at-risk infants were initially tested at 38 to 42 weeks conceptional age and were retested when they reached 4 mo and/or l yr corrected age. All at-risk infants tested in the neonatal period were medically stable and tested just before discharge.

Apparatus and Procedures

Each infant was tested using a Nicolet Compact Auditory Evoked Potential System. The click stimuli were generated by 100 μsec rectangular voltage pulses and delivered through a bone vibrator (Radioear Model B-70B) and an insert earphone (Nicolet Model TIP-300) coupled to an Immittance Tip Adapter (Nicolet Model 123-717900) and Infant Ear Tip (Nicolet Model 842-507300). Signal calibration of air- and bone-conducted click has been reported elsewhere (Stuart et al, 1990, 1993; Yang & Stuart, 1990; Yang et al, 1991, 1993). Click stimuli were presented at a rate of 57.7/sec with alternating initial phase. The stimulus intensity levels for bone conduction were 15 and 30 dB nHL, and for air conduction were 30, 45, and 60 dB nHL. In cases of at-risk infants, where no detectable response to air-conducted clicks at 60 dB nHL was evident, ABR threshold searches were undertaken.

For bone-conducted stimulus delivery, an elastic band with Velcro was used to hold the vibrator in place. The elastic band was adjusted to maintain a vibrator to head coupling force of 425 ± 25 g. This was achieved by first attaching a fine nylon monofilament under the single casing screw head at the distal end of the vibrator and then looping and tying it around the transducer cord adjacent to the proximal end of the vibrator. The elastic band was then positioned around the infant's head under the loop of nylon monofilament and against the bone vibrator. A spring scale (Ohaus Model 8014) was then attached to the monofilament and the vibrator was then manually pulled away from the scalp; coupling force was then measured at the point when the vibrator cleared and became flush with the scalp.

Three gold-plated cup electrodes, consisting of one (non-inverting) attached to the high forehead, one (inverting) attached to the inferior ipsilateral postauricular area, and one (common) attached to the inferior contralateral postauricular area, were used. Interelectrode impedance was maintained below 5 kohm. The recorded EEG was amplified 10^5 times and band-pass filtered (30-3000 Hz). EEG samples exceeding ±25 mV were rejected. A total of 2048 samples were averaged and replicated for each stimulus condition. Replication was defined as two or more waveforms with identifiable wave V peaks within 0.15 msec from one trial to the next. Analysis time was 15 msec poststimulus onset with a sampling frequency of 33 kHz.

Neonates were tested shortly after feeding while in natural sleep in quiet rooms adjacent to the newborn nurseries. Typical testing time was approximately 45 to 60 min. Follow-up ABR retests were performed in a

Table 1. Means (M), (SD), and upper limits of ABR wave V latencies (msec) from the normal control groups of neonates *(n = 140)*, 4 mo *(n = 34)*, and 1 yr olds *(n = 29)*.[a]

| | | Stimulus Intensity (dB nHL) | | | | |
| | | Bone Conduction | | Air Conduction | | |
		15	30	30	45	60
Neonates	M	9.36	8.67	8.59	8.07	7.62
	SD	(0.51)	(0.43)	(0.34)	(0.35)	(0.33)
	Upper limit	10.38	9.53	9.27	8.77	8.28
4 mo	M	8.39	7.76	7.68	7.18	6.76
	SD	(0.37)	(0.33)	(0.30)	(0.23)	(0.22)
	Upper limit	9.13	8.42	8.28	7.64	7.20
1 yr	M	8.20	7.44	7.26	6.79	6.28
	SD	(0.27)	(0.24)	(0.23)	(0.18)	(0.22)
	Upper limit	8.74	7.92	7.72	7.15	6.72

[a]Note: An upper limit was defined as the mean plus 2 SD.

quiet room while infants were in natural sleep or resting quietly. Visual reinforcement audiometry was performed in an audiometric test suite.

Results

Normative ABR Data

ABRs to air- and bone-conducted clicks were obtained from the left ear of all normal control infants. Absolute ABR wave V latencies were measured from all recordings. Normative ABR wave V latencies were collected from the normal full-term newborn infants (38-42 weeks gestational age), 4 mo (±2 weeks) old, and 1 yr (±1 month) old infants. The means of the ABR wave V latencies for each stimulus condition were calculated from the three normal control groups and are displayed in Table 1.

Risk Factors Among the SNCU and WBN Infants

Among 170 at-risk newborn infants who received an initial ABR assessment, 76 were recruited from the SNCU and 94 were from the WBN. An analysis of at-risk factors in infants of the SNCU and WBN is displayed in Figure 1. Four cases of multiply at-risk infants from the WBN involved a combination of both at-risk factors of family history and congenital anomaly. A breakdown of risk factors among the 13 multiply at-risk infants from the SNCU is displayed in Table 2.

Findings of Initial ABR Assessments for At-Risk Neonates

During the perinatal period, an infant was considered to pass the initial screening if his/ her ABR, elicit-

ed from air-conducted click stimuli at 30 dB nHL, showed an identifiable and replicable wave V with a latency within +2 SD of the mean of the age-appropriate norm in both ears. Ear-specific findings are reported because the technique used in the present study permitted the assessment of individual ears.

Initially, abnormal ABR findings in each ear were classified based on the ABR threshold to air-conducted click stimuli. The degree of auditory deficit was estimated as mild to moderate or severe to profound. Mild to moderate deficits were identified among ears that exhibited: (1) an identifiable and replicable ABR wave V at 30, 45, or 60 dB nHL with a latency exceeding normal limits; or (2) an identifiable and replicable ABR wave V at 45 and/or 60 dB nHL, but not at 30 dB nHL (i.e., the ABR threshold was equal to or better than 60 dB nHL). Severe to profound deficits were identified among ears with an unidentifiable ABR wave V at 60 dB nHL (i.e., the ABR threshold was worse than 60 dB nHL). Furthermore, based on the contrast of ABR findings between air- and bone-con-

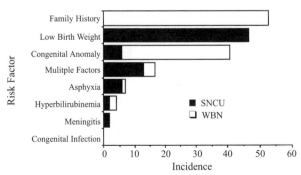

Figure 1. Incidence of at-risk factors (Joint Committee on Infant Hearing, 1982) among neonates from the SNCU and WBN.

Table 2. Incidence of risk factors in 13 multiply at-risk infants from the SNCU.

Risk Factor	Incidence
Family history	3
Congenital anomaly	4
Low birth weight	10
Hyperbilirubinemia	4
Meningitis	4
Congenital infection	1
Asphyxia	4

ducted stimuli (i.e., air-bone gap), the type of auditory deficit was classified as sensorineural, conductive, or mixed. Ears that exhibited severe to profound deficits with no detectable ABR to bone-conducted stimuli at the output limitation of the bone vibrator (approximately 45-50 dB nHL) were classified as severe to profound sensorineural deficits. It was recognized, however, that due to the limited dynamic range of the bone-conducted click stimuli, a conductive component could not be ruled out in these cases.

During the perinatal period, 35 at-risk infants failed ABR screening with air-conducted clicks at 30 dB nHL in at least one ear. This represented an initial failure rate of 20.6% by case. Ear-specific results indicated an initial failure rate of 15.0% (51/340). A summary of these findings, indicating type and estimated degree of auditory deficits, is displayed in Table 3.

Sensorineural, mixed, and conductive deficits represented 4.1, 1.5, and 9.4% of total ears tested, respectively. It is of particular interest that 32 of 51 ears, or approximately 63%, that failed the initial ABR exhibited purely conductive deficits. In contrast, the incidence of ears with sensorineural deficits during perinatal period was 5.6% (19/340 ears).

Findings of Follow-Up Assessments for At-Risk Infants

Among 170 at-risk infants who received initial ABR testings, 148 cases have received follow-up retests at 4 mo and/or 1 yr corrected age. This represents a follow-up rate of 87.1%. Retests were obtained from only one ear with two separate subjects, and, therefore, 294 of a possible 296 ears are represented. The summary at-risk infant follow-up status is displayed in Table 4.

Analyzed findings of follow-up assessments are presented with respect to the presence of conductive or sensorineural deficits. It should be noted that the following estimates of the incidence of hearing loss are conservative, as some infants lost to follow-up may have exhibited a hearing loss.

Conductive Deficits

During the perinatal period, 37 ears were found to exhibit a conductive component (i.e., conductive or mixed deficits) in at least one ear. Follow-up retests were performed in 33 of 37 involved ears. Varying results were found when comparing the initial test and follow-up retests.

Seventeen ears (51.5%) exhibited a conductive deficit upon follow-up retest. In one case, a conductive deficit that resolved at the 4 mo retest recurred at the 1 yr retest. Sixteen ears (48.1%) exhibited no conductive component upon follow-up retests. Thirty-seven of 294 ears (12.6%) receiving retests that presented with no conductive deficit during the perinatal period acquired conductive deficits.

Sensorineural Deficits

All 19 ears that presented with sensorineural deficits during the perinatal period received at least one follow-up retest. Follow-up results indicated that 17 (89.5%) ears showed persistent sensorineural deficits, whereas two (10.5%) ears from two separate cases exhibited apparent normal cochlear reserve. Of the infants showing apparent changes in cochlear, one presented with severe asphyxia during the perinatal

Table 3. Incidence of hearing deficits, by type and estimated degree, in total number of ears of at-risk newborn infants during the perinatal period ($n = 340$).

Estimated Degree of Deficit	Type of Deficit							
	Sensorineural		Mixed		Conductive		Total	
	n	(%)	n	(%)	n	(%)	n	(%)
Mild to moderate	10	(2.9)	3	(0.9)	30	(8.8)	43	(12.6)
Severe to profound	4[a]	(1.2)	2	(0.6)	2	(0.6)	8	(2.4)
Total	14	(4.1)	5	(1.5)	32	(9.4)	51	(15.0)

[a]Cannot rule out a conductive component.

Table 4. Summary of at-risk infant follow-up status.

Status	n	(%)
Complete data	148	(87.1)
Lost	13	(7.6)
Withdrew from study	3	(1.8)
Could not test	3	(1.8)
Repeated broken appointment	2	(1.2)
Deceased	1	(0.6)
Total	170	(100)

period and the other presented with low birth weight and suffered from fetal alcohol syndrome.

Follow-up retests in 275 ears, with no sensorineural deficits during perinatal period, indicate that three (1.1%) ears from three separate cases displayed sensorineural deficits. Ironically, these ears exhibited conductive deficits during the perinatal period. Test results from these ears are displayed in Table 5.

Tentative Operating Characteristics of ABRs to Air- and Bone-Conducted Clicks in Auditory Screening for Congenital Sensorineural Deficits

One hundred and forty-seven at-risk infants representing 294 ears were evaluated with initial ABR screening and follow-up retests. Based on these findings, the potential use of the ABR to air- and bone-conducted clicks as newborn screening tools for identification of congenital sensorineural deficits was evaluated. Thirty dB nHL was used as the pass/fail "cutoff" point in both cases. The findings regarding the tentative operating characteristics with ABRs to air- and bone-conducted clicks are presented in Tables 6 and 7, respectively.

Discussion

Findings from the present study suggest that the ABR to bone-conducted clicks is feasible and reliable in identification of congenital sensorineural deficits in at-risk neonates. The advantage of applying ABR to bone-conducted stimuli in testing newborn infants is obvious. First, such an approach can differentiate sensorineural from conductive deficits in neonates who fail an ABR screening using air-conducted stimuli, and hence, can provide valuable information regarding the strategy for further management. Second, the timing of identification of substantial sensorineural deficits can be advanced to the earliest stage of life, thus allowing clinicians a precious period for preparing and administering early intervention. This constitutes a substantial advantage in patient management compared to the sug-

gestion of initial testing at 3 to 5 mo corrected age (Durieux-Smith, Picton, Edwards, MacMurray, & Goodman, 1987; Hyde, Riko, Corbin, Moroso, & Alberti, 1984). Further, it may be psychologically less stressful for parents to be provided with more audiological information than to wait for follow-up or initial testing when at-risk infants are 3 to 5 mo corrected age.

The tentative operating characteristics provided from the present study offer an initial insight in the possible use of the ABR to bone-conducted clicks as opposed to air-conducted clicks in newborn auditory screening. It is recognized, however, that these figures need to be cautiously interpreted as "the practice of validating neonatal or infant ABR data using a subsequent ABR test as the 'gold standard' addresses the reproducibility of ABR results but not their accuracy as estimators of true hearing threshold" (Hyde, Riko, & Malizia, 1990, p. 60). The results of the comparison between ABRs to air- and bone-conducted clicks at 30 dB nHL for identification of sensorineural deficits in at-risk neonates suggest that the latter yielded better specificity, predictive value of positive results, and overall efficiency, albeit slightly worse sensitivity and predictive value of negative results. However, it is speculated that the 100% sensitivity obtained from ABRs to air-conducted stimuli may be a consequence of sampling bias. Specifically, all three ears with possible late onset sensorineural deficits happen to exhibit conductive deficits during the perinatal period.

Based on the findings of the present study, the ABR to bone-conducted clicks appears to be an ideal alternative for newborn auditory screening. It is suggested, however, that the ABR to bone-conducted stimuli be viewed as a valuable addition in the assessment of cochlear reserve in infants who fail newborn auditory screening to air-conducted stimuli. In this case, however, the ABR to bone-conducted stimuli does not fit the customary definition of a screening tool, but rather serves as an extremely powerful diagnostic tool.

Table 5. Test results of ears exhibiting sensorineural deficits upon follow-up retests with initial tests indicating normal cochlear reserve.[a]

		Auditory Status		
Case	Risk Factor	Perinatal	4 mo	1 yr
1	Congenital anomaly	SC	SC	SM
2	Congenital anomaly	MC	MS	MS
3	Family history	MC	MM	MM

[a]Note: SC, severe to profound conductive deficit; MC, mild to moderate conductive deficit; SM, severe to profound mixed deficit; MM, mild to moderate mixed deficit; MS, mild to moderate sensorineural deficit.

Table 6. Tentative operating characteristics of the ABR to air-conducted clicks at 30 dB nHL as decision criterion for sensorineural (SN) deficit in the auditory screening of at-risk newborn infants (*n* = 294).[a]

ABR Screening	Follow-Up Findings		
	SN Deficit	No SN Deficit	Total
Fail	20	27	47
Pass	0	247	247
Total	20	274	294

[a]Note: sensitivity = 100.0%; specificity = 90.1%; predictive value of positive result = 42.6%; predictive value of negative result = 100.0%; and overall efficiency of the test = 90.8%.

Table 7. Tentative operating characteristics of the ABR to bone-conducted clicks at 30 dB nHL as decision criterion for sensorineural (SN) deficit in the auditory screening of at-risk newborn infants (*n* = 294).[a]

ABR Screening	Follow-Up Findings		
	SN Deficit	No SN Deficit	Total
Fail	17	2	19
Pass	3	272	275
Total	20	274	294

[a]Note: sensitivity = 85.0%; specificity = 99.3%; predictive value of positive result = 89.5%; predictive value of negative result = 98.9%; and overall efficiency of the test = 98.3%.

In this capacity, it needs to be recognized that the bone conduction technique reported herein and elsewhere in the literature (Nousak & Stapells, 1992; Stuart et al, 1990, 1993; Yang et al, 1987, 1991, 1993; Yang & Stuart, 1990) requires an appreciation for and considerable attention paid to controlled stimulus delivery as well additional testing time.*

Two points need to be acknowledged further. The first is that ABRs elicited by click stimuli reflect auditory sensitivity up to the brain stem level in the frequency range between 1000 and 4000 Hz. Therefore, the use of click-evoked ABR cannot provide an estimation of low-frequency threshold nor information concerning hearing perception. Second, the recognized differences in amplitude spectra for air- and bone-conducted clicks may be problematic in differential diagnosis (Weber, 1983). It has been speculated that the differences in ABRs to air- and bone-conducted clicks may be attributed to these spectral differences and not a conductive deficit. "Marked differences in hearing sensitivity in the 1500 and 300 Hz regions can also produce similar differences between air and bone conducted ABRs" (Weber, 1983, p. 348). However, observations of: (1) air-conducted click spectra being altered by ear canal resonances (Johnson & Nelson, 1991) and residual tissue and fluid in the middle ear cavity (Yang et al, 1987); (2) filter effects of the infant cranium

toward bone-conducted stimuli (Nousak & Stapells, 1992); and (3) the questioned lack of high-frequency responsiveness of the cochlea (Rubel, Born, Dietch, & Durham, 1984) suggest that the observed amplitude spectra differences may be moot. Regardless, considering cautiously the above two points, one can easily recognize that a long-term follow-up program is indispensable so that reliable audiometric measures can be obtained and used as a gold standard to evaluate the effectiveness of early tests in the at-risk pediatric population (Durieux-Smith, Picton, Bernard, MacMurray, & Goodman, 1991; Hyde et al, 1990; Hyde, Malizia, Riko, & Alberti, 1991).

The finding of the incidence of sensorineural deficits of 5.6% is consistent with previous reports in the literature (Cox, Hack, & Metz, 1984; Dennis, Shelden, Toubas, & McCaffee, 1984; Galambos et al, 1984; Jacobson & Morehouse, 1984; Sanders, Durieux-Smith, Hyde, Jacobson, Kileny, & Murnane, 1985; Shannon, Felix, Krumholz, Goldstein, & Harris, 1984; Stein et al, 1983). Among initial failures, approximately two-thirds of ears exhibited conductive deficits. Such a finding supports the suggestion that middle ear involvement contributes to high initial failure rates during initial ABR screenings.

Findings from initial tests and follow-up assessments suggest that conductive deficits in at-risk infants may be either transient or persistent. It is unclear, however, whether those persistent conductive deficits that presented at the initial assessment and upon follow-up retest in fact persisted or resolved and recurred. Transient conductive deficits, on the other hand, may further be classified as resolved, acquired, or fluctuating. Conductive deficits that were present at initial tests and not at follow-up retests may be classified as resolved. However, these deficits may have recurred between the test periods, and consequently may not have been detected. Acquired conductive deficits were those that presented at retest among infants who initially displayed no conductive component during the initial ABR testing. Fluctuating conductive deficits were those that presented among infants who initially exhibited conductive components that were resolved at the 4 mo retest only to recur at the 1 yr retest.

Findings from the initial test and follow-up assessment also suggest that some ears may have shown a change in cochlear reserve with either an apparent recovery or deterioration. It is speculated that a number of factors may have attributed to such observations among these at-risk infants. The first is that these

---

*Acquiring ABRs to bone-conducted clicks typically requires approximately an additional 15 to 20 min with a cooperative infant. This includes testing both ears at two intensities (e.g., 15 and 30 dB nHL).

infants may have experienced true changes in cochlear reserve. The second is a possible technical error in the control of the delivery of the bone-conducted stimulus. That is, improper bone vibrator coupling force or placement (Stuart et al, 1990; Yang et al, 1991) may have led to a misinterpretation of the cochlear reserve at the initial assessment. However, during testing sessions, repeated measures and recordings were routinely performed in ears that exhibited abnormal findings of ABRs to bone-conducted clicks. Further, it has been shown that there is no significant difference in ABRs from test to retest with controlled bone-conducted signal delivery (Yang et al, 1993). Hence, it is argued that the likelihood of a technical error was minimal. Third, it may be the case that these newborn infants presented with an atypical oriented petrosal, squamosal, and/or petrosquamosal suture (see Stuart et al, 1990, for a review of underlying anatomical structures relevant to bone-conducted signal delivery in neonates). The structural variations may have led to ineffective (in the case of suspected abnormal cochlear reserve) or unusually effective (in the case of apparent normal cochlear reserve) bone-conducted stimulus delivery to the cochlear during the perinatal period. These phenomena may have also led to misinterpretations of cochlear reserve at the initial assessment. Finally, it may be an occurrence of type I or type II errors (i.e., false-positive or false-negative for sensorineural deficits) with ABR to bone-conducted clicks testing during the perinatal period.

In conclusion, findings of the present study suggest that sensorineural deficits in at-risk newborn and young infants may be detected using ABR to bone-conducted stimuli. When abnormal ABR to air-conducted stimuli from at-risk newborn infants is indicated, ABR to bone-conducted stimuli is recommended to assess the cochlear reserve, provided normative data are established in a particular clinical setting.

References

Alberti, P.W., Hyde, M.L., Riko, K., Corbin, H., and Abramovich, S. An evaluation of BERA for hearing screening in high-risk neonates. *Laryngoscope* 1983;93:1115-1121.

Balkany, T.J., Berman, S.A., Simmons, M.A., and Jafek, B.W. Middle ear effusion in neonates. *Laryngoscope* 1978;88:398-405.

Berman, S.A., Balkany, T.J., and Simmons, M.A. Otitis media in the neonatal intensive care unit. *Pediatrics* 1978;62:198-201.

Buch, N.H., and Jorgensen, M.B. Embryonic connective tissue in the tympanic cavity of the fetus and newborn. *Acta Otol* 1964;58:111-126.

Cox, L.C., Hack, M., and Metz, D.A. Auditory brainstem response audiometry in the premature infant population. *Int J Pediatr Otorhinolaryngol* 1981;3:213-224.

Cox, L.C., Hack, M., and Metz, D.A. Auditory brainstem response abnormalities in the very low birthweight infants: Incidence and risk factors. *Ear Hear* 1984;4:47-51.

Dennis, J.M., Shelden, R., Toubas, P., and McCaffee, M.A. Identification of hearing loss in the neonatal intensive care unit population. *Am J Otol* 1984;5:201-205.

Derkay, C.S., Bluestone, C.D., Thompson, A.E., Stephenson, J.S., and Kardtzke, D. Otitis media in the pediatric intensive care unit: A prospective study of its incidence, prevalence, bacteriology, etiology and treatment. *Am Otol Rhinol Laryngol* 1988;97(Suppl 133):56-57.

Durieux-Smith, A., Picton, T.W., Bernard, P., MacMurray, B., and Goodman, J.T. Prognostic validity of brainstem electric response audiometry in infants of a neonatal intensive care unit. *Audiology* 1991;30:249-265.

Durieux-Smith, A., Picton, T.W., Edwards, C., Goodman, J.T., and MacMurray, B. The Crib-O-Gram in the NICU: An evaluation based on brain stem electric response audiometry. *Ear Hear* 1985;6: 20-24.

Durieux-Smith, A., Picton, T.W., Edwards, C.G., MacMurray, B., and Goodman, J.T. Brainstem electric-response audiometry in infants of a neonatal intensive care unit. *Audiology* 1987;26:284- 297.

Galambos, R., Hicks, G.E., and Wilson, M.J. The auditory brainstem response reliably predicts hearing loss in graduates of tertiary intensive care nursery. *Ear Hear* 1984;5:254-260.

Groothius, J.R. Medical treatment of otitis media: The pediatrician's point of view. *Semin Speech Lang Hear* 1982;3:324-328.

Hall, J.W. ABR 20 years later: Answers to 5 common questions. *Hear J* 1992;45(2):22-27.

Hall, J.W., Kripal, J.P., and Hepp, T. Newborn hearing screening with auditory brainstem response: Measurement problems and solutions. *Semin Hear* 1988;9:15-32.

Hecox, K., and Galambos, R. Brainstem auditory evoked responses in human infants and adults. *Arch Otolaryngol* 1974;99:30-33.

Hooks, R.G., and Weber, B.A. Auditory brainstem responses of premature infants to bone conducted stimuli: A feasibility study. *Ear Hear* 1984;5: 42-46.

Hyde, M.L., Malizia, K., Riko, K., and Alberti, P.W. Audiometric estimation error with ABR in high risk infants. *Acta Otol* 1991;111:212-219.

Hyde, M.L., Riko, K., Corbin, H., Moroso, M., and Alberti P. A neonatal hearing screening research program using brainstem electric response audiometry. *J Otolaryngol* 1984;13:49-54.

Hyde, M.L., Riko, K., and Malizia, K. Audiometric accuracy of the click ABR in infants at risk for hearing loss. *J Am Acad Audiol* 1990;1:59-66.

Jacobson, J.T., and Morehouse CR. A comparison of auditory brainstem response and behavioral screening in high-risk and normal newborn infants. *Ear Hear* 1984;5:247-253.

Johnson, S.E., and Nelson, P.B. Real ear measures of auditory brain stem response click spectra in infants and adults. *Ear Hear* 1991;12:180-183.

Joint Committee on Infant Hearing. Position statement. *Asha* 1982;24:1017-1018.

McLellan, M.S., Strong, J.D., Johnson, Q.R., and Dent, J.H. Otitis media in premature infants: A histopathologic study. *J Pediatr* 1962;61:53-57.

Nousak, J.K., and Stapells, D. Frequency specificity of the auditory brain stem response to bone-conducted tones in infants and adults. *Ear Hear* 1992;13:87-95.

Paradise, J.L. Otitis media during early life: How hazardous to development? A critical review of the evidence. *Pediatrics* 1981;68:869-873.

Paradise, J.L., Smith, C.G., and Bluestone, C.D. Tympanometric detection of middle ear effusion in infants and young children. *Pediatrics* 1979;58:198-210.

Proctor, B. The development of the middle ear space and their surgical significance. *J Laryngol Otol* 1964;78:631-648.

Proctor, L.R., and Kennedy, D.W. High-risk newborns who failed hearing screening: Implications of otological problems. *Semin Hear* 1990;11(2): 167-176.

Rubel, E.W., Born, D.E., Dietch, J.S., and Durham, D. Recent advances toward understanding auditory system development. In Berlin, C.I., Ed. *Hearing Science*. San Diego: College Hill Press, 1984:109-158.

Sanders, R., Durieux-Smith, A., Hyde, M., Jacobson, J., Kileny, P., and Murnane, O. Incidence of hearing loss in high-risk and intensive care nursery infants. *J Otolaryngol* 1985;14:28-33.

Schreiner, R.L., and Kiesling, J.A., Eds. The Newborn with Respiratory Distress: *A Practical Approach to Management*. New York: Raven Press, 1981.

Schulman-Galambos, C., and Galambos, R. Brain stem evoked response audiometry in newborn hearing screening. *Arch Otolaryngol* 1979;105: 86-90.

Schwartz, D.M., and Schwartz, R.H. Acoustic impedance and otoscopic findings in young children with Down's syndrome. *Arch Otol* 1978;104:652-656.

Shannon, D.A., Felix, J.K., Krumholz, A., Goldstein, P.J., and Harris, K.C. Hearing screening of high-risk newborns with brainstem auditory evoked potentials: A follow-up study. *Pediatrics* 1984;73: 22-26.

Stapells, D.R. Auditory brainstem response assessment of infants and children. *Semin Hear* 1989; 10:229-251.

Stapells, D.R., and Ruben, R.J. Auditory brain stem responses to bone-conducted tones in infants. *Ann Otol Rhinol Laryngol* 1989;98:941-949.

Stein, L., Özdamar, O., Kraus, N., and Paton, J. Follow-up of infants screened by auditory brainstem response in the neonatal intensive care unit. *J Pediatr* 1983;103:447-453.

Stockard, J.E., and Curran, J.S. Transient elevation of threshold of the neonatal auditory brain stem response. *Ear Hear* 1990;11:21-28.

Stuart, A., Yang, E.Y., and Stenstrom, R. Effect of temporal area bone vibrator placement on auditory brainstem response in newborn infants. *Ear Hear* 1990;11:262-269.

Stuart, A., Yang, E.Y., Stenstrom, R., and Reindorp, A.G. Auditory brainstem response thresholds to air and bone conducted clicks in neonates and adults. *Am J Otol* 1993;14:176-182.

Weber, B.A. Masking and bone conduction testing in brainstem response audiometry. *Semin Hear* 1983;4:342-352.

Yang, E.Y., Rupert, A.L., and Moushegian, G. A developmental study of bone conduction auditory brainstem response in infants. *Ear Hear* 1987;8: 244-251.

Yang, E.Y., and Stuart, A. A method of auditory brainstem response to bone-conducted clicks in testing infants. *J Sp-Lang Path Audiol* 1990;14 (4):69-76.

Yang, E.Y., Stuart, A., Stenstrom, R., and Green, W.B. Test-retest variability of the auditory brainstem response to bone conducted clicks in newborn infants. *Audiology* 1993;32:89-94.

Yang, E.Y., Stuart, A., Stenstrom, R., and Hollett, S. Effect of vibrator to head coupling force on the auditory brain stem response to bone conducted clicks in newborn infants. *Ear Hear* 1991;12:55-60.

Acknowledgments

This work was supported by the National Health Research and Development Program, Health and Welfare Canada (Project No. 6603-1292-42). The authors wish to thank Dr. Walter Green, Dr. Andrée Durieux-Smith and Robert Stenstrom for their helpful comments, assistance, and consultation toward the completion this research project. Acknowledgment is also extended to nursery staffs of the Grace Maternity Hospital and Izaak Walton Killam Hospital for Children, and to the staff of the Nova Scotia Hearing and Speech Clinic. In particular, the assistance of Dr. Heather Cake and Ms. Doris Sampson of the Perinatal Follow-up Program and Ms. Barb Muldowney of the Transitional Care Nursery, Grace Maternity Hospital, is greatly appreciated.

Address reprint requests to Edward Y. Yang, School of Human Communication Disorders, Dalhousie University, 5599 Fenwick Street, Halifax, NS, Canada B3H 1R2.

Received July 14, 1992; accepted September 22, 1992.

Portions of this paper were presented at the American Auditory Society Meeting, Seattle, WA, November 15, 1990;

the 17th Annual Conference of the Canadian Association of Speech-Language Pathologists and Audiologists, Saskatoon, SK, May 8, 1992; and the XXI International Congress of Audiology, Morioka, Japan, September 4, 1992.

Auditory Steady-State Evoked Potential in Newborns

Field W. Rickards, Lesley E. Tan, Lawrence T. Cohen, Oriole J. Wilson, John H. Drew, and Graeme M. Clark

Human Communication Research Centre, Department of Otolaryngology, The University of Melbourne(F.W.R., L.E.T., L.T.C., O.J. W., G.M.C.), Deafness Studies Unit, Department of Educational Psychology and Special Education, The University of Melbourne, Parkville 3052 (F.W.R.), and Mercy Hospital for Women, East Melbourne 3002, Australia (J.H.D.)

Abstract

Steady-state evoked potential responses were recorded from 337 normal full-term sleeping newborns to combined amplitude and frequency modulated tones. Responses were automatically detected by statistical analysis of the response phase. Responses were most easily and consistently recorded at carrier frequencies of 500 Hz, 1500 Hz and 4000 Hz when the modulation frequency was between 60 Hz and 100 Hz. In this modulation frequency range, the response latencies were found to be between 11 ms and 15 ms, depending on carrier frequency, and the mean response thresholds for the three carrier frequencies were found to be 41.36 dB HL, 24.41 dB HL and 34.51 dB HL respectively. The results of this study suggest that steady-state evoked potentials at modulation rates in excess of 60 Hz may be useful for frequency specific, automated hearing screening in newborns.

Keywords: auditory steady-state evoked potentials; neonatal hearing; automated hearing screening.

INTRODUCTION

Auditory evoked potentials are important electrophysiological tools for the assessment of auditory function in difficult to test subjects. The auditory brainstem response (ABR) is particularly useful in infants because it is unaffected by sleep (Osterhammel et al., 1985). However, its usefulness in accurately measuring hearing threshold levels across the audiometric frequency range is limited by auditory threshold estimates at frequencies below 1-2 kHz (Gorga et al., 1988). Further, when using the ABR as a neonatal screening test, the use of broadband click stimuli has been shown to miss infants with frequency specific hearing losses (Durieux-Smith et al., 1991).

Auditory steady-state evoked potentials (SSEP) have been elicited by a wide variety of stimuli in both awake and sleeping adults (Galambos et al., 1981; Rickards and Clark, 1982; Rickards and Clark, 1984; Picton et al., 1987a; Cohen et al., 1991). The SSEP is a periodic response to a periodically changing stimulus (Fig. 1). Because of its periodic nature, it can be easily characterized by the amplitude and phase of the fundamental and second harmonic frequency components of the response. The response has the same period as the period of stimulus variation. Increased interest in auditory SSEPs followed the finding that at certain repetition rates the responses seemed to be quite strong (Rickards and Clark, 1984), particularly at 40 Hz (Galambos et al., 1981). While the "40 Hz" response has been used to obtain good estimations of behavioural thresholds in normal and hearing impaired adults at low and high frequencies (Lynn et al., 1984; Stapells et al., 1984), the response is considerably affected by sleep or sedation (Gallambos et al., 1981; Brown and Shallop, 1982; Shallop, 1983; Osterhammel et al., 1985). Response thresholds are reported to be elevated and less reliable during sleep (Picton et al., 1987b).

Cohen et al. (1991) showed that in sleeping adults SSEPs to amplitude modulated and combined amplitude and frequency modulated tones, were more easily detected at modulation rates above 70 Hz. This was particularly true for higher carrier frequencies. They also found latencies of approximately 30 ms and 10 ms at modulation frequencies of 30-60 Hz and 90-195 Hz respectively. In addition, the responses around 40 Hz were more affected by sleep than the responses recorded at higher modulation rates.

Portions of this paper were presented at the 8th and 9th National Conferences of the Audiological Society of Australia in 1988 and 1990.

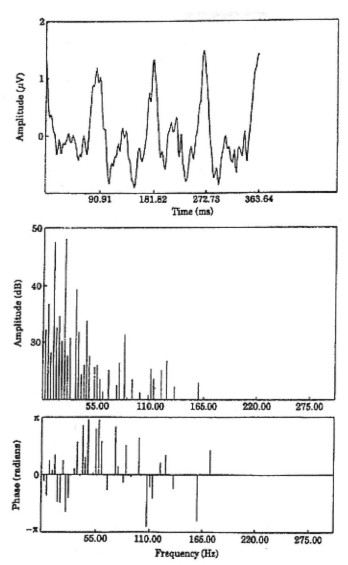

Fig. 1. Waveform and spectrum for an averaged steady-state evoked potential. The stimulus was a continuous 250 Hz tone modulated at 11 Hz presented at 65 dB HL. Segments of EEG, equivalent to four periods of modulation (363.64 ms) were averaged 1000 times to produce the waveform. The amplitude scale for the spectrum is logarithmic with an arbitrary reference. The principal components of this response are at 11 Hz, 22 Hz and 33 Hz.

The middle-latency response (MLR) and the "40 Hz" response have both been used in the assessment of hearing in infants and young children. The detection of the responses however, has been found to be inconsistent (Shallop and Osterhammel, 1983; Kraus et al., 1985; Stapells et al., 1988). Kraus et al. (1985) have shown that the detectability of the Pa wave (30 ms) of the MLR is dependent on the subject's maturation and decreases to less than 50% in very young children. The dependence of the detectability of the MLR on sleep stage in 4-9-year-old children (Kraus et al., 1989) could account in part for inconsistent detectability in previous studies. In contrast, the SN-10 transient response has been found to be consistently recorded in normally hearing newborns (Hawes and Greenberg, 1981; Shallop and Osterhammel, 1983) suggesting that the 10 ms response is less affected by maturation and sleep stage. Overall these findings suggest that the use of steady-state evoked responses in the assessment of hearing in sleeping infants and young children may be most effective when using responses with latencies of about 10 ms. The results of Cohen et al. (1991) indicate that modulation rates in excess of 70 Hz are required in order to produce these latencies. Aoyagi et al (1992) found modulation frequencies from 80-100 Hz to be most suitable for generating steady-state responses in sleeping young children (mean age 3.5 years). Similarly, in sleeping infants, Levi et al. (1993) demonstrated that 80 Hz was the optimal modulation frequency for detecting amplitude modulated tones at 500 and 2000 Hz. Our preliminary investigations have indicated that consistent SSEPs can be recorded from full term neonates at these higher modulation rates (Tan et al., 1988); Richards et al., 1990).

This study investigates steady-state evoked responses recorded from normal, healthy newborn infants to tones which have been sinusoidally amplitude and frequency modulated. In order to evaluate the applicability of these responses in neonatal hearing screening this study had three aims. Firstly, to determine the modulation frequencies at which responses are most efficiently detected. Secondly, to estimate the latencies of the responses at these modulation frequencies. Latency estimates will be useful in explaining the behaviour of these responses in this population during sleep and relating the results to other evoked potentials such as the more familiar ABR and MLR. Thirdly, to determine the evoked potential thresholds at three carrier frequencies for newborn infants.

METHODS

The stimuli and recording procedures are similar to those described previously (Cohen et al., 1991). They are summarized briefly below.

Subjects

All subjects were from a well-baby nursery and ranged in age from 1-7 days. Gestational ages ranged from 36-42 weeks. All weighed more at birth than 2500 g, an Apgar score of 7 or higher at 1 min of age and none had been in an Intensive Care Nursery. Written informed consent was obtained from at least one parent of all participating infants. Sixty-three babies participated in Experiment 1, 29 babies in Experiment 2 and 245 babies in Experiment 3.

Apparatus

The specifically designed evoked potential system allowed control of stimulus generation, had response measurement circuitry, and was controlled by an IBM-compatible XT-type micro-computer. The stimulus generation circuitry was designed to produce pure carrier tone which could be sinusoidally amplitude modulated (AM) and/or sinusoidally frequency modulated (FM). This section produced sinusoidal waveforms at the modulation frequency, one in phase with the modulation envelope and another shifted by 90 degrees. These waveforms were used in the response measurement section to perform a Fourier analysis on the electrical brain activity (EEG) being recorded.

The analysis section performed a Fourier analysis on the periodic evoked potential at the fundamental and the second harmonic of the modulation frequency, using analogue multiplication followed by low-pass filtering (Regan, 1966). For each harmonic, two multipliers and two low-pass filters were used to extract both amplitude and phase information. Each low-pass filter had a slope of 24 dB/octave and produced an effective time window of 64 modulation periods duration and of a similar shape to a Hanning window. This process is equivalent to mathematical Fourier analysis in which the usual integrand (the wave-form multiplied by cos $(2\pi ft)$ or sin $(2\pi ft)$ is multiplied by the time window function. In the present case, therefore, the integration time interval covered approximately 64 modulation periods prior to the instant that the low-pass filter was sampled. The computer sampled the output of the four lowpass filters every 32 modulation periods, resulting in an overlap of sample time windows, which obviated a loss of information which would otherwise have occurred. The analogue system is robust and reliable, and does not require frequent sampling. The computer is therefore free to do other processing.

Stimuli

Sound was delivered monaurally by Etymotic Research ER-3A Tube-phones with a funnel-shaped tip. Calibration levels for pure-tones were provisional levels provided by the manufacturer (Etymotic Research, 1985) and were acquired using a Phonic Ear HA-1 (2cc)coupler, a B&K 4144 condenser microphone, a B&K 2613 amplifier and a B&K 2120 frequency analyser.

The stimuli used were sinusoidally swept FM tones which were also sinusoidally amplitude modulated (AM/FM). The modulation frequencies for amplitude and frequency modulation were identical. AM/FM stimuli were used because they were found to evoke larger responses than AM tones in adults (Cohen et al., 1991). The depth of modulation was set to 100% for AM and 20% for FM. The amplitude spectra for the stimuli are described in Cohen et al. (1991) and are dependent on both modulation and carrier frequency. For the parameters used in this study, the stimuli have good audiometric frequency specificity.

A pure tone was used to calibrate the stimulus level. The introduction of frequency modulation did not change the peak-to-peak amplitude of the stimulus waveform. However the introduction of amplitude modulation increased the stimulus energy by 1.76 dB. This was confirmed for a group of 10 normal hearing adult subjects, where the mean behavioral thresholds for pure tones were found to reduce by less than 2 dB when combined amplitude and frequency modulation was introduced.

Responses were measured at carrier frequencies of 500 Hz, 1500 Hz and 4000 Hz. In Experiment 1, 10 modulation frequencies were used, varying from 40-190 Hz in intervals of 10-30 Hz. In Experiment 2 the modulation frequencies were set to 72 Hz, 85 Hz and 97 Hz respectively for the three carrier frequencies.

Recording

EEG activity was measured between silver-silver chloride disc electrodes placed at the mid-forehead and the ipsilateral mastoid process. An electrode placed on the cheek served as a ground electrode. Inter-electrode impedances were less than 10 kohms at 260 Hz. The signal was amplified by a specifically designed pre-amplifier with a bandwidth of 0.2-10.0 kHz.

In measuring a steady-state response to a particular stimulus, a 'run' comprised between 120 and 540 samples of amplitude and phase data. The number of samples collected in a 'run' depended in each case on the

Table 1. Background noise levels expressed in octave band levels and the corresponding effective masking.

Frequency (Hz)	63	125	250	500	1k	2k	4k	8k	16k
dB SPL	43	43	42	37	32	28	21	16	27
Masking (dB)	<	-	10	17	13	4	1	<-5	<-5

amplitude of the response and on the background EEG noise level. The 'run' was terminated when a detection criterion was satisfied.

Analysis

The samples of amplitude and phase taken during a 'run' allowed several statistical quantities to be calculated for both the fundamental and second harmonic responses. In particular, means for the amplitude and phase of the responses as well as the standard deviation of the sample phase angles were calculated. The residual EEG noise level was also calculated from these measures and was used to determine the noise floor. It was calculated by subtracting the mean vector amplitude derived from the samples within a run from the vector amplitude of each sample, and then calculating the rms of the corrected samples. The resulting noise value was dependent on the duration of the time window, and could also be related to the EEG noise spectral density. An estimation was then made of the standard errors for the amplitude and phase. This is defined as the mean amplitude measurement that would be expected with no true response present. An estimate was also made of the probability that the distribution of samples could have arisen from a random noise background.

Mean background EEG noise levels as a function of frequency were determined for the subjects in Experiment 1, using the method described in Cohen et al. (1991). The subjects in the present sutdy were found to have similar EEG noise levels to sleeping adults (Cohen et al., 1991). A noise criterion level was determined as the mean plus two standard deviations of the noise distributuions at each frequency. A single response sample was rejected if its noise level exceeded this value. The noise criterion level (in μ V p-p) was found to be approximated by the equation where N is the noise criterion level and *fm* the modulation frequency.

$$N = 56/fm + 50)$$

where N is the noise criterion level and *fm* the modulation frequency.

To estimate the probability that a set of samples measured during a run could have arisen from a random source, the distribution of phase angles relative to the modulation envelope was considered. The criterion for response detection was equivalent to the 'phase coherence' technique described by Jerger et al. (1986) and Stapells et al. (1987). This technique was used to determine whether a response was present. After the collection of each sample, and the associated calculation of the phase, the computer calculated the probabillity that the phase distributuion could have arisen by chance. The probability calculated is correct if it is calculated at any one time, such as the end of a fixed measuring time. However, for a random angle distribution, repeat-ed calculations of the probability during a run result in an increased percentage of low values, with a corresponding increase in the percentage of responses falsely detected. Therefore, in view of the considerable advantage in being able to stop a run, dependent on the signal-to-noise ratio before the maximum allotted time, an empirical criterion was established for the termination of a run. An initial false response rate of $P=0.05$ was obtained if the calculated probability was required to remain below 0.01 for a number of successive samples. Subsequent refinements to the electronics resulted in a slight reduction in artefact, and consequently the probability of a false response fell to $P<0.03$. At this time, a response was accepted, and the run terminated. The time taken to detect a response was typically in the range of 20-90s, depending on the signal-to-noise ratio of the response and the electroencephalographic noise.

In order to assess the relative detectability of responses for different stimulus conditions, a 'detection efficiency' function was used. This function was essentially proportional to the inverse of the time that would be taken to detect a response, and so it involved not only the response amplitude and the noise level, but also the modulation frequency. Its value was calculated from the mean response amplitude taken from all subjects for a given stimulus condition and from the mean noise level taken from all subjects and all carrier frequencies for a given modulation frequency. This assumed that the background EEG noise level was independent of the carrier frequency of the modulated tone. The function was given by:

Eff=(modulation frequency)
x (signal amplitude/EEG Noise Level)^2

The limitations of this function are described in Cohen et al. (1991).

Procedures

Babies were tested during natural sleep in a quiet room in a maternity ward of the Mercy Hospital for Women. The overall noise level near a baby's ear was found to be 39 dB(A). The levels found in an octave band analysis and the corresponding effective masking levels, determined from critical and masking theory (Hawkins and Stevens, 1960), are listed in Table 1. These values suggest that this noise could create a 10 to 20 dB masking effect in the freuqncy range 250 Hz to 1000 Hz based on data from normal adult ears. The effects of masking on neonate ears may be different. These estimates also ignore possible attenuation by the ear tips. The effective masking of background noise in thresholds at higher frequencies would be minimal.

RESULTS

Experiment I

Each baby was initially tested with a stimulus at 55 dB HL at the three carrier frequencies using a modula-

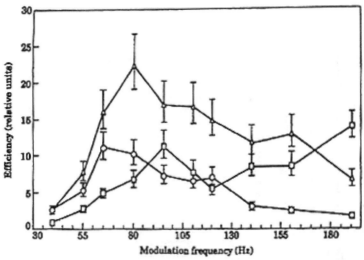

Fig. 2. Mean detection efficiency plotted against modulation frequency for the three carrier frequencies. Each data point was the average of 18–22 responses. The error bars represent one standard error of the mean. (—○—), 500 Hz; —△—, 1500 Hz; —□—, 4000 Hz).

tion frequency of 95 Hz. This modulation frequency was selected based on the results from sleeping adults (Cohen et al., 1991) and the moderate level was selected based on preliminary trials on a small group of babies which confirmed that consistent responses could be obtained at this level. These initial responses were used as a screen so that if the baby woke up early in the session some feedback could be given to the parent concerning the hearing status of the infant. In this experiment, three babies failed to give a response at 500 Hz at 55 dB HL. No further responses were recorded from these babies at this frequency.

Using 55 dB HL stimuli, modulation frequency was systematically varied for each carrier frequency in turn. Up to 17 trials were run with each baby, one trial being recorded for each condition. From the 63 babies tested in this experiment, 18-22 responses were obtained for each modulation-frequency/carrier-frequency condition.

Figure 2 shows the relative detection efficiencies as a function of modulation frequency for each of the three carrier frequencies. The error bars indicate one standard error of the mean to indicate detection efficiency variability. A significant increase in detection efficiency was observed at all carrier frequencies for modulation frequencies above 55 Hz followed by a general reduction beyond 110 Hz. In the case of 4000 Hz, a second increase was observed beyond 120 Hz.

On the basis of these findings, three modulation frequencies were selected as being appropriate for further testing of neonates. The values selected were 72 Hz, 85 Hz and 97 Hz for the carrier frequencies 500 Hz, 1500 Hz and 4000 Hz respectively. These values avoided simple harmonic relationships with mains electricity (50 Hz), and were felt to represent a central frequency for the main peaks in this figure, although the frequency producing the highest efficiency aat 4000 Hz was 190 Hz. The decision to select the lower peak at this carrier frequency was an arbitrary one which was influenced by a desire to keep the modulation frequencies in the same frequency region. It was recognized that the efficiency difference between the two frequen-

cy regions was not large (11.1 at 97 Hz and 13.8 at 190 Hz). The efficiencies at 40 Hz were all less than 2.6 and the maximum mean efficiency was found to be greater than the efficiency at 40 Hz by a factor of 4.20, 9.35 and 15.85 at the carrier frequencies 500 Hz, 1500 Hz and 4000 Hz respectively.

Experiment 2

With steady-state evoked potentials it is not possible to measure latencies in a conventional way. The periodic nature of the response and the stimulus make the assignment of response peak to stimulus peak ambiguous. In this experiment, latencies were estimated by dividing the gradient of the linear regression of phase on modulation frequency by 2π (Regan, 1972, 1977). The latencies are reported as the means of individual subject latencies. As with Experiment 1, each baby was screened at the three carrier frequencies, but at modulation frequencies selected at the completion of Experiment 1. The modulation-frequency/carrier-frequency combinations were 72/500 Hz, 85/1500 Hz, and 97/4000 Hz. Twenty-nine babies were tested in this experiment, all of whom passed the screen. Using 55 dB HL stimuli, responses were recorded for five modulation frequencies spaced at three Hz intervals around the selected best modulation frequency at each carrier frequency. As the number of responses recorded from each infant varied, it was not always possible to obtain estimates of latency at each of the three carrier frequencies.

Table 2. Means and standard deviations (SD) for the latencies of the evoked responses at each carrier frequency. The number of cases at each frequency is also reported.

Carrier Frequency (Hz)	Number	Mean (ms)	SD
500	21	14.82	3.22
1500	20	12.07	3.10
4000	27	11.19	3.55

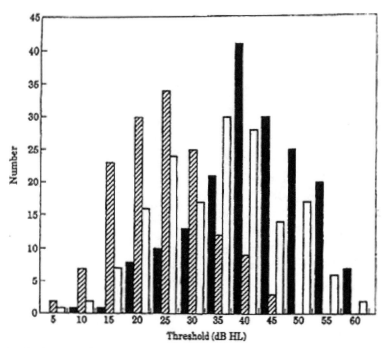

Fig. 3. Histograms for steady-state evoked potential thresholds at the three carrier frequencies. A total of 486 thresholds were obtained; 177 at 500 Hz (■), 145 at 1500 Hz (▨) and 164 at 4000 Hz (□).

Table 2 reports the mean latencies and standard deviations as a function of frequency. The latency at 500 Hz was found to be significantly longer than at 1500 Hz ($t = 2.78$, $P < 0.01$) and 4 kHz ($t = 3.62$, $P < 0.01$). The difference between 1500 Hz and 4000 Hz, however, was not significant.

Experiment 3

In this experiment electrophysiological thresholds were determined. The modulation frequency was selected and fixed for each carrier frequency based on the results in Experiment 1. As with Experiment 2, each baby was screened at the three modulation-frequency/carrier-frequency combinations determined in Experiment 1. The number of responses recorded from each infant varied, but typically ranged from 10 to 30 before the infant became restless. While no responses were recorded for 11 infants at the first attempt due to excessive EEG noise, these infants were successfully tested on a second occasion prior to discharge. At least one threshold could be established for each infant in the session but usually it was two to three. Seven infants failed to give a response to the initial screening tone at

Table 3. Means and standard deviations (SD) for the evoked response thresholds at each carrier frequency. The number of cases at each frequency is also reported.

Carrier Frequency (Hz)	Number	Mean (ms)	SD
500	177	41.36	10.40
1500	145	24.41	8.51
4000	164	34.51	11.33

55 dB HL at 500 Hz and two to the 55 dB HL tone at 4000 Hz. The nine babies who failed these initial screening levles were still included in this experiment and their thresholds were determined at the failed frequencies using the procedures described below. None of the babies in this experiment has been followed up with subsequent behavioural testing.

Following the initial screening, electrophysiological thresholds were recorded from each infant at one or more of the three carrier-frequencies using the modulation-frequencies selected. The threshold seeking technique used reductions of 10 dB in the stimulus level, usually from 55 dB HL, until a non-response was recorded. The stimulus level was then increased in 5-dB steps until a response was again recorded. The procedure continued until at least two non-responses had been recorded. The threshold was taken as the lowest level where a response had been recorded, with two non-responses at 5 or 10 dB below this level.

Figure 3 shows the frequency distributions for the evoked potential thresholds at the three carrier frequencies. Table 3 reports the mean thresholds and standard deviations as a function of frequency. The histograms in Fig. 3 were converted to cumulative distributions and were compared to a normal ogive with the same mean and standard deviation of each of the histograms. The Kolmogorov-Smirnov D-statistic was not significant in each case, indicating that these distributions were not different from normal. Figure 4 shows the observed and expected cumulative distributions for 500 Hz, 1500 Hz and 4000 Hz respectively. The results of an analysis of variance showed a significant difference for the mean thresholds across the three frequencies ($F2, 483 = 110.03$, $P < 0.001$). *Post hoc* analysis (Scheffe test)

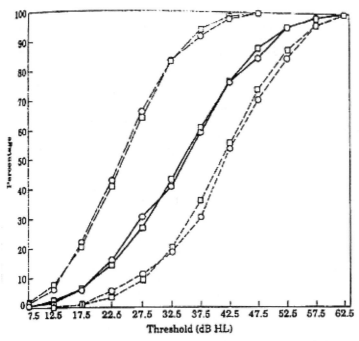

Fig. 4. Cumulative distribution and theoretical normal curve for the threshold data at 500 Hz (- - -); 1500 Hz (— — —); and 4000 Hz (———. (—○—, observed; —□—, expected).

revealed a significant difference for the mean thresholds between each frequency ($P < 0.001$).

DISCUSSION

This investigation has shown that SSEPs can be consistently recorded from young normal full-term sleeping infants in the first few days of life for the carrier frequencies 500 Hz, 1500 Hz and 4000 Hz. The efficiency of response detection, which in part was dependent on the evoked potential amplitude in EEG noise ratio, was found to be dependent on the modulation frequency of the stimulus. Furthermore, the maximum detection efficiency occurred above 60 Hz modulation and was significantly larger than at 40 Hz. This is consistent with the findings of Cohen *et al.* (1991) who found that in sleeping adults the most efficient response detection was usually above 70 Hz, although this depended on carrier frequency.

Responses could be recorded from all babies who participated in these experiments. On a small number of occasions, responses could not be recorded at the first attempt due to high electrophysiological noise. Responses were however recorded on these babies at a second test prior to discharge from the hospital. The ability to record responses from all babies in this normal population suggests that the response is reasonably well developed at birth, as is the case with the ABR (Hecox and Galambos, 1974; Starr *et al.*, 1977).

Other studies investigating SSEPs in infants and young children have found the detection of responses to

be inconsistent (Shallop and Osterhammel, 1983; Kraus *et al.*, 1985; Stapells *et al.,* 1988). These studies have used a stimulus rate of 40/s. The latency of the response at this rate is around 30 ms (Stapells *et al.*, 1984; Cohen *et al.*, 1991). In the present study, where higher modulation rates were used, the latency was found to be between 11.2 and 14.8 ms., depending on carrier frequency. This is consistent with recordings from adults at the same modulation rates where the range for the same carrier frequencies was 9.6 to 12. 6 ms (Cohen *et al.*, 1991). The transient SN-10 response, with similar latency to these steady-state responses, has also been consistently recorded in normally hearing sleeping newborns (Hawes and Greenberg, 1981; Shallop and Osterhammel, 1983). The decrease in latency for these steady-state responses from infant to adult is consistent with ABR latency changes observed from similar groups (Zimmerman, 1987). The decrease in latency from low to high carrier frequencies is likely to be due to the properties of the cochlea. The latency differences are similar to those found in adults by Gorga *et al.* (1988).

The threshold responses reported in this paper represent responses to frequency-specific stimuli and appear to originate from the appropriate region of the basilar membrane (Griffiths and Chamber, 1991). Further, some comparison of the thresholds obtained is possible with ABR studies using frequency specific stimuli. In the present study, the mean thresholds (in Table 3), when expressed in dB SPL, were found to be 52.9 at 500 Hz, 31.4 at 1500 Hz and 45.0 at 4000 Hz. Gorga *et al.* (1988) used tone bursts and found mean thresholds of approximately 48, 26 and 23 dB SPL respectively at the same frequencies in a group of young normally hearing sleeping adults with standard deviations of 14, 6 and 9 dB. With the exception of the mean threshold at 4000 Hz, the results from the two studies are similar. Hyde *et al.* (1987) determined ABR thresholds on a group of 230 four-month-old infants using 2-1-2 tones in notched noise at 500 Hz and 4000 Hz. They found that at 500 Hz, 59% gave responses at 40 dB nHL (approximately 65 dB SPL) and 95% at 60 dB nHL (85 dB SPL). In the present study, these percentiles were reached at 41 dB HL (52.5 dB SPL) and 56 dB HL (67.5 dB SLP). At 4000 Hz, 83% gave responses at 40 dB nHL (approximately 69 dB SPL) and 100% at 60 dB nHL (89 dB SPL). These values compare with 45 dB HL (54.5 dB SPL) and 62.5 dB HL (72 dB SLP) for the same percentiles in the present study. Although these comparisons suggest that the SSEP thresholds in babies are approximately 15 dB lower than the ABR thresholds on an equivalent SPL basis, some preliminary ABR results from Stapells (1989), also using tones in notched noise, suggest that lower thresholds in infants can be obtained, which would agree more closely with the findings of Gorga *et al.* (1988) for adults and also the steady-state thresholds reported in this study.

There has been no follow-up on most of the babies used in this study. The population may have included some children with mild or moderate hearing losses, but the nine children in experiment three who did not respond at 55 dB HL at the three carrier frequencies did respond at 60 dB HL, eliminating the possibility of severe or profound hearing loss in these babies. The exclusion of any children who were later found to have a hearing loss would probably lower the mean response levels. It should also be remembered that there was a 0.03 probability that EEG noise could be interpreted as a response. Thresholds were taken as the lowest response. Some of these may in fact have been non-responses which could underestimate the threshold. However in most threshold determinations, three or more responses were recorded over a narrow intensity range, thereby reducing the error caused by the occasional false positive response.

The mean thresholds in this study were significantly lower at 1500 Hz than at the other two frequencies. The higher thresholds at 500 Hz may in part be attributed to room background noise which has an effective masking level of about 20 dB at this frequency. The differences may also suggest different physiological mechanisms in the generation of the response. This may account in part for the difference between the low and the mid to high frequency stimuli, but does not easily account for the difference between 1500 and 4000 Hz. It is also possible that the intrameatal sound pressure levels generated by ipsilateral stimulation of neonatal ears are higher than expected. Measurements by McMillan *et al.* (1985) during ipsilateral acoustic reflex measurements of neonatal ears, showed sound pressure levels which were up to 25 dB higher than the manufacturer's specification in the mid frequencies. Future stud-ies should consider the use of probe tube monitoring of the sound pressure levels actually deliverd to neonates.

Overall, the findings of this study suggest that SSEPs may be an appropriate method for screening the hearing of neonates for a number of reasons. Firstly, when recorded at high modulation rates, the response can be consistently detected from full-term babies in the first four days of life. Second, the mean response threshold levels are similar to those obtained using unmasked tone bursts in sleeping adults. Third, the distribution of response thresholds appears to be normal which allows for appropriate selection of screening levels and prediction of false positive results. Fourth, response detection is totally automated thereby allowing for less skilled professionals to use the procedure. Fifth, the sinusoidally, continuously modulated tones have good audiometric frequency specificity, offereing the potential for selective hearing losses to be identified. Finally, the time taken to detect a response was normally less than the recording time for an ABR. Replications were rarely required. Aside from its appropriateness in screening, this procedure is seen as having a potential use in the estimation of threshold for diagnostic applications.

ACKNOWLEDGEMENTS

This research was supported in part by the National Health and Medical Research Council of Australia, The Deafness Foundation of Victoria, and the Australian Bionic Ear and Hearing Research Institute, Australia. The authors wish to thank Dr. Susan Roberts and Sandra De Vidi for their helpful comments and contributions in the preparation of this paper. The authors are also deeply indebted to the staff at the Mercy Hospital for Women for their co-operation during the data collection.

REFERENCES

Aoyagi, M., Kiren, T., Kim, Y., Suzuki, Y., Fuse, T., Koike, Y. Optimal modulation frequency for amplitude-modulation following response in young children during sleep. Hear Res 1993; 65:253-61.

Brown, D., Shallop, J.K. A clinically useful 500 Hz evoked response. Nicolet Potentials 1982; 1:9-12.

Cohen, L.T., Rickards, F.W., Clark, G.M. A comparison of steady-state evoked potentials to modulated tones in awake and sleeping humans. J Acoust Soc Am 1991; 90: 2467-79.

Durieux-Smith, A., Picton, T.W., Bernard, P., MacMurray, B., Goodman, J.T. Prognostic validity of brainstem electric response audiometry in infants of a neonatal intensive care unit. Audiology 1991; 30: 249-65.

Etymotic Research. Etymotic Research ER-3a Tubephone Insert Earphone Calibration Instructions. Elk Grove Village, IL: Etymotic Research, 1985.

Galambos, R., Makeig, S., Talmachoff, P.J. A 40 Hz auditory potential recorded from the human scalp. Proc Natl Acad Sci 1981; 78: 2643-7.

Gorga, M.P., Kaminski, J.R., Beauchaine, K.A., Jesteadt, W. Auditory brainstem responses to tone bursts in normally hearing subjects. J Sp Hear Res 1988; 31:87-97.

Griffiths, S.K., Chambers, R.D. The amplitude-modulation following response as an audiometric tool. Ear Hear 1991; 12:235-41.

Hawes, M.D., Greenberg, H.J. Slow brainstem responses (SN10) to tone pips in normally hearing newborns and adults. Audiology 1981; 20:113-22.

Hawkins, J.E., Stevens, S.S. Masking of pure tones and of speech by white noise. J Acoust Soc Am 1950; 22:6-15.

Hecox, K., Galambos, R. Brain stem auditory evoked responses in human infants and adults. Arch Otolaryngol 1974; 99:30-3.

Hyde, M.L., Matsumoto, N., Alberti, P.W. The normative basis for click and frequency-specific BERA in high-risk infants. Acta Otolaryngol 1987; 103:602.11.

Jerger, J., Chmiel, R., Frost, J.D., Jr., Coker, N. Effect of sleep on the auditory steady state evoked potential Ear Hear 1986; 7:240-5.

Kraus, N., McGee, T., Comperatore, C. MLRs in children are consistently present during wakefulness, Stage I, and REM sleep. Ear Hear 1989; 10:339-45.

Kraus, N., Smith, D.I., Reed, N.L., Stein, L.K., Cartee, C. Auditory middle latency responses in children:effects of age and diagnostic category. Electroencephalogr Clin Neurophysiol 1985; 62:343-51.

Levi, E.C., Folsom, R.C., Dobie, R.A. Amplitude-modulation following response (AMFR) effects of modulation rate, carrier frequency, age and state. Hear Res 1993; 68: 42-52.

Lynn, J.M., Lesner, S.A., Sandridge, S.A., Daddario, C.C. Threshold prediction from the auditory 40-Hz evoked potential. Ear Hear 1984; 5: 366-70.

McMillan, P.M., Bennett, M.J., Marchant, C.D., Shurin, P.A. Ipsilateral and contralateral acoustic reflexes in neonates. Ear Hear 1985; 6: 320-4.

Osterhammel, P.A., Shallop, J.K, Terkildsen, K. The effect of sleep on the auditory brainstem response (ABR) and the middle latency response (MLR). Scan Audiol 1985; 14:47-50.

Picton, T.W., Skinner, C.R., Champagne, S.C., Kellett, J.C., Maiste, A.C. Potentials evoked by the sinusoidal modulation of the amplitude or frequency of a tone. J. Acoust Soc Am 1987a; 82: 165-78.

Picton, T.W., Vajsar, J., Rodriguez, R., Campbell, K.B. Reliability estimates for steady-state evoked potentials. Electroencephalogr Clin Neurophysiol 1987b; 68:119-31.

Regan, D. Some characteristics of average steady-state and transient responses evoked by modulated light. Electroencephalogr Clin Neurophysiol 1966; 20:237-48.

Regan, D. Evoked potentials in psychology, sensory physiology, and clinical medicine. London: Chapman Hall, 1972.

Regan, D. Fourier analysis of evoked potentials; some methods based on Fourier analysis. In: Desmedt, J.E., ed. Visual evoked potentials in man: new developments. Oxford: Oxford UP, 1977; 110-7.

Rickards, F.W., Clark, G.M. Steady-state evoked potentials in humans to amplitude-modulated tones. J Acoust Soc Am 1982; 72 (Suppl I):S54.

Rickards, F.W., Clark, G.M. Steady-state evoked potentials to amplitude modulated tones. In: Nodar, RH, Barber C, eds. Evoked Potentials II. Boston, MA: Butterworth, 1984; 163-8.

Rickards, F.W., Wilson, O.J., Tan, L.E., Cohen, L.T. Steady-state evoked potentials in normal neonates. Aust J Audiol 1990; Suppl 4:21.

Shallop, J.K. Electric response audiometry: the morphology of normal responses. Adv Oto Rhino Laryngol 1983; 29:124-39.

Shallop, J.K., Osterhammel, P.A. A comparative study of measurements of SN-10 and the 40/sec middle latency responses in newborns. Scand Audiol 1983; 12:91-5.

Stapells, D.R. Auditory brainstem response assessment of infants and children. Semin Hear 1989; 10:229-51.

Stapells, D.R., Galambos, R., Costello, J.A., Makeig, S. Inconsistency of auditory middle latency and steady-state responses in infants. Electroencephalogr Clin Neurophysiol 1988; 71:289-95.

Stapells, D.R., Makeig, S., Galambos, R. Auditory steady-state responses: threshold prediction using phase coherence. Electroencephalogr Clin Neurophysiol 1987; 67:260-70.

Starr, A., Amlie, R.N., Martin, W.H., Saunders, S. Development of auditory function in newborn infants revealed by auditory brainstem potentials. Pediatrics 1977; 60:831-9.

Tan, L.E., Rickards, F.W., Cohen, L.T. Neonatal hearing screening using auditory steadystate evoked potentials. Aust J. Audiol 1988; Suppl 3:25.

Zimmerman, M.C., Morgan, D.E., Dubno, J.R. Auditory brain stem evoked response characteristics in developing infants. Ann Otol Rhinol Laryngol 1987; 96:291-9.

Evoked Otoacoustic Emissions in Normal-Hearing Infants and Children: Emerging Data and Issues*

Susan J. Norton and Judith E. Widen
Department of Hearing & Speech, University of Kansas Medical Center, Kansas City, Kansas 66103

Abstract

Evoked otoacoustic emissions (EOAEs) are a promising tool for evaluating cochlear status in children. Preliminary data from normal-hearing subjects ranging from birth to 29.9 years old are discussed. EOAEs are present and robust in infant ears. However, there is a statistically significant decrease in EOAE amplitude for a fixed stimulus level with increasing age even in a carefully screened sample. At the present time it is unclear if these age-associated changes are due to normal developmental changes in the external and/or middle ear acoustics, normal developmental changes in cochlear mechanics and/or everyday cochlear wear and tear. Issues related to further application of evoked emissions to pediatric populations are discussed.

Several investigators have suggested that transient evoked otoacoustic emissions (EOAEs) are potentially a valuable noninvasive, objective clinical, as well as research, tool for evaluating cochlear status in infants and young children (Bonfils, Uziel, & Pujol, 1988a, b; Elberling, Parbo, Johnsen, & Bagi, 1985; Johnsen, Bagi, & Elberling, 1983; Kemp, 1978, 1988; Kemp, Bray, Alexander, & Brown, 1986; Lutman, Mason, Sheppard, & Gibbin, 1989). There is considerable evidence that EOAEs are a property of the healthy, normal-functioning cochlea, generated by active, frequency-selective, nonlinear elements within the cochlear partition. These elements enhance the cochlear response to sound by a positive feedback mechanism, thus improving sensitivity and frequency selectivity. While the exact site and mechanisms of these elements are unknown, the outer hair cells are probably critical components (see Kemp, 1988 for a review).

In addition to elucidating aspects of normal cochlear function, potentially EOAEs could be used to assess cochlear function in a frequency-specific manner in infants and young children suspected of sensorineural hearing loss. They may be particularly valuable in monitoring the cochlear status of children who are very ill with diseases such as meningitis and/or children who are receiving ototoxic drugs. Emissions may also be valuable for separating cochlear from more central components of auditory dysfunction. However, techniques for measuring EOAEs and our understanding of them are still evolving. It is uncer-

tain, even in adults, which parameters of otoacoustic emissions are most appropriate for clinical applications. Questions include which evoking stimulus (tone pips or clicks) would be most useful clinically; which parameters of a given emission (threshold, latency, spectrum, or input-output function) will provide the most information; and how much analysis is needed and/or reasonable in order to judge an emission present and normal?

Basic research on these issues is occurring concurrent with the implementation of clinical applications of emissions. Most studies have focused on adult subjects (Elberling et al, 1985; Kemp, 1978; Kemp, 1988; Kemp et al, 1986; Probst, Coats, Martin, & Lonsbury-Martin, 1986; Probst, Lonsbury-Martin, Martin, & Coats, 1987). Since Johnsen et al (1983) demonstrated that neonatal ears generated evoked emissions, there has been relatively little study of the effects of age on emissions. If EOAEs are to be used as a clinical tool, age-related changes must be understood. EOAE characteristics as a function of age and their relationship to pure-tone thresholds and middle-ear status must be carefully determined in large populations of normal-hearing infants and young children. In addition, the validity of EOAEs as a screening tool for hearing loss in neonates must be established by longitudinal study of infants who pass and as well as those who fail EOAE "screening tests."

Depending upon the mechanisms underlying the generation of OAEs, two possible age-related cochlear changes could occur. If emission generation requires cochlear irregularities or imperfections (Ruggero, Rich, & Freyman, 1983) both spontaneous and evoked emissions could become more prevalent and/or stronger with increasing age. On the other hand, if OAEs are

Reprinted by permission of authors and Williams & Wilkins. Copyright 1990.
Ear & Hearing, 11, No. 2, pp. 121-127.
*Supported by NIH grant K08DC00011 to S.J.N.

related to normal active, physiologically vulnerable mechanisms whose efficiency and output are decreased by wear and tear, the incidence of spontaneous emissions and strength of evoked emissions should decrease with increasing age. Currently available data suggest that both hypotheses have some merit.

Early studies in neonates by Johnsen et al (1983) used a 2 kHz half-sinusoidal click at three intensities, –20, 50, and 70 dB pe SPL. Subjects were 20 normal, healthy full-term infants, 40 to 96 hours old. Johnsen et al reported amplitude input-output functions and group latencies. Clear responses were obtained at 50 and 70 dB pe SPL, approximately 10 to 15 and 25 to 35 dB SL re: normal adult subjective threshold, respectively, for the evoking stimulus. No attempts to identify EOAE threshold were reported. As in adults, there was significant variation in waveform morphology across subjects. The input-output functions displayed a saturating nonlinearity similar to adults, although inspection of their data (Johnsen et al, 1983, Fig. 4) suggests response magnitudes at 50 dB pe SPL were significantly larger for neonates than adults. They also reported that the latency of the first echo tended to be "shorter" than in adults, and that the "frequency content of the EOAE seemed so different from the stimulus" (p. 22). Although not discussed by the authors, these differences could be related to the higher incidence of high frequency spontaneous emissions (SOAEs) in neonates and infants (Bonfils, 1989; Strickland, Burns, & Tubis, 1985). In a later study, Elberling et al (1983) reported that they observed EOAEs in the 199 ears examined in 100 normal, full-term neonates. Strickland et al (1987) reported a higher incidence of SOAEs above 3 kHz in neonates 17 to 45 days old compared to adults and children 5 to 12 years old. They did not report a higher incidence of SOAEs per se. Bargones and Burns (1988) likewise found that the frequency distribution of SOAEs was skewed toward higher frequencies in neonates than in adults.

In a large survey of normal (148) ears and ears with sensorineural hearing loss (136) Bonfils (1989) reported an inverse correlation between age and incidence of SOAEs for subjects from 0 to 70 years old. He found SOAEs in 60.8% (15 of 22) ears in infants less than 15 months old. For subjects between 18 months and 9 years old the incidence of SOAEs decreased to 36.3%. In contrast to Burns and his colleagues, he found no differences in SOAE frequency as a function of age. This discrepancy may be due to differences in the age cohorts examined—Bonfils did not distinguish between neonates, infants, and toddlers. Significant changes are most likely occurring in the first 6 to 12 months. Bonfils also examined EOAEs in

most of the ears studied and found that SOAE incidence decreased as EOAE threshold increased for adults. Unfortunately, he did not obtain EOAEs for most of the infants and young children in his series because of noise problems.

In a related study, Bonfils et al (1988a) obtained both click-evoked auditory brain stem potentials (ABR) and EOAEs from 27 infants between 48 hours and 12 months old. Data from 30 ears of normal-hearing, full term infants were compared to data from 16 ears of infants considered high risk for hearing loss because they did not respond well to sound. While ABRs were obtained at several intensities ranging from 80 dB HL to threshold, EOAEs were measured at only one intensity, 20 dB HL re: normal adult subjective threshold. The normal group all had ABR thresholds below 30 dB HL and all had detectable EOAEs. In the high-risk group, ABR thresholds ranged from 30 to 100 dB HL and none showed an EOAE. Since EOAEs were measured at only one stimulus level the exact relationship between hearing loss, ABR thresholds, and EOAE thresholds cannot be discerned from these data. In addition, no information on middle ear status was provided.

Thus, current data indicates that all normal-hearing infants and children should have EOAEs. However, whether there are significant, consistent differences between EOAEs in children and adults is unclear.

Currently, we are conducting clinical trials on normal-hearing individuals from birth to old age using an EOAE technique developed by Kemp (Kemp et al, 1986; Kemp, 1988). The purpose of the study is to determine if there are significant, age-related changes in EOAEs in normal ears, and to provide a normative data base for studying clinical populations. Preliminary data from subjects 0 to 30 years old will be presented, with the emphasis on subjects below 10 years of age.

Methods

Procedures

Click-evoked emissions were measured using the IL088 hardware and software (Kemp et al, 1986; Kemp, 1988) controlled by a Zenith 159 computer with an 8087 math coprocessor. Stimuli were 80 μsec rectangular pulses presented at a rate of 50/sec at 80 dB pe SPL. Pulses were generated by a 12-bit digital to analog converter and presented to the subject through a miniature transducer housed in a probe fitted in the subject's external ear canal. Stimulus level was controlled by a digital attenuator. The sound pressure level in the ear canal was measured using a miniature microphone also housed within the probe. The output of the microphone was averaged in the time domain using a 12-bit analog to digital converter at a 25 kHz sampling rate. In order to cancel the stimulus artifact, a series of four pulses were subaveraged using an 80 msec time window. The first three pulses in a series were of equal amplitude and polarity. The fourth had opposite polarity and was 9.5 dB greater in amplitude than the previous three. In a linear system, the average of these four would be zero. The remaining response obtained in the ear canal represents the nonlinear EOAE generated by the cochlea. Responses to stimulus sets were averaged into two, 20 msec time-domain buffers. Next, each array was reverse high-pass filtered at 200 Hz to remove any remaining stimulus artifact. Each response was windowed, blanking the first 2.5 msec as seen in Figure 1. Last, the responses were band-pass filtered from 600 to 6000 Hz (IL088 User Manual, 1988). The rms amplitude of each averaged, windowed, and filtered waveform was then computed. The two overall amplitudes were averaged and the average converted to dB SPL using appropriate calibration values derived for the probe. In addition to overall average EOAE

amplitude, the "Reproducibility" using a simple cross-correlation of the two waveforms was computed. Kemp uses reproducibility as a way of determining the presence of an EOAE. It will be zero for two completely unrelated waveforms and 100% for identical waveforms. He argues that reproducibility of 50% or greater is associated with hearing sensitivity better than 30 dB HL from 300 to 3000 Hz. In addition to time-domain analysis, the spectra of each response and the background noise were computed. Overall response spectrum was determined by taking a 512 Fast Fourier Transform (FFT) of the two waveform buffers and then computing their cross-power spectrum.

Subjects older than about 3 years were seated in a comfortable reclining chair with their heads well supported. Infants and younger children were generally seated on the lap of a parent or other adult, also with the head well supported. The computer, printer, monitor, and interface box were in a separate room from the subject in order to minimize external noise. The monitor was situated so that the examiner could see it and control the testing sequence using the keyboard in the test room.

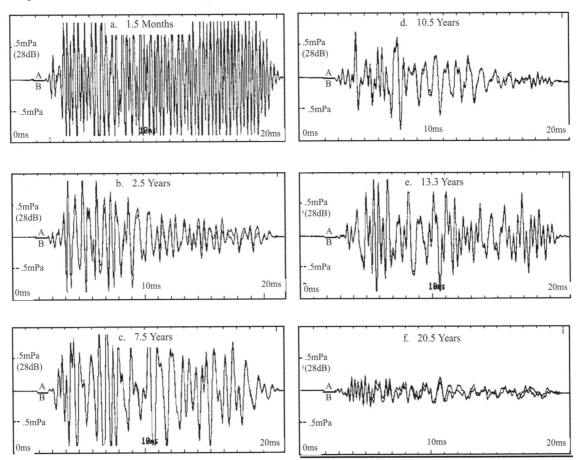

Figure 1. EOAE waveforms for normal-hearing subjects. Ages are a, 1.5 months; b, 2.5 years; c, 7.5 years; d, 10.5 years; e, 13.3 years; and f, 20.5 years old.

A small probe containing a microphone and transducer was fitted in the external ear canal using shortened acoustic immittance probe tips. Although it is not necessary to have a hermetic seal, the probe must fit well enough to block environmental noise. Probe fit was judged by presenting a series of stimuli and observing their averaged waveform and spectrum. If there was significant ringing in the waveform, its peak to peak amplitude was low or there were significant discontinuities in the stimulus spectrum the probe was refitted. With small ear canals the overall SPL of the stimulus in the ear canal can vary considerably. Therefore, care was taken to adjust the gain and attenuation so that the stimulus level was as close to 80 dB pe SPL as possible (mean = 79.8, SD = 1.6). A noise rejection level was set by the examiner. Any time the noise level in the trace exceeded this amount, the sample was not added to the running average. Responses to 260 stimuli per buffer were obtained. The time necessary to acquire the data ranged from 58 sec to 3.5 minutes depending upon subject noise.

Subjects

Subjects reported here ranged in age from 17 days to 30 years old. They were divided into three age groups; group 1: 0.0 to 9.9 years (mean = 5.4 years, SD = 2.7 years); group 2: 10.0 to 19.9 (mean = 12.6 years, SD = 1.9 years); and group 3: 20.0 to 29.9 years (mean = 23.7 years, SD = 2.1 years). All subjects over 3 years of age had normal pure-tone audiograms (thresholds better than or equal to 10 dB HL at the standard audiometric frequencies) and normal middle ear function, as measured by tympanometry and acoustic reflex thresholds. For younger subjects available audiological data varied, but all were within normal limits and had negative otologic and medical histories.

Results

Figure 1 shows time-domain averaged waveforms from six subjects ranging in age from one and one-half months (a) to 20.5 years old (f). In each trace the abcissa is 20 msec long, with the first 2.5 msec blanked or zeroed. The darker, heavier line on the abcissa simply represents the time window over which the cross-correlation and FFTs were computed. The one and one-half month old is a healthy, full-term female with a negative medical and family history for hearing loss and normal behavioral responses to sound. The 20.5 year old is a healthy female with a negative otologic and family history for hearing loss, no history

of noise exposure, and pure-tone thresholds of 5 dB HL or better for audiometric frequencies from 0.25 to 8.0 kHz. Clearly, the amplitude and temporal characteristics of the EOAEs are different across the six ears shown and these differences are, at least partially, age associated. The most dramatic differences are for the one and one-half month old and 20.5 year old versus the other subjects. Figure 2 shows overall EOAE rms amplitude (dB SPL) as a function of age. Individual data points represent different ears and the different symbol types represent different age groups. Although there is considerable scatter, there is a statistically significant decrease in EOAE amplitude as age increases. The mean for group 1 ($N = 32$ ears) was 20.0 dB SPL (SD = 5.4); for group 2 ($N = 37$ ears), 17.0 dB SPL (SD = 4.2); and for group 3 ($N = 37$), 10.9 (SD = 4.3) dB SPL. t-Tests indicated that each group was significantly different from the other at the 0.025 level or better. For group 1 versus group 3, $t = 6.69$ with df = 67 and $p < 0.0005$. For group 2 versus group 3, $t = 5.65$ with df = 72 and $p < 0.0005$. The least difference was observed for group 1 versus group 2, $t = 2.18$, df = 67 and $p < 0.025$. In the future, more ears will be added to the data base and the sample divided into smaller age groups.

For all ears tested, EOAEs were judged to be present by at least two independent observers, even when reproducibility was low. As seen in Figure 3, which shows EOAE amplitude as a function of reproducibility decreases as amplitude decreases. That is, smaller EOAEs are more affected by noise than larger ones. Mean reproducibility for group 1 was 90.4% (SD = 12.3); for group 2, 90.6% (SD = 10.4); and for group 3, 83.4% (SD = 14.8). None was statistically different from any other. Figure 4 shows EOAE *(lines only)* and background noise *(solid area)* spectra for the EOAEs shown in Figure 1. Note that only 128 points are displayed for each spectra. There is some trend for the upper frequency cut-off of the emission spectra to decrease with increasing age. However, for these healthy ears the differences are greatest for the one and one-half month old. EOAE spectral differences as a function of age will be investigated as the sample size increases.

Discussion

Preliminary data from our group and others indicate that EOAEs from the ears of neonates, infants, and young children are healthy and robust. In fact, they appear to be stronger and more robust than in adolescents and adults. There are several possible explanations for these differences, including changes in

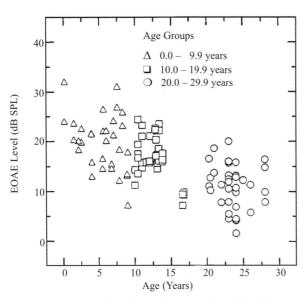

Figure 2. EOAE amplitude in response to 80 dB pe SPL clicks as a function of age.

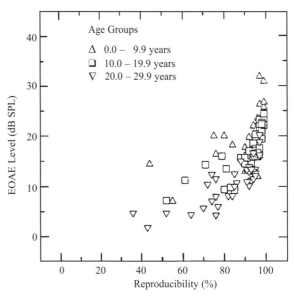

Figure 3. EOAE amplitude in response to 80 dB pe SPL clicks as a function of EOAE waveform reproducibility.

external and middle ear acoustics, developmental changes in cochlear mechanics, and age-associated cochlear changes due to normal wear and tear.

Humans are generally considered precocial with regard to auditory function in that most peripheral auditory system development is complete before birth (see Rubel, 1978, for a review). However, differences among neonates, infants, and young children are routinely observed and they may contribute to age-related EOAE differences in childhood.

The most basic differences are external and middle ear sound pressure transformations. There are obvious differences in the size, shape, and tissue of neonate and infant ear canals compared to adult ears. The tympanic membrane is more horizontal in neonates than adults and the tympanic ring is incomplete (Anson & Donaldson, 1981). The infant external ear is more cartilaginous than that the adult, making it more compliant (Margolis & Shanks, 1985). In addition, there are small differences in the average ear canal length, 25-26 mm for adults compared to 23 mm for neonates (Johansen, 1975). These physical differences are manifested as differences in the resonant frequency of the external ears of children. Kruger (Kruger, 1987; Kruger & Ruben, 1987) determined diffuse field to ear canal pressure transformations in children from birth to 3 years. She found that the resonant frequency of neonate ear canals ranged from 5.3 to 7.2 kHz, decreasing to the adult average of 2.7 kHz by 20 months of age. Conversely, the effective length of the ear canal increased over the same time period. In contrast to the small differences in physical length, Kruger

calculated that the effective length of the ear canal in neonates was 12 mm versus 32 mm for adults. The majority of changes in resonant frequency and length occurred in the first 6 to 12 months. Feigin, Kapin, Stelmachowicz, and Gorga (1989) measured sound pressure level generated in the ear canal using a probe microphone in children from 1 month to 5 years old. They were primarily interested in real ear coupler differences in children versus adults. They found that infants and children consistently demonstrated greater real ear coupler differences, that is, higher ear canal sound pressure levels, than adults. These differences, which averaged 4 dB, gradually decreased with age, but were still present at 5 years. Feigin et al predicted that the differences would disappear by 7.7 years, consistent with Nelson Barlow, Auslander, Rines, and Stelmachowicz (1988) who found no differences between 8 year olds and adults. While it has been suggested that the smaller ear canal volume of children may account for the higher sound pressure levels observed, Feigin et al found no correlation between real ear coupler differences and ear canal volume in their children.

Studies of acoustic impedance in neonates and infants have been concerned primarily with the application of tympanometry. Routinely, it has been reported that neonates show a high percentage of notched tympanograms, even for 220 Hz probe tones (Himelfarb, Popelka, & Shanon, 1979; Keith, 1973, 1975). Himelfarb et al reported that, for a 220 Hz probe tone, resistance was much higher than reactance and that reactance was often positive indicting that the

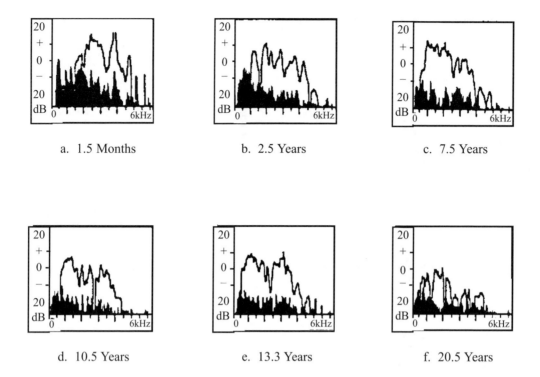

a. 1.5 Months   b. 2.5 Years   c. 7.5 Years

d. 10.5 Years   e. 13.3 Years   f. 20.5 Years

Figure 4. EOAE *(solid line)* and background noise *(shaded area)* spectra for waveforms shown in Figure 1.

ear was mass dominated. This resulted in double peaked tympanograms in about 50% of normal neonatal ears. These differences diminished by about 2 months of age, resulting in a net decrease in impedance and in typical single-peaked tympanograms for 220 Hz. Changes in ear canal volume due to the increased compliance of the wall of the external ear canal probably contributes significantly to these differences (Margolis & Shanks, 1985). However, there may be other middle ear maturational processes operating.

Although the probe used with infants and young children was designed to compensate for their smaller ear canals, differences in external and middle ear properties could affect both the evoking stimulus and the evoked emission. As noted earlier, the smaller ear canal volume does generate a higher stimulus level for a fixed voltage across the sound transducer, making it necessary to calibrate the stimulus level in the ear canal. The same increase in measured SPL of the cochlear output, that is, the EOAE, could occur. Likewise, the higher resonant frequency of the neonatal and infant ear canal could result in selective amplification of the higher frequency components of the EOAE in neonates and infants compared to adults. Persistence of some of these changes through the seventh year would be consistent with Nelson Barlow et al and the observation that the external ear canal continues to mature until about age 7 years (Northern &

Downs, 1978). We are currently studying the relationship between ear canal and middle ear characteristics and EOAE characteristics.

A second major source of age differences in EOAE characteristics could be cochlear differences. As noted above, the human is precocial with regard to the peripheral auditory system. By 26 to 28 fetal weeks, the human cochlea achieves a developmental status comparable to that found in other mammals when responses to sound can be reliably elicited (Rubel, 1978, 1985). This is consistent with strong EOAEs in neonates. However, why they should be stronger than in older infants, children, and adults is not obvious. It has been suggested that structural anomalies in humans and other primates may provide a basis for some spontaneous emissions and enhancement of evoked emissions (Lonsbury-Martin, Martin, Probst, & Coats, 1988; R. Pujol, personal communication; Wright, 1984). These include extra rows of outer hair cells and irregular stereocilia orientation. Such anomalies are routinely observed in human fetuses (R. Pujol, personal communication) and it may be that these subtle differences persist for some time after birth, contributing to enhanced spontaneous and evoked emissions in some neonates. This hypothesis will be difficult to test.

A third factor which may contribute to changes in EOAEs with age is normal cochlear wear and tear. The normal infant and young child is routinely exposed to high levels of sound and environmental toxins which may contribute to decreases in the output of the physiological vulnerable, active elements responsible for emissions (Norton, Mott, & Champlin, 1989). Although the group of individuals reported in the present study were carefully screened for noise exposure, they were undoubtedly exposed to noise in everyday situations.

Summary and Conclusions

Click-evoked otoacoustic emissions are present and robust in normal neonates, infants, and young children. Although there is individual variability, there are statistically significant decreases in EOAE amplitude in response to a fixed intensity stimulus with increasing age. This change may reflect changes in external and middle ear acoustics as well as cochlear changes. Changes in cochlear function may be normal developmental changes or represent normal wear and tear.

It is clear that, within the limits of individual variability and our present state of knowledge, EOAEs can be used (1) as a screening tool for cochlear dysfunction across individuals; and (2) to monitor changes over time in cochlear status within an ear.

Finally, while EOAEs are potentially a valuable clinical and research tool for assessing cochlear status in neonates, infants, and young children several questions must be answered. These include:

1. What is the relationship between normal changes in external and middle ear properties and EOAE characteristics?

2. Are there normal postnatal changes in the human cochlea which underlie changes in EOAEs?

3. What are the most significant and/or stable EOAE characteristics in relation to cochlear status? That is, is the presence or absence of an EOAE sufficient clinical information, or can significantly more information be known by examining evoked emission thresholds and growth functions across frequency?

Only by conducting both cross-sectional and longitudinal clinical trials of EOAEs in large numbers of infants and children will we be able to answer the above questions.

References

Anson, B.J., and Donaldson, J.A. *Surgical Anatomy of the Human Temporal Bone*. Philadelphia: WB Saunders, 1981.

Bargones, J.Y., and Burns, E.M. Suppression tuning curves for spontaneous otoacoustic emissions in infants and adults. *J Acoust Soc Am* 1988;83: 1809-1816.

Bonfils, P. Spontaneous otoacoustic emissions: clinical interest. *Laryngoscope* 1989;99:752-756.

Bonfils, P., Piron, J-P, Uziel, A., and Pujol, R. A correlative study of evoked otoacoustic emission properties and audiometric thresholds. *Arch Otorhinolaryngol* 1988;245:53-56.

Bonfils, P., and Pujol, R. Screening for auditory dysfunction in infants by evoked oto-acoustic emissions. *Arch Otolaryngol Head Neck Surg* 1988; 114:887-890.

Bonfils, P., Uziel, A., and Pujol, R. Evoked otoacoustic emissions from adults and infants: clinical applications. *Acta Otolaryngol* 1988a;105:445-449.

Bonfils, P., Uziel, A., and Pujol, R. Evoked otoacoustic emissions: a fundamental and clinical survey. *J Otorhinolaryngol Relat Spec* 1988b;50: 212-218.

Elberling, C., Parbo, J., Johnsen, J., and Bagi, P. Evoked otoacoustic emissions: clinical applications. *Acta Otolaryngol* (Stockh) 1985:421 (Suppl):77-85.

Feigin, J.A., Kopun, J.G., Stelmachowicz, P.G., and Gorga, M.P. Probe-tube microphone measures of ear-canal sound pressure levels in infants and children. *Ear Hear* 1989;10:254-258.

Himelfarb, M.Z., Popelka, G.R., and Shanon, E. Tympanometry in normal neonates. *J Speech Hear Res* 1979;22:179-191.

Johansen, P.A. Measurements of the human ear canal. *Acustica* 1975;33:349-351.

Johnsen, N.J., Bagi, P., and Elberling, C. Evoked otoacoustic emissions from the human ear. III. Findings in neonates. *Scand Audiol* 1983;12:17-24.

Keith, R.W. Impedance audiometry with neonates. *Arch Otolaryngol* 1973;97:465-467.

Keith, R.W. Middle function in neonates. *Arch Otolaryngol* 1975;101:376-379.

Kemp, D.T. Stimulated acoustic emissions from the human auditory system. *J Acoust Soc Am* 1978; 64:1386-1391.

Kemp, D.T. Developments in cochlear mechanics and techniques for noninvasive evaluation. *Adv Audiol* 1988;5:27-45.

Kemp, D.T., Bray, P., Alexander, L., and Brown, A.M. Acoustic emission cochleography-practical aspects. *Scand Audiol* 1986;25(Suppl):71-95.

Kruger, B. An update on the external ear resonance in infants and young children. *Ear Hear* 1987;8: 333-336.

Kruger, B., and Ruben, R.J. The acoustic properties of the infant ear. *Acta Otolaryngol* (Stockh) 1987;103:578-585.

Lonsbury-Martin, B.L., Martin, G.K., Probst, R., and Coats, A.C. Spontaneous otoacoustic emissions in non-human primate: II cochlear anatomy. *Hear Res* 1988;33:69-74.

Lutman, M.E., Mason, S.M., Sheppard, S., and Gibbin, K.P. Differential diagnostic potential of otoacoustic emissions: a case study. *Audiology* 1989;28:205-2110.

Margolis, R.H., and Shanks, J.E. Tympanometry. In Katz, J. Ed. *Handbook of Clinical Audiology*, 3rd ed. Baltimore: Williams & Wilkins, 1985.

Nelson Barlow, N.L., Auslander, M.C., Rines, D., and Stelmachowicz, P.G. Probe-tube microphone measures in hearing-impaired children and adults. *Ear Hear* 1988;9:243-247.

Northern, J.L., and Downs, M.P. *Hearing in Children*, 2nd ed. Baltimore: Williams & Wilkins, 1978.

Norton, S.J., Mott, J.B., and Champlin, C.A. Behavior of spontaneous otoacoustic emissions following intense ipsilateral acoustic stimulation. *Hear Res* 1989;38:243-258.

Probst, R., Coats, A.C., Martin, G.K., and Lonsbury-Manin, B.L. Spontaneous click- and toneburst-evoked otoacoustic emissions from normal ears. *Hear Res* 1986;21:261-275.

Probst, R., Lonsbury-Martin, B., Martin, G., and Coats, A. Otoacoustic emissions in ears with hearing loss. *Am J Otolaryngol* 1987;8:73-81.

Rubel, E.W. Ontogeny of structure and function in the vertebrate auditory system. In Jackson, M., (Ed). *Handbook of Sensory Physiology*. Vol. IX. Development of Sensory Systems. New York: Springer-Verlag, 1978.

Rubel, E.W. Strategies and problems for future study of auditory development. *Acta Otolaryngol* (Stockh), 1985;421:114-128.

Ruggero, M.A., Rich, N.C., and Freyman, R. Spontaneous and impulsively evoked otoacoustic emissions: indicators of cochlear pathology? *Hear Res* 1983;10:283-300.

Strickland, E.A., Burns, E.M., and Tubis, A. Incidence of spontaneous otoacoustic emissions in children and infants. *J Acoust Soc Am* 1985;78: 931-935.

Wright, A. Dimensions of the cochlear stereocilia in man and the guinea pig. *Hear Res* 1984;13:89-98.

Address reprint requests to: Susan J. Norton, Ph.D., CCC-A, Department of Hearing and Speech, University of Kansas Medical Center, 39th and Rainbow Blvd., Kansas City, KS 66103.

Distortion-Product and Click-Evoked Otoacoustic Emissions of Preterm and Full-Term Infants

Jacek Smurzynski, Marjorie D. Jung, Denis Lafreniere, D.O. Kim,
M. Vasudeva Kamath, Jonelle C. Rowe, Marlene C. Holman, and Gerald Leonard
Division of Otolaryngology, Department of Surgery (J.S., M.D.J., D.L., D.O.K., G.L.),
Center for Neurological Sciences (D.O.K.), Division of Neonatology,
Department of Pediatrics (M.V.K., J.C.R.), and Clinical Research Center (M.C.H.),
University of Connecticut Health Center, Farmington, Connecticut.

Abstract

Full-term and preterm infants were evaluated with click-evoked and distortion-product otoacoustic emissions (CEOEs and DPOEs). The CEOEs and DPOEs recorded from each individual ear were analyzed by calculating the root-mean-square levels within half-octave bands. The fail criterion of the OE tests was that the half-octave RMS DPOE or CEOE levels of an ear under test were below the 10th percentile of full-term newborns in two or more bands. The DPOE data were collected from 118 ears of 61 premature babies; 80 (68%) ears passed the DPOE test, 30 (25%) ears without middle ear effusions failed the test, and 8 (7%) ears with effusions also failed. The CEOE data were collected from 128 ears of 65 premature babies; 102 (80%) ears passed the CEOE test, 18 (14%) ears without middle ear effusions failed the test, 8 (6%) ears with effusions also failed. In 23 of 80 ears (29%) that passed the DPOE test and in 23 of 102 ears (23%) that passed the CEOE test, RMS OE levels of preterm infants were above the 90th percentile of full-term newborns. The analyses of the combined DPOE and CEOE data obtained from a group of 25 ears of full-term newborns and from a group of 72 ears of preterm babies showed statistically significant correlations between the DPOE and CEOE root-mean-square levels in each of the half-octave bands in the 1.4 to 4 kHz region. For 42 preterm infants tested with auditory brain stem response (ABR), specificity was 86% for CEOE and 74% for DPOE. All infants who failed the ABR also failed OE tests. To the best of our knowledge, this study is the first using combined DPOEs, CEOEs, and ABRs for preterm babies. It showed the feasibility of DPOEs and CEOEs for this population.

Since its initial discovery, the phenomenon of the otoacoustic emission (OE) (Kemp, 1978) has been studied by many investigators. Recent reviews may be found in studies by Shimizu (1990), Probst, Lonsbury-Martin, and Martin (1991), and Lonsbury-Martin, Whitehead, and Martin (1991). Evoked OEs come in different forms. Click-evoked otoacoustic emissions (CEOEs) are echo-like signals emitted after the presentation of a click. Distortion-product otoacoustic emissions (DPOEs) are continuous signals that appear at frequencies equal to some combination (e.g., $2f_1-f_2$, $2f_2-f_1$, f_2-f_1, etc.) of frequencies f_1 and f_2 of two continuous primary tones introduced to the ear canal. The mechanisms generating various types of OEs are not completely known. However, there is general agreement that OEs are produced under normal working conditions of the cochlea and indicate normal functioning of the outer hair cells (OHCs). When the cochlear mechanism of OHCs is impaired, hearing threshold is raised and OEs diminish. Therefore, OEs have been proposed as a means of detecting human sensorineural hearing impairment of cochlear origin. A large amount of information has been collected in normal-hearing and hearing-impaired adults using CEOEs (e.g., Avan, Bonfils, Loth, Narcy, & Trotoux, 1991; Bonfils, Bertrand, & Uziel, 1988a; Harris & Probst, 1992; Norton & Widen, 1990) and DPOEs (e.g., Kim, Leonard, Smurzynski, & Jung, 1992; Kimberly & Nelson, 1989; Martin, Ohlms, Franklin, Harris, & Lonsbury-Martin, 1990; Smurzynski, Leonard, Kim, Lafreniere, & Jung, 1990; Lonsbury-Martin et al, 1991).

Because early detection of hearing impairment is desirable, many investigators reported using CEOEs as a screening tool for auditory dysfunction in infants. Johnsen, Bagi, and Elberling (1983) reported CEOEs recorded in 20 full-term newborns at intensities near threshold. They concluded that CEOEs could be applicable as a screening procedure in newborns. Bonfils, Uziel, and Pujol (1988b) compared the CEOE and ABR results in 46 infant ears. The CEOEs were always present when ABR wave V threshold was equal to or below 30 dB HL. However, infants with ABR

Reprinted by permission of authors and Williams & Wilkins. Copyright 1993.
Ear & Hearing, 14, No. 4, pp. 258-274.

thresholds higher than 40 dB HL never had detectable CEOEs. Stevens, Webb, Hutchinson, Connell, Smith, and Buffin (1989) reported the CEOE and ABR data collected from 346 babies taken largely from a neonatal intensive care unit (NICU). They concluded that the CEOE test would make a good first screen to be followed by the ABR test if no CEOE was present. Norton and Widen (1990) presented CEOE data obtained from 106 ears of subjects ranging in age from 17 days to 30 years old. They found a statistically significant decrease in CEOE level as age increased and suggested that age-related changes in external and middle ear acoustics and developmental changes in cochlear mechanics might contribute to the effects of age on the CEOE level. A recent article by Bonfils, Francois, Avan, Londero, Trotoux, and Narcy (1992) presented results of spontaneous otoacoustic emissions and CEOEs for a group of 67 preterm infants not at risk for hearing loss. Their study found that there were no statistically significant variations of CEOE amplitude with postconceptional age and that the CEOE spectrum did not vary with postconceptional age.

Only limited DPOE data have been published concerning the pediatric population (e.g., Owens, McCoy, Lonsbury-Martin, & Martin, 1992). Studies of our group reported combined CEOE and DPOE data in children 4 to 10 years old (Spektor, Leonard, Kim, Jung, & Smurzynski, 1991) and in infants (Lafreniere, Jung, Smurzynski, Leonard, Kim, & Sasek, 1991). The latter study demonstrated the feasibility of DPOE among full-term newborns and provided a preliminary normal baseline for this age group. To our knowledge, no DPOE data have been published concerning preterm infants. The DPOE is believed to be generated in the organ of Corti in the region stimulated by the primary frequencies (e.g., Zurek, Clark, & Kim, 1982). Findings reported in the literature support the view that DPOE methods have the potential to test micromechanical properties of the inner ear in frequency-specific regions, including high frequencies (up to 8 kHz). The existing CEOE measuring system (i.e., the ILO88 system) does not allow to collect data for frequencies above 6 kHz. That frequency region was easily tested with DPOEs among adults (e.g., Lonsbury-Martin, Harris, Stagner, Hawkins, & Martin, 1990; Smurzynski & Kim, 1992) and among infants in our pilot study (Lafreniere et al, 1991). Therefore, exploring the feasibility of DPOEs among preterm infants is important.

An important consideration when testing babies is the possibility of middle ear pressure or fluid (Owens et al, 1992). Pressure imbalance has the effect of reducing CEOE energy below about 2 kHz and possibly increasing it above 3 kHz (Kemp, Ryan, & Bray, 1990). Middle ear fluid prevents the reception of OEs due to heavy loading of the tympanic membrane and ossicles. Failure to record OEs in an infant should be followed by otoscopy.

The goals of this study are: (1) to increase the data base of DPOEs obtained from healthy full-term newborns (reported preliminarily by Lafreniere et al, 1991) and, thus, to provide a normal baseline for this age group; (2) to measure CEOEs and to establish a normal baseline for full-term newborns; (3) to propose pass/fail criteria of DPOEs and CEOEs for infants; (4) to compare the CEOEs and DPOEs from the same newborn ears; (5) to obtain DPOEs and CEOEs from preterm infants and to compare their individual OE data to the normal baselines obtained from full-term newborns; (6) to compare the CEOEs and DPOEs from the same ears of preterm babies; (7) to investigate the influence of middle ear effusion on OEs; and (8) to compare OE data for preterm babies with their ABR results.

Methods

Procedures

The $2f_1-f_2$ DPOE measurements were conducted using a digital system based on an Ariel DSP-16 board in an IBM PC/AT computer. The waveforms corresponding to two pure tones with frequencies f_1 and f_2 were synthesized by the computer and were played out periodically by two separate channels of a 16-bit digital to analog converter on the Ariel board, which generated two sinusoidal signals, each 4.096 sec in duration. These signals were sent to a pair of Etymotic Research ER-2 insert earphones through two impedance-matching transformers. The primary tones were mixed acoustically and coupled via short tubes to an ear probe that was sealed into the external ear canal with an Etymotic Research infant eartip. The ear canal sound pressure was measured by a low-noise, miniature microphone system (Etymotic Research, ER-10B) with an internal amplifier providing an additional gain of +40 dB before the signal was delivered to a Krohn-Hite 3342 high-pass filter (48 dB/octave). The cutoff frequency was set at 100 Hz. The filtered signal was sampled by a 16-bit analog to digital converter of the DSP-16 board at a sampling rate of 50 kHz. The microphone signal was averaged in the time domain over the duration of the stimulus. Its fast Fourier transform (FFT) was performed yielding an amplitude and a phase spectrum represented with $f_0 = 48.8$ Hz. Because of the 4.096-sec average, the effective bandwidth around each component was approximately 0.25 Hz.

Multiple measurements were recorded for each frequency pair to obtain at least two results with consistent amplitudes and phases of the $2f_1$-f_2 DPOE and low background noise. These consistent data were averaged as vectors. The magnitude of that vector was taken as the DPOE magnitude for a particular frequency pair and was converted into DPOE level in dB SPL re 20 µPa. The level of the background noise was calculated as the average of the magnitudes of four FFT components adjacent to the $2f_1$-f_2 frequency (two above and two below the $2f_1$-f_2 frequency). Test parameters and FFT outputs were displayed on the computer monitor and stored on a disk for further analysis.

At the beginning of the DPOE measurement, the system was calibrated for each ear by applying a broadband chirp signal in each of the two ER-2 earphones sequentially. The chirp consisted of equiamplitude sine waves having a specified phase distribution. From this measurement, the system transfer function was obtained. The frequency characteristics of both ER-2 transducers placed in an ear canal were displayed graphically on the monitor and stored in the computer. The calibration data were used during the DPOE measurements to adjust the output voltage of the digital to analog converter signals at every frequency pair tested in order to obtain a specified value of sound pressure level in the sealed ear canal. The calibration curve was also used to check the fit of the probe in the ear canal. If the fit was good, the frequency characteristics of the ER-2 earphones were nearly flat for the low-frequency region (below 2 kHz). The sound pressure level was decreased below 1 kHz when a probe was loosely fit. We evaluated the lower limit of our system by measuring the level of the $2f_1$-f_2 signal in a rigid test cavity. The levels of the $2f_1$-f_2 signal obtained in the 2 cm^3 cavity after 10 repeated measurements were employed to determine the system distortion level at each frequency pair tested.

The DPOE data were collected using the iso-(f_2/f_1) paradigm, also called the "DPOE audiogram" paradigm. The primary tones were presented at 65 dB SPL. The f_2/f_1 ratio was kept at approximately 1.2 (varying from 1.18 to 1.23), whereas the frequencies f_1 and f_2 were varied in such a way as to produce the geometric mean of f_1 and f_2 at an equally spaced logarithmic frequency scale. The geometric mean of the frequencies f_1 and f_2 was varied in $\frac{1}{3}$ octave steps from approximately 8000 to 850 Hz (14 points). Table 1 gives details of the frequency range investigated.

The CEOEs were obtained using an ILO88 Otodynamic Analyzer (Kemp et al, 1990) that included a plug-in board for an IBM PC/AT computer. The standard default operational mode of the ILO88 was used as follows. Stimuli were 80 msec rectangular pulses presented at a rate of 50/sec. The gain of the ILO88 system was adjusted to present stimuli at a peak level of 82 ± 4 dB SPL. Pulses were generated by a 12-bit digital to analog converter and presented to the subject through a miniature transducer housed in a probe fitted in the subject's external ear canal. The sound pressure level in the ear canal was measured using a miniature microphone also housed within the probe. The output of the microphone was averaged in the time domain using a 12-bit analog to digital converter at a 25 kHz sampling rate. The ILO88 system used a nonlinear differential method by presenting four pulses in a block. Every fourth stimulus was inverted and was three times greater in amplitude. In a linear system, the sub-average of these four would be zero. The remaining response represented the nonlinear CEOE generated by the cochlea. The interval between the clicks within each block was 20 msec. Responses to stimulus blocks were averaged into two 20 msec buffers (A and B). Each response was windowed, blanking the first 2.5 msec. Then the responses were band-pass filtered from 600 to 6000 Hz. Responses to 260 stimulus blocks per buffer were obtained. A cross-correlation of the two averaged waveforms from buffers A and B was computed to obtain the reproducibility factor. It would be zero for two completely unrelated waveforms and 100% for identical waveforms. Kemp, Bray, Alexander, and Brown (1986) reported that reproducibility of at least 50% was associated with behavioral thresholds of 30 dB HL or better. Therefore, in the present study, a CEOE recording with the reproducibility greater than

Table 1. The f_1, f_2, and $2f_1$-f_2 frequencies in Hz, the geometric mean, $(f_1 \cdot f_2)^{fi}$, of f_1 and f_2 in Hz, and the f_2/f_1 ratio used in the DPOE audiogram measurements. The values of frequencies shown in the table are rounded to the integers.

f_1	f_2	$2f_1$-f_2	$(f_1 \cdot f_2)^{fi}$	f_2/f_1
781	928	634	851	1.19
928	1123	733	1021	1.21
1074	1269	879	1167	1.18
1269	1514	1024	1386	1.19
1514	1807	1221	1654	1.19
1807	2148	1466	1970	1.19
2197	2637	1757	2407	1.20
2588	3125	2051	2844	1.21
3076	3711	2441	3379	1.21
3662	4394	2930	4011	1.20
4346	5225	3467	4765	1.20
5176	6201	4151	5665	1.20
6152	7373	4931	6735	1.20
7324	8789	5859	8023	1.20

50% was one of the requirements to be accepted as a pass of the CEOE test. In addition to time-domain analysis, the spectra of each response and the background noise were computed. The overall CEOE spectrum was determined by taking 512-point FFTs of the two waveform buffers and then computing their cross-power spectrum. The noise spectrum was calculated by obtaining an FFT of the difference in the two waveforms (A-B). The frequency resolution of the CEOE and noise spectra was 48.8 Hz. The probe was fitted in the external ear canal using a shortened Etymotic Research infant eartip. Probe fit was judged by presenting a series of stimuli and observing their averaged waveform and spectrum. If needed, the probe was refitted (Kemp et al, 1990) to obtain a good seal without ringing in the waveform or internal probe blockage.

Most of the OE measurements were obtained in a single-walled, sound-treated booth in the audiology section of our center with the babies swaddled and placed in a bassinet. Some of the preterm infants were tested in a quiet room in the NICU with the babies placed in an isolette. At the time of the measurements, the infants were in natural sleep, usually after feeding. A typical session required approximately 45 min. The CEOE from one ear was recorded first (approximately 3 min), and then a complete "DPOE audiogram" from the same ear was obtained (during approximately 10-15 min) before testing was begun on the second ear. The noise produced by the subject during breathing, swallowing, and muscle and joint movement or by vascular pulsation was usually highest at the low frequencies—below 1.5 kHz. Therefore, a DPOE recording started with the geometric mean of primary tone frequencies at approximately 8 kHz. Then, the frequencies were gradually decreased in ⁄ octave steps for as long as detectable DPOEs could be recorded above the background noise. The interpretation of the individual DPOE data in terms of the DPOE detection was based on the level of noise itself and the signal (DPOE) to noise ratio. If the noise level was low and the level of the DPOE was at least 3 dB higher than the noise, we interpreted that measurement as a real emission detectable above the noise. If the noise was low but the signal to noise ratio was below 3 dB, we treated that measurement as an undetectable DPOE. If the noise was high, we interpreted the data as noisy measurements and invalid for further analysis. Usually, lower frequencies of primary tones required more presentations of two-tone stimuli to obtain two recordings with a relatively low background noise and consistent amplitude and phase of the DPOE. For some of the subjects, the noise floor was high and no detectable DPOEs could be recorded for frequencies below 2

kHz. Some other subjects were very quiet and some additional, clearly detectable DPOEs were recorded even in the 500 Hz region.

The ABR tests were conducted using a Grason-Stadler GSI 55 ABR screener. Electrodes were positioned at the high forehead and each mastoid. Impedance values were maintained below 5 kohm while bioelectric activity was recorded between the forehead and ipsilateral mastoid, with the contralateral mastoid serving as ground. Clicks of 100 μsec duration with negative polarity were presented at a rate of 20/sec through an insert earphone at the intensities of 60 and 30 dB nHL. Responses were amplified, with the filter setting at 150 to 2000 Hz (with 6 and 12 dB/octave) and averaged over 1024 sweeps. Each measurement was replicated at least once. The latency of wave V in milliseconds was obtained by placing the instrument's cursor on the peak of the wave and marking its position. Color-coded printouts of the two superimposed waveforms were obtained using a built-in printer.

Data Treatment

Several reports in the literature (e.g., Kemp et al, 1990; Lonsbury-Martin et al, 1990; Smurzynski & Kim, 1992) showed that the detailed characteristics of the OEs recorded from an ear are unique and depend on the individual. A CEOE spectrum often has "missing" frequency bands or notches, which are not believed to be associated with a hearing loss. Similarly, DPOE audiograms often show local peaks or troughs. An analysis of the DPOE and CEOE data described below was performed to smooth out individual data. The DPOEs recorded from each individual ear were converted into half-octave root-mean-square (RMS) levels in six frequency bands centered at approximately 1.0, 1.4, 2.0, 2.8, 4.0, and 5.6 kHz. The half-octave RMS level was computed from the data for three primary tone pairs falling within each of the half-octave bands, according to the standard definition of an RMS measure (e.g., Lapedes, 1978) as follows. The three DPOE levels, expressed in dB SPL (re 20 μPa), were converted into sound pressure amplitudes expressed in μPa. These were then squared, summed, and divided by three. Next, a square root of the result was taken and converted into dB SPL, which represented the half-octave RMS DPOE level. The half-octave RMS levels of the background noise and the system distortion were also computed in the six bands. Similarly, the CEOEs recorded from each individual ear were analyzed in five half-octave bands centered at approximately 1.0, 1.4, 2.0, 2.8, and 4.0 kHz. The RMS levels of the CEOE and the noise were calculated by averaging the CEOE and the noise levels at all 48.8 Hz intervals falling within each half-octave band. Those half-octave RMS OE levels were used to define the pass/fail criterion described under "Results."

Subjects

All subjects were selected from the neonatal population at John Dempsey Hospital, University of Connecticut Health Center, with full consent from the parents. Data were collected from two groups of subjects. The first group consisted of 48 ears of 30 full-gestation infants (13 males and 17 females) ranging in age from 2 to 4 days. The study of Kok, van Zanten, and Brocaar (1992) showed that the CEOE examination should not be done during first 24 hr postpartum. The full-term subjects were delivered naturally or by cesarean section and were not considered at risk for hearing impairment (i.e., normal prenatal history, normal bilirubin values, and no history of ototoxic drug use, anatomic malformation, bacterial meningitis, asphyxia, or familial history of childhood hearing impairment). All of the full-term subjects participated in both the DPOE and CEOE measurements. However, 15 ears were tested with DPOEs using a custom probe and 33 ears using the ER-10B probe. Our previous report (Lafreniere et al, 1991) suggested the influence of acoustical probe impedance on DPOE results. Therefore, only the DPOE data obtained using the ER-10B probe from 33 ears of 19 full-term infants were included in the present study. Bilateral DPOEs were collected for 14 of those infants. For two other subjects, poor OEs of one ear prompted otoscopic examinations that showed unilateral middle ear effusion and those data were excluded from the further analysis. Another three subjects woke up during the measurements and OE data were collected from one ear only. Bilateral CEOEs were collected for 18 full-term infants. In addition to two infants (described above) with unilateral effusion and three infants who woke up during the test, unilateral CEOE data of another seven infants were excluded from the normal database. Even though their CEOEs were clearly detectable, the test parameters were not consistent with our default values described in the procedure section. These included the number of averages with low noise less than 260 stimulus blocks, the unstable position of the probe during the test, or a stimulus peak level outside our range of 82 ± 4 dB SPL.

The second group consisted of 137 ears of 69 preterm neonates (35 males and 34 females). Birth weight ranged from 565 to 2380 g (mean = 1293 g; SD = 476 g), gestational age at birth ranged from 24 to 33 weeks (mean = 29.3; SD = 3.0 weeks), and postconceptional age, when tested, ranged from 33 to 44 weeks (mean = 37.5; SD = 3.2 weeks). Those subjects were tested at 2 to 14 weeks postpartum. Gestational age was assessed by estimated date of confinement, ultrasonic examination during pregnancy, and the modified Dubowitz examination (Ballard, Novak, & Driver, 1979; Dubowitz, Dubowitz, & Goldberg, 1970). If a difference of 2 or more weeks existed between the clinical assessment and the mother's dates, the clinical assessment (modified Dubowitz) was used. Hearing impairment risk factors for these infants (Joint Committee on Infant Hearing, 1991) included very low birth weight (<1500 g), hyperbilirubinemia, administration of ototoxic medications (aminoglycosides and loop diuretics used in combination with aminoglycosides), Apgar scores of 0 to 3 at 5 min, and prolonged mechanical ventilation. Before the OE evaluation, an otoscopic examination by an otolaryngologist was performed for every preterm infant. The DPOEs were collected from 118 ears of 61 preterm infants and the CEOEs from 128 ears of 65 preterm infants. Most of the subjects participated in both the DPOE and CEOE measurements. For others, only the CEOE or only the DPOE data were collected due to the subject's movement.

Results

The DPOE audiogram demonstrates the relationship between the level of the $2f_1$-f_2 DPOE and the geometric mean of f_1 and f_2. The results obtained from 33 ears of full-term infants are presented in Figure 1, which shows the median with the 10th, 25th, 75th, and 90th percentiles calculated for this group of ears. System distortion was determined as the 75th percentile of the level of the $2f_1$-f_2 obtained in a cavity, as described under "Methods." The 75th percentile of the background noise of the tested ears was calculated as described under "Methods." Analysis of the DPOEs from the 33 ears of healthy full-term newborns showed that all ears had detectable DPOEs that were above the noise floor of the system and above the background noise of the subjects in a frequency range of 850 to 8000 Hz. The median level of DPOEs was in the 6.5 to 11.4 dB SPL range for the geometric mean of primary tone frequencies below 3 kHz. There was a trough in the 3.4 to 4 kHz region with a minimum level of 0.7 dB SPL. A peak in the DPOEs was noted in a 4.8 to 6.7 kHz region where the maximal value of the median reached about 7 dB SPL. In general, the 10th percentile of the DPOE audiogram could be approximated by the value of 1 ± 3.5 dB SPL with the exceptions of -5.4 dB SPL in the 3.4 kHz trough region and -5.9 dB SPL in the 8 kHz region.

The 75th percentile of the system distortion (Fig. l) was below -20 dB SPL throughout the frequency range. It reflected the residual signal at the frequency of $2f_1$-f_2, resulting from the nonlinearity of the measuring system. The 75th percentile of the background noise (Fig. l) increased with decreasing frequencies below about 2 kHz, where the energy of the noise produced by the infant during breathing, swallowing, and movements is mostly concentrated. In the higher frequency region (above 2 kHz), the noise floor is below -13 dB SPL, but was above the system distortion. Thus, in most cases, the subject's noise limited the detection of DPOEs; however, for extremely quiet subjects, the system distortion determined the lower limit of our system.

Results of CEOE data collected from 48 ears of full-term newborns are presented in Figure 2. Figure 2A presents the median of CEOE spectra, with the 10th, 25th, 75th, and 90th percentiles calculated for this group. Each segment in Figure 2 corresponds to a frequency of the spectrum represented at every 48.8 Hz. All 48 ears of full-term newborns showed wideband CEOE spectra detectable above the background noise with the reproducibility factor greater than 70%. The median CEOE spectrum peaked in the 1.4 to 3.5 kHz region, where the CEOE level ranged from -6 to -2 dB SPL. For higher frequencies, the CEOE level

gradually decreased, reaching the level of -30 dB SPL at 5.3 kHz. The CEOE level also gradually decreased for frequencies below 1.3 kHz. Figure 2B presents the 25th percentile of CEOE spectra together with the 75th percentile of noise spectra for the same group of 48 ears shown in Figure 2A. This comparison shows that in general, the analysis of CEOE data was limited to a 1.3 to 4.5 kHz frequency region, where 75% of tested ears exhibited CEOEs detectable above the noise floor. This comment relates to the group data of CEOE and noise. In practice, the CEOEs from each ear should be treated individually in terms of signal to noise relations. Some of the ears tested showed low background noise, which did not obscure even low CEOEs. In some other ears with high CEOEs, even relatively high noise did not prevent acquisition of reliable CEOE recordings. The average overall CEOE level was 19.5 dB SPL (SD = 5.2 dB). The mean level of the A-B difference signal, which is the measure of the noise in the cochlear response, was 4.5 dB SPL (SD = 1.7 dB).

The analysis of individual DPOE and CEOE data showed that the detailed characteristics of the OEs recorded from an ear of a healthy newborn are unique and depend on the individual. An example of individual DPOE and CEOE data obtained from the left ear of a full-term boy (subject B33) are shown in Figure 3. The DPOE audiogram (Fig 3A) peaked in the 1 to 2 kHz region and showed a local trough at 2.4 kHz. The CEOE spectrum (Fig. 3B) had three narrow notches at the 1.8, 3, and 3.7 kHz regions. This spectrum also

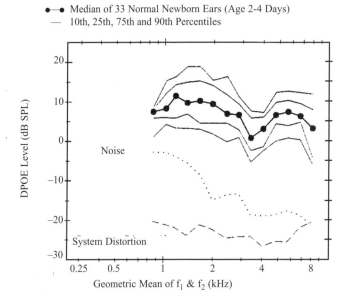

Median of 33 Normal Newborn Ears (Age 2-4 Days)
— 10th, 25th, 75th and 90th Percentiles

Figure 1. The "DPOE audiogram" showing $2f_1$-f_2 DPOE level versus geometric mean of f_1 and f_2 for 33 normal newborn ears. The *thick solid line with circles* represents the median, and the *thin solid lines* represent the 10th, 25th, 75th, and 90th percentiles. The *dashed line,* corresponding to the 75th percentile of multiple measurements of DPOE level in a test cavity, represents the system distortion. The *dotted line* corresponds to the 75th percentile of the background noise of the tested ears.

showed several narrow peaks. Figure 3C presents the half-octave RMS levels of the DPOE and noise derived from Figure 3A. The local peaks and notches were smoothed out. Please note that the noise level of that ear was very close to the system distortion. The half-octave RMS CEOE and noise levels derived from Figure 3B are shown in Figure 3D. All narrow notches and peaks that were present in the original CEOE spectrum (Fig. 3B) were removed by the half-octave band averaging.

The half-octave RMS calculations were performed for all individual OE data obtained from full-term newborns. Then, based on those RMS DPOE data obtained from a group of 33 ears of full-term newborns, the values corresponding to the 10th, 50th, and 90th percentiles were calculated for the six half-octave bands. Similar analysis was performed to obtain the 75th percentile of the half-octave RMS noise levels. Figure 4A presents the 10th, 50th, and 90th percentiles of half-octave RMS DPOE levels plotted versus the center frequency of half-octave bands. Also presented are the 75th percentile of half-octave RMS levels of noise and the 75th percentile of half-octave RMS levels of system distortion. The median of RMS levels peaked in the half-octave bands centered at the 1 to 2 kHz region and was in the 10 to 11 dB SPL range. A trough occurred in the 2.8 to 4.0 kHz region with an elevation of DPOEs in the 5.6 kHz band. The 10th percentile of the half-octave RMS DPOE levels could be approximated by the value of 4.7 ± 1.2 dB SPL, with the exception of 0.3 ± 0.6 dB SPL in the 2.8 to 4.0 kHz trough region. The 75th percentile of the half-octave RMS background noise levels was high at low frequencies (1-1.4 kHz) and then gradually decreased to approximately −19 dB SPL at 4 to 5.6 kHz.

Analogously, based on the half-octave RMS CEOE data obtained from a group of 48 ears of full-term newborns, the values corresponding to the 10th, 50th, and 90th percentiles were calculated for the five half-octave bands. A similar analysis was performed to obtain the 75th percentile of the RMS noise data. Figure 4B presents levels of half-octave RMS CEOE data obtained from full-term newborns plotted with the same logarithmic frequency scale as the DPOE data of Figure 4A. The 10th, 50th and 90th percentiles of the half-octave RMS CEOE levels and the 75th percentile of the half-octave RMS noise levels are presented. The median of RMS CEOE levels peaked in the 2.0 to 2.8 kHz region with a decrease for lower and higher frequencies. The 75th percentile of RMS noise level was the highest in the 1 kHz band and was higher than the median RMS CEOE level. For higher frequencies, the noise level dropped below the 10th percentile of the

RMS CEOE level. Therefore, further analysis of the RMS CEOE data is limited to the 1.4 to 4 kHz region. The 10th percentile of the half-octave RMS CEOE level could be approximated by the value of −10.4 ± 1.2 dB SPL in the 1.4 to 2.8 kHz region and by −14 dB SPL in the 4 kHz band.

The half-octave RMS OEs of full-term newborns shown in Figure 4 were used to evaluate OEs obtained from preterm infants. Figure 5 presents DPOE and CEOE data obtained from the left ear of subject P51, a preterm girl (born at 25 weeks gestational age, birth weight 740 g) tested at 40 weeks postconceptional age. Hearing impairment risk factors for this infant (Joint Committee on Infant Hearing, 1991) included very low birth weight, combined administration of aminoglycosides, and loop diuretics for 16 days and prolonged mechanical ventilation (47 days). Figure 5A presents the DPOEs of subject P51 plotted on top of the 10th and 90th percentiles of healthy full-term infants. The left ear of subject P51 exhibited high DPOEs, close to or even higher than the 90th percentile of normal new-

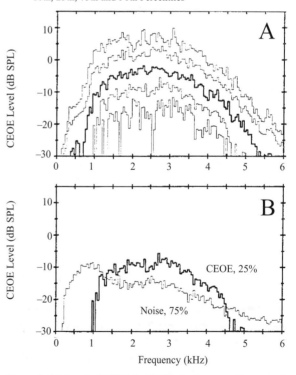

— Median of 48 Normal Newborn Ears (Age 2-4 Days)
— 10th, 25th, 75th and 90th Percentiles

Figure 2. (*A*) Level of CEOE in 48.8 Hz bands versus frequency for 48 normal newborn ears. The *thick line* represents the median, and the *thin lines* represent the 10th, 25th, 75th, and 90th percentiles. (*B*) The 25th percentile of CEOE spectra *(thick line)* and the 75th percentile of noise spectra *(thin line)* for the same group of 48 ears as shown in *panel A.*

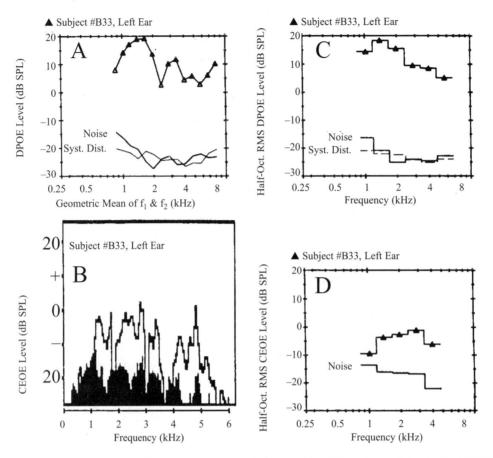

Figure 3. Individual DPOE and CEOE data obtained from the left ear of a full-term boy. (*A*) "DPOE audiogram" showing $2f_1$-f_2 DPOE level versus geometric mean of f_1 and f_2 n. The *thick solid line* corresponds to the background noise of the tested ear. The *dashed line* represents the system distortion. (*B*) CEOE *(unshaded area)* and noise *(shaded area)* spectra obtained using the ILO88 system.(*C*) Half-octave RMS levels of DPOE n, noise *(thick line)*, and system distortion *(thin line)* versus center frequency of the half-octave bands calculated from raw data presented in *panel A*. *(D)* Half-octave RMS levels of CEOE n and noise *(thick line)* versus center frequency of the half-octave bands calculated from raw data presented in panel B. Please note that *panels A, C,* and D have a logarithmic frequency scale, but *panel B* has a linear frequency scale as originally displayed by the ILO88 system.

borns for almost the entire frequency region. Figure 5B presents the CEOEs of subject P51 plotted on top of the 10th and 90th percentiles of healthy full-term infants. This ear exhibited high CEOEs in the 2 to 4 kHz region.

Figure 6 presents DPOEs (Fig. 6A) and CEOEs (Fig. 6B) obtained from the right ear of subject P28, a preterm girl (born at 30 weeks gestational age, birth weight 1420 g) tested at 34 weeks postconceptional age. Hearing impairment risk factors for this infant included very low birth weight and administration of aminoglycosides for 17 days. The DPOEs of the right ear of subject P28 (Fig. 6A) were within the normal range (between the 10th and 90th percentiles of normal newborns ears) in the 1 to 2 kHz region. For higher frequencies, the DPOEs decreased and dropped below the 10th percentile. However, those DPOEs were clearly detectable above the background noise (Fig. 6A).

During the test, the infant was very quiet and the subject's noise was close to the system distortion measured in the cavity (Fig. 6A). The half-octave RMS CEOE level recorded from this ear was high in the 1.4 kHz range (Fig. 6B). However, for higher frequencies, the CEOEs were below the noise. The CEOE test was repeated three times within 2 days and the results were consistent with those presented in Figure 6B. The results of otoscopy were normal for both ears. The CEOEs from the left ear of subject P28 were within the normal range for the entire frequency region. The ABR test performed for each ear showed normal latency-intensity functions in the 30 to 60 dB nHL range. The DPOE and CEOE results from the right ear of this subject suggested a possibility of a mild high-frequency sensorineural hearing loss with a decrease of hearing sensitivity in the region above approximately 3 kHz. If that is the case, we might still obtain normal

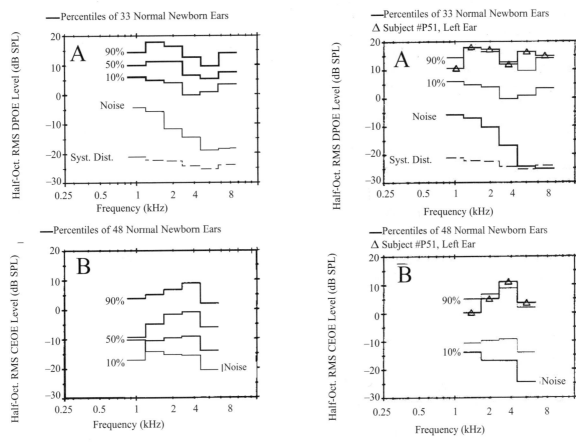

Figure 4. Half-octave RMS DPOE (*A*) and CEOE *(B)* levels versus center frequency of half-octave bands for a group of normal newborn ears. *Thick solid lines* correspond to the 10th, 50th, and 90th percentiles. (*A*) DPOE data for a group of 33 normal newborn ears. The thin *solid line* corresponds to the 75th percentile of the half-octave RMS levels of the background noise of the tested ears. The *dashed line* corresponds to the 75th percentile of the half-octave RMS levels of the system distortion *(B)* CEOE data for a group of 48 normal newborn ears. The thin *solid line* corresponds to the 75th percentile of the half-octave RMS levels of the noise of the tested ears.

Figure 5. Examples of individual RMS DPOE and CEOE data from the left ear of subject P51 (a preterm girl) superimposed on the 10th and 90th percentiles data. (*A*) The *thin solid lines* correspond to the 10th and 90th percentiles of the half-octave RMS DPOE levels obtained from 33 normal newborn ears. n, left ear of subject P51. The *thick solid line* represents the half-octave RMS noise levels of subject P51. (*B*) The *thin solid lines* correspond to the 10th and 90th percentiles of the half-octave RMS CEOE levels obtained from 48 normal newborn ears. n, left ear of subject P51. The *thick solid line* represents the half-octave RMS noise levels of subject P51.

results of the click ABR test reflecting neural activities in the 1 to 3 kHz region. Follow-up on this subject is planned by the audiology clinic of our center.

The results presented in Figure 6 illustrate a need of having systematic pass/fail criteria to analyze the OEs clinically. In our study, we used half-octave RMS levels of DPOEs and CEOEs as measures of individual OEs for preterm infants. Those data were compared to the normal ranges defined by the 10th and 90th percentiles of RMS levels obtained from a group of normal newborn ears, as illustrated in Figures 5 and 6. Our definition of "normal newborn ears" was based on several assumptions. The prevalence of hearing loss among newborns not considered at risk for hearing impairment is estimated as 0.1% (Turner, 1991). Therefore, the probability of including a hearing-

impaired newborn in our normal population was very low. The second assumption is based on OE results reported in the literature for adults with a known hearing status. Those data support the assumption that DPOEs clearly detectable above the background noise in a particular frequency region correspond to hearing sensitivity better than 35 to 40 dB HL in that region (e.g., Lonsbury-Martin et al, 1991). That was the case for all ears from the first group of our full-term subjects. However, it should be kept in mind that because our normal subjects had not yet been seen for behavioral tests, their true hearing status was not available at the time of the study. Nevertheless, we treated them as normal-hearing newborns as our first approach of defining pass/fail criteria. More OE data for this risk-free population combined with behavioral follow-up information would be needed to establish "perfectly normal OE ranges."

In the present study, if a preterm infant ear's half-octave RMS DPOE or CEOE level was below the 10th percentile of full-term newborns in a particular frequency band, we defined it to be an abnormal OE in that frequency band. If RMS DPOE or CEOE levels of an ear were below the 10th percentile in two or more bands, we defined the ear to be a failure in the DPOE or CEOE test. In addition, the CEOE pass criterion also included the requirement that the reproducibility was greater than 50%. According to our criteria, the right ear of subject P28 failed both the DPOE and CEOE tests. As depicted in Figure 6, the RMS DPOE and CEOE levels were below the 10th percentile in three half-octave bands. Figure 5 illustrates an example in which individual OE data obtained for a preterm infants were higher than the normal range.

Tables 2 and 3 present outcomes of the DPOE and CEOE tests, respectively, for each of the half-octave bands. As mentioned under "Methods," some of the subjects were not quiet enough to measure DPOEs in the low-frequency region. Qualitatively based on the noise data obtained from the full-term newborns (Fig. 1), we arbitrarily set the acceptance condition of the noise to be below 0 dB SPL for the primary frequencies at and below 2 kHz and below –10 dB SPL for higher frequencies. If the noise was higher than the above criterion, we interpreted the data as noisy measurements and invalid for further analysis. The last row of Table 2 shows the number of ears for which DPOEs with low noise were obtained in particular half-octave frequency bands. The DPOE data recorded from all 118 ears were available for the analysis at 2.8 kHz and above. The number of ears with valid data decreased as the primary tones decreased. Table 2 gives the number of ears of preterm infants that exhibited RMS DPOE levels below the 10th percentiles of normal newborn ears in the specified half-octave bands. Eight of the 118 ears were found to have middle ear effusions, as determined by otoscopy. Therefore, the number of failures is shown separately for ears with and without effusion. The top right part of Table 2 shows the number of ears that had RMS levels below the 10th percentiles in at least two half-octave bands, thus showing the number of ears that failed the DPOE test. All eight ears with middle ear effusions failed the DPOE test. Five of the eight ears exhibited RMS DPOE levels below the 10th percentiles for all frequency bands at which the DPOE data were available. Three of the eight ears had RMS DPOE levels above the 10th percentiles in one or two bands in the 2.8 to 5.6 kHz region, but below the 10th percentile in at least two

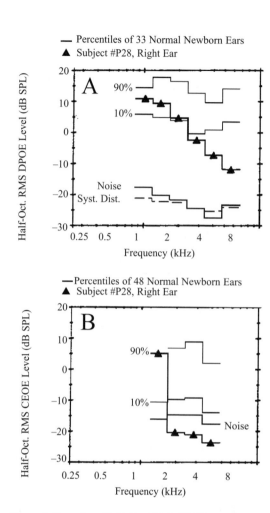

Figure 6. Examples of individual RMS DPOE and CEOE data from the right ear of subject P28 (a preterm girl) superimposed on the 10th and 90th percentile data. (*A*) The *thin solid lines* correspond to the 10th and 90th percentiles of the half-octave RMS DPOE levels obtained from 33 normal newborn ears. ▲, right ear of subject P28. The *thick solid line* represents the half-octave RMS noise levels of subject P28. (*B*) The *thin solid lines* correspond to the 10th and 90th percentiles of the half-octave RMS CEOE levels obtained from 48 normal newborn ears. ▲, right ear of subject P28. The *thick solid line* represents the half-octave RMS noise levels of subject P28.

other bands. The incidence of ears failing the DPOE test was 27.3% (30 out of 110 ears) among preterm infant ears without middle ear effusions. The incidence of abnormal DPOEs increased as higher frequencies of the half-octave band were analyzed and was the greatest at 5.6 kHz [i.e., 26 out of 110 ears without effusion (23.6%) exhibited the RMS DPOE level below the 10th percentile]. In terms of number of infants, 25 out of 61 infants (41%) tested for DPOEs failed the test. Thirteen of them failed bilaterally and 12 unilaterally. Table 2 also shows the number of ears of preterm infants that exhibited high DPOEs above the 90th percentile in each specified half-octave band. The inci-

Table 2. Number of ears of preterm infants that exhibited half-octave RMS DPOE levels below the 10th percentile or above the 90th percentile of normal full-term newborn ears in the specified frequency bands. The ears with low DPOEs are further categorized as to the presence of middle ear effusions. The number of ears that exhibited low or high DPOEs in two half-octave bands or more is listed in the far right column. The lowest row presents number of ears for which DPOE data with low noise were obtained at a particular frequency region.

	Center Frequency of Half-Octave Band (kHz)						Two Bands or More
	1.0	1.4	2.0	2.8	4.0	5.6	
<10%							
Total	2	17	24	24	31	33	38
With effusion	1	6	7	6	7	7	8
Without effusion	1	11	17	18	24	26	30
>90%	2	4	5	21	28	10	23
Total collected with low noise	23	85	108	118	118	118	

Table 3. Number of ears of preterm infants that exhibited half-octave RMS CEOE levels below the 10th percentile or above the 90th percentile of normal full-term newborn ears in the specified frequency bands. The ears with low CEOEs are further categorized as to the presence of middle ear effusions. Number of ears of preterm infants that exhibited low or high CEOEs in two half-octave bands or more is listed in the far right column. The lowest row presents number of ears for which CEOE data with low noise were obtained at a particular frequency region.

	Center Frequency of Half-Octave Band (kHz)				Two Bands or More
	1.4	2.0	2.8	4.0	
<10%					
Total	29	20	24	19	26
With effusion	9	5	7	4	8
Without effusion	20	15	17	15	19
>90%	9	15	20	27	23
Total collected with low noise	122	128	128	128	

dence of high DPOEs among preterm infants was the highest at the 4 and 2.8 kHz bands. As shown in the table, 23 ears had high DPOEs in at least two half-octave bands, which is 20.9% of all ears without effusion (23/110) or 28.7% (23/80) of all ears of preterm infants that passed the DPOE test.

Table 3 presents a summary of individual CEOE data for a group of preterm infants. Six ears (out of 128 tested) exhibited clearly detectable CEOEs for the higher frequencies, but no detectable emission in the lower frequencies. These subjects were noisy and their low-frequency noise obscured the CEOE in that region. This resulted in the noise RMS level being higher than the CEOE level in the 1.4 kHz half-octave band, which prevented the detection of any possible CEOE in this frequency region. In order to be accepted as a valid test in each halfoctave band, we required the half-octave CEOE level to be more than 3 dB above the RMS noise level in that band. Table 3 gives the number of ears of preterm infants that exhibited RMS CEOE levels below the 10th percentiles of normal newborn ears in the specified half-octave bands (with and without middle ear effusion). The far right column of Table 3 shows the number of ears that had RMS levels below the 10th percentiles in at least two half-octave bands, thus showing the number of ears that failed the CEOE test. Otoscopy determined the presence of middle ear effusion in 10 ears that were tested with CEOEs. Twelve ears (three with middle ear effusions) had absent CEOEs (i.e., the reproducibility factor was lower than 50% and the RMS CEOE levels were below the lowest values obtained among the normal newborn ears). Eight out of 10 ears with effusions

failed the CEOE test. Six ears with effusions exhibited RMS CEOE levels above the 10th percentile of normal newborn ears in the 4 kHz half-octave band. However, four of those ears had low CEOEs in at least two half-octave bands below 4 kHz and, thus, failed the CEOE test. One ear with effusion had RMS CEOEs below the normal range in the 1.4 kHz band, but within the normal range in 2 to 4 kHz region, thus passing the CEOE test. One ear with effusion had RMS CEOEs around the median of normal range. In summary, 2 ears out of 10 passed the CEOE test despite the presence of effusion. The incidence of failing the CEOE test was 16.1% (19 out of 118 ears) among those ears without effusions. The failure rate was rather equally distributed across the half-octave bands. Twenty-one out of 65 infants (32.3%) tested for CEOE failed the test; 5 of them bilaterally and 16 unilaterally. Table 3 also shows the number of ears that exhibited high CEOEs above the 90th percentile in the specified half-octave bands. The incidence of high CEOEs among preterm infants was the highest at the 2.8 and 4 kHz regions. As shown in the table, 23 ears had high CEOEs in at least two half-octave bands, which is 19.5% of all ears without effusions (23/118) or 22.5% (23/102) of all ears of preterm infants that passed the CEOE test.

One of the goals of the present study was to compare the OE data to the ABR results among infants at risk for hearing impairment. Even though it is generally agreed that the ABR is not a direct measurement of hearing sensitivity, ABR testing is the recommended evaluation for the initial neonatal hearing screening (Joint Committee on Infant Hearing, 1991). Because several authors suggested that the OE tests would provide important additional information (e.g., Stevens et al, 1989), the OE data were compared to the ABR results. The ABR screening was performed on 42 preterm infants (84 ears) who were evaluated with OE tests. The fail criterion for the ABR was an undetectable wave V at 30 dB nHL stimulus level. Three of the 42 infants (four ears) passed the ABR even though otoscopy determined the presence of the middle ear effusions. The comparison of the ABR and OE data for the ears of preterm infants without effusions is presented in Table 4. All ears that failed the ABR also failed the OE tests. There was a group of ears that passed the ABR but failed the CEOE and/or DPOE tests. The right ear of subject P28 (Fig. 6) is an example of such a case. The specificity of the DPOE and CEOE tests determined on the basis of the ABR test results (i.e., percentage of OE passes among all ABR passes) was 73.9 and 86.3%, respectively. When the frequency range of the DPOE data analysis was limited to the 1.4 to 4 kHz region (the same as for the CEOE data), its specificity increased to 78.3% (54/69).

A tendency we observed during this study was that an ear exhibiting high DPOEs also exhibited high CEOEs. The OEs of the left ear of subject P51 presented in Figure 5 illustrate this tendency. Some other ears exhibiting low DPOEs also showed low CEOEs. An analysis of the combined DPOE and CEOE data collected for preterm and full-term infants was performed to verify the hypothesis that the two types of OEs are correlated. The combined DPOE and CEOE data obtained from 25 ears of full-term newborns were analyzed in four half-octave bands centered at approximately 1.4, 2.0, 2.8, and 4.0 kHz. The relationship between individual RMS DPOE levels versus RMS CEOE levels was plotted for each half-octave band. The results are presented in Figure 7. The linear regression was performed for the data obtained from the 25 ears (Fig. 7). The slope of the regression line and the correlation coefficient (r) are listed in Table 5. The regression analysis showed statistically significant correlation between the half-octave RMS values of DPOEs and CEOEs in the 2 and 4 kHz regions at the 0.005 level of significance. The level of significance was 0.05 for the 2.8 kHz region and 0.01 for the 1.4 kHz band. A similar analysis was performed for the OE data obtained from preterm infants who passed both DPOE and CEOE tests according to the criteria described above. As mentioned before, low-frequency DPOE data could not be collected for some of the preterm infants due to high background noise. Therefore, the number of ears included in the correlation analysis was 55 for the 1.4 kHz region and 72 for higher frequencies. The results are plotted in Figure 8

and the details of the regression analysis are listed in Table 6. The regression analysis showed statistically significant correlation between the RMS values of DPOEs and CEOEs in the 1.4 kHz region at the 0.01 level of significance. The level of significance was 0.001 for the remaining three regions. In general, the data presented in Figures 7 and 8 showed a trend for the level of the two types of OEs to be correlated. However, there was also some scatter in the data. Therefore, a statistical model more complex than a linear one might provide more insight into the relationship between the two measurements. In should be also kept in mind that the data presented in Figures 7 and 8 were obtained for one stimulus condition of CEOE and one stimulus condition of DPOE. It is still possible that other conditions for either or both OE types might provide different insights into the relationship between them.

The RMS OE regression data obtained from two groups of subjects (i.e., full-term and preterm infants), presented in Figures 7 and 8 were tested for homogeneity of the two groups. An F-test in an analysis of covariance was used (Steel & Torrie, 1980) to compare the regression data separately for each of the four half-octave bands. Between the two populations, no statistically significant differences were found in any of the bands ($F_{1,78} = 0.62$ for 1.4 kHz band; $F_{1,95} = 1.19$ for 2 kHz; $F_{1,95} = 1.03$ for 2.8 kHz; $F_{1,95} = 0.01$ for 4 kHz). Therefore, the null hypothesis of equality of two regression lines of the data from preterm and full-term infants could not be rejected for any of the four half-octave bands.

Discussion

All ears in our sample of full-term newborns showed detectable DPOEs for the frequency range of the geometric mean of primary tones varying from approximately 0.8 to 8 kHz, with the level of primary tones kept at 65 dB SPL. This finding is consistent with our previous newborn study (Lafreniere et al, 1991) and with studies of DPOEs for normal-hearing children (Spektor et al, 1991) and adults (e.g., Lonsbury-Martin et al, 1990; Smurzynski & Kim, 1992). The DPOE data obtained for full-term newborns (Fig. l) are qualitatively similar to those of adults measured previously using the same equipment and procedure (Smurzynski & Kim, 1992). Both age groups showed a dip in the DPOE audiograms. However, the frequency of the dip for newborns (3.4 kHz) was higher than that obtained for adults (2.8 kHz). The newborns showed a higher level of DPOEs in the middle frequency region (1.6-2.8 kHz) and a lower level in the

Table 4. Comparison of the ABR and the OE tests for preterm infants without middle ear effusions. Each entry represents the number of ears. The fail criterion for ABR was an undetectable wave V at 30 dB nHL stimulus level. The fail criteria for the DPOE and CEOE tests were that half-octave RMS levels were below the 10th percentile of normal full-term newborns in two or more bands.

		ABR				ABR	
		Pass	Fail			Pass	Fail
	Pass	51	0		Pass	63	0
DPOE				CEOE			
	Fail	18	5		Fail	10	7

Specificity = 51/(51 + 18) = 73.9%	Specificity = 63/(63 + 10) = 86.3%

higher frequencies (3.4-6.7 kHz) than the adults. Lonsbury-Martin et al (1990), analyzing their own DPOE data for adults, speculated that the middle frequency decline in DPOE level could be caused by an interaction of the resonances common to a particular individual's middle ear and cochlea. If that is the case, changes of the resonances of the outer and middle ear occurring during the maturation processes could affect the frequency of the dip in the DPOE audiogram, as illustrated in Figure 1 and our previous adult data (Smurzynski & Kim, 1992). As expected, the noise level of the full-term infants (dotted line in Fig. 1) was higher than that of the previously tested adults over the entire frequency range.

All ears in our sample of full-term newborns also showed detectable CEOEs. This finding is consistent with several previous studies. Johnsen, Bagi, Parbo, and Elberling (1988) showed detectable CEOEs in all 199 newborn ears tested. Bonfils, Dumont, Marie, Francois, and Narcy (1990) reported the presence of CEOEs in 98 out of 100 ears of full-term newborns. Uziel and Piron (1991) identified a clear and reproducible CEOE at a stimulus level of 30 dB nHL in 105 out of 108 ears of normal newborns. The CEOE spectrum of some of the ears in our sample was limited to 4.5 kHz, as shown by the 10th percentile curve in Figure 2A. A comparison of the median CEOE spectrum from newborn ears (Fig. 2, present study) to that of adults (Smurzynski & Kim, 1992) depicts several differences between the two age groups. The CEOE level of newborns was higher than that of adults for frequencies above 1.5 kHz. For frequencies below 1.5 kHz, the level of CEOE was higher in adults than in newborns. The differences between the CEOE spectra for low and high frequencies could be due to different stimulus spectra observed for the two age groups (Kemp et al, 1990; Lafreniere et al, 1991). The spectrum of click stimulus in newborns' ears exhibited a

band-passed shape with a decline below about 2 kHz and above about 4.5 kHz, whereas that in adults' ears exhibited a low-passed shape with a flat spectrum in the low-frequency range and a decline above about 4 kHz. The noise level of newborns (Fig. 2B) was higher than that of the adults (Smurzynski & Kim, 1992) over the entire frequency region.

Some individual DPOE audiograms recorded from ears of full-term newborns were not smooth curves, but had peaks and troughs obtained for consecutive pairs of primary tones (e.g., Fig. 3A). Some of those ears produced a low-level DPOE for a particular pair of primary tones. When the frequencies of primaries were shifted up or down by as little as 48.8 Hz from a trough condition, the DPOE level increased to a normal level in some ears. Therefore, in a clinical application, an unusually low-level DPOE obtained from an infant ear with one stimulus frequency would require additional measurements surrounding this frequency to avoid a false interpretation. The unique type of individual DPOE audiograms was also illustrated by the inter-subject DPOE variability. The distance between the 10th and the 90th percentiles of DPOE audiograms collected from normal newborn ears (Fig. 1) was in the 10 to 18 dB range except for the lowest pair of primary tones at 850 Hz region, where that value was 8 dB. Similarly, detailed CEOE characteristics of individual newborn ears showed unique patterns often exhibiting distinct peaks and notches (e.g., Fig. 3B). The unique pattern of each CEOE spectrum led to a high degree of intersubject variability of the CEOE data. The distance between the 10th and the 90th percentiles of 48.8 Hz CEOE spectra collected for normal newborn ears (Fig. 2A) was in the 14 to 30 dB range in the 1.4 to 4.5 kHz region except for two narrow bands (at around 1.7 and 2.5 kHz), where the 10th percentile level dropped below −30 dB SPL. The greater distance between the 10th and 90th percentiles of the CEOEs than the DPOE counterpart represents a greater intersubject variability of the CEOEs than the DPOEs. Among full-term infants, the higher degree of intersubject variability seen in the CEOE data when compared to the DPOEs was also observed when the results were averaged over half-octave bands (Fig. 4). In addition, the slopes of the linear regression lines for the data collected from full-term newborns (Fig. 7) and from preterm infants (Fig. 8) were < 1 for all four half-octave bands. Slopes < 1 indicated that the range of RMS CEOE variability was greater than the range of RMS DPOE variability for both groups of infants. The irregular, local DPOE and CEOE behaviors observed for some newborn ears suggested that using a smoothing technique on the raw data could be useful in forming

FULL-TERM INFANTS

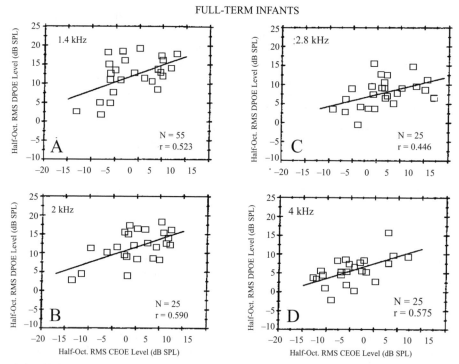

Figure 7. The relationship between RMS DPOE levels versus RMS CEOE levels of 25 ears of full-term newborns calculated in half-octave bands centered at approximately 1.4 kHz (*A*), 2.0 kHz (*B*), 2.8 kHz (*C*), and 4.0 kHz (*D*). The *straight thick lines* correspond to the linear regression lines obtained for 25 ears. Correlation coefficients (r) are shown within each panel.

DPOE and CEOE baselines and in defining the pass/fail criteria of DPOE and CEOE tests. We decided to use RMS values averaged over half-octave bands to smooth out local irregularities (Fig. 3). Those RMS data transformed into the 10th and 90th percentiles of full-term infant ears established the normal ranges for DPOEs and CEOEs and were used to compare the OEs obtained from preterm infants (Fig. 4). As a result of this data transformation, we were able to establish pass/fail criteria for OE tests in specified half-octave frequency bands.

Table 5. Details of the correlation analysis for the DPOE and the CEOE data of full-term infants (25 ears). The RMS values of both DPOE and CEOE levels were computed over half-octave bands, 3 points for DPOEs and 10 to 29 points for CEOEs. All frequencies are in Hz.[a]

Center Frequency of the Band	$(f_1 \cdot f_2)^{fi}$ for DPOEs	Frequency Range of CEOE	Linear Regression	
			Slope	r
1386	1167;1386;1654	1172-1660	0.45	0.523
1970	1654;1970;2407	1660-2393	0.42	0.590
2844	2407;2844;3379	2393-3369	0.31	0.446
4011	3379;4011;4765	3369-4785	0.39	0.575

[a]The critical values for the correlation coefficient r are: $N = 25$, $r_{0.05} = 0.396$, $r_{0.01} = 0.505$, $r_{0.005} = 0.543$.

The incidence of hearing loss among newborns in the high-risk registry for hearing impairment has been reported to be around 1.5% (Northern & Gerkin, 1989). Many infants at risk for hearing loss are preterm neonates. To the best of our knowledge, this study is the first one using combined DPOEs, CEOEs, and ABRs for preterm infants. The results showed the feasibility of DPOEs and CEOEs among preterm infants. Most of the infants were quiet enough to perform the OE recordings. Some of the infants were restless and had to be settled down before the recordings could be completed. As expected, the subject noise was highest in the low frequencies, as illustrated in Figures 1, 2B, and 4 for a group of full-term infants. The low-frequency noise prevented collection of DPOEs in the 1 kHz region for many of the subjects, as illustrated in Table 2. However, DPOEs were collected for 72% (85 of 118) of the ears in the 1.4 kHz region and for 91% (108 of 118) of the ears in the 2 kHz region. Some of the infants were extremely quiet and the subject's noise was comparable to the system distortion, as illustrated by the DPOE data of subject P28 (Fig. 6A).

There were several previous reports on using CEOEs in neonatal screening for NICU infants and comparing the CEOE data to the ABR results. For example, Stevens, Webb, Hutchinson, Connell, Smith, and Buffin (1990) tested 723 NICU infants and

PRE-TERM INFANTS

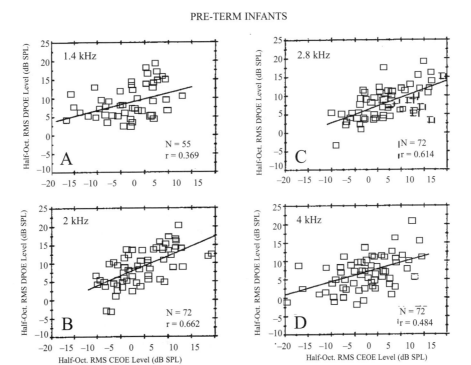

Figure 8. The relationship between RMS DPOE levels versus RMS CEOE levels of ears of preterm newborns calculated in half-octave bands centered at approximately 1.4 kHz (*A*), 2.0 kHz *(B)*, 2.8 kHz *(C)*, and 4.0 kHz *(D)*. The *straight thick lines* correspond to the linear regression lines obtained for 55 ears (*A*) and 72 ears *(B, C,* and *D)*. Correlation coefficients (r) are shown within each panel.

showed that 80% of the subjects produced recordable CEOEs. The sensitivity and specificity with regard to the ABR results in the period up to 3 months post due date was 93 and 84%, respectively. The criterion of passing the CEOE test used by Stevens, Webb, Smith, Buffin, and Ruddy (1987) was based on visual scoring of the cochlear response and the correlation value between the two average waveforms. In our study, the 10th percentile of the half-octave RMS CEOE level was used to establish the pass/fail criterion. Any ear

Table 6. Details of the correlation analysis for the DPOE and the CEOE data of preterm infants (55 ears for 1.4 kHz region and 72 ears for 2-4 kHz region) who passes both DPOE and CEOE tests. The RMS values of both DPOE and CEOE levels were computed over half-octave bands, 3 points for DPOEs and 10 to 29 points for CEOEs. All frequencies are in Hz.

Center Frequency of the Band	$(f_1 \cdot f_2)^{fi}$ for DPOEs	Frequency Range of CEOEs	Linear Regression	
			Slope	r
1386	1167;1386;1654	1172-1660	0.31	0.369
1970	1654;1970;2407	1660-2393	0.54	0.662
2844	2407;2844;3379	2393-3369	0.45	0.614
4011	3379;4011;4765	3369-4785	0.35	0.484

[a]The critical values for the correlation coefficient r are: $N = 55$, $r_{0.01} = 0.345$, $N = 72$, $r_{0.001} = 0.380$.

exhibiting the RMS CEOE levels below the 10th percentile in at least two half-octave bands was classified as a failure. Using that criterion, the specificity of the CEOE test was 86.3%. Eight of the 10 ears that failed the CEOE test (according to our criterion), but passed the ABR, had detectable CEOEs with the reproducibility factor (correlation between two averaged cochlear response waveforms) above 50%. The right ear of subject P28 (Fig. 6B) is an example of such a case. If we use the presence of CEOEs with a Reproducibility factor 50% as an acceptable CEOE, the specificity would be 97.3% (71/73 ears). However, applying this criterion would pass ears regardless of spectral content of CEOEs, like the right ear of subject P28.

Otoscopy performed for the preterm infants revealed the presence of middle ear effusions in 10 out of 137 ears tested (7.3%). A number of authors have reported a higher prevalence of otitis media in preterm infants than in full-term babies. Berman, Balkany, and Simmons (1978) reported abnormal tympanic membrane mobility in 22% of premature infants. Pestalozza, Romagnoli, and Tessitore (1988) reported that the incidence of otitis media was 21.1% among infants from NICU, whereas the incidence among unselected newborns was only 3.3%. In our study, all eight of the ears with effusions that were tested with DPOEs failed the test. The DPOEs recorded from those ears were below the normal range in at least two half-octave bands. We observed the tendency that their DPOEs were mostly reduced or even absent for the low-frequency region (below 2 kHz). Those DPOEs were below the lowest values obtained from full-term newborns. However, the DPOE levels exhibited the tendency to get closer to the normal range for the higher frequencies. Among 10 ears that had effusions, three of them had absent CEOEs. Another five ears failed the CEOE test. However, four of them had a normal-range CEOE level in the 4 kHz half-octave band. Two ears passed the CEOE test despite the presence of the middle ear effusions. Our finding of a close-to-normal type of response in the high-frequency region for ears with middle ear effusions is consistent with Kemp et al (1990), who showed an example of the CEOE recorded from a newborn ear with middle ear negative pressure. That ear exhibited a detectable CEOE only in the 3 to 4.5 kHz region without low-frequency response. Similarly, Bonfils et al (1992) reported a specific CEOE pattern with a reduced emission energy below approximately 2 kHz for preterm infants with flat tympanogram. A comparison of our DPOE and CEOE data obtained from the ears of preterm infants with effusions suggests that the DPOE test is more sensitive for a middle ear disorder than the CEOE test. However, more data are needed to explore and explain this tendency.

There were four ears of preterm infants with middle ear effusions that passed the ABR test. All of them failed the DPOE test and three of them failed the CEOE test. This finding suggests that the ABR test is less sensitive in detecting a middle ear problem than are OEs. Two ears without effusions passed ABR, but had absent CEOEs. A comparison of ABR and OE data for preterm infants without effusions shown in Table 4 suggests a higher passing rate with the ABR test than with the OE tests. One possible explanation of this finding is that OEs are more sensitive to middle ear disorders than ABR. When performing an ABR test, the middle ear must be normal to support the forward transmission of acoustic signals. This is also true for the OE tests. Moreover, a normal middle ear is essential to record low-level energy of the OEs propagated in the reverse direction. Experiments in rabbits reported by Whitehead, Lonsbury-Martin, and Martin (1991) showed that an abnormal middle ear had a greater effect on the level of the reversely transmitted DPOEs than on the forward transmission. Our data suggest that the effect of middle ear disorders seems to be more visible in the DPOEs than in the CEOEs. There were 12 ears of preterm infants without middle ear effusions (as judged by otoscopy) for which the results of CEOE and DPOE tests disagreed. Nine of those ears passed

the CEOE test according to our criterion, but failed the DPOE test, and three ears passed the DPOE test, but failed the CEOE test. One possible explanation of these findings is that those ears may have had a minimal middle ear disorder not detected by otoscopy. If the DPOEs are more sensitive to the middle ear status than the CEOEs, the incidence of passing the CEOE test would be higher than that of the DPOE test. More data are needed to explore this suggestion.

Eggermont and Salamy (1988) and Samani, Peschiulli, Pastorini, and Frior (1990) studied ABRs in preterm and full-term infants. In both studies, preterm infants showed longer wave latencies than full-term infants of the same postconceptional age. Our OE data described in Tables 2 and 3 indicated that about 20% of preterm infant ears (without middle ear effusions) had OEs higher than the 90th percentiles of full-term newborns in at least two half-octave bands. Those differences between the two populations were mostly observed in the 2.8 to 4 kHz region. These findings suggest that the maturation of the peripheral auditory system of preterm infants may possibly pursue a different time course than that of full-term babies. The OEs are believed to reflect the functional status of the cochlea. However, the mechanism of the antero- and retrograde transmission of the signal may also affect OE measurements. The transmission mechanism can be influenced by the properties of the probe sealed in the ear canal, the canal itself, and the characteristics and developmental changes of the outer, middle, and inner ear. All these structural characteristics are possible factors influencing signal transmission and thus influencing OEs. Bonfils et al (1992), who presented spontaneous otoacoustic emission and CEOE data obtained from preterm infants of 32 to 41 weeks gestational age (not considered at risk for hearing impairment), reported statistically nonsignificant changes of CEOE level with gestational age. They also analyzed the highest and the lowest frequency of detectable CEOEs. There was no statistical difference in either the highest frequency response or in the lowest frequency response between age groups. We did not break our data into different postconceptional age groups because all of our preterm infants were considered at risk for hearing impairment. In our opinion, we need more subjects to form age groups that would include infants with similar medical history (e.g., similar gestational age at birth, similar birth weight, comparable duration of ototoxic drug administration, etc.). Using our current data, a statistical analysis was performed to find possible correlations between OE data and several medical factors that could potentially influence OE behaviors of preterm infants. The only parameter that showed statistically significant correlation was the duration of stay in the NICU. This finding seems to be rather straightforward, as the less healthy the infant, the longer he/she stays in the NICU, and, therefore, the higher the incidence of multiple hearing impairment risk factors. More data are needed to perform more precise analyses.

The analysis of the OE data (Figs. 7 and 8) showed a statistically significant correlation between the DPOEs and the CEOEs obtained from the same ears of full-term and preterm infants. A similar finding was reported earlier for a group of normal-hearing adults (Smurzynski & Kim, 1992). These data suggest that some common mechanisms underlie the generation of CEOEs and DPOEs in the human cochlea at different stages of development. Even though the two types of OEs exhibit some differences, they are both believed to reflect active biomechanical properties of OHCs. Subtle differences in the middle ear transmission characteristics might be another element that can potentially influence the correlation between DPOEs and CEOEs. This possibility was reflected, for example, by the fact that some ears that passed the CEOE test failed the DPOE test. The comparison of the DPOE/CEOE regression data (Figs. 7 and 8) did not show any statistically significant differences between data of the two groups. This finding suggests that the relationship between DPOEs and CEOEs is similar among full-term and preterm infants.

The two types of OE tests have advantages and disadvantages. The CEOE test is performed quickly. Once the probe is fitted correctly and the infant is still, it takes about a minute to complete the test in a quiet subject. However, the spectral information is limited to a region of approximately 1.3 to 4.5 kHz. For lower frequencies, the noise interferes with the CEOE measurement (Fig. 2B). The high-frequency region is limited by the stimulus spectrum, decreasing gradually above 4.5 kHz. The signal to noise ratio is relatively low, in general, as illustrated by Figure 2B for a group of full-term newborns. The signal to noise ratio for the DPOEs in the present system is higher than that of the CEOEs. The 10th percentile of the DPOEs among full-term newborns was above the noise floor (Fig. 1). The DPOEs were relatively easy to measure above 2 kHzm and high-frequency DPOE data in the 5 to 8 kHz region can be obtained. The feasibility of the DPOE test for low frequencies depends on the infant's noise level, as illustrated by the data in Table 2. The DPOE test requires collecting data at several frequency regions and, in general, it takes longer to complete this test than the CEOE test. However, the DPOE audiogram is frequency specific, as shown for hearing-impaired adults (e.g., Kim et al, 1992; Martin et al, 1990) and children (Spektor et al, 1991).

The results of this study suggest that the CEOE test can be used as a quick hearing screening for infants with some frequency-specific information in the 1.3 to 4.5 kHz range. More frequency-specific information, including frequencies around 1 kHz and above 5 kHz, can be obtained from the DPOE data. Several authors (e.g., Bonfils et al, 1990; Uziel & Piron, 1991) suggested that OEs might be the initial choice for screening auditory function in infants considered at risk for hearing impairment. In cases when an infant fails the OE test, this test should be complemented by behavioral test, tympanometry, and ABR. Because the use of OEs broadens the range typically available from click-evoked ABR measures, this information is of increased value not only in terms of speech and language development, but for the preliminary fitting of hearing aids.

References

Avan, P., Bonfils, P., Loth, D., Narcy, P., and Trotoux, J. Quantitative assessment of human cochlear function by evoked otoacoustic emissions. *Hear Res* 1991;52:99-112.

Ballard, J.L., Novak, K.K., and Driver, M. A simplified score for assessment of fetal maturation of newly born infants. *J Pediatr* 1979;95:769-774.

Berman, S.A., Balkany, T.J., and Simmons, M.A. Otitis media in the neonatal intensive care unit. *Pediatr* 1978;62:198-201.

Bonfils, P., Bertrand, Y., and Uziel, A. Evoked otoacoustic emissions: Normative data and presbycusis. *Audiology* 1988a;27:27-35.

Bonfils, P., Dumont, A., Marie, P., Francois, M., and Narcy, P. Evoked otoacoustic emissions in newborn hearing screening. *Laryngoscope* 1990;100: 186-189.

Bonfils, P., Francois, M., Avan, P., Londero, A., Trotoux, J., and Narcy, P. Spontaneous and evoked otoacoustic emissions in preterm neonates. *Laryngoscope* 1992;102:182-186.

Bonfils, P., Uziel, A., and Pujol, R. Screening for auditory dysfunction in infants by evoked oto-acoustic emissions. *Arch Otolaryngol Head Neck Surg* 1988b;114:887-890.

Dubowitz, L.M.S., Dubowitz, V., and Goldsberg, C. Clinical assessment of gestational age in the newborn infant. *J Pediatr* 1970;77:1-10.

Eggermont, J.J., and Salamy, A. Maturational time course for the ABR in preterm and full term infants. *Hear Res* 1988;33:35-48.

Harris, F.P., and Probst, R. Transiently evoked otoacoustic emissions in patients with Meniere's disease. *Acta Otolaryngol* (Stockh)1992;112:36-44.

Johnsen, N.J., Bagi, P., and Elberling, C. Evoked acoustic emissions from the human ear. III. Findings in neonates. *Scand Audiol* 1983;12:17-24.

Johnsen, N.J., Bagi, P., Parbo, J., and Elberling, C. Evoked acoustic emissions from the human ear. IV. Final results in 100 neonates. *Scand Audiol* 1988;17:27-34.

Joint Committee on Infant Hearing. 1990 position statement. *Am Speech Hear Assoc* 1991;33(Suppl 5):3-6.

Kemp, D.T. Stimulated acoustic emissions from within the human auditory system. *J Acoust Soc Am* 1978;64:1386-1391.

Kemp, D.T., Bray, P., Alexander, L., and Brown, A.M. Acoustic emission cochleography: Practical aspects. *Scand Audiol Suppl* 1986;25:71-95.

Kemp, D.T., Ryan, S., and Bray, P. A guide to the effective use of otoacoustic emissions. *Ear Hear* 1990;11:93-105.

Kim, D.O., Leonard, G., Smurzynski, J., and Jung, M.D. Otoacoustic emissions and noise-induced hearing loss: Human studies. In Dancer, A.L., Henderson, D., Salvi, R.J., and Hamernik, R.P., Eds. *Noise-Induced Hearing Loss*. St. Louis: Mosby Year Book, 1992:98-105.

Kimberly, B.P., and Nelson, D.A. Distortion product emissions and sensorineural hearing loss. *J Otolaryngol* 1989;18:365-369.

Kok, M.R., van Zanten, G.A., and Brocaar, M.P. Growth of evoked otoacoustic emissions during the first days postpartum. *Audiology* 1992;31: 140-149.

Lafreniere, D., Jung, M.D., Smurzynski, J., Leonard, G., Kim, D.O., and Sasek, J. Distortion-product and click-evoked otoacoustic emissions in healthy newborns. *Arch Otolaryngol Head Neck Surg* 1991;117:1382-1389.

Lapedes, D.N., Ed. *McGraw-Hill Dictionary of Physics and Mathematics*. New York: McGraw-Hill, 1978.

Lonsbury-Martin, B.L., Harris, F.P., Stagner, B.B., Hawkins, M.D., and Martin, G.K. Distortion product emissions in humans. I. Basic properties in normally hearing subjects. *Ann Otol Rhinol Laryngol* 1990;99:3-14.

Londsbury-Martin, B.L., Whitehead, M.L., and Martin, G.K. Clinical applications of otoacoustic emissions. *J Speech Hear Res* 1991;34:964-981.

Martin, G.K., Ohlms, L.A., Franklin, D.J., Harris, F.P., and Lonsbury-Martin, B.L. Distortion product emissions in humans. III. Influence of sensorineural hearing loss. *Ann Otol Rhinol Laryngol* 1990;99:30-42.

Norton, S.J., and Widen, J.E. Evoked otoacoustic emissions in normal-hearing infants and children: Emerging data and issues. *Ear Hear* 1990;11:121-127.

Northern, J.L., and Gerkin, K.P. New technology in infant hearing screening. *Otolaryngol Clin North Am* 1989;22:75-87.

Owens, J.J., McCoy, M.J., Lonsbury-Martin, B.L., and Martin, G.K. Influence of otitis media on evoked otoacoustic emissions in children. *Semin Hear* 1992;13:53-66.

Pestalozza, G., Romagnoli, M., and Tessitore, E. Incidence and risk factors of acute otitis media and otitis media with effusion in children of different age groups. *Adv Otol Rhinol Laryngol* 1988;40:47-56.

Probst, R., Lonsbury-Martin, B.L., and Martin, G.K. A review of otoacoustic emissions. *J Acoust Soc Am* 1991;89:2027-2067.

Samani, F., Peschiulli, G., Pastorini, S., and Frior, R. An evaluation of hearing maturation by means of auditory brainstem response in very low birthweight and preterm newborns. *Int J Pediatr* 1990;19:121-127.

Shimizu, H., Ed. Otoacoustic emissions: Clinical implications. *Ear Hear* 1990;11:81-167.

Smurzynski, J., and Kim, D.O. Distortion-product and click-evoked otoacoustic emissions of normally-hearing adults. *Hear Res* 1992;58:227-240.

Smurzynski, J., Leonard, G., Kim, D.O, Lafreniere, D.C., and Jung, M.D. Distortion product otoacoustic emissions in normal and impaired adult ears. *Arch Otolaryngol Head Neck Surg* 1990; 116:1309-1316.

Spektor, Z., Leonard, G., Kim, D.O., Jung, M.D., and Smurzynski, J. Otoacoustic emissions in normal and hearing-impaired children and normal adults. *Laryngoscope* 1991;101:965-976.

Steel, R.G.D., and Torrie, J.H. *Principles and Procedures of Statistics*. New York: McGraw-Hill Book Co., 1980.

Stevens, J.C., Webb, H.D., Hutchison, J., Connell, J., Smith, M.F., and Buffin JT. Click evoked otoacoustic emissions compared with brain stem electric response. *Arch Dis Child* 1989;64:1105-1111.

Stevens, J.C., Webb, H.D., Hutchison, J., Connell, J., Smith, M.F., and Buffin, J.T. Click evoked otoacoustic emissions in neonatal screening. *Ear Hear* 1990;11:128-133.

Stevens, J.C., Webb, H.D., Smith, M.F., Buffin, J.T., and Ruddy, H. Comparison of otoacoustic emissions and brain stem electric response audiometry in the normal newborn and babies admitted to a special care baby unit. *Clin Phys Physiol Meas* 1987;8:95-104.

Turner, R.G. Modeling the cost and performance of early identification protocols. *J Am Acad Audiol* 1991;2:195-205.

Uziel, A., and Piron, J.P. Evoked otoacoustic emissions from normal newborns and babies admitted to an intensive care baby unit. *Acta Otolaryngol* (Stockh) 1991;(Suppl 482):85-91.

Whitehead, M.L., Lonsbury-Martin, B.L., and Martin, G.K. Effects of the crossed acoustic reflex on distortion-product otoacoustic emissions in rabbit. *Hear Res* 1991;51:55-72.

Zurek, P.W., Clark, W.W., and Kim, D.O. The behavior of acoustic distortion products in the ear canals of chinchillas with normal or damaged ears. *J Acoust Soc Am* 1982;72:774-780.

Acknowledgments

This work was supported by grants from the Deafness Research Foundation, and the Department of Surgery, Division of Otolaryngology, and Clinical Research Center, University of Connecticut Health Center. We would like to thank the staff of the Neonatal Intensive Care Unit and the newborn nursery at the University of Connecticut Health Center, without whom this project could not have been completed.

Portions of this article were presented at the 15th Midwinter Research Meeting of the Association for Research in Otolaryngology, February 2-6, 1992, St. Petersburg Beach, Florida, and at the joint meeting of the American Pediatric Society and the Society for Pediatric Research, May 4-7, 1992, Baltimore, Maryland.

Address reprints requests to Dr. Jancek Smurzynski, Division of Otolaryngology, University of Connecticut Health Center, 263 Farmington Avenue, Farmington, CT 06030-1110.

Received September 17, 1992; accepted November 24, 1992.

IV. Screening for Auditory Function

Early identification of hearing loss in children has been advocated for more than four decades (Ewing and Ewing, 1947; Murphy, 1962; Wedenberg, 1963; Downs and Sterritt, 1964; Eisenberg, Griffin, Coursin, and Hunter, 1964; Downs, 1967). Despite the persistent efforts of professionals in hearing health care, it has been only recently that newborn hearing screening has become accepted practice. In the last decade, however, considerable progress has been made toward the widespread implementation of newborn hearing screening. As of 2003, 86.5% of all births in the United States are now screened on an annual basis. Consequently, the age of identification has decreased from an average of 18 months to below 3 months.

Interest in the early identification of hearing loss among young children increased markedly in the decade of the nineties and beyond. Several professional organizations developed position statements concerning the need for early identification as well as proposed recommended screening protocols. Moreover, the Joint Committee on Infant Hearing (1994) revised and expanded the high-risk register. The National Institute on Deafness and other Communication Disorders (NIDCD) sponsored a national meeting (March 1-3, 1993) on early identification of hearing loss in infants and young children. An important outgrowth of this meeting was the development of a collective opinion statement on early identification of hearing loss in children (NIH Consensus Statement, 1993).Finally, JCIH (2000) provided principles and comprehensive guidelines for early hearing detection and intervention (EHDI) programs.

The articles that appear in this section represent the historical evolution of important issues surrounding early identification. Newborn hearing screening is the focus of this section primarily because much of the research on early identification has centered on this area. There is, however, a need for us to begin to divert at least some of our enthusiasm from newborn screening to develop effective screening programs for infants and young preschool children.

Section IV begins with an article by Turner on modeling the cost and performance of early identification. A full evaluation of the costs involved in establishing a screening program is essential. Such an evaluation needs to include not only the direct costs of screening but also the follow-up costs for services initiated as a result of the screening. Of special concern are the monetary costs associated with false positive tests: both the monetary costs of parents' lost time from work, transportation to care facilities, unnecessary tests, and unnecessary treatments; and the human and probably more consequential costs of attendant parental anxiety, frustration, distraction, stress, and potential misunderstanding.

Although the work of Downs (e.g., 1967) who advocated the "arousal" technique for newborn screening, was considered seminal, behavioral observation audiometry with newborns was fraught with limitations, and consequently, more objective, reliable measures of audition were pursued. The article by Galambos and coworkers highlights the value of using auditory brainstem response (ABR) in the neonatal intensive care unit for detecting significant hearing loss. The work by Galambos brought about an abundance of research on the use of ABR for newborn screening. Herrmann and colleagues discuss the application of one automated ABR device for screening infants. The use of an automated system is much quicker, simpler, and less expensive than the traditional diagnostic ABR. Nevertheless, concerns about cost, sophistication of equipment, the need for electrodes, and the reported high failure rates in many of the earlier studies gave momentum to evoked otoacoustic emissions (EOAEs) as another objective alternative for screening newborns.

In a multicenter clinical trial supported by the NIH, Norton and colleagues examined the performance of three tests used for hearing screening; transient evoked otoacoustic emissions, distortion product OAEs, and the auditory brainstem response. Behavioral audiometry at 8 to12 months of age, which was completed on all neonates regardless of test outcome, was used as the gold standard. All three methods were similar in performance for the identification of moderate degrees of hearing loss and greater. A series of excellent papers resulting from the project were published in the same issue of *Ear and Hearing* and will provide readers with a wealth of information regarding multiple topics relevant to the identification of congenital hearing loss in the neonatal period.

The report of Prieve and colleagues is one of a series of fine articles on the New York State Newborn Hearing Screening Demonstration Project. This four-year project examined the feasibility of instituting universal newborn hearing screening within a state with great geographic and socioeconomic diversity and a high annual birth rate. One of the important results of the New York project was that it provided evidence that well-coordinated hospital-based universal hearing screening and subsequent aggressive follow-up on infants who failed or missed the test was a practical and efficient method for achieving the goals of early identification, confirmation, and intervention by 6 months of age for infants with hearing loss.

The conference sponsored by NIDCD of the NIH developed a consensus statement that supported universal hearing screening within an infant's first 3 months of life, preferably prior to hospital discharge. A two-stage screening protocol was recommended; all infants would first be screened with EOAEs. Those who failed the EOAE test would receive an ABR test at 40 dB nHL. Failure at this second stage would lead to a comprehensive diagnostic hearing assessment within six months. Because at least 20 to 30 percent of all hearing loss in children occurs later during infancy or early childhood, infant hearing screening was also recommended at periodic intervals throughout early childhood.

The NIH consensus recommendation was met with some controversy. Some of the advocates of early identification believed that the implementation of a universal screening program was premature because of the limited data at that time on screening healthy newborns in well-baby nurseries and because there was insufficient evidence on the performance of the two-tier screening protocol. Bess and Paradise delineated their concerns about universal newborn hearing screening and questioned the practicability, effectiveness, cost, and harm-benefit ratio associated with the NIH recommendation. Various replies to the Bess and Paradise position are provided, followed by a response by Bess and Paradise. This series of articles/letters illustrates that universal newborn screening, although popular, is not without controversy, highlights the multitude of complicated issues associated with implementing a universal newborn hearing program, and demonstrates the need for continued research on all phases of an early identification program that includes follow-up, comprehensive assessment, and appropriate and timely management.

References

Downs, M.P. 1967. Testing hearing in infancy and early childhood. In F.E. McConnell, and P.H. Ward, (Eds.), *Childhood deafness.* Nashville, TN:Vanderbilt University Press.

Downs, M.P., and Sterritt, G. 1964. Identification audiometry in neonates: A preliminary report. *Journal of Auditory Research* 4:69-80.

Eisenberg, R.B., Griffin, E.J., Coursin, D.B., and Hunter, M.A. 1964. Auditory behavior in the human neonate: A preliminary report. *Journal of Speech and Hearing Research* 7:245-269.

Ewing, A.W.G., and Ewing, I.R. 1947. *Opportunity and the deaf child.* London: University of London Press.

Joint Committee on Infant Hearing. 1994. Position statement. *Audiology Today* 6(6):6-9. (JCIH: www.jcih.org).

Joint Committee on Infant Hearing. 2000. JCIH Year 2000 Position Statement: Principles and guidelines for early hearing detection and intervention programs. *American Journal of Audiology,* 9:9-29. (JCIH: www.jcih.org).

Murphy, K.P. 1962. Development of hearing in babies. *Child and Family* 1:16-20.

NIH Consensus Statement. 1993. *Early identification of hearing impairment in infants and young children.* 11(1):1-24.

Wedenberg, E. 1963. Auditory tests on newborn infants. *Acta Otolaryogologica Suppl.* 175:1-32.

Additional Readings

Cadman, D., Chambers, L., Feldman, W., and Sackett, D. 1984. Assessing the effectiveness of community screening programs. *Journal of the American Medical Association* 251(12Z):1580-1585.

Clayton, E.W. 1992. Issues in state newborn screening programs. *Pediatrics* 90:641-646.

Clayton, E.W., and Tharpe, A.M. 1998. Ethical and legal issues associated with newborn hearing screening. In Bess, F.H. (Ed.) *Children with hearing impairment: Contempory trends.* (pp. 33-44). Nashville, TN: Vanderbilt Bill Wilkerson Center Press.

Galambos, R., Wilson, M.J., and Silva, P.D. 1994. Identifying hearing loss in the intensive care nursery: A 20-year summary. *Journal of the American Academy of Audiology* 5:151-162.

Holtzman, N.A. 1991. What drives neonatal screening programs? *New England Journal of Medicine* 325:802-804.

Jacobson, J., Jacobson, C.A., and Spahr, R.C. 1990. Automated and conventional ABR screening techniques in high-risk infants. *Journal of the American Academy of Audiology* 1:187-195.

Kenworthy, O.T. 1990. Screening for hearing impairment in infants and young children. *Seminars in Hearing* 11(4):315-332.

Turner, R.G. 1992. Comparison of four hearing screening protocols. *Journal of the American Academy of Audiology* 3:200-207.

Modeling the Cost and Performance of Early Identification Protocols

Robert G. Turner
University of California, San Francisco, California

Abstract

This is the first in a series of three papers concerned with the early identification of hearing loss. In this paper, a simple model is presented that permits the calculation of the performance and cost of early identification protocols. In the second paper (Turner, in press), this model is used to compare four early identification protocols that differ in hearing screening strategies. The third paper (Turner, in press) examines the factors that influence the early identification protocol. The model described in this paper is sufficiently general to accommodate most early identification strategies including those that meet the goal of identification and habilitation by 6 months. The model measures protocol performance using hit rate, false alarm rate, and selected posterior probabilities. The model also calculates two measures of the financial cost. One measure reflects the cost of implementing the protocol; the other reflects the cost-effectiveness of the protocol. The parameters required by the model are also specified and are based on published clinical data. The model is provided to help audiologists design and select early identification protocols that are optimum for their particular clinical situation.

Key Words: Hearing loss, early identification, infant, model, cost-benefit analysis

It is generally accepted that hearing-impaired children benefit from the early detection and habilitation of hearing loss. The Joint Committee on Infant Hearing (1982) has recommended that hearing loss be identified and habilitation begun by 6 months of age. The need for such an effort is clear to most audiologists, but how does one determine the most appropriate early identification (EID) protocol?

One approach is to rely entirely on intuition and clinical experience. This, however, is only appropriate with extremely complex problems that defy any type of quantitative analysis. Unfortunately, this strategy is often used because it is the least demanding. While it has a certain appeal, such a subjective approach is often vulnerable to bias and undetected error. Decisions may be based on inappropriate assumptions that result from atypical or limited clinical experience. Also, it is difficult to evaluate and validate the decision making process because it is seldom explicitly known.

Another strategy is to quantify every variable and then perform a detailed cost-benefit analysis. Theoretically, this is the best approach, but often it is too difficult to be practical. With this strategy it is necessary to assign some quantitative measure of cost to errors and benefit to correct decisions. The problem is that some important variables may be difficult or near impossible to quantify. For example, what are the actual financial and societal costs of not identifying a hearing-impaired infant?

There is a third strategy that is a compromise between the two described above. A simplified model can be developed to serve as an objective, defensible starting point. With this model, certain issues can be evaluated quantitatively. Factors that can not be included in the model can then be considered to yield the ultimate decision. Thus, the cost-benefit analysis combines objective data derived from a quantitative model with a subjective evaluation of important factors. While there is a subjective component to this strategy, at least the decision process begins with a more rigorous, objective foundation.

What factors would we want to quantify in a model? There are many important factors to consider when selecting an EID protocol, but the two most fundamental are performance and cost. By performance, we mean how many hearing-impaired (IH) infants will be detected. It would also be useful to know how many normal hearing (NH) infants will be incorrectly called hearing impaired. Since resources are limited, some measure of the cost of implementing an EID protocol is essential, as well as some measure of cost-effectiveness. Thus, reasonable measures of performance and cost are the minimum information we would want when evaluating and selecting EID protocols. It is dif-

Reprinted by permission of authors and Decker Periodicals Inc. Copyright 1991. *Journal of the American Academy of Audiology*, 2, pp. 195-205.

ficult to see how an appropriate decision can be made without this basic information Fortunately, performance and cost, the most basic factors, are also the easiest to quantify in a model.

Prager et al (1987) used a simple model to compare the cost-effectiveness of newborn hearing screening with the Crib-O-Gram and auditory brainstem response techniques. This paper extends their work and presents a more general and detailed model for EID protocols. The techniques for calculating the cost and performance of EID protocols are described in detail. Essential data for the implementation of these techniques is also provided.

This model is easy to implement and can be used by audiologists to develop their own EID protocols. The quantitative results of this model can be considered along with more subjective local factors to evaluate different EID strategies. Each program can design an EID protocol that is optimum to its particular need instead of relying on one universal recommendation.

Protocol Design

The first step in developing the model is to specify the basic design of the EID protocol (Fig. 1). This design is sufficiently general to accommodate many actual protocols. With certain implementations, it is consistent with the goal of identification and habilitation by 6 months. The model does not consider the identification of progressive loss.

Nursery

The first component is the hospital nursery. This can be either a well baby nursery (WBN) or an intensive care nursery (ICN). It is necessary to distinguish between the types of nurseries because prevalence of hearing loss can be very different. In addition, screening tests may perform very differently on infants from the two nurseries. In general, infants in either nursery are referred to a screening protocol; however, this is not essential.

Screening Protocol

The primary purpose of any screening protocol is to reduce the cost of identification. The screening protocol identifies infants at risk, that is, infants with a higher probability of disease than the general population. This reduces the infants who must be followed and tested with the diagnostic procedures, reducing the cost of identification. Usually, the result of screening is either pass or fail; the screening is not diagnostic. Infants that fail are referred for diagnostic testing. Infants that pass are not followed. Experience has shown that with some screening protocols, all infants cannot be tested before discharge. A provision for this is incorporated in the model.

Follow-Up

Technical limitations prevent the diagnostic testing of newborns; therefore, infants must be followed until they are sufficiently old for diagnostic procedures. Both infants who fail the screening and infants who were not screened before discharge must be followed. The reason that this component must be explicitly shown in the model is that there is some expense in following infants until diagnostic testing. In addition, experience has demonstrated that some infants will be lost from follow-up. Both factors will have a significant impact on the cost and performance of EID protocols.

Diagnostic Protocol

The final component in the EID process is the diagnostic protocol. It is this component that actually

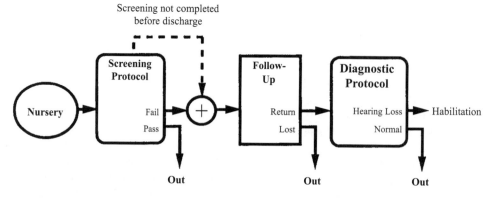

Figure 1. Basic early identification protocol design. "Out" means that an infant is no longer tested or followed by the protocol.

identifies hearing loss. Infants with hearing loss are referred for additional evaluation, habilitation, and management.

Measures of Performance and Cost

Simple, but adequate, measures of test performance are hit rate (HT) and false alarm rate (FA). These same measures can be applied to test protocols (Turner et al, 1984). Hit rate for the EID protocol (HTp) is the percentage of hearing-impaired infants in the nursery who are identified by the protocol. False alarm rate for the protocol (FAp) is the percentage of normal hearing infants in the nursery who are incorrectly called hearing impaired by the protocol.

Also of interest are the posterior probabilities. One posterior probability (PPf) is the probability of hearing loss in an infant who fails screening. PPf indicates how much confidence we can have that an infant who fails is actually hearing impaired. A second posterior probability is PPp. This is the probability of hearing loss in an infant who passes screening.

There are many different measures of financial and societal costs that could be used. For our purposes, we will restrict our calculations to two basic measures of financial cost. These are the dollar cost of the EID protocol per infant in the nursery (CPIN) and the dollar cost of the EID protocol per hearing-impaired infant identified (CPHL). These two measures reflect different aspects of protocol costs. CPIN is a measure of what it costs to implement the program, whereas CPHL is a measure of cost-effectiveness. A program could be inexpensive to implement, but could identify few IH infants. In this case, CPIN would be low but CPHL would be large. On the other hand, an expensive program could identify many IH infants. CPIN would be large, but CPHL small.

Model Parameters

To calculate performance and cost for an EID protocol, it is necessary to specify the parameters that are used in the model. For calculating performance, the parameters are disease prevalence, HT/FA of the individual tests in the protocol, and test correlation (Turner et al, 1984).

To determine CPIN and CPHL we must know the cost of each component of the EID protocol plus protocol performance. Hit rate and false alarm rate of the total protocol are not sufficient; we must also know the number of infants processed by each component. This means tracking the infants, in detail, all the way through the EID protocol.

For EID protocols, two additional factors must be considered. First, the percentage of infants who cannot be screened in the nursery are combined with the screening failures to constitute the infants to be followed. Second, it is necessary to specify a follow-up percentage. This is the percentage of infants who remain in the program until diagnostic testing.

In general, the model parameters will be derived from published clinical data. This is not without some problems. For many parameters the reported values can vary significantly. A parameter will be selected that is the average of the reported values or is within the approximate middle of the reported range. An additional problem is that some of the parameters have received little attention in the literature. In this case a best guess will be made based on available information. A summary of the selected model parameters is shown in Table 1.

Prevalence

Prevalence (Pr) is the percentage of infants in a nursery with hearing loss at the time of testing. Determining prevalence is more complex than it may seem. The first problem is defining hearing loss in terms of degree of loss, type of loss, and unilateral versus bilateral hearing loss. Historically, most prevalence data, particularly for the general population, have been for moderate to profound sensorineural loss. Newer techniques in the ICN have made possible the detection of milder losses, conductive losses, and unilateral losses. For our purposes, we will focus on the identification of moderate to profound sensorineural loss, unilateral or bilateral.

A number of studies provide estimates of prevalence for the ICN. Some good reviews of relevant studies are provided in Murry et al (1985), Jacobson and Hyde (1986), and Stein (1986). Estimates of prevalence vary from about 1 to 8% with the generally accepted range being 2 to 4 percent (Committee on Infant Hearing, 1989). If conductive loss was included, then the prevalence would be higher. Three percent will be used as the model parameter for prevalence in the ICN.

We are also interested in the prevalence in the WBN. In general, this figure has not been determined directly; we must estimate this from data for the general population. Reported prevalence has varied from less than 0.1 to more than 0.3 percent, but the most frequent reports are 0.1 to 0.2 percent (see Peckham, 1986; Riko et al, 1985 for reviews). We would expect the prevalence in the WBN to be smaller than the general population for two reasons. In many studies preva-

Table 1. Base Parameters Used with Model

	Performance		Cost	
	ICN	WBN	Min./Test	$/Test
Pr: Prevalence (%)	3.0	0.1		
CNT: Can Not Test Before Discharge (%)	10	10		
HRR: High Risk Register			10	13
Hit rate (%)	95	60		
False alarm rate (%)	65	10		
ABR: Auditory Brainstem Response Screening		45	60	
Hit rate (%)	95	95		
False alarm rate (%)	15	10		
FU: Follow-Up Success (%)	50	50	10	13
Diagnostic Protocol			120	160
Hit rate (%)	100	100		
False alarm rate (%)	0	0		
Test Correlation	Zero	Zero		

lence is based on hearing loss in children from 5 to 8 years of age. Some of the measured hearing loss would be progressive and not present in the WBN. Also, the general population consists of infants from the WBN and the ICN where the prevalence of hearing loss is greater. We will use 0.1 percent (1 per 1000) as the model parameter for prevalence in the WBN.

Screening Test Performance

A variety of different tests have been used to screen infants for hearing loss. Today, the only tests in extensive use are the high-risk register (HRR) and auditory brain stem response (ABR) screening; therefore, we will concentrate on these two tests for the model. As new screening tests are developed, these can be incorporated into the model as long as the hit rate and the false alarm rate can be specified.

The performance of some screening tests can be quite different in the two nurseries; therefore, the nurseries must be considered separately. Remarkably, there is little information in the literature on the performance of the HRR in the ICN even though the HRR has been employed in many studies. Frequently, the HRR has been used to determine which infants receive ABR screening without any attempt to evaluate the performance of the HRR. One study (Simmons et al, 1979) found HT/FA = 96/ 64 percent for the HRR in the ICN.

Several studies do report failure rate (FR) for the HRR. These rates have varied significantly from 20 to more than 90 percent (Alberti, 1986; Hosford-Dunn et al, 1987; Swigonski et al, 1987; Kramer et al, 1989). FR can provide an estimate of false alarm rate. When prevalence is low, the FA will be only a few percent

smaller than FR. With a FR of 20 percent, a 3 percent prevalence would yield a FA of almost 18 percent. Thus, the FA for the HRR in the ICN will vary as the FR varies. In general for a diagnostic test, as false alarm rate decreases so does hit rate. Thus, a low FR means a low FA, which may indicate a low HT. Unfortunately, there is no information on the HT of the HRR when FR is low. We will use as a model parameter, HT/FA = 95/65 percent, consistent with the results of Simmons et a (1979).

There is information on the performance of the HRR in the WBN and the general population (Mencher, 1974; Feinmesser and Tell, 1976; Downs, 1978; Simmons et al, 1979; Feinmesser et al, 1982; Mencher and Mencher, 1982; Stein et al, 1983; Alberti, 1986; Coplan, 1987; Elssmann et al, 1987; Kramer et al, 1989). The results of the two populations are similar, although we would theoretically expect a slightly higher HT and FA for the general population because that would include ICN infants. HT varies from approximately 50 to 75 percent; FA from approximately 7 to 12 percent. We would expect some variation because different high-risk items have been employed. In general, the more restricted the HRR, the lower the HT and FA. Feinmesser and Tell (1976) found the performance of the HRR reduced from HT/FA = 72/20 percent to 60/7 percent when fewer items were used. We will use HT/FA = 60/10 percent for the model parameter for the HRR in the WBN.

There is limited information on the HT of ABR screening in the ICN. To determine hit rate, it is necessary to know how many hearingimpaired infants were missed by the screening. This means that infants who *pass* the screening must be followed; unfortunately, this is seldom done. Three studies attempted to follow all infants that had been screened with ABR (Shannon et al, 1984; Bradford et al,1985; Swigonski et al, 1987). In all studies, HT = 100 percent for the ABR screening, but in each case the number of infants tested was relatively small. In the largest relevant study, over 700 infants were followed (Hyde et al, 1990). HT for ABR screening varied from 98 to 100 percent depending on criterion for passing the screen. It is important to note that in this study, infants were tested under ideal conditions at 3 months of age or later, not in the ICN. In addition, this study did not consider low frequency loss that can be missed by ABR testing with a click stimulus. These studies indicate a high HT for ABR screening; however, we would not expect HT = 100 percent. A small number of hearing-impaired infants could be missed because they have low frequency loss or because a high click level (e.g., 40 dB nHL) was used for the criterion (Riko et al, 1985; Durieux-Smith et al, 1987; Kramer et al, 1989). For the model parameter, we will use HT = 95 percent for the ABR in the ICN.

There are extensive data on the failure rate of the ABR in the ICN. A number of studies have been summarized by Murry et al (1985), Jacobson and Hyde (1986), and Stein (1986). In general, FR varies from 10 to 25 percent in these reviews with an average FR (as calculated from Murry et al and Jacobson and Hyde) of about 17 percent. As discussed previously, the FA will be several percent below the FR. A FA of 15 percent will be used as the model parameter so as to reflect general experience, not optimum performance. Recent improvements in technique may consistently improve the FR for ABR. Gorga et al (1988) tested ICN infants under ideal conditions, including insert earphones, and found that only 5 percent of the ears failed the screening. This corresponds to a failure rate of 5 to 10 percent depending on the distribution of impaired ears among the infants.

There is little information on the performance of ABR screening in the WBN. This strategy has seldom been used because of the large number of infants to be tested and the low prevalence of hearing loss. There is no obvious reason to expect the HT in the WBN to be much different than in the ICN. As for the ICN, we will use HT = 95 percent as the model parameter. We would expect the FA in the WBN to be lower than the ICN. There would be fewer infants in the WBN with developmental delays or transient conductive loss. A lower limit on false alarm rate is indicated by the work of Hyde et al (1987). They tested more than 200 normal infants who were not at-risk for a hearing loss. The infants were screened at approximately 4 months with ABR under ideal conditions, except that insert phones were not used. They found a FR of 7 percent

for a 30 dB nHL click stimulus. Assuming no hearing-impaired infants in this population, the FA would be identical to the FR. We would expect the FR to be slightly higher in newborns, as opposed to 4 months; therefore, FA = 10 percent will be used as the model parameter.

Cannot Test

Certain screening tests such as ABR require physical access to the newborn in the nursery. In the ICN, testing is most reliable when the infant is less ill, that is, right before discharge. This significantly reduces the time available for testing. In the WBN, infants may be hospitalized for only 2 or 3 days, again reducing the opportunity for testing. A certain percentage of infants (CNT) will be discharged before testing can be accomplished. This issue is seldom discussed in published studies, but conceivably could impact on the cost and performance of EID protocols. Durieux-Smith et al (1987) reported that 21 percent of the infants could not be screened with ABR before discharge. On the other hand, Kramer et al (1989) were able to test 95 percent of infants with ABR before discharge. For screening protocols that use ABR, we will use CNT = 10 percent as the model parameter; otherwise, CNT = 0 percent.

Follow-Up Percentage

Another important parameter that has received little attention in the literature is followup percentage (FU). This is the percentage of infants that are successfully followed until diagnostic testing. There has been no specific study of follow-up rates or the factors that influence follow-up success. Several studies do give some indication of follow-up, but usually without much detail as to the procedure for following infants (Mencher, 1974; Simmons et al, 1979; Stein et al, 1983; Durieux-Smith et al, 1987; Elssmann et al, 1987; Swigonski et al, 1987; van Zanten et al, 1988; Kramer et al, 1989). In these studies, follow-up percentages varied from 40 to 90 percent. Jacobson and Hyde (1986) summarize about a dozen studies (Table 5-2, pg. 93) and indicate the number of infants tested at follow-up. Follow-up percentages ranged from 32 to 100 percent with an average of 50 percent.

The author was involved with an EID program that included initial diagnostic testing at several months. Long-term follow-up success to that appointment was about 50 percent with a modest effort to recall infants for testing (Jacobson et al, 1990). Based on this very limited information, FU = 50 percent will be used for the model parameter.

Diagnostic Protocol

We would expect the performance of any reasonable diagnostic protocol to be quite good, although not necessarily perfect. Hyde et al, (1990) found ABR screening at several months to have excellent performance (HT/FA = 98/4 percent). More comprehensive ABR testing combined with other procedures should yield a performance as good as, or better than, ABR screening. Behavioral testing at an appropriate age should also have excellent performance. For this model, it is reasonable to assume that the diagnostic testing is definitive, that is, HT/FA = 100/0 percent. This simplifies calculations and should not introduce much error. In reality, we would expect an occasional miss or false alarm. The number, however, would be so small as to have little effect on the cost and performance of the EID protocol. In addition, the diagnostic protocol would usually be the same when comparing different screening protocols. Any errors would impact on all protocols and have little impact on their relative cost or performance.

Costs

To determine protocol costs, it is necessary to specify the cost of the individual components in the protocol. This would include the screening and diagnostic tests and follow-up. Specifying these costs is difficult; actual expense could vary significantly with institution. Also, there is little information in the literature as to the expense of testing and follow-up.

Costs were determined based on the time required to provide the service. It was assumed that there was a general expense of $80 per hour for any activity. What we assume for this rate is not particularly critical if our primary interest is in comparing the relative costs of different protocols. The time required per infant for each activity is given in Table 1. This was multiplied by $80/hour to determine the cost per infant tested or followed.

There is a tendency to ignore the cost of a HRR. Some minimum time is required to review charts and identify those infants to be followed or screened. Ten minutes per infant was assumed for a cost of $13. A time of 45 minutes per infant was assumed for ABR screening. This would include testing time, set-up time, travel time to the nursery, reports, and record keeping. The cost for ABR screening is $60 per infant.

A follow-up of 50 percent was specified for the model. This was based, in part, on the author's own experience with an EID program. In that program, all record keeping was performed by computer. Infants were automatically identified for follow-up with minimum labor expense. The effort to retrieve infants for testing was modest. On this basis, 10 minutes per infant was assumed for follow-up to the first visit for a cost of $13.

The final component is diagnostic testing. The actual composition of this protocol could vary significantly, thus producing a significant variation in cost. To illustrate the techniques, we will assume a particular diagnostic strategy that consists of ABR threshold testing plus some limited behavioral and immittance audiometry. Infants that demonstrate hearing loss would return for additional audiologic testing and evaluation by other professionals. This is a streamlined strategy; 2 hours are specified for this protocol resulting in a cost of $160 per infant.

Test Correlation

Test correlation is the tendency of two tests to identify the same patients the same way. Test correlation can have a significant impact on protocol performance. Limited clinical data suggest that audiologic tests that distinguish cochlear from retrocochlear site of lesion have a mid-positive correlation (Turner et al, 1984). There is essentially no information on correlation for the tests commonly used in an EID protocol.

For this model, we will assume a test correlation of zero. This means that the tests are independent; the results on one test do not influence the other. To illustrate, consider two tests, A and B. Test A evaluates a group of infants. Test B evaluates the infants that fail Test A. If the tests have zero correlation, then the hit rate and false alarm rate of Test B would be the same on the original population of infants as on the subpopulation that failed Test A. If correlation was not zero, this would not be true.

An assumption of zero correlation simplifies the calculation for the model. This assumption is reasonable for several reasons. Test correlation is only an issue when two or more tests are combined. If one of the tests has perfect performance (HT/FA = 100/0 percent), then test correlation does not matter. We have assumed perfect performance for the diagnostic protocol; thus, correlation between the screening protocol and the diagnostic protocol is not an issue. The only time we must worry about test correlation is when the screening protocol consists of two or more tests. We have limited our interest to just two screening tests, HRR and ABR. The mechanics of these two tests are so different that there may, in fact, be little correlation between these tests. When these two tests are combined into a screening protocol, we will assume zero correlation.

Example

There are two ways to determine protocol performance and cost. It is possible to derive explicit equations for the EID protocol in Figure 1 that would permit the direct calculation of HTp, FAp, CPIN, and CPHL using model parameters. These equations, however, would be fairly complex. In addition, there would be no information as to the characteristics of a protocol other than the calculated measures of cost and performance.

A second technique is to track infants through the EID protocol by calculating performance and cost at each component. Ultimately, HTp, FAp, CPIN, and CPHL are calculated, but there is much additional information provided as to the contribution of each component to the overall cost and performance of the protocol. This strategy will be illustrated by an EID protocol that uses ABR as the screening component. The model parameters from Table 1 are used.

Protocol Performance

Protocol performance is calculated first (Fig. 2). We assume that there are 100 infants in the nursery. The actual number of infants is not important because hit rate and false alarm rate are relative measures independent of the number of infants tests. The infants in the nursery are divided into 3 IH infants and 97 NH, consistent with a prevalence of 3 percent.

Ten percent of the infants are discharged before screening (CNT). This 10 percent is applied to both subpopulations of infants. Thus 0.3 IH infants and 9.7 NH infants are not screened. For convenience, there is some rounding of the number of infants. Thus, the 9.7 NH infants are rounded to 10.

A total of 89.7 infants (2.7IH/87NH) will be screened. The HT/FA of the screening protocol is 95/15 percent. The next step is to calculate the number of hits, misses, false alarms, and correct rejections that result from the screening protocol. The number of hits (2.6) is the number of IH infants who are screened (2.7) times the hit rate of the screening protocol (95% = 0.95). The remaining 0.1 IH infants (2.7 − 2.6 = 0.1) constitute the misses. Likewise, the false alarms (13) equal the number of NH infants screened (87) times the false alarm rate (15%). The remaining 74 NH infants (87 − 13 = 74) are the correct rejections.

The posterior probabilities can also be calculated. PPf, the probability of hearing loss in an infant who fails

the screening, is simply the prevalence of hearing loss in the population of infants who fail. This is the number of IH infants (2.6) divided by the total number of infants who fail (2.6 + 13). For this protocol, PPf is 17 percent. PPp, the probability of hearing loss in an infant who passes the screen, is the prevalence of hearing loss in the infants who pass. This is less than 1 percent.

The misses and correct rejections (0.1/74) are the infants who pass the screening protocol and are no longer followed. The hits and false alarms (2.6/13) are the infants who have failed the screening protocol and are referred for follow-up. These are combined with the infants who were not screened before discharge to generate a total of 2.9 IH infants and 23 NH infants who are to be followed.

The follow-up percentage (FU) is assumed to be 50 percent for both IH and NH infants. The number that return for diagnostic testing is the number followed times FU. In this example, half the infants are followed and half are lost from follow-up. The actual number followed are rounded to 1.4 IH and 11 NH infants.

The diagnostic protocol is assumed to have perfect performance (i.e., HT = 100% and FA = 0%). Again, the number of hits (1.4) is the number of IH infants tested (1.4) times the diagnostic protocol hit rate (100% = 1.0). This means that all IH infants will be correctly identified as hearing impaired; there are no misses. The number of false alarms (0) will be the number of NH infants tested (11) times the false alarm rate (0%). All NH infants will be correctly identified as normal hearing; thus, there are 11 correct rejections and no false alarms.

The EID protocol hit rate (HTp) is the number of diagnostic protocol hits (1.4) divided by the number of IH infants in the nursery (3). Thus, we have

$$HTp = \frac{1.4}{3} = 46\%.$$

The protocol false alarm rate (FAp) is the number of diagnostic protocol false alarms (0) divided by the number of NH infants in the nursery (97). Thus,

$$FAp = \frac{0}{80} = 0\%$$

As we would expect, the protocol false alarm rate will always be zero if the diagnostic protocol has FA = 0%.

Protocol Costs

Protocol costs for the example protocol (Fig. 3) are calculated next. To determine CPIN and CPHL, it

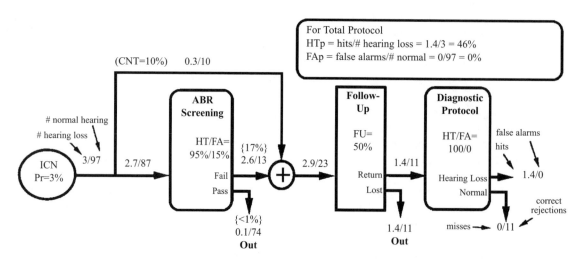

Figure 2. Calculations of performance for example protocol when used in the intensive care nursery (ICN). In this example, the screening protocol consists of auditory brainstem response (ABR) screening. The 17 percent in brackets is the posterior probability that an infant who fails screening actually has a hearing loss. The <1 percent is the probability that an infant who passes screening has a hearing loss. Pr = prevalence of hearing loss; HT/FA = hit rate/false alarm rate; CNT = percentage not screened before discharge; FU = follow-up success; and HTp/FAp = hit rate/false alarm rate of early identification protocol.

is first necessary to calculate the total cost of the EID protocol (see Fig.3). The parameters are the same in this example as in Figure 2. The costs of the individual components are from Table 1. Again it is assumed that 100 infants will be tested. While total cost is a function of the number of infants tested, CPIN and CPHL are relative measures independent of the number of infants. When calculating cost, it does not matter if an infant is hearing impaired or has normal hearing. Unlike when calculating performance, it is not necessary to separate the infants into an IH subpopulation and a NH subpopulation. What is important is the total number of infants processed by each component of the protocol.

There are 89.7 infants to be screened by ABR at a cost of $60 per infant. The total cost of the screening protocol ($5382) would be the number of infants screened (89.7) times the cost per infant ($60). The next component is follow-up. From the performance calculations (see Fig. 2), we see that a total of 25.9 infants are to be followed. The total cost of follow-up ($337) is the number of infants followed (25.9) times the cost per infant ($13). A total of 12.4 infants receive diagnostic testing. The total cost of diagnostic protocol ($1984) is the number of infants tested (12.4) times the cost of diagnostic testing ($160).

The total cost of the EID protocol is the sum of the cost of the individual components ($5382 + $337 + $1984 = $7703). The cost per infant (CPIN) equals the total cost of the EID protocol divided by the number of infants in the nursery ($7703/100 = $77). The cost per impaired infant identified (CPHL) equals the total pro-

tocol cost divided by the number of total protocol hits. From Figure 2, there are 1.4 protocol hits; thus,

$$CPHL = \frac{\$7703}{1.4} = \$5500.$$

Discussion

Modeling EID protocols serves several important purposes. It forces us to consider all components of the EID process and the factors that influence performance and cost. It is easy to focus on one aspect, such as screening, and lose sight of the ultimate objective, which is the identification of hearing-impaired infants. There is a tendency to choose an EID protocol on the basis of the screening component, not the total protocol. The model forces us to consider total protocol cost and performance, the most basic factors, when developing an EID strategy.

With this model, we have identified issues, such as follow-up, that have been largely over-looked, but that can have a significant impact on the EID process. In addition, this work has revealed deficits in the published literature as to information essential for the evaluation of EID protocols. For example, the HRR is used extensively in the ICN, but there is little information as to its performance.

With this model, it is possible to explore the relationship between model parameters and the ultimate cost and performance of the EID process. This can be accomplished by using the model to calculate cost and performance while a model parameter is varied within a range that reflects actual clinical experience. For example, how does prevalence of hearing loss influence the design of a protocol? Would we want a different protocol if follow-up percentage was low instead of high? Consideration of such issues helps provide a better theoretical foundation for the development and selection of EID protocols.

An important feature of this model is the ability to compare different potential EID protocols on the basis of cost and performance. This would be particularly useful for hospitals that are going to establish an EID program and have no previous clinical experience. While actual experience may ultimately be somewhat different than indicated by the model, the model would still provide essential information as to the advantages and disadvantages of different protocols. This type of model is the only way to generate reasonable estimates of cost and performance when clinical data are not available.

Many hospitals have implemented EID programs. This model could be used to better estimate the expense and cost-effectiveness of an existing program. The accuracy of these estimates would be a function of the parameters that were specified for the model. Care was taken when reviewing the clinical literature to derive reasonable estimates of these parameters; however, some model parameters could vary significantly with institution. The accuracy of the model could be improved by using parameter values that better reflect local experience.

Tests other than the HRR and ABR may be used for screening. Otoacoustic emissions is one technique that is currently being evaluated for this purpose (Stevens et al, 1990). Any procedure can be incorporated into the model provided there are reasonable estimates available for hit rate, false alarm rate, and cost of testing.

This model provides a more objective basis for the selection of an EID protocol. It generates a quality and quantity of information that is not available elsewhere. This information can be combined with other important factors, not considered in the model, to produce a reasonable, defensible cost-benefit analysis.

Summary

Ideally, the selection of an early identification (EID) protocol should be based on a detailed, quantitative cost-benefit analysis. Practical considerations make this impossible. A good alternative to a totally subjective decision process is one based on a combination of quantitative data and qualitative factors. The quantitative data can be supplied by a simple model for the EID protocol. With this model, useful measures of protocol performance and cost can be easily calculated. The model is sufficiently general to accommodate most early identification strategies including those that meet the goal of identification and habilitation by 6 months. The parameters required by the model are also specified and are based on published clinical data.

This model is provided to help audiologists select an EID protocol that is optimal for their particular situation. If local experience indicates parameter values different than those specified in this paper, then the more appropriate values should be used. Hopefully, the concepts described in this paper will result in a more rigorous, defensible strategy for the selection of EID protocols.

Acknowledgment

Presented in part at the meeting of the American Academy of Audiology, New Orleans, LA, April, 1990.

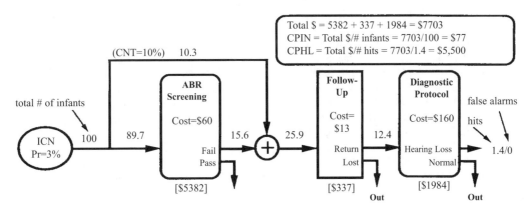

Figure 3. Calculations of costs for example protocol when used in the intensive care nursery (ICN). Dollar amount in brackets is the total cost for each component in the early identification protocol. Cost = expense of testing or follow-up for each infant; CPIN = cost per infant in nursery; CPHL = cost per hearing-impaired infant identified.

References

Alberti, P.W. (1986). An evaluation of hearing screening in high risk infants using BERA. *Audiol Pract* 2:3-4.

Bradford, J.B., Baudin, J., Conway, M.J., Hazell, J.W.P., Stewart, A.L., and Reynolds, E.O.R. (1985). Identification of sensory neural hearing loss in very preterm infants by brainstem auditory evoked potentials. *Arch Dis Child* 60:105-109.

Committee on Infant Hearing. (1989). Audiologic screening of newborn infants who are at risk for hearing impairment. *Asha* March: 89-92.

Coplan, J. (1987). Deafness: Ever heard of it? Delayed recognition of permanent hearing-loss. *Pediatrics* 79:206-213.

Downs, M.P. (1978). Auditory screening. *Otolaryngol Clin North Am* 11:611-629.

Durieux-Smith, A., Picton, T., Edwards, C., MacMurray, B., and Goodman, J. (1987). Brainstem electric response audiometry in infants of a neonatal intensive care unit. *Audiology* 26:284-297.

Elssmann, S., Matkin, N., and Sabo, M. (1987). Early identification of congenital sensorineural hearing impairment. *Hear J* 40:13-17.

Feinmesser, M.D., and Tell, L.T. (1976). Neonatal screening for the detection of deafness. *Arch Otolaryngol* 102:297-299.

Feinmesser, M., Tell, L., and Levi, H. (1982). Follow-up of 40000 infants screened for hearing defect. *Audiology* 21:197-203.

Gorga, M., Kaminski, J., and Beauchaine, K. (1988). Auditory brain stem responses from graduates of an intensive care nursery using an insert earphone. *Ear Hear* 9:144-147.

Hosford-Dunn, H., Johnson, S., Simmons, B., Malachowski, N., Low, K. (1987). Infant hearing screening: Program implementation and validation. *Ear Hear* 8:12-20.

Hyde, M.L., Matsumoto, N., and Alberti, P.W. (1987). The normative basis for click and frequency-specific BERA in high-risk infants. *Acta Otolaryngol (Stockh)* 103:602-611.

Hyde, M.L., Riko, K., and Malizia, K. (1990). Audiometric accuracy of the click ABR in infants at risk for hearing loss. J *Am Acad Audiol* 1:59-66.

Jacobson, G.P., Burtka, M.J., Wharton, J.A., Newman, C.W., Shepard, N., and Turner, R.G. (1990). Infant hearing screening 1984 to 1989: The Henry Ford Hospital experience. *Henry Ford Hosp Med* J 38(1):39-43.

Jacobson, J.T., and Hyde, M.L. (1986). The auditory brainstem response in neonatal hearing screening. In: Swigart, E.T., ed. *Neonatal Hearing Screening.* San Diego: College-Hill Press, 67-95.

Joint Committee on Infant Hearing. (1982). Position statement. *Asha* 24:1017-1018.

Kramer, S., Vertes, D., and Condon, M. (1989). Auditory brainstem responses and clinical follow-up of high-risk infants. *Pediatrics* 83:385-392.

Mencher, G.T. (1974). Infant hearing screening: State of the art. *Maico Audiological Library Series* 12(7).

Mencher, G.T., and Mencher, L.S. (1982). Report of a three year early identification of hearing loss program. *Paper presented at the Biannual Meeting of the International Society of Audiology, Helsinki.*

Murry, A.D., Javel, E., and Watson, C.S. (1985). Prognostic validity of auditory brainstem evoked response screening in newborn infants. *Am J Otolaryngol* 6:120-131.

Peckham, C.S. (1986). Hearing impairment in childhood. *Br Med Bull* 42:145-149.

Prager, D.A., Stone, S.A., and Rose, D.N. (1987). Hearing loss screening in the Neonatal Intensive Care Unit: Auditory brain stem response versus Crib-O-Gram; A cost-effectiveness analysis. *Ear Hear* 8:213-216.

Riko, K., Hyde, M.L., Alberti, P.W. (1985). Hearing loss in infancy: Incidence, detection, and assessment. *Laryngoscope* 95:137-144.

Shannon, D.A., Felix, J.K., Krumholz, A., Goldstein, P.J., and Harris, K.C. (1984). Hearing screening of high-risk newborns with brainstem auditory evoked potentials: A follow-up study. *Pediatrics* 73:22-26.

Simmons, F., McFarland, W., and Jones, F. (1979). An automated hearing screening technique for newborns. *Acta Otolaryngol* 87:1-8.

Stein, L.K. (1986). Follow-up of infants in a neonatal hearing screening program. In: Swigart, E.T., ed. *Neonatal Hearing Screening.* San Diego: College-Hill Press, 67-95.

Stein, L., Clark, S., and Kraus, N. (1983). The hearing-impaired infant: Patterns of identification and habilitation. *Ear Hear* 3:232-236.

Stevens, J.C., Webb, H.D., Hutchinson, J., Connell, J., Smith, M.F., and Buffin, J.T. (1990). Click evoked otoacoustic emissions in neonatal screening. *Ear Hear* 11:201-205.

Swigonski, N., Shallop, J., Bull, M., and Lemons, J. (1987). Hearing screening of high risk newborns. *Ear Hear* 8:26-30.

Turner, R. (In press). Comparison of four hearing screening protocols. *J Am Acad Audiol.* In press.

Turner, R. (In press). Factors that determine the cost and performance of early identification protocols. *J Am Acad Audiol.* In press.

Turner, R., Shepard, N., and Frazer, G. (1984). Formulating and evaluating audiological test protocols. *Ear Hear* 9:177-189.

van Zanten, G.A., Brocaar, M.P., Fetter, W.P.F., and Baerts, W. (1988). Brainstem electric response audiometry in preterm infants. *Scand Audiol [Suppl]* 30:31-97.

Reprint requests: Robert G. Turner, 400 Parnassus, Room A 706, UCSF, San Francisco, CA 94143-0340

The Auditory Brain Stem Response Reliably Predicts Hearing Loss in Graduates of a Tertiary Intensive Care Nursery*

Robert Galambos, Gayle E. Hicks, and Mary Jo Wilson
Speech, Hearing and Neurosensory Center, San Diego, California

Abstract

Babies *(N = 642)* were tested for auditory disorder, using the auditory brain stem response (ABR), at the time of their discharge from a tertiary intensive care nursery (ICN). Of those with ABR threshold elevation in one or both ears *(N = 97)*, 61% *(N = 59)* were retested some months later by a battery of audiological tests; 21 (*N = 3.3%* of the 642) suffered binaural peripheral loss and 11 (1.7%) now wear hearing aids. These new data, when combined with similar data previously reported from the same ICN, yield a sample of 1613 babies examined during a 5.8-year period from which these conclusions emerge: (1) About 16% of our ICN babies leave the hospital with reduced sensitivity in one or both ears; (2) the hearing deficiency is permanent for 8 to 10%; (3) the loss is sensorineural, bilateral, and so severe for about 4% that hearing aids will be required to optimize their language and psychosocial development. Use of the ABR procedure for neonatal hearing testing is the target of several criticisms: it is being applied too early in life; its predictions about permanent hearing loss are unacceptably inaccurate; or/and it is too costly. We discuss these and still other objections that have been raised.

The use of the auditory brain stem response (ABR) as a tool for detecting transient and permanent hearing disorders in newborn infants has burgeoned during the past several years.[3,4,8-13,15,17-21,23,25-28] We deal here mainly with how well the procedure has predicted temporary and permanent hearing loss in infants treated in our intensive care nursery (ICN), reporting first some new data, then adding these to a study already published from the same ICN.[11]

As we will show, the ABR is for us a practical and realistic way to identify a very large percentage of those patients discharged from our hospital with peripheral hearing disorders; in particular, and most importantly, it plays a crucial role in our ability to identify and treat those babies who need to be fitted with hearing aids during the first year of life. The conclusions of certain other investigators, however, seem not to coincide with ours, and we describe and discuss the points at issue.

Method

We attempt to apply the ABR test (Test) to every baby a day or so prior to his/her discharge from the ICN at the Children's Hospital in San Diego. (Many of these babies had already had one or more ABR tests

Reprinted by permission of authors and Williams & Wilkins. Copyright 1984. *Ear & Hearing*, 5, No. 4, pp. 254-260.

*This work was supported by Grants NS11707, 11154, and 17490 from the National Institutes of Health.

for medical-neurological reasons.) The Test procedure, already described in detail,[9,11] involves delivering 1000 to 2000 monaural clicks to the sleeping baby and recording the resulting ABR through vertex to mastoid electrodes using a CA 1000 averager. Each ear received 60 and 30 dB nHL clicks; if either stimulus did not elicit a response, an attempt was then made to estimate the threshold of that ear (±5 dB). The parent of every baby showing no response at 30 dB in one (or both) ears was told the infant "might have a hearing problem and should be returned for a retest in 6 weeks." All returned babies were retested by ABR (Retest) and, where indicated and feasible, by other standard audiological procedures (e.g., behavioral, tympanometry). Every baby found at Retest to have a monaural or binaural loss then entered a clinical follow-up program. Those with conductive losses were referred to a physician and returned for another Retest. Parents of babies with nonconductive losses below 40 dB were asked to return the baby in 6 months for another assessment. Babies with binaural losses greater than 40 dB were considered to be candidates for hearing aids; as illustrated in the case studies that follow, Board-certified audiologists decided whether these should be placed after applying behavioral, tympanometric, and reflex tests, and after observing the patient during a period of trial amplification and therapy.

The patient population is divided into three groups, each of which contains 80 to 85% of the infants discharged alive. Group I includes the 890 previously reported[11] to which is added the 81 discharged between September and December 1980. Groups II and III contain the dischargees for 1981 and 1982, respectively. Since no data obtained since December 31, 1982, are included here, Retest statistics for group III are obviously incomplete.[†]

Results

In what follows we emphasize use of the ABR both in identification audiometry of neonates and in the audiological test battery administered to small infants and children. In the broader context, however, these ABR tests have played only a part, albeit a very important part, in moving us toward our main goal, which is to identify, diagnose, and treat newborns with hearing loss.[8,20] The assistance provided by ABR data in the achievement of these objectives can be illustrated here through some representative case studies.

Case Histories

Case 1 illustrates successful identification of a severe bilateral hearing disorder and outlines the follow-up procedures we employ. This baby was discharged after 13 days in the ICN with the Test ABR shown in Figure 1. Born at home at an estimated gestational age of 34 weeks, she required tracheal intubation for 6 days and treatment for symptoms of respiratory distress syndrome; her pH on admission was 7.23 but was never measured below 7.25 thereafter.[5,9] Retest ABRs at 13 days, 1 mo, and 2 mos similarly estimated thresholds to be at or beyond 80 dB bilaterally. By 3 mos the infant was enrolled in our aural rehabilitation program where she received definitive diagnosis and therapy, including amplification. Loaner aids were used until 8 mos when the baby was fitted with her own binaural aids; routine aural rehabilitation sessions continued thereafter. At 13 mos a reliable behavioral audiogram indicated thresholds in the 55 to 65 dB HL range for frequencies 250 to 1000 Hz, and 80 to 90 for 2000 to 4000 Hz; these values were reconfirmed in subsequent audiological evaluations over a 2-yr period. Her most recent speech and language evaluations (aged 3 yrs) indicate she is about 6 mos behind her age group in expressive and receptive language skills. In keeping with a policy of this Center, the patient's younger sibling, a normal term boy, was tested by ABR at 2 mos, found to have no response bilaterally, and is currently also enrolled in the auditory rehabilitation program. His disorder raises the possibility that the patient's

hearing loss is of genetic origin (neither parent has a hearing problem) and not in fact related to any of the complications of prematurity for which she received treatment in the ICN.

Case 2 illustrates neonatal detection of a permanent monaural hearing loss. This baby was the product of a full term pregnancy complicated by mild pre-eclampsia and a flu-like illness at 4 mos. During delivery, a markedly irregular fetal heart rate prompted an emergency cesarean section; the baby was not asphyxiated. At 4 days cardiac catheterization revealed life threatening cardiac anomalies; following open heart surgery at age 5 days, her condition improved and she was discharged 16 days after birth. Test ABRs obtained 1 day prior to discharge (Fig. 1) revealed responses to a 30-dB HL click through the right ear and no response until 80 dB HL for the left. At age 2 mos the Retest ABR revealed 20 dB HL responses on the right but again not until 80 dB HL on the left. Since one normal ear is sufficient for normal development of speech and language, intervention in this case (e.g., hearing aids,

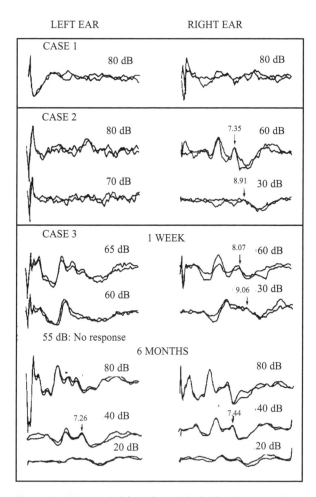

Figure 1. ABRs recorded from three of the babies whose case histories are described in the text.

[†]When this article was submitted, 72% of the group III Test failures known to be alive had been Retested.

aural rehabilitation) was not indicated. Biannual audiological evaluations were, however, recommended and behavioral audiological tests at age 16 mos, 2fi yrs, and 3fi yrs have all indicated normal hearing for the right ear and a severe hearing loss for the left.

Case 3 is an example of an apparently transient unilateral hearing loss associated with neurological ABR abnormalities. This term baby girl, the product of an uncomplicated pregnancy and delivery, was transferred to the ICN at 1 day because of tachypnea, possible necrotizing enterocolitis, and tonic-clonic motions of the foot due perhaps to hypocalcemia. She was placed on phenobarbital when on day 2 the EEG showed isolated sharp waves in the left central area. Neurological examination on day 5 revealed only minor motor weakness. On day 7 the EEG was normal and the patient was discharged home with a diagnosis of focal seizures of unknown etiology. ABRs on this day (Fig. 1) show prolonged I-V interval, reduced wave V amplitudes, and no response on the left below about 60 dB nHL. At 5 weeks the ABR was still abnormal neurologically but responses through the left ear now appeared at 40 dB and above. At 6 mos the ABR was essentially normal neurologically and audiologically with click threshold at 20 dB or better through each ear; conditioned localization of sound field stimulation showed consistent behavioral responses to voice in the 20 dB range. Developmental evaluation at 10 and 13 mos revealed above average mental and cognitive abilities, borderline psychomotor skills, and no auditory problems.

Case 4. An elective operation was performed on this term boy several days after birth, following which he was sent to recover in the ICN. As part of the discharge routine the Test ABR was automatically ordered for him; it revealed no response below 45 dB bilaterally. His private physician, on discovering that the Test had been performed and before knowing the results, objected to the routine Testing of babies who, like this one, were not at-risk for hearing loss by any known criteria. The Retest, when finally performed at 5 mos, gave identical ABR results, and tympanometry showed reduced compliance bilaterally consistent with middle ear pathology. The child then received regular treatment for otitis media and when last seen at 15 mos gave normal responses during behavioral audiometry.

Data Presentation and Analysis

Table l assembles under 4 columns the Test and Retest threshold estimates made between April 1977, and December 31, 1982, on 1613 ICN graduates. Group I includes, with recent additions, information from the 890 babies already reported;[11] groups II and III present entirely new data. Column IV shows the grand totals. Certain estimates consistently recur in the table and we will deal with them below in the following order: (1) Test failures (babies who show threshold elevation by ABR) amount to about 16%; (2) Retest failures are fewer in number; i.e., the threshold elevation at Test disappears for many babies; (3) Retest failures usually predict permanent monaural or binaural losses, of which some are so severe as to require hearing aids.

1. The number of Test failures, 16.1% at 30 dB nHL in Table l, resembles estimates ranging between 12 and 25% for somewhat smaller populations of tertiary ICN patients.[3,4,9, 13,15,24] The only major disagreement is the claim that 50% of term babies, and 44 of 75, or 57% of ICN graduates, fail at 40 dB nHL.[17]

2. Retest failures are always fewer in number than Test failures. Table 2 shows the direction and magnitude of all the threshold changes that took place in the Test-Retest interval. The change was relatively small, within ±15 dB, for nearly two-thirds of the ears, and within 30 dB for almost 90% of them. By far the majority of the changes were in the direction of improvements in the threshold estimate, but only 8% of the ears ($N = 23$) improved by more than 30 dB. From these facts it seems clear that a hearing loss identified at the time of discharge tends also to be found at the time of Retest, and that when there is an important threshold change, one greater than ±15 dB, it is highly likely to be in the direction of an improvement.

Of particular interest are those improvements that move the ear from above the 30-dB nHL to below it, for according to the criteria we arbitrarily follow[11,19]

Table 1. ABR Test-Retest results on ICN graduates.

	Group[a]			
	I	II	III	Totals
Test at discharge				
Babies tested	971	316	326	1613
Babies failed (F)	162	38	59	259
% failures 16.7	12.0	18.1	16.1	
Retest				
Babies retested	80	27	32	139
% of F above	49.4	71.1	54.2	53.7
Estimated loss				
None 33	10	17	60	
Unilateral	13	5	6	24
Bilateral	34	12	9	55
Now wear aids	24	6	5	35

[a]Patients in group I were tested April 1977 through December 1980, and groups II and III throughout 1981 and 1982, respectively.

Table 2. ABR Test-Retest difference by individual ears, in dB.

		Retest Better by			Same	Worse
	N	>46	31-45	16-30	±15	16-30
Group						
I	140	2	11	36	83	8
II	50	1	2	15	32	0
III	59	4	3	14	33	0
Totals	247	7	16	65	148	8
Percent	100	2	6	26	59	3

this changes its classification from an abnormal ear to a normal one. Table 1 shows that 1 out of every 2 or 3 babies who failed the Test has at least one ear that falls into this category.

Are these instances to be called "false positives" of the ABR method, i.e., patients erroneously identified as having a hearing problem at the time of discharge[4,17,23] or did the Test ABR actually correctly identify a disorder at discharge and then equally correctly show it to have disappeared by Retest?

Hearing disorders, due to middle ear effusion, exists in perhaps 30% of the infants in a typical ICN.[1,16] The Stockard group[25,26] have studied this problem; Stockard and Westmoreland[27] serially examined 23 ICN babies with ABR abnormalities consistent with a diagnosis of middle ear disorder. The ABR abnormalities disappeared in 19 by the time they left for home, and of the remaining 4 only 1, a confirmed case of otitis media, displayed them when retested some months later. These authors thus established that ICN babies have middle ear problems as patients and at the time of discharge, and that perhaps as many as 3 out of 4 who suffer the disorder at discharge will have recovered spontaneously when retested some time later.

If this were also to be true of our population, the amount of threshold elevation estimated at the Test should be consistent with a conductive loss, that is, the threshold should be elevated to no more than perhaps 50 or 60 dB nHL. Table 3 shows that 67 of the 100 babies in our series who passed the Retest after failing the Test had improvements of 20 dB or less (i.e., failed the Test with a threshold estimate of 50 dB nHL or better). These figures thus suggest that perhaps 2 out of 3 of our babies with normal Retest scores were in fact "true" positives who simply had recovered from middle ear conductive losses in the Test-Retest interval, as did those of Stockard and Westmoreland.

To test the claim[27] that "in the presence of brain stem disorders BAEP threshold is not a reliable index

of hearing sensitivity," we have evaluated the audiological status of those babies who showed neurologically abnormal Test ABRs. Altogether, 83 (156 ears) produced Test ABRs (at 60 or 80 dB nHL) with no wave V, or in which the I-V interval, or the V-I amplitude ratio, or both, deviated from the norms for age (see case 3, Fig. l, for examples of these ABR abnormalities). However, fully 66% of these patients with neurologically abnormal Test ABRs also yielded ABRs to 30 dB nHL clicks (Table 4) through one or both ears, which makes it clear that in our population normal peripheral auditory sensitivity can certainly coexist with central ABR abnormalities.

Unfortunately, neurologists do not regularly estimate the threshold ABR response and so the relationship between threshold elevation (both transient and permanent) and such factors as elevated intracranial pressure and intracranial hemorrhage largely remains to be worked out (but see Refs. 4 and 25 to 27). As for our data, in each neurological case in Table 4 where a measurement of wave I latency is available, the existence of a peripheral auditory disorder can be estimated directly. (Wave I latency measures cochlear output and is found to be prolonged in both conductive hearing loss and some cases of high frequency sensorineural damage at the cochlear level.[10,26]) Table 4 shows normal wave I latency for all but four of the neurologically abnormal patients without hearing loss, whereas wave I was prolonged for about two-thirds of those showing threshold elevations, which suggests that these patients may be like those without neurological abnormality in that their auditory problems very often lie in the periphery.

Finally, the idea has been advanced that "immaturity" is responsible for the Test failures who pass the Retest (that is, the "false positives"), and so the threshold norms presently in use incorrectly estimate the probability a given baby will respond to a 30-dB click.[7,17] Most published data agree, however, that the probability of a 30-dB response is already high for prematures at 35 weeks, and that it approaches 1.0 for

Table 3. Hearing loss at Test for ears with normal threshold at Retest.

		Threshold at Test (dB nHL)		
	N	31-50	51-60	>61
ABR abnormality				
Audiological	77	54(70)[a]	15 (19)	8 (10)
Neurological	23	13(57)	6 (26)	4 (17)
Totals	100	67(67)	21(21)	12(12)

[a]Numbers in parentheses, percent of N.

Table 4. Wave I Latency values, by ear, for patients with neurologically abnormal ABRs ($N = 156$ ears, 83 babies).

	ABR Threshold (in dB nHL)		
	30 or below	31-50	>50
Normal latency 100	18	0	
Prolonged latency	4	17	17

normal 40-week babies, both the newly born and those many weeks postnatal.[3-5,8-11,13,15,18,19,24-28] As for the babies reported here, Figure 2 assembles data from over 2900 ears of 1482 individuals; nearly 90% of these ears generated ABRs to the 30-dB click. Since five of the six babies aged 30 weeks generated ABRs to the 30-dB nHL clicks delivered to at least one ear, we may conclude that even at that early age the cochlea and central pathways cannot usually be "too immature" to do so.

3. Clinical outcome. As Table 1 shows, Retest failures total 79, which is 57% of those retested. This is the cohort that received a complete audiological assessment and clinical follow-up. Our case histories illustrate the main types of outcome. Case 1 represents those babies, on the average about one every 2 mos, subsequently fitted with hearing aids; her response to these has obviously been excellent. Case 2 shows, among other things, how accurate the Test ABR prediction can sometimes be: no other method known to

us has ever predicted so precisely which ear of a newborn will suffer permanent hearing loss, and how severe it will be. Case 3 illustrates a failure of the Test ABR to predict the final audiological status of a given ear although, interestingly, it also correctly predicted the status of the opposite ear. This case shows, as does Table 3, that the incidence of these failures is not highly correlated to whether the patient displays neurological abnormalities as well. Case 4, finally, shows the unreliability of conclusions about hearing loss based on clinical observation alone, and illustrates how the ABR consistently identifies even modest losses needing attention in the postnatal period.

If Retests were available for all babies who failed the Test, and if the results for them were those shown in Table l, the incidence of peripheral hearing disorders would be that shown in Table 5. We have discussed the propriety of these assumptions[12] and offer Table 5 tentatively, as our best current summary of the auditory pathology we have found, and expect to continue to find in our population of ICN graduates.

Discussion

Since 1971, when a California conference deplored the lack of a satisfactory method for newborn hearing screening,[2] the ABR has become a major candidate for filling this gap.[4,11,15,16,24,28] The present account

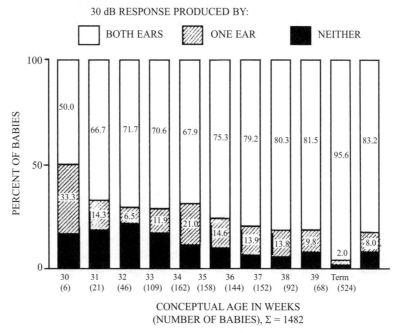

30 dB RESPONSE PRODUCED BY: □ BOTH EARS ▨ ONE EAR ■ NEITHER

At least one ear of all infants tested (for years 1977 to 1982) produced a response to 60 dB HL clicks.

Figure 2. Sensitivity to sound stimulation versus age for 1482 neonates. The majority of ears to which weak clicks (30 dB nHL) were delivered initiated ABRs, regardless of the baby's age.

Table 5. Incidence (%) of peripheral hearing disorder in ICN graduates.

At discharge (F)[a]	16.1
At Retest[b]	
No loss	6.9
Monaural	2.8
Binaural	6.0
Need hearing aids	4.0

[a]No ABR response to 30 dB nHL click in a least one ear.
[b]Numbers entered assume 100% retest of the failures (F) at discharge; actual percentage was 53.7 in this study.

illustrates how we use the ABR both as a screening device and as a diagnostic tool. The Test establishes whether a given ear passes the screen (i.e., responds to a 30-dB nHL click); when it does not, the Test then attempts to estimate the type and amount of its loss. Babies who fail the Test are recalled for the Retest some weeks or months later where a battery of audiological tests, including a repeat ABR, then separately reclassifies the patient and provides the basis for a definitive clinical evaluation. As Table 1 shows, the reclassification agrees with the initial classification about two times out of three and defines a cohort of babies highly likely to suffer permanent hearing disorders.

From time to time a variety of criticisms has been leveled at use of the ABR in newborn hearing assessment. We list the major ones and then discuss them in order.

1. Too many babies identified by the Test turn out not to have hearing loss (the "false positives").
2. No one knows the number of deaf newborns the Test fails to identify (the "false negatives").
3. An ABR test is expensive and the procedure is inefficient; only about 15 of every 100 Tests identifies a baby with hearing loss, and perhaps one-third of these passes the Retest.
4. The total number of babies helped does not justify the total expense (the system is "not cost-effective").

1. We define false positives as those babies who fail the Test but in fact had no hearing loss at the time. Table 3 assembles the ears ($N = 100$) that failed the Test but passed the Retest during 1981-1982. As discussed above, the ones that recovered from real but transient conductive losses in the Test-Retest interval should be removed from the list. Assuming that these ears are the ones that improved 20 dB or less, the candidate false positive ears number 33 in 20 babies (the

left ear of case 3, Fig. 1, is one of these). This gives (highly speculative) false positive rates of 0.032 (i.e., 20 babies for 624 tested) or 0.026 (33 ears for 1248 tested).

Whether or not this estimate is wide of the mark, false positives must exist; before their true number can be known, however, the threshold sensitivity of the neonate will have to be measured by some second test, ideally a behavioral one, that equals or exceeds the ABR in sensitivity and reliability. Such second tests as have been proposed and used during the past 50 years are generally considered to be unacceptably limited by comparison to the ABR.[20] Strictly speaking, therefore, to classify a baby like the one in case 3 as a true or a false positive must be considered merely a guess until this second test becomes available.

2. The false negative baby would yield a normal ABR but nevertheless suffer a real hearing loss at the time of the Test. The only patients known to be in this category show exclusively low frequency (below 1 kHz) hearing losses, and these are rare. This suggests that the true number of ABR false negatives is likely to be so small as to be of academic interest only. Furthermore, to establish it in any meaningful way will require that second newborn hearing test just described, both in order to demonstrate that a hearing loss did indeed exist at the time of Test and to prove that any loss measured at Retest did not in fact result from infection, trauma, genetic expression, or some of those other hazards to hearing every baby encounters in a Test-Retest interval. One might add, parenthetically, that any second test meeting these specifications would probably make use of the ABR superfluous in neonatal hearing testing.

3. Increasing Test efficiency. In our data (and in most test series others report) the ABR is applied unnecessarily to about 85% of all ICN graduates (because they pass the Test) and to one out of every two or three who fail the Test (because they pass the Retest). Is there some way to identify these normal babies before-hand and so limit testing to only that 9 or 10% to of ICN graduates who show a hearing loss when they are a few months old?

A common suggestion is to prescreen in some inexpensive but accurate manner and then Test only those who fail. Asking the staff (nurses, physicians, audiologists) to do this prescreening would, in our view, yield quite unreliable results; as previously reported[20] one of four babies found to need hearing aids in a particular study was judged by the staff to need no testing, and on occasion the staff is still surprised when a baby patient unexpectedly fails (or passes) the ABR Test (see case 4 above). Prescreening by such behavioral tests as the Crib-o-Gram[14] or Linco-Bennett Cradle[22] is a second possibility. The sensitivity of most such tests is inherently poor, however, and the reliability of all of them still remains to be established;[11,12,29] furthermore, no one has as yet validated their accuracy in separating normal from hearing-impaired newborns. Until a satisfactory prescreen procedure is developed, then, we see no alternative to applying the ABR Test to all ICN graduates if the ones with modest or monaural, as well as those with severe and bilateral hearing losses are to be identified reliably.

To eliminate retesting a baby whose hearing loss is conductive and transient, one might raise the Test criterion of failure from no response at 30 (or 40) dB nHL to, say, no response at 60 dB.[24] If groups II and III in Table 1 had been handled this way, the procedure would have precluded retesting 46 normal ears (28 babies) and also 29 permanently pathological ears in 19 babies, one of whom now wears a hearing aid. These numbers show that too great an elevation in the criterion for pass will eliminate testing of patients now being identified as seriously needing audiological attention. Changing the Test criterion by a smaller amount would of course eliminate fewer Retests, both the needed and the unnecessary, but what the optimal criterion change should be is not possible to say, given existing data. A final possibility is to apply the test not at the time of discharge but "three to six months later."[7] This would eliminate testing the ears with conductive losses that resolve, and the false postives, if any. In exchange, this plan would defeat a major goal our program now often attains, namely, to deliver definitive treatment for a diagnosed hearing loss by the time the baby is 3 to 6 mos old (see case 1). It would also preclude testing all members of the group; every baby is now accessible as an inpatient, but only a fraction of them would ever be returned for testing as outpatients. Unfortunately, then, we cannot suggest an acceptable plan that would eliminate any of either the Tests or Restests which, in hindsight, turn out to have been unnecessary to perform.

4. Cost-effectiveness. Whether ABR screening is cost-effective has been questioned.[7,17] Technically, a cost-effectiveness analysis has as its purpose "the identification of those programs that are effective in achieving a particular goal and those that are not."[6] Preconditions for performing the analysis include (1) a quantifiable and verifiable statement of the health goal to be achieved, along with (2) two or more programs having the same goal that can be compared with respect to efficiency, the resources each consumes (cost), and the types and amounts of benefits delivered. Given comparable data on each of two (or more) pro-

grams, one then estimates the effectiveness with which each of them has met the specified health goal.[6]

As a first step toward cost effectiveness analysis we can examine our program within this framework. As already stated, the program aims (1) to identify every infant who leaves the hospital with a hearing disorder, (2) to establish its magnitude and type, and (3) to begin to treat it, with hearing aids if necessary, during the first few months of life. The case histories above show the key diagnostic role played by the ABR at several points in the program, and Table 1 quantifies the degree to which this use of the ABR (along with many other procedures) has allowed us to approach the stated goals.

We can estimate the dollar cost of our program as follows: every 100 babies requires 100 Tests (at $65 each) and 16 Retests (at $130), for a total of $8580. According to Table 5 this expenditure yields, on average, 9 or 10 babies with diagnosed hearing problems brought under treatment during the first year of life, or about $1000 per baby identified. If only the 3 or 4 who do, or should, wear hearing aids is considered, the cost to identify each approaches $2500. Estimating program benefits is a more difficult problem: the dollar issue awaits a clear statement of any economic benefits that accrue to society from discovering a newborn hearing impairment and then reducing to an absolute minimum its potentially disastrous effect on language acquisition. Intangible benefits also accrue: the child begins very early to communicate with parents and peer; concerned adults (parents, teachers, physicians) are satisfied the best possible therapy is being administered, etc. What other benefits should be listed and then quantified are matters critical for a cost-effectiveness analysis but beyond the scope of the present discussion.

Roberts et al.,[17] using a loose, nontechnical definition, question whether ABR screening is cost-effective, stating: "Major concerns are the difficulty of adequate follow-up, the cost of equipment, administrative problems, the time required, and finally the large proportion of 'false failures'." Because they were unable to solve their problems and surmount their difficulties, Roberts et al. have abandoned use of the ABR in the ICN and "For early detection. . . depend on increased awareness of the possibility of hearing impairment in infants, on alert clinical observation, and on the guidance provided by attention to the high-risk factors for auditory impairment." Programs like the one they now use, and presumably recommend to others, have of course demonstrably failed to identify many deaf newborns in the past. We therefore consider their plan unacceptable, and based on the experiences summarized in this report, recommend continued use of the ABR as a screening and diagnostic tool, convinced that when properly used by skilled professionals it will almost never fail to supply information crucial for the early diagnosis and rational treatment of the hard-of-hearing infant.

References

1. Balkany, J.J., S.A. Berman, M.A. Simmons, and B.W. Jafek. 1978. Middle ear effusions in neonates. *Laryngoscope* 88, 398-405.

2. California State Department of Public Health. *Conference on Newborn Hearing screening: Proceeding, Summary, and Recommendations.* San Francisco, February 23-25, 1971.

3. Cox, L.C., M. Hack, and D.A. Metz. 1982. Longitudinal ABR in the NICU infant. *Int. J. Pediatr. Otorhinolaryngol.* 4, 225-231.

4. Cox, C.C., M. Hack, and D.A. Metz. 1984. Auditory brain stem response abnormalities in the very low birth-weight infant: incidence and risk factors. *Ear Hear.* 5, 47-51.

5. Despland, P.A., and R. Galambos. 1980. The auditory brainstem response (ABR) is a useful diagnostic tool in the intensive care nursery. *Pediatr. Res.* 14, 154-158.

6. Dittman, D.A., and K.R. Smith. 1979. Consideration of benefits and costs: A conceptual framework for the health planner. *Health Care Management Rev.* 4, 45-64.

7. Downs, D.W. 1982. Auditory brainstem response testing in the neonatal intensive care unit: A cautious response. *Asha* 24, 1009-1015.

8. Galambos, R. 1978. Use of the auditory brainstem response (ABR) in infant hearing testing. pp. 245-256. *in* S.E. Gerber, and G.T. Mencher, eds. *Early Diagnosis of Hearing Loss.* Grune and Stratton, New York.

9. Galambos, R., and P.A. Despland. 1980. The auditory brainstem response (ABR) evaluates risk factors for hearing loss in the newborn. *Pediatr. Res.* 14, 159-163.

10. Galambos, R., and K. Hecox. 1978. Clinical applications of the auditory brainstem response. *Otolaryngol. Clin. North Am.* 11, 709-722.

11. Galambos, R., G. Hicks, and M.J. Wilson. 1982. Hearing loss in graduates of a tertiary intensive care nursery. *Ear Hear* 3, 87-90.

12. Galambos, R., G.E. Hicks, and M.J. Wilson. 1982. Identification audiometry in neonates: A reply to Simmons. *Ear Hear* 3, 189-190.

13. Jacobson, J.T., M.R. Seitz, G.T. Mencher, and U. Parrott. 1978. Clinical applications of the auditory brainstem response. pp. 702-722. *in* S.E. Gerber, and G.T. Mencher, eds. *Early Diagnosis of Hearing Loss.* Grune and Stratton, New York.

14. Marcellino, G.R. 1981. Neonatal hearing screening utilizing microprocessor technology—a progress report. *Hear. Instrum.* 32, 12-14.

15. Mjoen, S. 1971. ABR in pediatric audiology. *Scand. Audiol. Suppl.* 13, 141-146.

16. Recommendations of the Saskatoon Conference. 1978. pp. 1-32. *in* S.E. Gerber, and G.T. Mencher, eds. *Early Diagnosis of Hearing Loss.* Grune and Stratton, New York.

17. Roberts, J.L., H. Davis, G.L. Phon, et al. 1982. Auditory brainstem responses in pre-term neonates: maturation and follow-up. *J. Pediatr.* 101, 257-263.

18. Schulman-Galambos, C., and R. Galambos. 1975. Brainstem auditory evoked responses in premature infants. *J. Speech. Hear. Res.* 18, 456-465.

19. Schulman-Galambos, C., and R. Galambos. 1979. Brainstem evoked responses in newborn hearing screening. *Arch. Otolaryngol.* 105, 86-90.

20. Schulman-Galambos, C., and R. Galambos. 1979. Assessment of hearing. pp. 91-119. *in* T.M. Field, A.M. Sostek, S. Goldberg, and N.H. Shuman, eds. *Infants Born at Risk*, Spectrum. NY.

21. Shannon, D.A., J.K. Felix, A. Krumholz, et al. 1984. Hearing screening of high-risk newborns with brainstem auditory evoked potentials: a follow-up study. *Pediatrics* 73, 22-26.

22. Shepard, N.T. 1983. Newborn hearing screening using the Linco-Bennett auditory response cradle: A pilot study. *Ear Hear.* 4, 5-10.

23. Simmons, F.B. 1983. Comment on "Hearing loss in graduates of a tertiary intensive care nursery." *Ear Hear.* 3, 188.

24. Stein, L., O. Ozdamar, N. Kraus, and J. Paton. 1983. Follow-up results with NICU infants screened by auditory brainstem response in the neonatal intensive care unit. *J. Pediatr.* 103, 447.

25. Stockard, J.E., J.J. Stockard, and R.W. Coen. 1983. Auditory brainstem response variability in infants. *Ear Hear.* 4, 11-23.

26. Stockard, J.E., and J.J. Stockard. 1981. Brainstem auditory evoked potentials in normal and otoneurologically impaired newborns and infants. pp. 421-466. *in* C. Henry (ed). *Current Clinical Neurophysiology*, Elsevier/North Holland, Amsterdam.

27. Stockard, J.E., and B.F. Westmoreland. 1981. Technical considerations in the recording and interpretation of the brainstem auditory evoked potential for neonatal neurologic diagnosis. *Am. J. EEG Technol.* 21, 31-54.

28. Weber, B.A. 1982. Comparison of auditory brain stem response latency norms for premature infants. *Ear Hear*, 3, 257-262.

29. Wright, L.B., and L.R. Rybak. 1983. Accuracy of Crib-O-Gram as a screening test on high risk newborns (abstract). *J. Acoust. Soc. Am.* (Suppl. 1) 73, 79.

Acknowledgments

The authors thank many friends and colleagues for ideas and help, and wish especially to recognize the contributions of the following persons at the Children's Hospital and Health Center at San Diego: the nursing staff of the Intensive Care Nursery; its staff neonatologists, Drs. M. Cohen, R. Henderson, L. Johnsgard, M. Segal, and Alan Schumacher; and Donald F. Krebs, Vice President, Ambulatory Services.

Address reprint requests to Robert Galambos, M.D., Speech, Hearing and Neurosensory Center, 8001 Frost St., San Diego, CA 92123.

Received July 1, 1983; accepted April 23, 1994

Automated Infant Hearing Screening Using the ABR: Development and Validation

Barbara S. Herrmann, Aaron R. Thornton, and Janet M. Joseph
Massachusetts Eye and Ear Infirmary, Boston

The recent endorsement of universal newborn hearing screening by the NIH Consensus Development Panel (March, 1993) has stimulated debate on the preferred technology for screening tests. Discussion of the suitability of auditory brainstem response (ABR) procedures has focused on ABR hearing screening as it is commonly done in the neonatal intensive care nursery (NICU), where the relatively high incidence of handicapping hearing loss has justified the time and highly trained personnel associated with conventional ABR testing. In discussing more efficient procedures needed because of the lower incidence of hearing loss in the well-baby nursery, little reference is made to an automated ABR instrument, the ALGO-I, specifically developed for infant hearing screening. This paper reports the results of three investigations that were undertaken during the development of the ALGO-I. While some descriptions and accounts of experiences with the ALGO-I have been published (Jacobson, Jacobson, & Spahr, 1990; Kileny, 1988; Peters, 1986), the data used in its development and initial validation have not been reported and are pertinent to its applicability in infant screening.

The focus of the three investigations was to determine the suitability of ABR for low-cost infant hearing screening by investigating the limits of ABR reliability and determining whether accurate ABR testing could be sufficiently optimized and automated to reduce costs to a practical level. Several steps were important in achieving this goal. First, the best possible performance of ABR hearing screening under ideal conditions was investigated, and the critical factors for obtaining accurate screening results were identified. Second, automatic control of many of those factors was designed into a prototype screening device, and the validity of the screener's performance was compared with the standard methods of ABR screening on the same infants. Finally, the screener's performance was evaluated under field conditions in the NICU.

Experiment I

The first priority in developing an independent ABR hearing screener was to determine the best possi-

ble performance of the ABR in identifying neonatal hearing loss. Unless the maximal performance of the ABR in infant hearing screening was adequate, its application to low-cost screening would be futile. Fria (1985) summarized the performance of clinical ABR hearing screening programs in several NICUs using general purpose ABR equipment. Most studies estimated the prevalence of hearing loss in NICU graduates to be between 1.5% and 5%. ABR screening failure rates, however, ranged between 5.3% and 59% with about 30% of the failures having normal hearing sensitivity on follow-up tests. Factors responsible for this variation in hearing screening performance divide into two categories (Table 1): factors associated with the baby and factors associated with screening technique (Murray, Javel, & Watson, 1985). Little can be done to control factors associated with babies, but factors associated with screening techniques such as myogenic activity, electrical artifact, masking noises, earphone placement, electrode montage, adequate averaging, and operator experience can be controlled.

In the first experiment, factors associated with screening technique were addressed in order to explore the limit of ABR hearing screening performance in an NICU population. In addressing these factors, the type of screening was limited to the identification of handicapping hearing loss. No attempt was made to measure

Table 1. Possible factors influencing the outcome of ABR hearing screening. Taken from Murray, Javel, and Watson, 1985.[a]

Baby Factors

Transient neurologic abnormalities
Poor health
Transient conductive problems
Poorer threshold sensitivity than adults

Technical Factors

Poor control of muscle artifact
Poor control of sound environment
Variable stimulus calibrations
Variable earphone placement
Collapsing ear canals
Mixed purpose for screening
Variable criteria for a pass

[a] Reprinted from the *American Journal of Otolaryngology, 6,* A. Murray, E. Javel, and C. Watson, Prognostic validity of auditory brainstem evoked response screening in newborn infants, pp. 120–131. Copyright 1985, with permission from Elsevier.

the neurologic status of the baby as is commonly included in NICU ABR screenings. Screening procedures for this first experiment were optimized for accuracy rather than cost-effectiveness because the goal was to determine the best possible performance of the ABR in order to recognize its inherent limitations for infant hearing screening.

Methods

Four hundred and fifty-one neonates from a tertiary neonatal intensive care unit were screened over a 46-month period. Screening was performed as close to discharge as possible in order to optimize the health of the infants. Conceptional age at the time of screening ranged from 30 to 58 weeks.

Babies were transported to an electrically shielded, sound-treated room in our laboratory where the ABR was recorded for each ear using a 30-dB HL 100-microsecond click at a rate of 37/second. Electroencephalic activity was filtered from 50 to 2,000 Hz with 6-dB per octave filter slopes. A vertex-to-nape electrode montage was used with a forehead ground. This montage was chosen because we had observed wave V to be significantly larger than with a vertex-to-mastoid electrode montage, making the response easier to detect. Most of the testing was done during natural sleep, but chloral hydrate was occasionally used to induce a satisfactory recording state.

Two audiologists screened; one operated the evoked potential system (Amplaid Mark 6) while the other monitored the baby. Each operator had at least 2 years experience with evoked-response-threshold audiometry. Two averages were recorded simultaneously, one to rarefaction phase clicks and one to condensation phase clicks. These simultaneous averages were visually evaluated to judge the repeatability of responses and to estimate residual noise levels. Responses were averaged until the noise was half the size of the response or until the residual noise level was less than 20 nV. Although 4,000 to 8,000 sweeps were used in the majority of screenings, averages of 16,000 sweeps were not unusual. Myogenic activity was controlled by a custom artifact-rejection system (Thornton, 1984; Thornton & Obenour, 1981) that allowed greater control over myogenic activity than is possible with conventional instruments. The system uses separate channels for signal averaging and artifact rejection, permitting the use of a higher high-pass filter cutoff and a steeper filter slope for the artifact-rejection channel. By reducing the relatively large slow-wave activity of the EEG, smaller changes in the background EMG can be detected more precisely. We also used a

minimum pause in averaging following each trigger of the rejection system, which more effectively prevents sporadic averaging during and immediately following a state of heightened EMG activity.

Screening results were categorized three ways: pass, fail, or could not test. The pass or fail decision was determined solely by the presence or absence of the response as judged by the operator. A baby was judged to be untestable if the conditions necessary for an adequate test could not be met. In most instances this meant that the baby presented too high a level of electrophysiologic noise for an accurate test.

Bilateral failures were followed as soon as possible with a comprehensive evoked response evaluation in which evoked response thresholds to tone bursts were obtained by air and bone conduction. Unilateral failures were not immediately retested. Because of the proportionally lesser risk of handicap to speech and language development, parents of babies who failed unilaterally were counseled to have their baby's hearing tested in 6 to 12 months.

Results

Examples of ABR waveforms from some of the infants passing the screening are shown in Figure 1. These pass responses have a similar configuration, with the most characteristic feature being a large negativity at approximately 12 ms. Wave V is either at the apex of the initial slow positive portion or falls on the downslope of the negative wave. This general configuration is robust across the wide 28-week range of conceptional ages.

The results of the NICU screenings are shown in Table 2. The total failure rate of 8% is equally divided between unilateral (4%) and bilateral (4%) failures. Very few babies (1%) were untestable. Follow-up evaluation of the bilateral failures (Table 3) indicated that the majority had sensorineural or mixed hearing losses. The incidence of conductive hearing loss was very low, and only one baby had normal hearing sensitivity on follow-up. This baby was in the NICU because of hyperbilirubinemia, and his bilirubin was still elevated when screened just before discharge to another nursery. Both his bilirubin level and his hearing sensitivity were normal 1 month later.

The total failure rate of 8% is much lower than failure rates reported by other programs (Fria, 1985), even though the percentage of infants with bilateral sensorineural hearing loss (2.4%) is similar to previous reports. Despite the fact that these infants were very sick babies from a tertiary-care nursery, their ABRs were

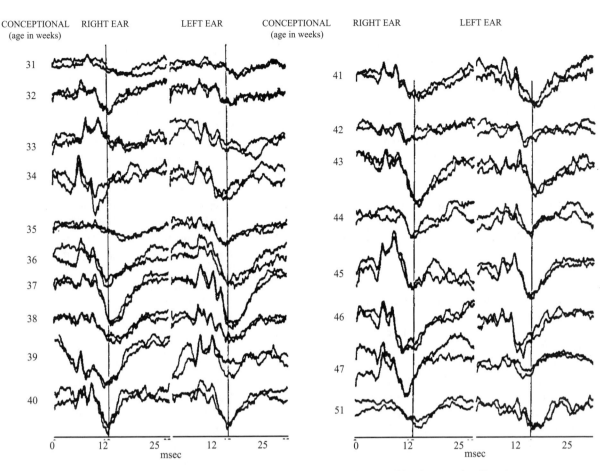

Figure 1. Representative waveforms from some of the infants passing the ABR signal-averaged hearing screening. Experiment I.

remarkably stable and homogeneous. These results indicate that the endogenous characteristics of neonates (Table 1) are not the limiting factors in ABR screening, leaving technical and methodologic factors as the major sources of variability. Because ABR hearing screening performance in this investigation was found to be robust, we proceeded to build and validate an ABR-based infant hearing screener, employing the necessary technical controls to ensure adequate performance in difficult testing environments such as the NICU.

Experiment II

Based on the experience from Experiment I, we designed an automated hearing screener to detect the neonatal ABR to a 35-dB HL click during unattended operation, incorporating previously developed techniques for automated AER detection (Sprague & Thornton, 1979; Thornton, 1978; Thornton & Obenour, 1981). The design concepts were incorporated into a reliable battery-operated instrument by Algotek, Inc.,

Table 2. Results of ABR hearing screening of NICU infants in Experiment I.

Screening Outcome	Percent of Infants ($N = 451$)
Pass	91%
Fail	8%
Bilateral—	4%
Unilateral—	4%
Could not test	1%

Table 3. Follow-up results on bilateral failures in Experiment I.

Total percentage of bilateral failures	4.0%
Bilateral hearing loss	
Sensorineural	2.4%
Conductive	0.4%
Mixed	0.6%
Normal hearing	0.2%
Lost to follow-up	0.2%

under the direction of Maurizzio Liverani, and the ALGO-I Infant Hearing Screener was commercially introduced in 1985. It is now produced by NATUS Medical, Inc.

The screener's function was limited to the single purpose of identifying handicapping hearing loss in infants in order to optimize the design and best control the essential test factors identified in Experiment I. Disposable, noise-attenuating earphones were designed with a clear faceplate to facilitate accurate placement and with an adhesive circumaural cushion to prevent changes in earphone position and prevent ear canal collapse. Ambient noise is monitored under the earphone, and screening is paused whenever the signal-to-noise ratio is less than 6 dB. Electrical artifacts are minimized by battery operation, shielded electrode leads, and an acoustic delay line. Myogenic activity is controlled by an improved artifact reject system, similar to that described in Experiment I, that effectively limits testing to myogenically quiet sleep. Electrode impedances are measured, and testing cannot begin or continue unless they are less than 12 kΩ and balanced.

The screener samples the post-stimulus EEG during intervals that meet the criteria for ambient noise under the earphone and myogenic noise or electrical artifact in the EEG, and calculates the likelihood of a response using a weighted-binary template-matching algorithm (Thornton & Obenour, 1981). The response template is modeled after the infant responses obtained in Experiment I. By emphasizing the large negativity near 12 ms, which has the least variance with age and signal intensity, and by sweeping the template through an appropriate range of latencies, the same template can be used with both pre-term and term infants. The binary detection algorithm is based on the use of a temporal matching filter in conjunction with a maximum likelihood ratio test using a Neyman-Pearson criterion (Schwartz & Shaw, 1975; Thornton, 1991; Thornton & Obenour, 1981). This technique directly assesses signal-to-noise ratio and permits an exact statistical test for detection.

The binary algorithm used in the ALGO-I was chosen because it is particularly robust with regard to assumptions of stationarity and stochasticity of the EEG, which are more critical for statistical tests that depend on estimated variances. Variance-ratio, maximum-likelihood tests (with or without templates) are optimal for signals in Gaussian noise, but they can become unpredictably inaccurate when the noise conditions change over time or include relatively strong periodic components, resulting in both Type I and Type II errors, falsely indicating a response or failing to show one. While the accuracy of the binary (Neyman-

Pearson) algorithm is also dependent on the amplitude distribution of the noise, it provides exact control over Type I errors or false-negative results (passing a deaf baby), which is the most serious error that can be made. Type II errors, or false-positives (failing a hearing baby), are controlled by the maximum number of response intervals sampled in the test. Varying noise characteristics can decrease the screener's sensitivity, but they cannot increase the probability of a false detection.

The screener runs automatically, without operator intervention, calculating the likelihood ratio for response detection after the first 1000 sweeps (500 for the prototype) and again at every increment of 500 accepted sweeps. When the probability that a response has been detected exceeds the criterion of 0.99997, the test of that ear is terminated and the outcome is reported as a PASS. When 15,000 sweeps are cumulated without meeting the PASS criterion, the test is stopped and reported as a REFER. The test then continues with the opposite ear. In the case that myogenic activity or ambient noise prevent reaching the PASS or REFER criteria, the outcome is categorized as COULD NOT TEST. Under favorable conditions, the screener can report a PASS (the most frequent outcome) for both ears in less than a minute of testing, whereas a REFER will take at least 7 minutes per ear.

Automated control over the factors essential for accurate testing combined with automatic response detection eliminates the need for an expensive, experienced operator, which greatly lowers the cost of ABR infant hearing screening. The purpose of the second experiment was to validate the performance of the automated screener by comparing the outcome of the screener to ABR results obtained from conventional signal-averaging procedures on the same infants.

Methods

The prototype ALGO-I screener was validated on 153 babies sampled in three settings: the neonatal intensive care nursery, a normal newborn nursery, and the clinic population of our laboratory. Conceptional ages ranged from 31 to 131 weeks, with a mean of 43 weeks (Table 4). Each ALGO-I screening was validated in one of two ways: (a) Output of the screener's EEG amplifier and signal trigger were recorded with an FM tape recorder (Teac R80), and the raw EEG data were reprocessed with conventional signal-averaging techniques (Amplaid Mark 6). (b) An additional ABR test of hearing threshold sensitivity, using the instrumentation and methods described for Experiment I, was done on the same day using tone bursts (1000,

Table 4. Subject breakdown for subject source and validation technique in Experiment II.

Subject Source	NICU	87
	Well-baby nursery	13
	Clinic	53
Validation	Screener taped	90
	Signal-averaged only	43
	Both techniques	20

2000, or 4000 Hz, 2-cycle rise-fall) or clicks (100 microsecond). Again, operators had at least 2 years' experience in evoked response audiometry, and a vertex-to-nape electrode montage was used for all tests.

Results

Results of the validation are in Table 5. Each of the 127 infants passing the screening had a visually detectable response to a click at 35-dB HL or lower. Examples of the signal-averaged responses for these babies are shown in Figure 2. The top traces are some of the largest responses detected by the screener, and the bottom traces are some of the smallest. The bottom response is the average of about 40,000 repetitions taken from the FM tape, and, although it is small, it had been detected by the screener in each of three successive trials ranging from 7,500 to 14,500 sweeps. Disagreements between the screener outcome and the results of signal-averaging occurred only for four babies that failed the screening. Of the 25 babies failed by the screener, 21 of them had no detectable response at 35-dB HL. On further follow-up, these 21 babies had hearing poorer than 25-dB HL in the ear that failed. Four of the screener failures had detectable signal-averaged ABRs. Two of these four had small amplitude responses, but actually had mild, conductive hearing losses. One child's response was clear but markedly different from the ALGO-I detection template. Examples of signal-averaged responses from screener failures are shown in Figure 3.

Experiment III

The results from the second experiment indicate very good agreement between the results of signal-averaged ABRs and those of the automated infant hearing screener. The screener's performance was, therefore, capable of high-quality infant hearing screening with greatly reduced demands on the operator. The prototype screener was further refined and subsequently manufactured. In this last experiment, we used the commercial ALGO-I to screen the hearing of

babies from the same NICU described in Experiment I, and we compared the performance of the screener in this less-than-ideal setting to the best performance of ABR screening under the ideal conditions described in Experiment I. This comparison independently verified the validation of the screener prototype reported in Experiment II.

Methods

The ALGO-I Infant Hearing Screener was used to screen the hearing of 398 babies from the tertiary intensive care nursery (NICU) over a 23-month period. Screenings were done in the NICU close to the baby's discharge by audiologists, including CFYs, who had little experience in evoked response audiometry. Babies failing the screening were followed as described in Experiment I. Bilateral failures were seen as soon as possible for a comprehensive evoked response evaluation, often before discharge. Parents of unilateral failures were notified by letter and followed less aggressively.

Results

Table 6 shows the screening results from those babies tested only with the ALGO-I. The proportions of babies passing and failing are not significantly different from those of Experiment I (Chi-square Test of Proportions, $p > 0.05$; Snedecor & Cochran, 1967). Follow-up of bilateral failures (Table 7) indicates a similar incidence of hearing loss and a false-positive rate of 1%.

These results indicate that performance of the automated ALGO-I screener used in the NICU by minimally trained staff is similar to the best performance of ABR hearing screening using signal-averaging under ideal conditions. Because it can produce accurate results within the NICU environment without the need for an experienced and skilled operator, which is the most expensive component of ABR infant screening, the cost of the automated screening is minimized.

Table 5. Automated screener validation results in Experiment II.

Screening Outcome (N= 153)	Automated Screener Outcome	Validation Results	
		Agree	Disagree
Pass	127	127	0
Fail	25	21	4
Bilateral	11	9	2
Unilateral	14	12	2
Could not test	1	—	—

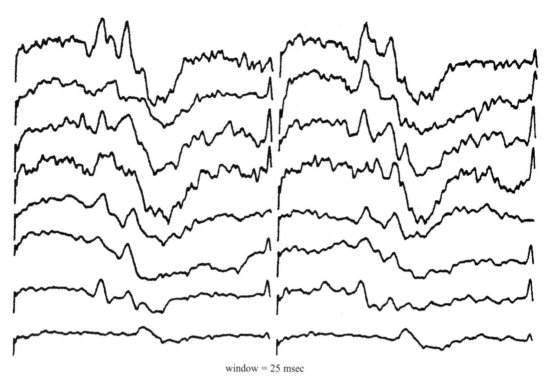

window = 25 msec

Figure 2. Examples of signal-averaged responses for babies passing the automated ABR infant hearing screening in the validation studies of Experiment II. (Representative sample from 153 infants screened.)

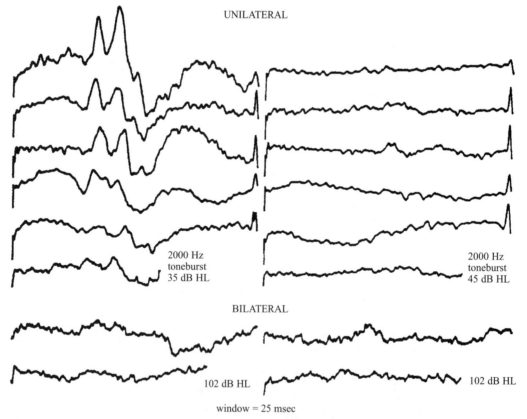

UNILATERAL

2000 Hz
toneburst
35 dB HL

2000 Hz
toneburst
45 dB HL

BILATERAL

102 dB HL

102 dB HL

window = 25 msec

Figure 3. Examples of signal-averaged responses for babies failing the automated ABR infant hearing screening in the validation studies of Experiment II.

Additional program savings are realized by the low false-positive referral rate, which reduces the number of costly follow-up tests on normal-hearing babies.

Discussion

The results of our studies demonstrate that ABR can be used to accurately screen the hearing of infants and that the factors critical for accurate screening were successfully automated in the ALGO-I infant hearing screener. These findings are similar to the experiences reported by other investigators (Hall, Kileny, Ruth, & Kripal, 1987; Jacobson et al.,1990; Von Wedel, Schauseil-Zipf, & Doring, 1988) who compared the ALGO-I performance against their own signal-averaging protocols for ABR hearing screening (Table 8). Their averaging protocols, developed for clinical feasibility, were not reported to have been specifically optimized for maximum performance of ABR hearing screening, nor were the protocol performances reported. Consequently, the performance standard against which the ALGO-I was compared in these other studies is unknown. In addition, some investigators used suboptimal electrode placements on the forehead and mastoid, which would be expected to increase the false-positive rate.

Even so, previously reported performance of the ALGO-I is good. Hall et al. (1987) found disagreements in only 3% of the ears, with no ear passing the ALGO-I that failed the signal-averaged screening. Jacobson et al. (1990) found disagreements in 5% of the ears in the first of two conventional signal-averaging ABR hearing screenings. Four of these ears passed the ALGO-I but failed the first screening with signal-averaging. These four ears, however, passed the second ABR signal-averaged screening and were normally hearing on follow-up, indicating that the ALGO-I produced a lower false-positive rate. Von Wedel et al. (1988) had a 12% disagreement rate with 4% (two infants) passing the ALGO but failing the signal-averaged screening. Findings of follow-up evaluations for those infants were not reported so it cannot be deter-

Table 7. Comparison of follow-up results between conventional signal-averaging ABR hearing screening and automated ABR hearing screening.

	Signal-Averaged Screening (N = 451)	Automated Screening (N = 393)
Total bilateral failures	4.0%	4.7%
Bilateral hearing loss		
Sensorineural	2.4%	1.5%
Conductive	0.4%	1.0%
Mixed	0.6%	0.0%
Undetermined	0.0%	0.8%
Normal hearing	0.2%	1.0%
Lost to follow-up	0.2%	0.5%

mined by follow-up results which technique was more accurate. Von Wedel et al. (1988) did find that the ALGO-I screening was twice as fast as the screening with signal-averaging, with an average time-to-pass of 2-3 minutes versus 6-8 minutes and an average time-to-fail of 7 minutes versus 10 minutes. This time savings is also a cost savings.

Table 9 contains the combined performance data on the ALGO-I compared to conventional signal-averaging hearing screenings for all studies. The specificity of the ALGO-I from the combined data is 96%, and the sensitivity is 98%, performance statistics that are quite acceptable for universal newborn hearing screening. It should be noted that three of the four studies reported sensitivities of 100%. Only the Von Wedel et al. study indicated a sensitivity under 100%, and the long-term follow-up results of the two discrepant ears in this study were not reported. It is not known if these ears were normal or hearing-impaired upon follow-up. The low false-negative rate of the ALGO-I indicated by the high sensitivity of the ALGO-I performance reflects the design emphasis on not passing a deaf baby. An infant hearing screening may likely be the only hearing test a child receives before entering school, making it imperative to accurately identify hearing loss. Because passing a test tends to create a sometimes false security in parents and caregivers, the false-negative rate must be kept negligible. The costs of false-negative error may be associated with delayed development and socioeconomic consequences.

Because screening failures can be immediately evaluated for accurate determination of hearing threshold sensitivity by present ABR technology, false-positive results tend to be self-correcting, making them more tolerable than the false-negative errors. However, the false-positive rate is a significant determinant of the total cost of a screening program, and the high specificity of the ALGO-I performance means that few

Table 6. Comparison of results between conventional signal averaging ABR hearing screening, from Experiment I, and automated ABR hearing screening.

Screening Outcome	Signal-Averaged Screening (N = 451)	Automated Screening (N = 393)
Pass	91%	87%
Fail	8%	11%
Bilateral	4%	5%
Unilateral	4%	7%
Could not test	1%	2%

Table 8. Comparison of ALGO-I automated ABR hearing screening with conventional signal-averaged ABR hearing screening.

Hall, Kileny, Ruth, and Kripal (1987)
N = 336 ears

ALGO-I	Signal-Averaging Pass	Fail	
Pass	307	0	307
Fail	11	18	29
	318	18	336

Specificity 97%
Sensitivity 100%

Jacobson, Jacobson, and Spahr (1990)
N = 447 ears

ALGO-I	Signal-Averaging[a] Pass	Fail	
Pass	397	0	397
Fail	17	33	50
	414	33	447

Specificity 96%
Sensitivity 100%
[a]Results of second signal-averaged screening

Von Wedel, Schauseil-Zipf, and Doring (1988)
N = 100 ears

ALGO-I	Signal-Averaging Pass	Fail	
Pass	86	2	88
Fail	4	8	12
	90	10	100

Specificity 96%
Sensitivity 80%

Herrmann et al. (Experiment II)
N = 304 ears

ALGO-I	Signal-Averaging Pass	Fail	
Pass	256	0	256
Fail	6	42	48
	262	42	304

Specificity 98%
Sensitivity 100%

babies will be referred for unnecessary follow-up testing. A low false-positive rate, such as the 1% obtained in Experiment III (Table 7) for the ALGO-I or the 3.2% indicated by the combined data (Table 9), is essential to control the costs associated with infant hearing screening (Goldstein & Tait, 1971; Turner, 1992).

The reduced costs and high accuracy of the automated ALGO-I makes universal hearing screening a practical option for the early identification of hearing loss. Many in health care have become accustomed to the strategy of preselecting infants for hearing screening according to the high-risk registers recommended by the Joint Committee (1982, 1990). Few, however, remember that the high-risk approach was a strategy taken by the Joint Committee to reduce the cost of early identification at a time when the diagnosis of childhood hearing loss was accomplished by a long drawn-out series of costly behavioral evaluations, and culminated when the child matured enough for accurate testing (Goldstein & Tait, 1971). The Joint Committee recommended that testing be limited to those children with a higher probability of hearing loss until such time that screening and follow-up methods were sufficiently improved (Joint Committee, 1974).

Studies of the efficacy of the high-risk register have shown that only 50 to 75% of infants with hearing loss are identifiable by high-risk criteria (Mauk, White, Mortensen & Behrens, 1991; Stein, Clark, &

Kraus, 1983). Given the 90% attrition rate for the follow-up testing of high-risk infants (Mahoney, 1987), at best only 7.5% of the babies with hearing loss are actually tested in infancy. It is not surprising that in the 20-year history of using the high-risk register, the average age of identification for a child with hearing loss is close to 36 months (U.S. Department of Health and Human Services, 1990). Implementation of the high-risk registry is also expensive. Personnel time is needed for chart review to determine which babies are high-risk. Then parents are informed, permissions are obtained, appointments are made, tests are performed, and follow-up is monitored. With the automated screener, an infant's hearing can be screened in less time than it takes to determine whether the baby is

Table 9. Combined data from all studies comparing ALGO-I automated ABR hearing screener with conventional signalaveraged ABR hearing screening.

N = 1,187 ears

ALGO-I	Signal-Averaging Pass	Fail	
Pass	1,046	2[a]	1,048
Fail	38	101	139
	1,084	103	1,187

Specificity 96%
Sensitivity 98%
[a]Follow-up on these ears not known.

high-risk. Costs are decreased, and all babies with hearing loss identified.

The best way to achieve early identification of hearing loss is to test all babies when they are already in the hospital. Technological development over the last 30 years has solved the problems of test sensitivity and over-referral that made newborn hearing screening unaffordable in the late 1960s. ABR audiometry has not only eliminated the need for extensive and repetitive behavioral follow-up of all screening failures, but automation of ABR hearing screening, such as that represented by the ALGO-I, further decreases the costs for hearing screening in the nursery. The ALGO-I may be used now to implement universal hearing screening at an affordable cost, making early identification of hearing loss a reality. Similar instruments for newborn hearing screening, whether based on ABR or otoacoustic emissions, must meet the criteria of a negligible false-negative rate, a low false-positive rate, and affordability to be successfully used in universal newborn hearing screening.

Acknowledgments

The authors gratefully thank the staff of the neonatal intensive care nursery at the Massachusetts General Hospital, specifically I. David Todres, A.K. Krishnamorthy, and the NICU nursing staff, and Roland Eavey of the Massachusetts Eye and Ear Infirmary, without whose help and support this work would not have been possible. In addition, we acknowledge and thank Dr. Maurizzio Liverani and Jeff Harrison, who designed and built the prototype and commercial instruments used in this work.

References

Fria, T.J. (1985). Identification of congenital hearing loss with the auditory brainstem response. In J.T. Jacobson (Ed.), *The auditory brainstem response* (pp. 317-336). San Diego, CA: College-Hill Press.

Goldstein, R., & Tait, C. (1971). Critique of neonatal hearing evaluation. *Journal of Speech Hearing Disorders, 26,* 3-18.

Hall, J.W., Kileny, P.R., Ruth, R.A., & Kripal, J.P. (1987). Newborn auditory screening with ALGO-I vs. conventional auditory brainstem response. *Asha, 29,* 120.

Jacobson, J.T., Jacobson, C.A., & Spahr, R.C. (1990). Automated and conventional ABR screening techniques in high-risk infants. *Journal of the American Academy of Audiology, 1,* 187-195.

Joint committee on infant hearing screening: Supplementary statement. (1974). *Asha, 16,* 160.

Joint committee on infant hearing screening: Position statement. (1982). *Asha, 24,* 1017.

Joint committee on infant hearing screening: Position statement. (1990). *American Academy of Otolaryngology–Head and Neck Surgery Bulletin, 10,* 15.

Kileny, P.R. (1988). New insights on infant ABR hearing screening. *Scandinavian Audiology,* Suppl 30:81-88.

Mahoney, T. (1987). The ups and downs of high-risk hearing screening: The Utah statewide program. *Seminars in Hearing, 8,* 155.

Mauk, G.W., White, K.R., Mortensen, L.B., & Behrens, T.R. (1991). The effectiveness of screening programs based on high-risk characteristics in early identification of hearing impairment. *Ear and Hearing, 12*(5), 312-319.

Murray, A., Javel, E., & Watson, C. (1985). Prognostic validity of auditory brainstem evoked response screening in newborn infants. *American Journal of Otolaryngology, 6,* 120-131.

NIH Consensus Statement. (March 1-3, 1993). Early identification of hearing impairment in infants and young children. 11, 1-24.

Peters, J.G. (1986) An automated infant screener using advanced evoked response technology. *Hearing Journal, 39,* 25-30.

Schwartz, M., & Shaw, L. (1975). *Signal processing: Discrete spectral analysis, detection and estimation.* New York: McGraw Hill.

Snedecor, G.W., & Cochran, W.G. (1967). *Statistical methods* (6th ed.). Ames, IA: Iowa State University Press.

Sprague, B.H., & Thornton A.R. (1979). Simplified infant screening using middle component auditory evoked responses. *Asha (A), 21,* 735.

Stein, L., Clark, S., & Kraus, N. (1983). The hearing-impaired infant: Patterns of identification and habilitation. *Ear and Hearing, 4,* 232-236.

Thornton, A.R. (1978). Improved detection of auditory evoked potentials. *Asha (A), 20,* 765.

Thornton, A.R. (1984). Technical consideration in recording the ABR. In A. Starr, C. Rosenberg, M. Don, & H. Davis (Eds.), *Sensory evoked potentials 1. An international conference on standards for auditory brainstem response (ABR) testing.* Milan: Centro Ricerche e Studi Amplifon, 183-184.

Thornton, A.R. (1991). Detection algorithm for hearing sensitivity screening. *IERASG XII Biennial symposium (A), 36,* 18.

Thornton, A.R., & Obenour, J.L. (1981). Auditory response detection method and apparatus. United States patents #4,275,744, 1981. Reviewed in *Journal of the Acoustical Society of America, 70,* 1814.

Turner, R.G. (1992). Modeling the cost and performance of early identification protocols. *Journal of the American Academy of Audiology, 2,* 195-205.

U.S. Department of Health and Human Services. (1990). *Healthy people* 2000: *National health promotion and disease prevention objectives.* Washington, DC: Public Health Service.

Von Wedel, H., Schauseil-Zipf, U., & Doring, W.H. (1988). Horscreening bei Neugeborenen and Sauglingen. *Laryng. Rhinol. Otol.,* 67, 307-311.

Contact author: Barbara Herrmann, Ph.D., Department of Audiology, Massachusetts Eye and Ear Infirmary, 243 Charles Street, Boston, MA 02114

Received August 18, 1993; accepted July 20, 1994

Key Words: infant hearing screening, auditory brainstem response (ABR), newborn

Identification of Neonatal Hearing Impairment: Evaluation of Transient Evoked Otoacoustic Emission, Distortion Product Otoacoustic Emission, and Auditory Brain Stem Response Test Performance

Susan J. Norton, Michael P. Gorga, Judith E. Widen, Richard C. Folsom, Yvonne Sininger, Barbara Cone-Wesson, Betty R. Vohr, Kelley Mascher, and Kristin Fletcher

Children's Hospital and Regional Medical Center, Seattle, Washington [S.J.N., K.M., K.F.]
Boys Town National Research Hospital, Omaha, Nebraska [M.P.G.]
University of Kansas Medical Center, Kansas City, Kansas [J.E.W.]
University of Washington, Seattle, Washington [R.C.F.]
House Ear Institute, Los Angeles, California [Y.S.]
LAC-USC Medical Center, Los Angeles, California [B.C.-W.]
Women and Infants' Hospital, Providence, Rhode Island [B.R.V.]

Objectives: The purpose of this study was to compare the performance of transient evoked otoacoustic emissions (TEOAEs), distortion product otoacoustic emissions (DPOAEs), and auditory brain stem responses (ABRs) as tools for identification of neonatal hearing impairment.

Design: A totoal of 4911 infants including 4478 graduates of neonatal intensive care units, 353 well babies with one or more risk factors for hearing loss (Joint Committee on Infant Hearing, 1994) and 80 well babies without risk factor who did not pass one or more neonatal test were targeted as the potential subject pool on which test performance would be assessed. During the neonatal period, they were evaluated using TEOAEs in response to an 80 dB pSPL click, DPOAE responses to two stimulus conditions (L1=L2=75 dB SPL and l1=65dB SPL L2=50 dB SPL), and ABR elicited by a 30 dB nHL click. In an effort to describe test performance, these "at-risk" infants were asked to return for behavioral audiologic assessments, using visual reinforcement audiometry (VRA) at 8 to 12 mo corrected age, regardless of neonatal test results. Sixty-four percent of these subjects returned and reliable VRA data were obtained on 95.6% of these returnees. This approach is in contrast to previous studies in which, by necessity, efforts were made to follow only those infants who "failed" the neonatal screening tests. The accuracy of the neonatal measures in predicting hearing status at 8 to 12 mo corrected age was determined. Only those infants who provided reliable, monaural VRA test results were includeded in the analysis. Separate analyses were performed without regard to intercurrent events (i.e., events between the neonatal and VRA tests that could cause their results to disagree), and then after accounting for the possible influence of intercurrent events such as otitis media and late-onset or progressive hearing loss.

Results: Low refer rates were achieved for the stopping criteria used in the present study, especially when a protocol similar to the one recommended in the National Institutes of Health (1993) Consensus Conference Report was followed. These analyses, however, do not completely describe test performance because they did not compare neonatal screening test results with a gold standard test of hearing. Test performance, as measured by the area under a relative operating characteristic curve, were similar for all three neonatal tests when neonatal test results were compared to VRA data obtained at 8 to 12 mo corrected age. However, ABRs were more successful at determining auditory status at 1 kHz, compared with the otoacoustic emission (OAE) tests. Performance was more similar across all three tests when they were used to identify hearing loss at 2 and 4 kHz. No test performed perfectly. Using either the two- or three-frequency pure-tone average (PTA), with a fixed false alarm rate of 20%, hit rates for the neonatal tests, in general, exceeded 80% when hearing impairment was defined as behavioral thresholds ≥30 dB HL. All three tests performed similarly when a two-frequency (2 and 4 kHz) PTA (adding 1 kHz) was used as the gold standard definition. For both PTA and all three neonatal screening measures, however, hit rate increased a the magnitude of hearing loss increased.

Conclusions: Singly, all three neonatal hearing screening tests resulted in low refer rates, especially if referrals for follow-up were made only for the cases in which stopping criteria were not met in both ears. Following a protocol similar to that recommended in the National Institutes of Health (1993) Consensus Conference report resulted in refer rates that were less than 4%. TEOAEs at 80 dB pSPL, DPOAE at L1=65, L2=50 dB SPL and ABR at 30 dB nHL measured during the neonatal period, and as implemented in the current study, performed similarly at predicting behavioral hearing status at 8 to 12 mo corrected age. Although perfect test performance was never achieved, sensitivity for each measure increased

Reprinted by permission of authors and Lippincott, Williams and Wilkins. Copyright 2000. *Ear and Hearing,* 21, No. 5, pp. 508–528.

with themagnitude of hearing loss. This latter finding is important because it suggests that all three tests performed better at identifying hearing losses for which intervention would be immediately recommended.

(Ear and Hearing 2000; 21; 508-528.)

The primary goal of the Identification of Neonatal Hearing Impairment study wa to compare the performance of transient evoked otoacoustic emissions (TEOAEs), distortion product otoacoustic emissions (DPOAEs), and auditory brain stem responses (ABRs) as tools for identification of neonatal hearing impairment. The most common measures of test accuracy in health care are sensitivity and specificity, and their compliments, the false negative and false positive rate. Sensitivity indicates the proportion of time patients who have a disease or disorder (i.e., hearing impairment) do not pass the screening test. It is synonymous with hit or true positive rate. False negative (miss) rate is the proportion of time patients with a disorder pass a test. The sum of sensitivity and false negative rates equals 100%. Specificity is the proportion of time patients not having a disease or disorder (i.e., patients with normal hearing) are passed by the screening test. It is synonomous with the correct rejection or true negative rate. False positive (false alarm) rate is the proportion of time subjects without the disorder are failed by the test. The sum of specificity and false positive rates also must equal 100%.

Table 1A shows a typical two-by-two decision matrix often used to describe test performance. True hearing status (impaired or normal) is compared with screening test outcome (not pass or pass). The use of a single two-by-two matrix implies that both hearing loss and the screening tool are binary entities (i.e., hearing loss is present or absent as defined by a "gold standard") and the response being measured is present in all normal-hearing newborns and absent in all hearing-impaired newborns. Unfortunately, neither of these assumptions is completely true.

First, hearing status is a continuous tow-dimensional variable (e.g., threshold as a function of frequency), and the majority of responses to auditory stimuli are continuous, multi-dimensional variables. Therefore, when evaluating the performance of a neonatal hearing-screening test, several variables must be defined to interpret the results. For example, the target hearing loss must be selected, including degree, configuration, and type of hearing loss. If five degrees (normal, mild, moderate, severe, and profound), three within-ear configurations (flat, high-frequency, and low-frequency), two between-ear configurations (unilateral and bilateral), and three types (conductive, sensorineural, or mixed) of hearing loss are considered, there would be 90 possible definitions of haring impairment. It is not reasonable, at least for hearing screning, to use 90 definitions of hearing loss. The low prevalence of neonatal hearing loss requires that the number of hearing loss categories be kept to a minimum.

The definition of hearing loss has a significant effect on test performance as well as test construction (e.g., screening level, pass criterion). The definition of hearing loss, in large measure, is determined by the goal of hearing screening. Two goals are generally cited: 1) identify all infants at risk for significant hearing loss; and 2) enroll all infants with significant hearing loss in early intervention by 6 mo of age. Recent studies by Yoshinaga-Itano, Sedey, Coulter, and Mehl (1998) and by Moeller (Reference Note 1) indicate that intervention by 6 mo benefits children with any degree of hearing loss, from mild to profound. If standard clin-

TABLE 1. A. Two-by-two table defining the four cells derived from the comparison of results of a gold standard test to an experimental measure when both measures are available on all subjects. Note that the sum of the true positive and false negative rates and the sum of the false positive and true negative must each equal 100%. B. Two-by-two table showing the case when only those patients who did not pass the experimental measure are followed. Thus, the false negative and the true negative rates cannot be known exactly. By extension, estimates of true positive and false positive rates also cannot be known exactly.

		A. True Hearing Status				B. True Hearing Status	
Neonatal Test Results		Hearing Impaired	Normal Hearing		Neonatal Test Results	Hearing Impaired	Normal Hearing
	Not Pass	True Positive (Hit)	False Positive (False Alarm)			Not Pass	True Positive?	False Positive?
	Pass	False Negative (Miss)	True Negative			Pass	Unknown	Unknown

ical descriptors are used, a pure-tone average (PTA) greater than 20 dB HL represents a hearing impairment (Bess, Gravel, & Tharpe, 1996). However, previous studies (e.g., Hyde, Riko, & Malizia, 1990) have shown that the lower the target degree of hearing loss, the greater the mumber of false alarms and the more expensive the screening program. The fact that several ABR screening programs use 35 or 40 dB nHL clicks (e.g., Hermann, Thorton, & Joseph, 1995; Hyde et al., 1990) may be related to this issue.

Once criteria for normal and impaired hearing are determined, the distribution of the response variable being measured for both normal-hearing and hearing-impaired ears must be described. If a response is present in all infants meeting the definition of normal hearing and absent in all infants not meeting the definition, the screening tool accuracy will be 100%. However, if the response is continuously distributed in both groups and these distributions are not completely separated, errors will occur. In these circumstances, it is possible to emphasize one error at the expense of the other (i.e., reduce misses at the cost of an increase in the false positive rate), but it would be impossible to eliminate all errors. A common measure of accuracy for a continuously distributed response is the relative operating characteristic (ROC) curve (Swets, 1988; Swets & Pickett, 1982). These curves can be used to describe test performance because they display the true positive rate as a function of false positive rate for different pass-fail criteria for a fixed definition of hearing loss. Each point on a ROC curve represents a single two-by-two decision matrix. As the pass criteria become more stringent, both the true and false positive rates increase if the underlying distributions of responses from normal and impaired ears are not completely separated. Thus, ROC curves provide a unified description of the underlying distributions of responses from normal and impaired ears, and can be used to describe the extent to which these two distributions overlap.

There are several metrics that can be used to describe the overlap between two distributions of responses. Standard scores (d') can be used as a measure of the distance between the means of two distributions, assuming that both distributions are normally distributed and have the same variance. If the response distributions for normal-hearing and hearing-impaired ears are identical, d'=0, and the ROC curve would fall along the positive diagonal. This means that true positives and false positives are equally likely to occur regardless of the criterion value. As the distributions of responses from normal and impaired ears become more distinct, d' would increase and the ROC curve would move toward the upper left corner of the plot.

Another measure of the separation between the responses of ears with normal and impaired hearing is the area under the ROC curve. The area under the ROC curve is the probability that the test result for a randomly chosen hearing-impaired ear exceeds that for a randomly chosen normal-hearing ear (Swets & Pickett, 1982). Depending on how ROC curve area is estimated, it is less dependent on assumptions of equal variance and normal distribututions, compared with d'. Area under the ROC curve can vary from 0.5, when normal and impaired distributions are completely separated. These analysis approaches have been applied to data from older subjects in efforts to describe the extent to which DPOAEs and TEOAEs accurately identify auditory status (Gorga, Neely, Bergman, Beauchaine, Kaminski, Peters, & Jesteadt, 1993; Gorga, Neely, Bergman, Beauchaine, Kaminski, Peters, Schulte, & Jesteadt, 1993; Gorga, Neely, & Dorn, 1999; Harrison & Norton, 1999; Hussain, Gorga, Neely, Keefe, & Peters, 1998; Kim, Paparello, Jung, Smurzynski, & Sun, 1996; Prieve et al., 1993). One goal of the present study is to apply a similar approach in efforts to determine how well screening tests performat identifying auditory status in infants. In addition to requiring gold standard data on all infants tested during the neonatal period, this approach also requires that a range of criterion measures be available for analyses.

Typically, a single "pass" criterion is chosen for a screening tool. These criteria (e.g., a TEOAE signal to noise ration [SNR]>3 dB in response to an 80 dB pSPL click or ABR Wave V presence in response to a 30 dB nHL click) presumably are based on responses from individuals with known audiograms, the majority of whom are cooperative, healthy, and tested under ideal conditions. Such approaches may be limited for several reasons, especially when applied with neonates. First, the extent to which these criteria are applicable with neonates has not been investigated thoroughly. Second, evaluation of a single criterion value limits the extent to which test performance can be described. It also runs the risk of missing the results achieved by other criteria, which may result in superior performance. Third, many reports describe test performance by following only infants who do not pass the neonatal tests. These studies assume a priori that all infants who "passed" the screen had normal hearing. This is a completely understandable approach because it would be prohibitively expensive and practically infeasible to follow all newborns, both passes as well as refers, under ordinary circumstances. Still, to determine the true accuracy of neonatal tests, it is necessary to follow all infants evaluated during the neonatal period, regardless of neonatal test outcome. Because the true hearing status of those

TABLE 2. Hypothetical demonstration that estimates of screening test performance depend on who receives follow-up evaluation with the gold standard.

True Auditory Status	Screening Test Results	Follow-Up All Ears	Follow-Up Only Fails
Hearing impaired	Fail	90	90
Hearing impaired	Pass	10	0
Normal hearing	Fail	360	360
Normal hearing	Pass	5540	5550
Sensitivity		0.90	1.0
Specificity		0.935	0.939

In this example, a total of 6000 ears at risk for hearing loss were screened, the overall refer rate was set to 7.5%, and it was assumed that there were 17 infants per 1000 with true hearing loss. In the first scenario, all infants, passes as well as refers, were followed to determine true hearing status. In the second scenario, only those ears failing the screening test were followed. If only those infants who "fail" the screening test are followed, the false negative responses are underestimated and, thus, the sensitivity is overestimated.

infants who "pass" the screening test is not known, true positive rate cannot be calculated as signified by the question marks in Table 1B. Errors made among infants with normal hearing (false positives) can be known, presumably because these false positives are evaluated with additional testing. The fact that the passes may include infants with hearing loss will have little influence on the true negative rate because the vast majority of infants have normal hearing. Unfortunately, the errors among ears with hearing loss (misses or false negatives) cannot be known if only those infants failing the newborn hearing test are followed. This is because misses (incorrectly identifying a hearing-impaired infant as normal) are not followed. Passing even a small number of babies with hearing loss can have a large effect on estimates of the true positive rate because of the overall small number of babies with hearing loss.

Table 2 illustrates the effects of these assumptions on performance estimates of a hypothetical test. Calculations are based on 6000 at-risk ears, 5550 of which "passed" the screening test and 450 of which "failed," resulting in an overall refer rate of 7.5%. If only those ears that "failed" were evaluated using the gold standard, test "sensitivity" is 100% and specificity is 94%. However, if all ears screened are reevaluated, including the 10 with hearing loss who passed the screening test, test "sensitivity" is 90%. In essence, if all infants who pass the screening test are assumed to have normal hearing, the overlap of response distributions for normal and impaired hearing is underestimated. Notice that whether or not the 10 false negatives are included had little effect on specificity because the number is small relative to the number of babies with normal hearing.

In addition to the influences of analysis approach on estimates of test outcome, it may be important to recognize that newborn hearing screening frequently occurs under less than ideal conditions. For example, if an infant does not display an otoacoustic emission (OAE) or an ABR, the infant could have a peripheral conductive and/or sensorineural hearing loss, a transient or permanent neurologic deficit, test conditions could be less than ideal, or other aspects of the infant's medical status could be preventing accurate assessment of peripheral hearing status.

Finally, it is important to establish an appropriate "gold standard" against which newborn hearing tests can be evaluated. Whether presented in terms of sensitivity and specificity, derived from a single two-by-two decision matrix, or estimated on the basis of the area under an ROC curve, determination of test accuracy is predicted on the assumption that there is a "gold standard," independent of the screening tool, which defines "true" hearing status. For screening tests such as the PSA test used to screen for prostate cancer, the gold standard is a biopsy to determine if cancerous cells are present (e.g., Fishman & deVere White, 1994). The biopsy can be performed soon after the PSA test and there are few (if any) intervening events that could alter prostate status between the PSA test and the biopsy.

The situation is quite different for newborn hearing screening. Typically, infants who fail a screening ABR or an OAE test receive "diagnostic" ABR and OAE testing and a medical evaluation. Neither OAE nor ABR tests, however, evaluate hearing or describe how an individual will use their hearing. They are physiologic responses related to peripheral hearing status, but indirect measures of hearing. The ideal gold standard is one based on the disease for which the screening measure is being performed.and should be independent of the screening measures themselves. In the context of hearing screening, behavioral threshold measurements meet this need directly. Unfortunately, neonates are incapable of performing the voluntary tasks necessary for a behavioral assessment of auditory function, making comparisons between screening and gold standard results more difficult.

The present article provides a description of newborn hearing screening tests' performance when thse tests are evaluated against behavioral audiometric data, obtained when infants were 8 to 12 mo corrected age and, thus, capable of performing behavioral tasks. All infants "at risk" for hearing loss were followed, regardless of the outcomes on neonatal tests. This design was chosen to provide more complete descriptions of sensitivity and specificity for three neonatal tests, namely TEOAEs, DPOAEs, and ABRs.

Methods

Target Sample

The target neonatal sample size was based on detecting a true difference between test performance of 10%. In the planning this project, a 10% difference was chosen somewhat arbitrarily on the assumption that this would represent a clinically significant difference between tools. Neonatal hearing impairment is a low prevalence condition, with moderate-to-profound hearing loss occurring in 1 to 6 per 1000 healthy neonates with no risk factors. However, among infants who have spent time in the neonatal intensive care unit (NICU), estimates range from 2.5% (e.g., Durieux-Smith, Picton, Edwards, MacMurray, & Goodman, 1987; Jacobson & Morehouse, 1984) to as high as 8 to 14% (e.g., Cox, Hack, & Metz, 1982; Galambos & Despland, 1980; van Zanten, Brocaar, Fetter, & Baerts, 1988) with a mean of about 5%. Thus, by concentrating on the NICU population it was possible to evaluate signifiantly fewer infants than would be necessary if only a well baby population was targeted. Although precise estimates for the prevalence of congenital hearing loss are not available, for the purposes of determining sample size, a prevalence rate of 2.5% in NICU high-risk infants was used. More recent data suggest that the prevalence among NICU graduates may be closer to 6.4/1000 (e.g., Prieve, et al., 2000). It was estimated that a minimum of 90 hearing-impaired and 90 normal-hearing subjects would be required to detect a true difference of 0.10 or larger between the areas under two ROC curves ($p=0.05$) with 90% probability or power (Hanley & McNeil, 1982, 1983). Assuming a 2.5% prevalence of hearing impairment among NICU graduates and well babies with one or more risk factors for hearing loss, and 20% loss to follow-up, it was estimated that 4800 infants at risk for hearing loss needed to be enrolled during the neonatal period. Based on these assumptions, it was estimated that a randomly selected sample of 4800 NICU and well babies at risk for hearing loss would yield 120 true hearing-impaired and 4680 true normal-hearing infants. An estimated loss to follow-up rate of 20% by 12 mo of age would result in

TABLE 3. Target and actual study sample. The number of infants targeted for neonatal enrollment and follow-up testing is shown in the left column. The actual number of infants enrolled and seen for behavioral testing is shown in the right column.

	Target	Actual
Neonatal enrollment	4800	4911
Returned for follow-up	3864 (80%)	3134 (64%)
Reliable VRA results	3477 (90%)	2995 (95.6%)
HL ≥30 dB HL confirmed by VRA	96 (infants)	56 (infants)

VRA = visual reinforcement audiometry; HL = hearing level.

approximately 96 hearing-impaired and 3744 normal-hearing infants.

Final Sample

Table 3 summarizes the target and actual study samples. The entire sample of babies is described in detail by Vohr et al. (2000) and the final sample of children returning for visual reinforcement audiometry (VRA) is described by Widen et al. (2000). Briefly, the neonatal sample consisted of 7179 infants, 4911 of whom were considered to be at risk for hearing loss. All of these at-risk infants were targeted for follow-up behavioral hearing testing, which includes NICU graduates, well babies with one or more risk indicators, and well babies without risk indicators who did not pass the neonatal tests.

As discussed by Folsom et al. (2000) and Widen et al. (2000), only 64% of the at-risk infants tested as neonates returned for behavioral testing, but 95.6% of these infants produced reliable VRA data. Folsom et al. (2000) discusses factors thought to influence the less-than-expected follow-up reate. Notably, confirmed "permanent, congenital" hearing loss was found in only 86 ears of 56 infants in spite of efforts to bias the sample in favor of infants in whom it was assumed that hearing loss would be more likely. The small number of infants with confirmed hearing loss must be kept in mind when considering the test performance outcomes summarized in this article. The number of infants with hearing loss, when combined with the small differences among ROC curve areas (for example, see Table 8 below), limited the extent to which statistical analyses of differences in test performance could be performed.

The goal was to obtain all neonatal measures on both ears of all babies. In reality, this was sometimes difficult due to either infant or environmental factors. Complete neonatal data sets were obtained from 14,243 ears, representing 87.3% of the no-risk group and 93.9% of the high-risk group.

Problems associated with the small number of ears with hearing loss were compounded by the fact that complete sets of data were not always available, and

TABLE 4. Good response stopping criteria used during neonatal testing. For each measure, meeting one or more of these criterion was classified as a hearing screening "pass" for that measure. These criteria were chosen to ensure that good quality neonatal data would be obtained.

Measure	Criterion
TEOAE	
Good SNR in four out of five ½-octave bands centered at 1.0, 1.5, 2.0, 3.0, and 4.0 Hz	3 dB at 1.0 and 1.5 kHz; 6 dB at 2.0, 3.0, and 4.0 kHz
DPOAE	
SNR at four out of five F2 frequencies	3 dB re +2 SD above the mean noise for F2 = 1.0, 1.5, 2.0, 3.0, and 4.0 kHz
ABR—30 dB nHL	
Before protocol change	F_{sp} = 2.4
After protocol change	F_{sp} = 3.1

TEOAE = transient evoked otoacoustic emission; DPOAE = distortion product otoacoustic emission; SNR = signal to noise ratio; ABR = auditory brain stem response.

this was a more frequent occurrence among ears not meeting "passing" stopping criteria for individual neonatal tests. This occurrence was a consequence of the protocol. The protocol was designed to assure that each test was aforded full opportunity to result in a "pass". As a result, averaging was allowed to continue for extended periods of time and measures were repeated if stopping criteria were not met (Gorga et al., 2000; Norton, Vohr, Widen, Cone-Wesson, Sininger, Gorga, & Folsom, 2000; Sininger et al., 2000). In a baby with no response on any test (as happened in cases when hearing loss existed), the full protocol could take approximately 2 hr to complete under ideal conditions. If artifact rejection was engaged on any measure and/or if the baby was fussy for any portion of the protocol, test time would increase further. For obvious reasons, it was not always possible to complete the entire protocol in these cases. Unfortunately, this had the effect of reducing the number of infants on whom all neonatal test data were available, with greater effect among infants with hearing loss. Whether due to a lower-than-expected prevalence of hearing loss among at-risk infants or a consequence of incomplete testing, caution should be exercised when interpreting the outcomes to follow. These factors highlight the difficulty in accurately assessing screening test performance, which requires rigourous research paradigms, in a target population made up of subjects with who time-consuming, rigourous paradigms cannot always be applied.

Stopping Criteria

Table 4 provides a summary of the stopping criteria used for each of the three neonatal tests. SNR was used for both OAE tsts (although the definitions for TEOAEs and DPOAEs differed) and the Fsp (a quantity similar to an SNR) was used for the ABR. The rationales for selecting these criteria are provided in previous articles describing each of these tests (Gorga et al., 2000; Norton, Vohr, Widen, Cone-Wesson, Sininger, Gorga, & Folsom, 2000; Sininger et al., 2000). Briefly, these criteria are more stringent than those in current clinical

use, but allowed us to evaluate less stringent criteria after the fact.

Gold Standard

Neonatal screening tests were compared with behavioral audiometric data obtained when infants were 8 mo corrected age or older. Widen et al., (2000) provide a complete description of these data. For the purposes of the analyses summarized in this article, minimum response levels (MRLs) at 1, 2, and 4 kHz (pulsed warble tones) and speech awareness (SAT) served as the gold standard. Gold standard MRLs were defined for each of these foud stimuli singly. In addition, two- (2 and 4 kHz) and three- (1, 2, 4 kHz) frequency PTA thresholds were used. In all cases, MRLs were specified in dB HL (American National Standards Institute, 1996). Normal hearing was defined as an MRL <30 dB HL. MRLs ≥ 30 dB HL were defined as hearing loss. If a response was reliably measured at 20 dB HL, lower levels were not assessed. This is a typical definition for MRL. On the other hand, "threshold" is perhaps the more appropriate term to describe data when responses were not observed at 20 dB HL (see Widen et al., 2000). For the purposes of simplicity, however, the term "MRL" is used throughout this article to describe VRA measurements.

Slight differences in the definition of hearing loss were used in the present article, compared with the summaries provided in either Widen et al. (2000) or Cone-Wesson et al. (2000). The change in definition in the present article was necessitated by a desire to examine test performance for each VRA stimulus individually. Thus, an MRL of 30 dB HL for one stimulus (e.g., 4 kHz) would be viewed as hearing loss at that frequency, even if the MRLs at 1 and 2 kHz were 20 dB HL. This contrasts with the approach used in Widen et al. and Cone-Wesson et al., where two MRLs of 30 dB HL were necessary for a hearing-impaired classification. Furthermore, we were interested in evaluating test performance as a function of the magnitude of hearing loss, not only for individual frequencies, but also for "average" thresholds across frequency. Such an evaluation is more straightforward when criterion thresholds are based on averages. These differences in definitions of hearing loss also cause slight differences in the number of subjects with "hearing loss" across these articles.

Experimental Measures

SNR was used as the experimental criterion for OAE tests, and Fsp was used as the experimental measure for the ABR test. Whenever predictions about auditory status were based on the ABR, the maximum Fsp (channel A or channel B) was used. See previous articles in this series for complete descriptions of the procecures and criteria for ABR (Sininger et al., 2000), TEOAE (Norton, Vohr, Widen, Cone-Wesson, Sininger, Gorga, & Folsom, 2000), and DPOAE (Gorga et al., 2000) data.

Results

Pass Rates Referenced to Stopping Criteria

Without regard to the VRA data, the neonatal data can be analyzed relative to the stopping criteria described in Table 4. This analysis is provided in Table 5 where "pass" rates are listed separately for the well babies without risk factors and babies at risk for hearing loss. If one were to refer only babies not meeting criteria bilaterally, "pass" rates for all tests would be between 94% and 98%, for babies at risk for hearing loss (NICU and well babies) and for babies without risk indicators, respectively. ABRs resulted in slightly higher pass rates than either OAE test. These findings are not surprising, given the hypothesis that OAEs may be more affected by transient middle-ear conditions because of their reliance on reverse enery transmission into the ear canal. Although pass rates were high for most tests, one exception was the high-level DPOAE test for babies at risk for hearing loss, where the pass rate was under 90% for either one or both ears. There is no reason why high-level stimuli should result in lower pass rates, compared with lower-level stimuli. Indeed, one would predict that such stimuli would result in higher pass rates. It is also unlikely that this result is due to sampling error, given the size of this subject group. Thus, there is no obvious explanation for this outcome.

More importantly, pass rates for the present set of criteria were in the range of values recently reported among newborn hearing screening programs (e.g., Barsky-Firsker & Sun, 1997, 1997; Mason & Hermann, 1998; Mehl & Thomson, 1998; Meyer et al., 1999; Spivak et al., 2000; Van Kershaver, 1998; Watkin & Baldwin, 1999). It is important to remember, however, that these data only describe the refer rate they do not provide information relative to test sensitivity. Although specificity also cannot be estimated precisely, errors in

TABLE 5. Percentages of subjects meeting good response (stopping) criteria in both or one ear for each neonatal test.

	No Risk Factors for HL	NICU and Risk Factor for HL
ABR 30 dB	%	%
Passed both ears	86.8	85.7
Passed only one	11.4	10.6
Passed either one or both ears	98.2	96.3
DPOAE 75/75		
Passed both ears	91.2	82.8
Passed only one	7.3	6.8
Passed either one or both ears	98.5	89.6
DPOAE 65/50		
Passed both ears	83.9	81.6
Passed only one	11.9	12.2
Passed either one or both ears	95.8	93.8
TEOAE 80 dB		
Passed both ears	84.9	85.4
Passed only one	11.7	9.9
Passed either one or both ears	96.6	95.3

NICU = neonatal intensive care unit; HL = hearing loss; ABR = auditory brain stem response; DPOAE = distortion product otoacoustic emission; TEOAE = transient evoked otoacoustic emission.

these estimates are much smaller because the vast majority of newborns do not have hearing loss (see discussion of Table 2 above).

Pass Rates Relative to the National Institutes of Health (1993) Consensus Conference Recommended Protocol

Another way to evaluate the data without regard to hearing status is shown in Table 6. Newborn hearing screening test outcomes were evaluated in a manner that would provide results relative to the recommendations in the National Institutes of Health (1993) Consensus Conference Report. That report recommended that all newborns be screened first with an OAE test, followed by an ABR test on those babies not passing the OAE test. an equivalent condition can be obtained for the present study by examining the "pass" rates for the ABR test or an OAE test (either TEOAEs or DPOAEs). Table 6 provides this summary for the entire sample of infants. Pass rates range from 96.6% to 98.7% when the National Institutes of Health protocol is applied to our data.

Test Time

Table 7 shows test time for each of the neonatal tests. Recall that there was one change in the protocol after the first 9 mo of subject enrollment (Gorga et al., 2000; Norton, Vohr, Widen, Cone-Wesson, Sininger, Gorga, & Folsom, 2000; Sininger et al., 2000). The changes in the ABR protocol involved doubling the stimulus presentation rate, thus resulting in a reduction in test time. Changes in the other tests were qualitative (such as probe removal and reinsertion if stopping criteria were not met for at least one frequency after the min-

TABLE 6. Refer rates when the National Institutes of Health Consensus Conference (1993)-recommended hearing screening protocol is followed.

Acceptable Screening Tests Completed	Well Babies w/o RFs			NICU and Well Babies w/RFs		
	N (ears)	N passed	(%)	N (ears)	N passed	(%)
ABR 30 dB or TEOAE 80 dB	4400			8747		
Overall pass rate		4269	97.0		8451	96.6
Overall fail rate		131	3.0		296	3.4
ABR 30 dB or DPOAE 75/75	4372			8868		
Overall pass rate		4314	98.7		8643	97.5
Overall fail rate		58	1.3		225	2.5
ABR 30 dB or DPOAE 65/50	4218			8483		
Overall pass rate		4134	98.0		8264	97.4
Overall fail rate		84	2.0		219	2.6

W/O RFs = without risk factors; W/RFs = with risk factors; NICU = neonatal intensive care unit; ABR = auditory brain stem response; TEOAE = transient evoked otoacoustic emission; DPOAE = distortion product otoacoustic emission.

imum number of sweeps) and thus had little effect on mean or mode estimates of test time. Each OAE test required less time than ABR, particularly when the set-up time (electrode application) is considered, which typically required about 6 minutes. The differences among measures in data acquisition time, particularly after the protocol change, is statistically significant, but perhaps of less clinical interest. For all tests, however, there were outliers in which test time for individual tests ranged from about 6 to 60 minutes. This occurred as a result of poor test conditions (such as an agitated baby) and/or when stopping criteria were not met. Unfortunately, this latter event occurred more frequently among infants with hearing loss. As a result, complete data were not always available on these infants because it was not possible to test these infants for the extended periods of time that would be required to complete all tests.

Comparison of Neonatal and VRA Outcomes

To this point, ABR, DPOAE, and TEOAE neonatal test results were reviewed without reference to the VR data. However, true sensititivy and specificity can be estimated only when the neonatal hearing screening tests are compared with this gold standard.

Only ears with reliable VRA data were included in the description of test performance to follow. As detailed in Widen et al. (2000), 43 babies died after the neonatal period and 1734 infants were lost to follow-up. Sixty-four percent (3134/4911) of the targeted at-risk sample returned for VRA. Reliable VRA data were obtained on 95.6% (2995/3134) of these returning infants. Only 4.4% of the returning infants could not be tested reliably with VRA. This latter group included infants who had neurodevelopmental deficits that precluded reliable

TABLE 7. Neonatal test times in seconds for each of the four individual neonatal screening tests.

	Well Babies w/o RFs Seconds		NICU and Well Babies w/RFs Seconds	
	Before protocol change	After protocol change	Before protocol change	After protocol change
ABR 30 dB acquisition				
Mean	299.15	149.96	297.23	141.41
SD	215.52	131.39	218.47	124.51
Mode	138.00	59.00	124.00	58.00
DPOAE 75/75				
Mean	83.83	85.84	94.91	97.23
SD	66.87	66.69	67.47	71.77
Mode	34.40	34.40	34.40	34.40
DPOAE 65/50				
Mean	109.68	111.24	118.03	121.19
SD	77.09	79.24	76.19	81.02
Mode	34.40	34.30	34.40	34.30
TEOAE 80 dB				
Mean	114.61	115.44	125.02	129.09
SD	126.66	122.49	118.13	134.62
Mode	29.00	42.00	27.00	40.00

For ABR, the testers were required to hit a carriage return for each step. If the tester entered two carriage returns, the time for the "skipped" step was recorded as zero. This resulted in unequal numbers for the three ABR steps.
W/O RFs = without risk factors; W/RFs = with risk factors; NICU = neonatal intensive care unit; ABR = auditory brain stem response; DPOAE = distortion product otoacoustic emission; TEOAE = transient evoked otoacoustic emission.

VRA testing, and those who could not be conditioned reliably. A small percentage of infants would not tolerate insert earphones, providing only sound field VRA data. These two groups of infants were excluded from the analysis of test performance because individual ear, gold standard data were not available.

The neonatal screening and VRA data were analyzed for three different subsets of subjects with elevated MRLs. In the first, most inclusive category, all ears with an individual frequency or PTA greater than or equal to 30 dB HL were included in the analysis. In the second analysis, ears with hearing loss (based on the VRA) were excluded if data were available suggesting that transient conductive hearing loss might be present (i.e., typanometry, medical history and/or otologic examination) at the time of the VRA testing. This choice was based on the view that the screening tests could not be expected to detect transient conductive hearing loss whose onset likely occurred after the neonatal period. Ears having evidence of middle-ear dysfunction but producing normal MRLs at the VRA evaluation were not excluded. Ears in which late-onset or progressive sensorineural hearing loss existed were included in the second analysis. It was hypothesized that these hearing losses existed in nine ears of seven children because they had robust responses on all neonatal tests, but then revealed hearing loss at the VRA assessment. Although admittely circular, we reasoned that the chances of "passing" stopping criteria on four separate tests (two DPOAEs, TEOAEs, ABR) in the presence of hearing loss was highly unlikely. In the third analysis, both ears with transient middle-ear pathology and elevated MRLs at the time of VRA testing and those with putative late-onset or progressive sensorineural hearing loss were excluded. Excluding these two groups of infants was based on the assumption that the losses did not exist at the time of the screening tests. Presumably, this left only ears with permanent neonatal sensorineural or conductive hearing loss. A summary of results for all three groups is provided in Table 8 in the form of ROC curve areas. ROC curve areas can be interpreted such that the higher these values, the better the test performed.

 ABR performance was similar for all gold standard definitions, whereas OAE tests tended to provide poorer performance when MRLs at 1 kHz were used either singly or in combination with other frequencies. This result occurs because of the high levels of acoustical noise (and, therefore, less reliable measurements) associated with OAEs at this frequency (see Norton, Vohr, Widen, Cone-Wesson, Sininger, Gorga, & Folsom, 2000 and Gorga et al., 2000 for a more complete description of noise levels as a function of frequency).

Test performance, as defined by the ROC curve areas, was lowest for the most inclusive subject group, although ABRs performed better than other measures. Higher areas were observed when ears with middle-ear dysfunction and elevated MRLs at the time of the VRA were removed from the analyses. The best performance was achieved when both ears with middle-ear dysfunction and presumptive late-onset or progressive hearing loss were excluded. These findings make sense because the screening measures cannot be expected to detect hearing loss before a time when the hearing loss exists. Eliminating these cases, in the context of clinical decision theory, reduces the false negative rates and, thus, increases the area under the ROC curve. In the analyses to follow, the sample of ears with hearing loss includes only those ears on which reliable VRA data were obtained, excluding ears with middle-ear dysfunction (in combination with elevated MRLs) and/or late-onset and progressive hearing losses.

ROC Curves

ROC curves for each neonatal test are shown in Figure 1. These are the ROC curves from which the areas for the least inclusive group, provided in Table 8, were derived. True positive and false positive rates were estimated for all possible values of the criterion measure (SNR for OAEs and the Fsp for ABRs) within the range observed during data collection. Each panel represents the results for a single stimulus used during behavioral assessments (1, 2, 4 kHz, or SAT). The gold standard definition for normal hearing was an MRL <30 dB HL. With a minimum step size of 10 dB during VRA testing (Widen et al., 2000), an ear with an MRL of 20 dB HL was defined as normal and an ear with an MRL ≥30 dB HL was defined as impaired. Within each panel, the parameter is the neonatal measure. For all three OAE measurements (TEOAEs at 80 dB pSPL and DPOAEs at 65/50 and 75/75 dB SPL), comparisons between MRL and OAE were made at the same frequency. For the SAT, the "best" SNR of the three frequencies (1, 2, and 4 kHz) was used on the assumption that the SAT should correlate with the frequency at which hearing was best. For the ABR, Fsp at 30 dB nHL was used for all four VRA stimuli. The diagonal dashed line in each panel represents chance performance (i.e., equal likelihood of a true positive or a false positive). An excellent screening test would be characterized by a ROC curve displaced into the upper left corner of each panel. Under these circumstances, the true positive (hit) rate would be high and the false positive (false alarm) rate would remain low.

TABLE 8. Area under the relative operating characteristic (ROC) curves for individual frequencies, the speech awareness threshold (SAT), and the two- and three-frequency pure-tone average (PTA). The hearing loss criteria is 30 dB HL or greater.

	MRL 1.0 kHz	MRL 2.0 kHz	MRL 4.0 kHz	SAT	PTA (2 and 4 kHz)	PTA (1, 2, and 4 kHz)
1. All MRLs ≥30 dB HL						
DPOAE 75/75 dB SPL	0.62	0.67	0.63	0.68	0.65	0.67
DPOAE 65/50 dB SPL	0.60	0.69	0.66	0.71	0.66	0.65
TEOAE 80 dB pSPL	0.56	0.63	0.60	0.67	0.65	0.66
ABR 30 nHL	0.68	0.69	0.69	0.75	0.70	0.69
2. ME pathology excluded						
DPOAE 75/75 dB SPL	0.72	0.82	0.77	0.85	0.79	0.79
DPOAE 65/50 dB SPL	0.67	0.84	0.80	0.88	0.79	0.79
TEOAE 80 dB pSPL	0.67	0.80	0.76	0.90	0.84	0.85
ABR 30 nHL	0.85	0.85	0.83	0.90	0.84	0.85
3. Progressive loss and ME pathology excluded						
DPOAE 75/75 dB SPL	0.75	0.89	0.81	0.87	0.86	0.84
DPOAE 65/50 dB SPL	0.70	0.92	0.89	0.92	0.88	0.83
TEOAE 80 dB pSPL	0.74	0.92	0.88	0.94	0.90	0.84
ABR 30 nHL	0.90	0.89	0.87	0.91	0.88	0.87

Data are shown for three different hearing loss groups: 1) all ears with MRL, SAT, or PTA ≥30 dB HL; 2) ears with MRLs ≥30 dB HL excluding only ears with transient middle-ear pathology; and 3) ears with MRLs ≥30 dB HL excluding those with transient middle ear pathology at the time of VRA and those with assumed progressive hearing loss.
MRL = minimum response level; VRA = visual reinforcement audiometry; DPOAE = distortion product otoacoustic emission; TEOAE = transient evoked otoacoustic emission; ABR = auditory brain stem response.

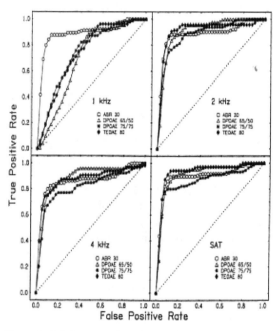

Figure 1. Relative operating characteristic (ROC) curves in which true positive rate is plotted as a function of the false positive rate, both of which are represented as proportions. Each panel represents results when a different visual reinforcement audiometry stimulus served as the gold standard. Within each panel, the parameter is screening measure. The dashed line represents the ROC curve that would be observed for chance performance. For the purposes of these analyses, normal hearing was defined as a minimum response level (MRL) <30 dB HL. Ears with MRLs ≥30 dB HL were classified as hearing impaired. ABR = auditory brain stem response; DPOAE = distortion product otoacoustic emission; TEOAE = transient evoked otoacoustic emission.

The results summarized in Figure 1 indicate that ABR test performance was similar when MRLs at 1, 2, and 4 kHz and the SAT served as the gold standard. The SAT generally correlates with the threshold(s) for the frequency(ies) at which hearing sensitivity is best. These results may suggest, therefore, that it was equally likely that the best sensitivity occurred at any of the three test frequencies. The ABR results in superior performance at identifying auditory status at 1 kHz, compared with either OAE test. In contrast to the ABR, performance for the OAE tests was frequency dependent. TEOAEs and DPOAEs at both stimulus levels performed poorest when attempting to describe auditory status at 1 kHz. Performance improved at both 2 and 4 kHz, and achieved similar performance in predicting auditory status defined by the SAT. The poorer performance at 1 kHz is expected, given the higher levels of acoustic noise at these frequencies. These results are similar, at least in form, to what has been observed in older children and adults when either TEOAEs or DPOAEs were used to predict auditory status (e.g., Gorga, Neely, Bergman, Beauchaine, Kaminski, Peters, & Jesteadt, 1993; Gorga, Neely, Bergman, Beauchaine, Kaminski, Peters, Schulte, & Jesteadt, 1993; Gorga et al., 1997; Harrison & Norton, 1999; Hussain et al., 1998; Kim et al., 1996; Prieve et al., 1993; Stover, Gorga, Neely, & Montoya, 1996). Although infants produce larger responses, the influence of frequency on test performance is similar to what has been observed in older subjects. Except for 1 kHz, high-level DPOAEs provided poorer performance (lower hit rates for similar false alarm rates), compared with either the moderate level DPOAE test or with TEOAEs. This result is consistent with previos findings from older patients that showed that high-level DPOAE stimuli were less sensitive to hearing loss (Stover et al., 1996; Whitehead, McCoy, Lonsbury-Martin, & Martin, 1995).

With the exceptions of the better ABR performance predicting auditory status at 1 kHz and the overall poorer performance for the DPOAE 75/75 dB SPL condition, ABR, TEOAE and DPOAE 65/50 dB SPL conditions result in similar test performance. Thus, for the frequencies at which concerns for early identification of hearing loss may be greatest, all three screening measures performed similarly. However, no test resulted in perfect performance. This means that there was no test condition for which the true positive (hit) rate was 100% while the false positive (false alarm) rate was zero. In fact, only for criteria associated with unacceptably high false alarm rates do the hit rates achieve 100%.

The fact that there were no conditions in which the false positive rates were zero indicates that some ears with normal hearing (defined as an MRL <30 dB HL) did not produce measurable OAE and/or ABR responses at the time of testing as neonates. These observations are consistent with the observations made in older children and adults for whom middle-ear status was normal, for whom the pure-tone audiogram was known, and for whom the experimental and gold standard procedures were performed in close temporal proximity. It is important to point out that before these data, little information was available that described test performance for neonatal screening tests. Thus, few data exist to which the present data can be compared.

Figure 2 shows the area under each ROC curve as a function of the criterion MRL used to separate normal and impaired hearing. With the exception of the SAT, there appears to be little influence of criterion MRL on area under the ROC curve, and, by extension, little influence on test performance. The effect of MRL on ROC curve area, even for the SAT, was small. In total, this means that, in a dichotomous decision, test performance for the four measures (TEOAEs, DPOAEs at two levels, ABRs) did not depend on the criterion for normal hearing. The interactions between test measure and frequency, evident in Figure 1, are also evident here. Specifically, ABRs provide superior performance in determining auditory status at 1 kHz, regardless of the criterion MRL. For other VRA stimuli, differences in test performance (as measured by area under the ROC curve) were observed but were small. ABRs, TEOAEs, and DPOAEs at 65/50 dB SPL resulted in larger areas under the ROC curve compared with high-level DPOAEs, which provided poorer performance for any gold standard at most MRLs. The most parsimounious hypothesis to explain this finding is that some ears with hearing loss produce DPOAEs at high levels, but not at lower levels. Thus, the high-level stimuli would increase the false negative rate (decrease the hit rate) because some hearing-impaired ears would

produce a response in excess of test criteria. This result is consistent with previous findings suggesting that, at least among older subjects, high level conditions do not result in optimal separation between response properties from normal or impaired ears (Stover et al., 1996; Whitehead et al., 1995).

There are two possible explanations for the greater frequency dependence of test performance for OAEs compared with the ABR. As stated previously, acoustical noise was higher at 1 kHz for all OAE tests (see Norton, Vohr, Widen, Cone-Wesson, Sininger, Gorga, & Folsom, 2000 and Gorga et al., 2000). Higher noise levels resulted in lower SNRs. Second, there may have been some middle-ear attenuative effects early in life that might affect reverse OAE energy transmission more in the lower frequencies (i.e., 1 kHz) than at higher frequencies. This hypothesis is based on what is known about the tendency for middle-ear dysfunction to affect behavioral thresholds at lower frequencies more than at higher frequencies.

ABRs, TEOAEs, and DPOAEs for the lower-level stimulus condition performed more similarly in determining auditory status when the SAT was used as the gold standard. Differences were observed for other stimuli, but the differences were small and inconsistent. Again, the exception to this was for 1 kHz, where the ABR provided superior performance.

Figure 3 shows ROC curves for each neonatal test using two PTA definitions of hearing status. In the left column, hearing impairment is defined as a two-frequency (2 and 4 kHz) PTA ≥30 dB HL. In the right column, data are shown using the three-frequency (1, 2, and 4 kHz) PTA. In the top row, results are summarized for ABR, the second row shows results for DPOAEs at 65/50 dB SPL, the third row shows results for DPOAEs at 75/75 dB SPL, and the bottom row shows results for TEOAEs. For the ABR, the Fsp was used to predict auditory status.

When auditory status was defined as the PTA at 1, 2, and 4 kHz, OAEs were evaluated at 1, 1.5, 2, 3, and 4 kHz. SNRs were incremented across all five frequency bands, using as the criteria the worst SNR. For example, if the SNR criterion was 2 dB, a pass would occur only if the SNR was 2 dB or greater at all five f2 frequencies (DPOAEs) or in all five frequency bands (TEOAEs). The SNR was incremented over its entire range to generate the ROC curves. When OAEs were used to predict auditory status defined by the PTA of 2 and 4 kHz, the SNR was considered only at 2, 3, and 4 kHz. In either case, SNR was incremented over its entire range, and SNR criteria had to be met at all frequencies to pass the test. The results shown here are similar to those described in Figure 1. Specifically, 1) all four measures perform well above chance (dotted

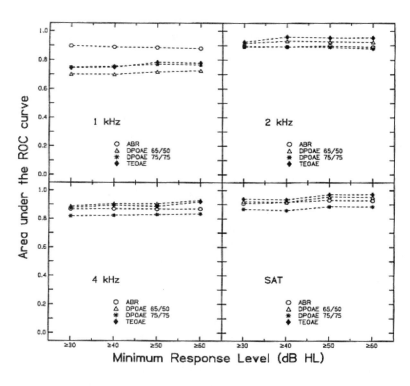

Figure 2. Area under the relative operating characteristic (ROC) curve as a function of minimum response level that was used to define normal hearing. Each panel represents results when a different visual reinforcement audiometry stimulus served as the gold standard. Within each panel, the parameter is neonatal hearing screening measure. Chance performance in this coordinate system would be represented as an area of 0.5. ABR = auditory brain stem response; DPOAE = distortion product otoacoustic emission; TEOAE = transient evoked otoacoustic emission.

diagonal line); 2) the ROC curve for high-level DPOAEs were closer to the diagonal line compared with the other three screening tests; 3) the placement of the ROC curve for the ABR test was similar for both PTAs; and 4) the ROC curves for OAE tests were displaced further toward the upper left corner of the plot when the analyses were restricted to frequencies at and above 2 kHz.

In Figure 4, the area under the ROC curve is shown for the two PTAs as a function of the MRL criteria used for hearing loss. Within each panel, the parameter is test type, of which there are four; TEOAE at 80 dB pSPL, DPOAE at 65/50 and 75/75 dB SPL, and ABR at 30 dB nHL. Performance is essentially equivalent regardless of the MRL criterion used to separate normal and impaired ears. The results seen here are similar to those described for the single-frequency comparisons (Fig. 2) in other ways as well. The high-level DPOAE condition consistently resulted in the poorest performance, although the differences between the ROC curve areas achieved for it and for other measures were small. Areas for the ABR test were about the same for both PTA gold standards, whereas the OAE tests resulted in better performance for the 2 and 4 kHz PTA, compared with the case when the gold standard and experimental measures included data at 1 kHz. These frequency effects also are consistent with previously described results. Whether singly (Fig. 2), or when combined with other frequencies (Fig. 4), OAE test performance generally was poorest whenever 1 kHz was included.

Having reviewed test performance,, based onROC curve analyses, it may be important to describe a possible limitation of this approach, imposed by using response-based stopping criteria during neonatal data collection. Recall that tests stoped when a predetermined Fsp (ABR) or SNR (TEOAEs and DPOAEs) was achieved. Thus, for subjects with normal hearing, the test would stop when these criteria were reached. In the construction of ROC curves, each symbol represents the true positive and the false positive rates for a single criterion value within the range produced by the test. Because the test stopped when the stopping criteria were reached, the false alarm rate would be expected to increase rapidly for criterion values exceeding the stopping criteria. This would have the effect of reducing the "height" of the ROC curve and, therefore, its area. Thus, there is the possibility that the present estimates, based on ROC curve analyses, underestimates test performance.

Having identified this potential limitation in ROC curve analyses, the influence of this problem is likely minimal for the present study. For example, an examination of the distributions of SNR for DPOAEs and TEOAEs (see Figs. 4 and 5 of both Gorga et al., 2000, and Norton, Vohr, Widen, Cone-Wesson, Sininger, Gorga, & Folsom, 2000) reveals that, with the exception of the lowest frequencies, distributions were normal and/or skewed toward values greater than the stopping criteria. Although not shown in the ABR article (Sininger et al., 2000), a similar pattern was observed in

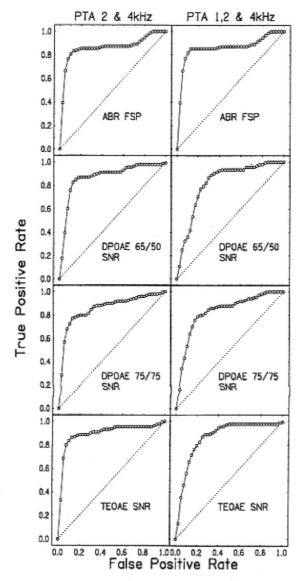

Figure 3. Relative operating characteristic (ROC) curves for each neonatal test using the pure-tone average (PTA) to define hearing status. Again, a PTA ≥30 dB HL defines an ear as hearing impaired. Data in the left column use a two-frequency PTA (2 and 4 kHz), and data in the right column use the three-frequency PTA (1, 2, and 4 kHz). Different neonatal tests are shown in separate panels within each column. Chance performance is represented by the positive diagonal line within each panel. ABR = auditory brain stem response; DPOAE = distortion product otoacoustic emission; TEOAE = transient evoked otoacoustic emission.

Response Distributions

Figure 5 presents a summary of the distribution of neonatal responses for normal-hearing and hearing-impaired ears in the form of "box and whisker" plots. Again, the definition of impaired hearing is a PTA ≥30 dB HL. Separate panels show ABR, DPOAE (one for each level), and TEOAE results. Within each paenl, data are plotted for the two PTA gold standards (PTA at 2 and 4 kHz, and PTA at 1, 2, and 4 kHz). Open boxes represent distributions for subjects with normal hearing, and the shaded boxes represent the distributions for ears with hearing loss. The middle line in the box represents the median value (50th percentile) for each group. The upper box limit represents the 75th percentile, and the lower box limit represents the 25th percentile from the respective distributions. Thus, each box represents the interquartile range. The whiskers are drawn at a value equal to 1.5 times the box length. Outliers are defined as values either above or below the whiskers, and are shown as individual data points.

From these box and whisker plots, it can be seen that there is separation between response properties for normal and impaired ears for all neonatal test measures. The differences between distributions, however, are less for DPOAEs measured in response to high-level stimuli, compared with DPOAEs at lower levels, TEOAEs, and ABRs. For all tests, overlap in the response distributions occurs among the "whiskers." These plots reiterate the points made in previous figures, namely that no criterion value can be selected for any test measurement that results in complete separation between responses from normal and impaired ears.

Figures 6 through 9 provide alternative representations of the data shown in Figure 5, showing ABR, TEOAE, DPOAE 65/50 and 75/75 dB SPL data as cumulative distributions. Cumulative distributions plot the cumulative percent as a function of the measured variable, in the present cases, SNR for OAE tests and Fsp for the ABR. In each figure, the left panel shows results when the PTA at 2 and 4 kHz wa used as the gold standard, and the right panel shows results when the PTA at 1, 2, and 4 kHz was used as the gold standard. Within each panel, two cumulative distributions are shown, one for hearing-impaired ears (dashed lines) and one for normal-hearing ears (solid lines). The definition for normal hearing was a PTA <30 dB HL; responses from ears exceeding this value were included in the impaired distributions.

In every case, there is separation between the cumulative distributions of response properties for normal-hearing and hearing-impaired ears. Unfortunately, the tails of these distributions are not completely sepa-

the distribution of Fsp. For both OAE and ABR tests, this means that the stopping criteria were frequently exceeded during data collection, and thus, the stopping criteria should not have had a large "negative" influence on ROC curve estimates of test performance.

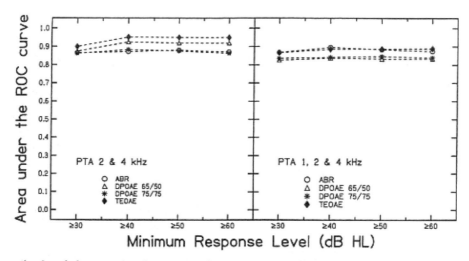

Figure 4. Area under the relative operating characteristic (ROC) curve as a function of the minimum response level used to define normal hearing. Results for the two- and three-frequency pure-tone averages (PTAs) are shown in the left and right panels, respectively, following the same convention that was used in Figure 2. ABR = auditory brain stem response; DPOAE = distortion product otoacoustic emission; TEOAE = transient evoked otoacoustic emission.

rated for any measure. No criterion SNR or Fsp could be selected that was exceeded by all normal ears (i.e., 100% specificity or 0% false alarm rate) that would not also be passed by a percentage of ears with hearing loss (false negatives). However, from these distributions, it is possible to pick combinations of hit and false alarm rates within the entire range of values produced by each individual test. For example, if one wished to achieve a hit rate of 80%, one would draw a horizontal line at the 80th percentile that intercepted the distribution of responses from impaired ears, and then drop a vertical line from this point to the X axis. This point of intersec-

tion would describe the criterion value (SNR or OAE tests, Fsp for the ABR test) that would result in a hit rate of 80%. The point at which the vertical line intersected the distribution of responses from normal ears would be the expected false alarm rate associated with that criterion value.

This approach may be followed in reverse order by selecting a target false alarm rate first. In that case, the horizontal line would be drawn at the percentage that represents the desired false alarm rate until it intersects the distribution of responses from normal-hearing ears. The vertical line drawn from that point to the X-axis

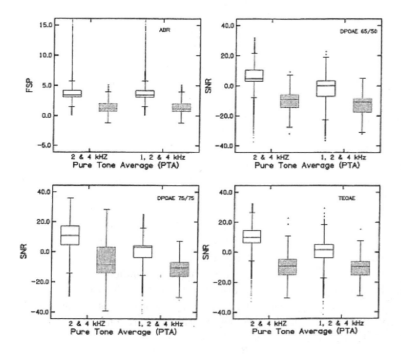

Figure 5. Box and whisker plots showing the distribution of responses (Fsp for the auditory brain stem response test; signal to noise ratio [SNR] for otoacoustic emission tests) for normal-hearing (open boxes) and hearing-impaired (shaded boxes) ears. Within each panel, data are shown for both the two- and the three-frequency pure-tone average (PTA). Hearing impairment is defined as PTA ≥30 dB HL. Different neonatal tests are shown in the different panels. The line within each panel represents the median (50th percentile) from each distribution. Upper and lower box limits represent the 75th and 25th percentiles, respectively. Upper and lower whiskers are drawn 1.5 box lengths above and below the box limits, respectively. Outliers, defined as values exceeding the whiskers in either direction, are shown as individual data points.

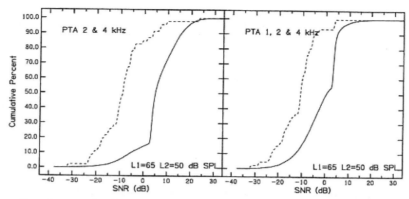

Figure 8. Same as Figure 6, except that data are shown for distortion product otoacoustic emissions at L1 = 65 dB SPL and L2 = 50 dB SPL. PTA = pure-tone average; SNR = signal to noise ratio.

provides the criterion value for that false alarm rate. The intersection of the vertical line with the distribution of responses from hearing-impaired ears provides an estimate of the expected hit rate for that same criterion value. Whether one followed an approach in which hit rate was fixed or false alarm rate was fixed, it is important to recall the same number of ears (86) on which sensitivity estimates are based.

Although the patterns across these four figures are similar, there are some details worth noting. In Figure 7, TEOAE SNR is defined as the dBdifference between mean response and mean noise level. In Figures 8 and 9, where DPOAE measurements are represented, SNR values represent the mean DPOAE level minus the mean noise level +2 SDs above the mean (see Gorga et al., 2000 for a more complete description of this definition of SNR).

Figure 6 shows cumulative distributions of the Fsp for the ABR. The Fsp was constrained to a smaller range of values, although the results from normal and impaired ears were well separated by this test. In many ways, Fsp can be viewed as an SNR. To make visualization easier and to convert these data to a ration not unlike dB, the Fsp is presented on a log scale. This conversion, of course, has no influence on test performance, and only serves to make the figure more readable.

Failure Rates in Relation to the Magnitude of Hearing Loss

To this point, we have described test performance dichotomously. That is, an ear either had normal hearing or had hearing loss. Even when the effects of MRL

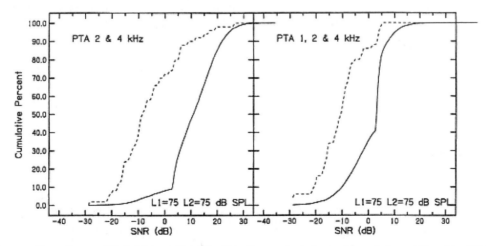

Figure 9. Same as Figure 6, except that data are shown for distortion product otoacoustic emissions at L1 = L2 = 75 dB SPL. PTA = pure-tone average; SNR = signal to noise ratio.

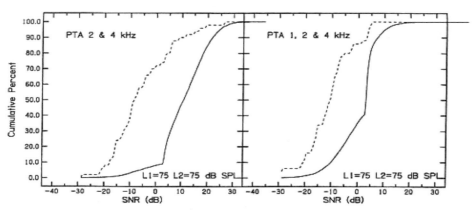

Figure 9. Same as Figure 6, except that data are shown for distortion product otoacoustic emissions at L1 = L2 = 75 dB SPL. PTA = pure-tone average; SNR = signal to noise ratio.

were evaluated (Figs. 2 and 4), a dichotomous decision was made. For example, an MRL <30 dB HL, in terms of clinical decision theory, means that every ear with MRLs <30 dB HL is classified as normal and every ear with MRLs ≥30 dB HL is classified as hearing-impaired. Ears with any degree of hearing loss, ranging from mild to profound, are all placed in one category for the purposes of evaluating test performance. An alternative to this approach, which has been applied todata from older subjects (Gorga et al., 1999), is to evaluate failure rates in relation to the magnitude of hearing loss. Although previous analyses have demonstrated that errors in diagnosis are inevitable, it is possible that test sensitivity increases with hearing loss, meaning that false negative errors occurred less frequently for more significant hearing losses.

Figure 10 shows failure rate as a function of hearing loss category for each neonatal test. The left column represents the case when thresholds were averaged at 2 and 4 kHz, and the three-frequency average (1, 2, and 4 kHz) was used to define thresholds for the right column. As in previous figures, normal hearing is defined

as a PTA <30 dB HL. The following definitions were used for the remaining four categories: mild hearing loss, 30 to 40 dB HL; moderate hearing loss, 41 to 60 dB HL; severe hearing loss, 61 to 89 dB HL; profound hearing loss, ≥90 dB HL. For the purposes of this figure, a false alarm rate of 20% was arbitrarily selected. That is, the criterion value that produced a 20% failure rate among ears with normal hearing was selected for each measure (SNR for TEOAEs and DPOAEs; Fsp for the ABR). That criterion value was then applied to ears with hearing loss. For OAE tests, the same approach that was taken for previous analyses, in which SNRs were used at multiple frequencies, was applied here (see, for example, Fig. 3 and its discussion).

As expected, failure rate increases as the magnitude of hearing loss increases, although some irregularities exist in some panels (severe hearing loss for DPOAEs at 65/50 dB SPL for the three-frequency PTA). Best performance for all measures was obtained using a PTA for 2 and 4 kHz. The failure rates for OAE measures in the moderate and severe hearing loss categories were 100%, but dropped for profound losses. In general,

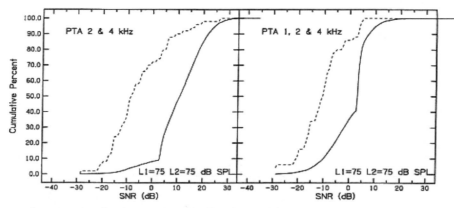

Figure 9. Same as Figure 6, except that data are shown for distortion product otoacoustic emissions at L1 = L2 = 75 dB SPL. PTA = pure-tone average; SNR = signal to noise ratio.

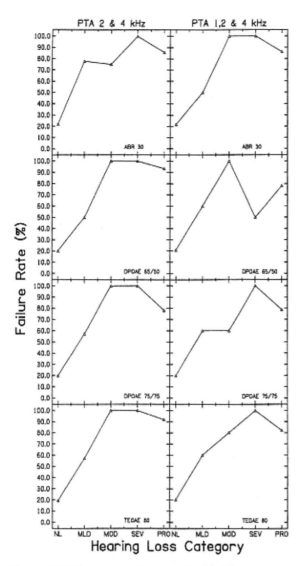

Figure 10. Failure rate as a function of hearing loss category: NL = minimum response levels (MRLs) <30 dB HL; MLD = MRLs of 30–40 dB HL; MOD = MRLs of 41–60 dB HL; SEV = MRLs of 61–89 dB HL; PRO = MRLs ≥90 dB HL. Data in the left column use a two-frequency pure-tone average (PTA) (2 and 4 kHz), and data in the right column use the three-frequency PTA (1, 2, and 4 kHz). Different neonatal tests are shown in separate panels within each column. ABR = auditory brain stem response; DPOAE = distortion product otoacoustic emission; TEOAE = transient evoked otoacoustic emission.

should be viewed cautiously because there were so few ears with hearing loss, especially when divided among four categories of hearing loss (Cone-Wesson et al., 2000). Although special effort was made to target infants for whom the prevalence of hearing loss was presumably greater (see Norton, Gorga, Widen, Folsom, Sininger, Cone-Wesson, Vohr, & Fletcher, 2000; Vohr et al., 2000), there still were few impaired ears in the sample.

An additional factor may have influenced estimates of test performance, especially the results summarized in Figure 10. It was decided to exclude from the analyses any ear with evidence of middle-ear dysfunction AND elevated MRLs at the time of VRA. Ears with evidence of middle-ear dysfunction that had normal MRLs were NOT excluded. Thus, our "normal" sample included ears with middle-ear dysfunction and potentially a conductive overlay to their MRLs that was insufficient to elevate their MRLs above 20 dB HL. It may have been the case that forward and (for OAE measurements) reverse middle-ear energy transmission was less efficient in these ears at the time of the neonatal tests. If this hypothesis is true, one would expect smaller neonatal responses in these "normal" ears. This would shift the distributions of response properties in "normal" ears closer to those achieved in ears with hearing loss. Selecting a criterion value that produces a specific false alarm rate would be expected to be less stringent if these ears are included in the "normal" sample, compared with the case if they were excluded. Our inclusion of them, therefore, would be expected to make the criteria less sensitive to hearing loss, thus resulting in an increase in the false negative rate.

Discussion

This study represents the culmination of efforts to provide estimates of test performance for three neonatal hearing screening tests, namely TEOAEs, DPOAEs, and ABRs. Details of each of these measures, including comprehensive descriptions of their properties in neonates and how these properties are affected by other factors, can be found in previous articles in this volume (Gorga et al., 2000; Norton, Vohr, Widen, Cone-Wesson, Sininger, Gorga, & Folsom, 2000; Sininger et al., 2000). In response to the request for applications issued by the National Institute on Deafness and Other Communication Disorders, a study was designed in which neonatal tests were compared with behavioral audiologic assessments. By necessity, the neonatal (experimental) measures were separated by 8 to 12 mo or more. Efforts were taken to assure that families would remain enrolled in the study and would return for

these trends are similar to recently reported results for older children and adults, in which DPOAE failure rates of nearly 100% were observed once hearing loss exceeded 40 dB HL (Gorga et al., 1999). Having demonstrated higher failure rates as the magnitude of the hearing loss increases, however, the present data follow-up behavioral testing, regardless of the outcomes on neonatal screening tests (Folsom et al., 2000). In spite of special efforts, only 2/3 of the targeted infants returned for follow-up testing. Still, 3134 infants returned for follow-up, and reliable VRA data were obtained on 95.6% (2995) of these children (Widen et al., 2000).

In addition, information was gathered that helped to identify any events that have occurred between the experimental and gold standard measurements that might have exerted an influence on the extent to which these measures agreed. As expected, the single most frequent intercurrent event was otitis media. Middle-ear dysfunction, more likely among children 6 to 12 mo of age and older than among neonates, could result in elevated thresholds at the time of the gold standard test, but not during the screening measures. Consequently, a decision was made to perform initial analyses on three different groups of subjects. Test performance was best when ears with middle-ear dysfunction and elevated MRLs at the time of VRA, and/or babies with presumptive late-onset or progressive hearing loss were not included in the analyses (see Table 8). This approach seems reasonable because the hearing screening measures should not be expected to detect hearing loss that presumably did not exist at the time the screening tests were performed.

Relatively low refer rates would have been achieved based on the present stopping criteria for each individual measurement (Table 5) or if the National Institutes of Health (1993) Consensus Conference protocol had been followed (Table 6). It is likely that the refer rates achieved under either of these conditions would be considered acceptable in most universal newborn hearing screening programs. Indeed, recent studies using an automated ABR system are reporting refer rates as low as 0.8% (Van Kershaver, 1998) when screening is done between 23 and 30 days in the home and 5.3% when done in hospital at time of discharge (Meyer et al., 1999). Studies using a two-stage screen (an OAE test, followed by an ABR screen for those infants not passing the OAE screen) report refer rates of 3% (e.g., Mehl & Thomson, 1998; Watkin & Baldwin, 1999).

Before the discussion of test performance, it is important to reiterate that, in spite of efforts to recruit infants at risk for hearing loss, the sample with hearing loss was small. The present estimates of specificity are probably reliable, as they are based on large samples of subjects who subsequently were demonstrated to have normal hearing. In contrast, estimates of sensitivity must be viewed more cautiously because so few infants had hearing loss. In addition, it was not possible to

obtain all neonatal data on every infant because of time constraints. This problem occurred more frequently among ears that did not meet protocol stopping criteria, and, thus, likely included a disproportionate number of ears with hearing loss. Our interpretations, therefore, should be viewed cautiously because of the limitations imposed by the small number of ears with hearing loss confirmed by VRA.

A final cautionary note related to the gold standard may be appropriate. To assess experimental test performance, a gold standard was needed. We chose a behavioral assessment of hearing, which is a common approach when "objective" measures are being evaluated. Given the ages of subjects, VRA was selected and a protocol was developed that increased the reliability of these measurements. Like all other audiologic measurements, however, VRA is not error free. Although we expect this to be a rare occurrence (given the VRA protocol), there may have been cases in which the gold standard was in error.

The most important observation from the present study is that several neonatal hearing tests can be used to identify infants with hearing loss. However, none of these tests performs without error. That is, no criterion value could be selected for which the hit rate was 100% while the false alarm rate remained at 0%. This result is similar to a recent report in which ABR screening test sensitivity was estimated at 82% for bilateral, PTA thresholds (0.5, 1, 2, 4 kHz) of 50 dB HL or greater (Mason, Davis, Wood, & Farnsworth, 1998). The present findings also are consistent with other previous evaluations of the performance of these tests, which typically were based on data from older subjects, for whom the experimental and gold standard tests were performed in close temporal proximity, and who were "demonstrably" free from middle-ear dysfunction at the time of test.

The present results should not be viewed as a negative commentary on universal newborn hearing screening. In spite of the small number of ears with hearing loss, the neonatal hearing tests performed well at identifying ears with significant hearing loss. Test performance was poor when hearing loss was between 30 and 40 dB HL, which is unfortunate because hearing losses, even of this magnitude, can affect speech and language development (Yoshinaga-Itano et al., 1998). Criteria can be selected that would detect mild losses more frequently, but the cost would be an increase in the false alarm rate to levels that may not be acceptable. It should be noted, however, that more than half of the ears with mild hearing loss failed the criteria used in Figure 10. Furthermore, intervention may be less critical for these ears and the form of intervention less obvious, compared with ears with greater loss. No screening test, whether for hearing loss or some other disorder, can be expected to detect a disorder that does not exist at the time of the measurement. Thus, it should be no surprise that several ears with progressive or late-onset hearing loss (perhaps due to cytomegalovirus or genetic factors) were "missed" by the neonatal tests.

These data, however, demonstrate that assumptions about screening tests must be evaluated more critically than has previously been the case. A common approach clinically is to assume that passing newborn hearing screening criteria indicates that hearing is normal. The present data suggest that such an assumption should be qualifed. The baby producing positive SNRs on OAE tests or positive Fsps (or ABRs however quantified) on the ABR test do not necessarily have normal hearing. That is, there are ears with hearing loss that will produce OAEs and/or ABRs. This observation is consistent with previous demonstrations in older subjects (e.g., Dorn, Piskorski, Gorga, Neely, & Keefe, 1999; Gorga et al., 1997, 1999; Hussain et al., 1998; Musiek & Baran, 1997; Prieve et al., 1993), although these previous studies demonstrated better performance than observerd here.

The decision to include data only for children on whom reliable monaural VRA estimates were obtained was motivated by a desire for a gold standard measure independent of the neonatal screening tests. As a result of this decision, however, several infants with developmental disabilities AND confirmed hearing loss (based on diagnostic ABR and OAE tests), of necessity, were fitted with amplification and enrolled in habilitation programs in a timely fashion as a result of their participation in this project. Thus, for them, the screening measures identified hearing loss early in life. On the other hand, excluding them from the sample included in the analyses of test performance potentially would have had a greater negative impact on hit rate, compared with false alarm rate, based on the assumption that the incidence of hearing loss is greater among infants with multiple disabilities. If this is true, then the effect would be compounded further because there were so few infants with hearing loss (confirmed by VRA) in the present sample. If the infants with confirmed hearing loss who were unable to perform VRA were included in the analyses, test sensitivity for all measures may have increased.

Conversely, all normal ears do not produce these responses. Indeed, criticism about neonatal hearing screening tests often focus on the false positive or refer rate. Obviously, there is a need to keep the failure rate among normal-hearing ears as low as possible. There are many nonauditory factors that may result in "abnor-mal" ABRs and OAEs in neonates. However, failing a newborn hearing screening test is not a catastrophic event, and testers and clinicians who convey screening test results to families should be sensitive to this fact. Oftentimes, inexpensive follow-up testing soon after the initial failure results in a pass.

Finally, one needs to determine the magnitude of the loss for which intervention will be initiated. For infants with moderate or greater hearing loss, there is little debate that intervention needs to occur quickly to optimize the development of speech, language, and social behavior. However, decisions about intervention for infants with mild losses may not be as straightforward. Given the general proximity between parent/caregiver and infant, the mild magnitude of the loss, the rapid growth of the external ear and ear canal (necessitating frequent replacements of ear molds), and the practical issues of keeping a hearing aid in place, the timing and course of intervention is not as clear for babies with mild hearing losses. Test sensitivity was better for children with greater losses, for whom intervention is more straightforward, namely infants with moderate or greater hearing loss.

Acknowlegments:

The authors thank Dawn Konrad-Martin and Wendy Harrison for assistance with data analysis and figure preparation, as well as many helpful discussions. We would also like to thank Margaret Pepe for sharing her biostatistical expertise and may helpful discussions concerning this project in general and data analysis in particular. We thank Steve Neely for many helpful discussions over the course of this project. Finally, we would like to thank Judy Gravel and four anonymous reviewers for the careful reading of this manuscript and their many helpful suggestions. This work was supported by the NIH (NIDCD R10-001958).

Address for correspondence: Susan J. Norton, Ph.D., Children's Hospital and Regional Medical Center, 4800 Sand Point Way N.E., P.O. Box 5371, CH-78, Seattle, WA 98105.

Received January 28, 2000; accepted May 26, 2000

References

American National Standards Institute (1996). *Specification for Audiometers S3.6.*

Barsky-Firsker, L., & Sun, S. (1997). Universal newborn hearing screening: A three-year experience. *Pediatrics, 99,* E-4.

Bess, F.H., Gravel, J.S., & Tharpe, A.M. (1996). *Amplification for Children with Auditory Deficits.* Bill Wilkerson Center Press: Nashville, TN.

Cone-Wesson, B., Vohr, B.R., Sininger, Y.S., Widen, J.E., Folsom, R.C., Gorga, M.P., & Norton, S.J. (2000). Identification of neonatal hearing impairment: Infants with hearing impairment. *Ear and Hearing, 21,* 488-507.

Cox, L.C., Hack, M., & Metz, D. (1982). Longitudinal ABR in the NICU infant. *International Journal of Pediatric Otorhinolaryngology, 4,* 225-231.

Dorn, P.A., Piskorski, P., Gorga, M.P., Neely, S.T., & Keefe, D.H. (1999). Predicting audiometric status from distortion product otoacoustic emissions using multivariate analyses. *Ear and Hearing, 20,* 149-163.

Durieux-Smith, A., Picton, T.W., Edwards, J.T., MacMurray, B., & Goodman, J.T. (1987). Brainstem electric-response audiometry in infants of a neonatal intensive care unit. *Audiology, 26,* 284-297.

Fishman, J.R., & deVere White, R.W. (1994). Prostrate cancer screening, diagnosis and staging. In M.B. Siroky & J.M. Fitzpatrick (Eds.) *Clinical Urology* (pp. 9393-955). Philadelphia: J.B. Lippincott Co..

Folsom, R.C., Widen, J.E., Vohr, B.R., Cone-Wesson, B., Gorga, M.P., Sininger, Y.S., & Norton, S.J. (2000). Identification of neonatal hearing impairment: Subject recruitment and follow-up. *Ear and Hearing, 21,* 462-470.

Galambos, R., & Despland, P.A. (1980). The auditory brainstem response (ABR) evaluates risk factors for hearing loss in the newborn. *Pediatric Research, 14,* 159-163.

Gorga, M.P., Neely, S.T., Bergman, B.M., Beauchaine, K.L., Kaminski, J.R., Peters, J., & Jesteadt, W. (1993). Otoacoustic emissions from normal-hearing and hearing impaired ears: Distortion product responses. *Journal of the Acoustical Society of America, 93,* 2050-2060.

Gorga, M.P., Neely, S.T., Bergman, B.M., Beauchaine, K.L, Kaminski, J.R., Peters, J., Schulte, L., & Jesteadt, W. (1993). A comparison of transient-evoked and distortion product otoacoustic emissions in normal hearing and hearing-impaired ears. *Journal of the Acoustical Society of America, 94,* 2639-2648.

Gorga, M.P., Neely, S.T., & Dorn, P.A. (1999). Distortion product otoacoustic emission test performance for a priori criteria and for multifrequency audiometric standards. *Ear and Hearing, 20,* 345-362.

Gorga, M.P., Neely, S.T., Ohlrich, B., Hoover, B., Redner, J., & Peters, J. (1997). From laboratory to clinic: A large scale study of distortion product otoacoustic emissions in ears with normal hearing and ears with hearing loss. *Ear and Hearing, 18,* 440-455.

Gorga, M.P., Sininger, Y.S., Cone-Wesson, B., Folsom, R.C., Vohr, B.R., Widen, J.E., & Norton, S.J. (2000). Identification of neonatal hearing impairment: Distortion product otoacoustic emissions during the perinatal period. *Ear and Hearing, 21,* 400-424.

Hanley, J.A., & McNeil, B.J. (1982). The meaning and use of the area under a receiver operating characteristic (ROC) curve. *Radiology, 143,* 29-36.

Hanley, J.A., & McNeil, B.J. (1983). Method for comparing the area under two ROC curves derived from the same cases. *Radiology, 148,* 839-843.

Harrison, W.A., & Norton, S.J. (1999). Characteristics of transient evoked otoacoustic emissions in normal-hearing and hearing-impaired children. *Ear and Hearing, 20,* 75-86.

Herrmann, B.S., Thornton, A.R., & Joseph, J.M. (1995). Automated infant hearing screening using the ABR: Development and validation. *American Journal of Audiology, 4,* 6-14.

Hussain, D.M., Gorga, M.P., Neely, S.T., Keefe, D.H., & Peters, J. (1998). Transient evoked otoacoustic emissions in patients with normal hearing and in patients with hearing loss. *Ear and Hearing, 19,* 434-449.

Hyde, M.L., Riko, K., & Malizia, K. (1990). Audiometric accuracy of the click ABR in infants at risk for hearing loss. *Journal of American Academy of Audiology, 1,* 59-66.

Jacobson, J.T., & Morehouse, C.R. (1984). A comparison of auditory brainstem response and behavioral screening in high risk and normal newborn infants. *Ear and Hearing, 5,* 247-253.

Joint Committee on Infant Hearing (1994). Joint Committee on Infant Hearing 1994 Position Statement. *Pediatrics, 95,* 152-156.

Kim, D.O., Paparello, J., Jung, M.D., Smurzynski, J, & Sun, X. (1996). Distortion product otoacoustic emission test of sensorineural hearing loss: Performance regarding sensitivity, specificity, and receiver operating characteristics. *Acta Otolaryngologica, 116,* 3-11.

Mason, S., Davis, A., Wood, S., & Farnsworth, A. (1998). Field sensitivity of targeted neonatal hearing screening using the Nottingham ABR screener. *Ear and Hearing, 19,* 91-102.

Mason, J.A., & Herrman, K.R. (1998). Universal newborn hearing screening by automated auditory brainstem response measurement. *Pediatrics, 101,* 221-227.

Mehl, A.L., & Thomson, M.A. (1998). Newborn hearing screening: The great omission. *Pediatrics, 101,* E4.

Meyer, C., Witte, J., Hildman, A., Hennecke, K., Schunck, K., Maul, K., Franke, U., Fahnenstich, H., Rabe, H., Rossi, R., Hatmann, S., & Gortner, L. (1999). Neonatal screening for hearing disorders in infants at risk: incidence, risk and follow-up. *Pediatrics, 104,* 900-904.

Musiek, F.E., & Baran, J.A. (1997). Distortion product otoacoustic emissions: Hit and false-positive rates in normal-hearing and hearing-impaired subjects. *American Journal of Otology, 18,* 454-461.

National Institutes of Health (1993). Early identification of hearing impairment in infants and young children. *NIH Consensus Statement, 11,* 1-24.

Norton, S.J., Gorga, M.P., Widen, J.E., Folsom, R.C., Sininger, Y.S., Cone-Wesson, B., Vohr, B.R., & Fletcher, K.A. (2000). Identification of neonatal hearing impairment: A multi-center investigation. *Ear and Hearing, 21,* 348-356.

Norton, S.J., Vohr, B., Widen, J., Cone-Wesson, B., Sininger, Y.S., Gorga, M.P., & Folsom, R. (2000). Transient otoacoustic emissions during the perinatal period. *Ear and Hearing, 21,* 425-442.

Prieve, B., Dalzell, L., Berg, A., Bradley, M., Cacace, A., Campbell, D., DeCristofaro, J., Gravel, J., Greenberg, E., Gross, S., Orlando, M., Pinheiro, J., Regan, J., Spivak, L., & Stevens, F. (2000). The New York State universal newborn hearing screening demonstration project: Outpatient outcome measures. *Ear and Hearing, 21,* 104-117.

Prieve, B.A., Gorga, M.P., Schmidt, A., Neely, S., Peters, J., Schultes, L., & Jesteadt, W. (1993). Analysis of transient-evoked otoacoustic emissions in normal-hearing and hearing-impaired ears. *Journal of the Acoustical Society of America, 93,* 3308-3319.

Sininger, Y.S., Cone-Wesson, B., Folsom, R.C., Gorga, M.P., Vohr, B.R., Widen, J.E., Ekelid, M., & Norton, S.J. (2000). Identification of neonatal hearing impairment with the auditory brain stem response. *Ear and Hearing, 21,* 383-399.

Spivak, L., Dalzell, L., Berg, A., Bradley, M., Cacace, A., Capbell, D., DeCristofaro, J., Gravel, J., Greenberg, E., Gross, S., Orlando, M., Pinheiro, J., Regan, J., Stevens, F., & Prieve, B. (2000). New York State universal newborn hearing screening demonstration project: Inpatient outcome measures, *Ear and Hearing 21,* 92-103.

Stover, L., Gorga, M.P., Neely, S.T., & Montoya, D. (1996). Towards optimizing the clinical utility of distortion product otoacoustic emission measurements. *Journal of the Acoustical Society of America, 100,* 956-967.

Swets, J.A. (1988). Measuring the accuracy of diagnostic systems. *Science, 240,* 1285-1293.

Swets, J.A., & Pickett, R.M. (1982). *Evaluation of Diagnostic Systems: Methods from Signal Detection Theorgy.* New York: Academic Press.

Van Kershaver, E. (1998). General ALGO-screening for newborn babies an integrated project for prevention of hearing impairment in Flanders. *WWH, 2,* 25-29.

van Zanten, G.A., Brocaar, M.P., Fetter, W.P.F., & Baerts, W. (1988). Brainstem electric response audiometry in preterm infants. *Scandinavian Audiology,* (Suppl.) *30,* 91-97.

Vohr, B.R., Widen, J.E., Cone-Weson, B., Sininger, Y.S., Gorga, M.P., Folsom, R.C., & Norton, S.J. (2000). Identification of neonatal hearing impairment: Characteristics of infants in the neonatal hearing impairment: Characteristics of infants in the neonatal intensive care unit and well-baby nursery. *Ear and Hearing, 21,* 373-382.

Watkin, P.M., & Baldwin, M. (1999). Confirmation of deafness in infancy. *Archives of Disease in Childhood, 81,* 380-389.

Whitehead, M.L., McCoy, M.J., Lonsbury-Martin, B.L., & Martin, G.K. (1995). Dependence of distortion product otoacoustic emissions on primary levels in normal and impaired ears. I. Effects of decreasing L2 below L1. *Journal of the Acoustical Society of America, 97,* 2346-2358.

Widen, J.E., Folsom, R.C., Cone-Wesson, B., Carty, L., Dunnell, J.J., Koebsell, K., Levi, A., Mancl, L., Ohlrich, B., Trouba, S., Gorga, M.P., Sininger, Y.S., Vohr, B.R., & Norton, S.J. (2000). Hearing status at 8 to 12 months corrected age using a visual reinforcement audiometry protocol. *Ear and Hearing, 21,* 471-487.

Yoshinaga-Itano, C., Sedey, A.L., Coulter, D.K., & Mehl, A.L. (1998). Language of early- and later-identified children with hearing loss. *Pediatrics, 102,* 1161-71.

Reference Notes

1. Moeller, M.P. (1998). Paper Presented at the National Symposium on Hearing in Infants, Denver, CO.

The New York State Universal Newborn Hearing Screening Demonstration Project: Outpatient Outcome Measures

Beth Prieve, Larry Dalzell, Abbey Berg, Mary Bradley, Anthony Cacace, Deborah Campbell, Joseph DeCristofaro, Judith Gravel, Ellen Greenberg, Steven Gross, Mark Orlando, Joaquim Pinheiro, Joan Regan, Lynn Spivak, and Frances Stevens

Syracuse University, Syracuse, New York (B.P.),
Strong Memorial Hospital, Rochester, New York (L.D., M.O.),
Pace University, New York (A.B.),
Babies' and Children's Hospital of New York/New York Presbyterian Hospital (A.B., E.G., J.R.),
State University of New York at Stony Brook, East Setauket, New York (M.B.),
Albany Medical Center, Albany, New York (A.C., J.P.),
Montifiore Medical Center, Bronx, New York (D.C.),
State University of New York at Stony Brook, Stoney Brook, New York (J.D.),
Albert Einstein College of Medicine, Bronx, New York (J.G.),
Crouse Hospital, Syracuse, New York (S.G.),
North Shore-Long Island Jewish Health System, New Hyde Park, New York (L.S.),
New York State Department of Health, Albany, New York (F.S.)

Objective: To investigate outpatient outcome measures of a multi-center, state-wide, universal newborn hearing screening project.

Design: Eight hospitals participated in a 3-yr, funded project. Each hospital designed its own protocol using common criteria for judging whether an infant passed a hearing screening. Infants were tested in the hospital, and those either failing the in-hospital screening or who were not tested in the hospital (missed) were asked to return 4 to 6 wk after hospital discharge for outpatient rescreening. Those infants failing the outpatient rescreening were referred for diagnostic auditory brain stem response testing. Each hospital used its own audiological equipment and criteria to determine whether a particular infant had a hearing loss. All data were collected and analyzed for individual hospitals, as well as totaled across all hospitals. Data were analyzed in terms of year of program operation, nursery type, and geographic region.

Results: Seventy-two percent of infants who failed the in-hospital screening returned for outpatient testing. The percentage of in-hospital fails returning for retesting was significantly higher than the percentage of in-hospital misses returning for retesting. The percentage of infants returning for retesting increased with successive years of program operation. Some differences were noted in the percentage of infants returning for retesting among hospitals and geographic regions of the state. Some differences in outpatient outcome measures also were noted between infants originally born into the neonatal intensive care unit (NICU) and the well-baby nursery (WBN). The percentage of infants from the NICU who returned for retesting was slightly higher than that for infants from the WBN. The percentage of infants from the WBN passing the outpatient rescreening was higher than that for the NICU infants. The overall prevalence of hearing loss was 1.96/1000, with that in the NICU being 8/1000 and that in the WBN being 0.9/1000. Positive predictive value for permanent hearing loss based on inpatient screening was approximately 4% and based on outpatient rescreening was approximately 22%.

Conclusions: Several outpatient outcome measures changed with successive years of program operatin, suggesting that programs improve over time. Also, some outpatient outcome measures differ between NICU and WBN populations. The differences noted across regions of the state in the percentage of infants returning for outpatient retesting require further research due to demographic and/or procedural diffferences. (*Ear & Hearing* 2000;21;104- 117).

....

Most universal newborn hearing screening programs involve an inpatient screening and an outpatient rescreening. Those infants not meeting the criteria set by the hospital to pass the inpatient screening are brought back as outpatients at 3 to 6 wk of age. At that time, infants are retested using the same screening tool and criteria for passing as those used in the hospital. There are several important outpatient outcome measures to assess the success of screening programs. One of these outcome measures is the percentage of infants who returned for the outpatient screening. Published percentages of infants returning for rescreening from programs referring unilateral and bilateral inpatient fails range from 48% (Mehl & Thompson, 1998) to 85% (Vohr, Carty, Moore, & Letourneau, 1998). Vohr et al. (1998), the only published study that reports the percentage of infants passing the outpatient rescreening, found that 86.3% of infants passed the rescreening. Reports of the percentage of infants referred for costlier diagnostic testing range from 0.4% to 2.9% (Finitzo, Albright, & O'Neal, 1998; Watkin, 1996).

Although some issues have been addressed by these studies, other important data are needed to determine the efficacy of screening programs. For example, there are sparse data to indicate what percentage of infants who did not get tested as inpatients ("missed") returned for outpatient hearing screening. Only one study based in a single hospital made an attempt to screen, as outpatients, those infants who were missed as inpatients (Mason & Herrmann, 1998). In this program, only bilateral inpatient fails (infants who were tested in the hospital and did not meet pass criteria in both ears) were referred for outpatient testing. These researchers found that only 53% of in-hospital misses returned for outpatient screening, whereas 91% of in-hospital fails returned for outpatient rescreening. To further explore this issue in a multi-center study, the New York State project tracked both misses and fails (newborns who completed the inpatient screening and did not meet the criteria for passing). Data such as these are important because they provide insight into how universal hearing screening may fare if it were performed only as an outpatient test. If there are no differences in the percentage returning for those failing and missing an inpatient screen, it could affect inpatient procedures and protocols.

Another important consideration is whether outpatient outcome measures improve with year of program operation. Analysis such as this allows other researchers/clinicians to obtain realistic estimates of how well their own screening programs might do in the first year of operation, and the variability they might expect. Inpatient data from the project indicate that some outcome measures show considerable improvement with year of program operation, such as decreases in the percentage of infants failing the in-hospital screening and the percentage of infants missed before hospital discharge (Spivak et al., 2000). No other published studies provide outpatient outcome data by year of program operation in this manner; however, two studies include data about the percentage of infants returning for screening as a function of calendar year. Vohr et al. (1998) indicate that, across several hospitals, the percentage of infants returning for rescreening rose from 76% to 88% between the first and third years of data collection. Finitzo et al., (1998) found that, for aggregate data from 11 hospitals, the percentage of infants returning for rescreening rose from 66.3% to 76.7% over a 2½ yr period. Data from individual hospitals indicated that seven of the hospitals showed increased percentages of infants returning for outpatient screening from one year to the next. Only Vohr et al. (1998) report the percentage of infants passing the outpatient rescreen as a function of calendar year. There was an increase in the percentage of infants who passed the outpatient screening from 70% to 88% between the first and second years of data collection. These data suggest that, like inpatient outcome measures, there is a "learning curve" to optimal program operation. Clearly, more data are needed to determine which outpatient outcome measures change with year of program operation, for individual hospitals as well as for groups of hospitals.

Other critical outpatient outcome measures pertain to the nursery type of the infant. Inpatient outcome measures indicate that there are large differences in the percentage of infants missed for in-hospital screening and failure rates based on nursery type (Spivak et al., 2000). In light of these data, there also may be differences in the outpatient outcome measures between nursery types. No currently published data have reported outpatient measures with regard to nursery type other than the number of infants identified with hearing loss in each nursery.

Finally, it would be helpful to explore whether outpatient outcome measures vary among regions that are different in demographics and population density. Although the current data should be viewed as preliminary, because it cannot be determined precisely whether differences noted between geographic regions can be attributed only to that geographic region, they could elucidate areas for further research. For the inpatient data, it was found that the percentage of neonatal intensive care unit (NICU) misses was higher in New York City than in the other regions of New York State (Spivak et al., 2000). Therefore, it is possible that some outpatient measures differ among regions as well.

The purpose of this article is to describe the outpatient outcome measures of the New York State universal newborn hearing screening demonstration project during the first 3 yr of funding.

Methods

The conception of the project, names and locations of hospitals (Prieve & Stevens, 2000), and inpatient protocols and pass criteria (Spivak et al., 2000) are detailed elsewhere. Briefly, an inpatient pass meant that the infant met screening criteria in both ears. Transient evoked otoacoustic emissions (TEOAEs) and auditory brain stem responses (ABRs) were used either alone or in combination as screening tools. TEOAEs were measured using click stimuli. Acceptable levels ranged from 78 to 83 dB pSPL. At least 50 averages were collected, and an infant met passing criteria if the TEOAE energy in one-half octave bands centered at 2, 3, and 4 kHz was at least 3 dB higher than the residual noise. Passing criteria for ABR was wave V latency within developmental norms in response to 35 dB nHL clicks. In most hospitals, infants failing TEOAEs were tested using ABR before hospital discharge. Those infants not meeting criteria in one or both ears were considered inpatient fails and were referred for outpatient testing. Those infants who did not get tested in the hospital for any reason (missed before discharge, too ill to test before transfer) wer considered inpatient misses and were referred for outpatient testing as well.

The project was fully funded from 1995 to 1997. Data were organized into year of program operation. Year 1 (Y1) was the start-up year for each program, and year 2 (Y2) and year 3 (Y3) were the subsequent years. Two of the hospitals (3 and 8) started their programs in 1996, so they have no data for Y3.

Outpatient Screening

All sites chose to rescreen infants who failed or missed the inpatient screening at 4 to 6 wk after hospital discharge. Each hospital had its own protocol for informing parents that the newborn did not pass the inpatient screening. For example, at one hospital, parents were told before hospital discharge that their newborn had not passed the screening and were given an outpatient appointment. At another hospital, parents were contacted by phone approximately 2 wk after the infant's birth and asked to return for outpatient testing. The initial outpatient test used by all sites was TEOAEs using the same pass criteria as the in-hospital screening. However, some sites also had ABR available (either screening ABR or conventional ABR) at the time of retesting, and, if needed, ABR also was performed. The infants at all sites were tested in a quiet room in an outpatient or audiology clinic. At some sites, a few infants having indicators for increased risk of hearing loss were referred directly for diagnostic ABR (DxABR). This constituted 7% of NICU infants referred for outpatient testing and 0.8% of infants from the well-baby nursery (WBN). The term outpatient retesting is used in this article to accurately portray that, although the majority of infants were screened as outpatients, a small number were referred directly for DxABR. The word "screening" is used when newborns actually were screened as outpatients.

Outpatient rescreening was conducted by audiologists at all sites. If infants did not pasws the outpatient rescreen, they were referred to an audiologist for DxABR. Each local audiologist followed his or her clinic's protocol for DxABR procedures and determination of hearing status. In the majority of cases, reports of hearing loss were based on elevated ABR thresholds evoked by click stimuli. Therefore, hearing loss is defined as estimated hearing threshold at any one frequency between 1000 and 4000 Hz of greater than 20 dB HL. Some sites also may have used visual reinforcement audiometry to diagnose hearing loss. In that case, hearing thresholds also may have been tested at 500 Hz. For hearing loss due to transient conductive hearing loss (TCHL), sites used various criteria, such as bone-conducted ABR threshold better than air-conducted ABR threshold and wave V latency-intensity functions outside developmental age limits concomitant with delayed wave I latency and normal interpeak wave I-V. Although abnormal wave V latency-intensity functions

do not, in themselves, measure conductive hearing loss, they are an accepted means by which to infer probable conductive hearing loss (Fowler & Durrant, 1994). Some sites also used tympanometry to test for extremely reduced middle ear admittance. Significantly reduced middle ear admittance has been documented to be a sensitive indicator of ititis media with effusion (Margolis & Hunter, 1999), which often produces conductive hearing loss.

Outpatient data were analyzed in terms of infants who failed the in-hospital screen (fails) and those infants who were not screened in the hospital and were considered misses. All hospitals organized the infants returning for outpatient retesting in terms of misses and fails, except for hospital 2, which was not able to separate which infants were misses or fails in Y1. Therefore, miss and fail data for Y1 for hospital 2 are not shown.

Statistical Analyses

Chi-square tests were performed to analyze pooled data for statistical significance. Data were pooled across sites and nurseries as a function of program year. Cochran's test of linear trend was performed to determine whether there was a linear increase or decrease with year. To test for differences between nursery types, data were pooled across nursery types for each region (New York City, Long Island, and Upstate). The resulting Chi-square test provided whether there were significant diffferences among regions, but not which particular region(s) were significantly different from one another.

Calculation of Prevalence of Hearing Loss

Because approximately 28% of infants born in 1997 were still in process for DxABR testing at the time the data were compiled for this article, diagnostic data are being reported for infants born in calendar years 1995 and 1996. Prevalence of hearing loss was calculated by dividing the number of infants with permanent hearing loss (PHL) or hearing loss due to TCHL by the total number of infants screened during 1995 and 1996. These measures of prevalence are believed to be a low estimate because 1) not all infants who failed the inpatient screening returned for outpatient rescreening; and 2) some infants who were referred for DxABR testing were lost or refused testing. Infants in either of these groups were at higher risk for hearing loss than nonscreened newborns because they had failed either one or two hearing screenings. Therefore, an attempt was made to estimate the prevalence of hearing loss accounting for these lost newborns using a multi-step process.

First, calculations were made only for those infants failing the inpatient screening. Because hospital 2 could not analyze their 1995 data into misses and fails, their 1995 data (including infants identified with hearing loss) were excluded from the calculations. In step one, the proportion of infants who were identified with hearing loss compared with the number of infants having completed DxABRs was calculated. As a reminder, infants referred for DxABR had failed both inpatient

TABLE 1. Outpatient outcome measures pooled across sites as a function of program year.

	Year 1	Year 2	Year 3	Combined Totals
Number of fails referred for outpatient testing	1107	1055	551	2713
Percentage fails returning	66%	72%	85%	72%
Number of misses referred for outpatient testing	644	646	269	1559
Percentage misses returning	17%	38%	46%	31%
Percentage total returning (miss and fails)	48.6%	59.5%	71.8%	56.6%
Percentage refusing outpatient screen	13.7%	14.2%	12.0%	13.7%
Percentage lost before outpatient screen	36.3%	24.3%	11.1%	27.6%
Percentage died before outpatient screen	1.1%	2.0%	1.0%	1.4%
Percentage pass rescreen	83%	80%	75%	79%
Percentage refer DxABR (out of total screene d)	10.5%	0.88%	0.75%	0.89%
Percentage in process of rescreen as of 9/1/98	0%	0.1%	5.8%	1.3%
Percentage in process for DxABR as of 9/1/98	0%	1.%	28.0%	10.4%

DxABR = diagnostic auditory brain stem response.

and outpatient screenings or had risk indicators for hearing loss (Joint Committee on Infant Hearing, 1994) that prompted a decision to bypass the rescreen and refer directly for DxABR. That proportion was applied to the number of infants who also failed inpatient and outpatient screening tests but did not return for DxABRs. This procedure estimated the number of infants with hearin gloss in the group who did not comply with DxABR testing. This estimate was added to the number of infants identified with hearing loss. In the second step, the newly estimated number of infants was set in proportion to the number of infants who returned for retesting (these infants failed an inpatient screening). That proportion was used to estimate the hearing loss in the number of infants not returning for the outpatient retesting. The number of infants with estimated hearing loss from this calculation was added to the previous estimate of the number of infants with hearing loss. The estimated prevalence of infants with hearing loss was then complete for those infants who received and failed inpatient screening.

The second calculation was performed to determine how many infants had hearing loss in the group who

were inpatient misses. For this case, the proportion of infants with estimated hearing loss simply was applied to the number of infants who were inpatient misses. The final step was to add the number of infants with estimated hearing loss from the inpatient misses and fails. The estimated number of infants with hearing loss was divided by the total number of births/admissions. The corrected values may more truly represent the prevalence of hearing loss in the newborn population.

Results

Table 1 reports outpatient outcome measures pooled across sites as a function of program year. Totals for all 3 yr appear in the last column. The number of infants who failed inpatient testing who were referred for outpatient testing and the percentage who returned for outpatient retesting are shown in the first and second rows, respectively. The percentages of infants returning for outpatient testing increased significantly from 66% in Y1 to 85% in Y3 ($X^2 = 85.8$, $p < 0.005$). Across all years, the percentage of infants who failed inpatient screening and returned for outpatient retesting was 72%.

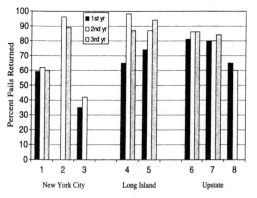

Figure 1. The percentage of inpatient fails returning for outpatient retesting for each individual hospital. Each bar represents a different year of program operation. The black bar represents data for Y1, the white bar represents data for Y2, and the gray bar represents data for Y3.

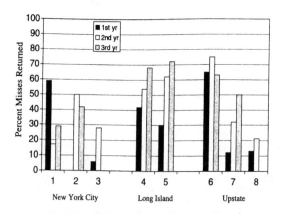

Figure 2. The percentage of inpatient misses returning for outpatient retesting for each individual hospital. Bar representation is the same as that used for Figure 1.

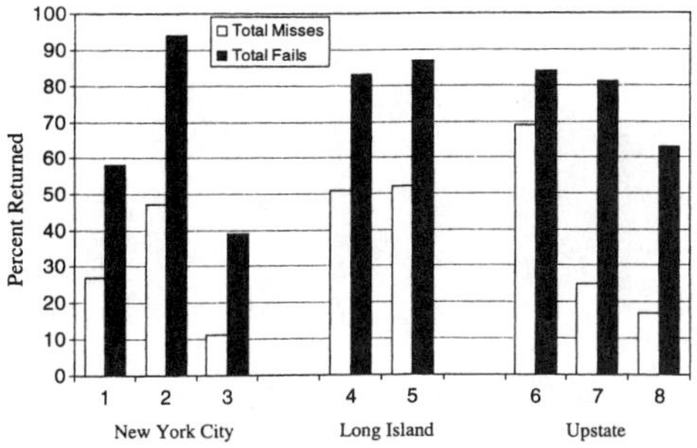

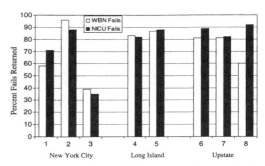

Figure 3. The percentage of infants returning for retesting for each hospital based on whether they were an inpatient miss or fail. The return of inpatient misses is represented by the open bar, and that for inpatient fails is represented by the black bar. At every hospital, the percentage of inpatient fails returning for retesting is higher than that for inpatient misses.

Figure 4. The percentage of infants returning for retesting for each hospital based on nursery type—neonatal intensive care unit (NICU) or well-baby nursery (WBN). Data for WBN are represented by open bars, and data for NICU are represented by black bars. Slightly more NICU infants returned for retesting than WBN infants.

It is also important to determine whether the trend of increasing percentages of infants returning for outpatient testing with program year is true for individual hospitals as well. Figure 1 illustrates the percentages of inpatient fails returning for outpatient retesting for each of the sites. The black bar represents the data for the start-up year of the program at each site (Y1), the white bar represents data for Y2, and the gray bar represents data for Y3. Among the individual hospitals, there was a wide range of percentage of infants returning for retesting. The percentage of infants returning for retesting during Y1 ranged from 35% to 81%. For Y3, the variability among hospitals was less, with percentages of infants returning for retesting ranging between 60% and 95%. Across all years of program operation, five of the hospitals had return rates of more than 80% (numbers 2, 4, 5, 6, and 7), two hospitals had return rates of approximately 60% (numbers 1 and 8), and only one hospital (number 3) had an extremely low return rate (38%). In general, the percentage of infants returning for outpatient retesting increased with year of program operation, although there was some variability among hospitals. Five of the hospitals (numbers 3, 4, 5, 6, and 7) showed increasing percentages of returning inpatient fails between at least 2 yr of program operation.

The number of misses referred for outpatient testing and the percentages of inpatient misses who returned for outpatient retesting are shown in Table 1, rows three and four, respectively. The percentage of misses reeturning for outpatient retesting significantly increased from 17% in Y1 to 46% in Y3 ($X^2 = 109.0$, $p < 0.0005$). The total percentage across all years is 31%. For individual hospitals, there was also a trend for increasing percentages of misses returning for outpatient retesting by year, as shown in Figure 2. Year of program operation is represented by a different colored bar, with bar color the same as that used in Figure 1.

TABLE 2. Outpatient outcome statistics—differences between nursery types.

	NICU	WBN
Number of fails referred for outpatient testing[a]	597	2116
Percentage of fails returning	80%	70%
Number of misses referred for outpatient testing[a]	780	779
Percentage misses returning	34%	27%
Percentage total returning[b]	52.6%	58.6%
Percentage pass re-screen[c]	70%	84%
Percentage refer DxABR[d]	3.1%	0.5%
Percentage in process of rescreen	0.5%	0.8%
Percentage in process for DxABR	7.9%	7.3%
Percentage refusing outpatient screen	11.9%	14.6%
Percentage lost before outpatient screen	30.8%	25.9%
Percentage died before outpatient screen	4.1%	0.03%

[a] Data from hospital 2 not included because data were not reported in terms of misses/fails.
[b] Data from hospital 2 are included.
[c] This number reflects the percentage rescreened and excludes those infants who were not screened as outpatients but were referred directly for DxABR.
[d] Denominator for total tested is the number tested as inpatients plus the number of misses tested as outpatients. This total is slightly low because hospital 2 misses were not included in the misses for 1995 but is the best approximation for the number of infants tested. NICU = neonatal intensive care unit; WBN = well-baby nursery; DxABR = diagnostic auditory brain stem response.

The percentage of inpatient misses returning for rescreening varies widely mong hospitals, from approximately 15% (numbers 3 and 8) to approximately 70% (number 6). Five hospitals were able to increase the percentage of infants returning for retesting with each successive year (numbers 3, 4, 5, 7, and 8).

The middle section of Table 1 reports the reasons for infants not returning for the outpatient screening. The percentage of infants refusing outpatient retesting was similar across year and totaled to 13.7% ($X^2 = 1.3$, $p = 0.26$). The percentage of infants who died before outpatient retesting ranged from 1 to 2%. Although the percentage of infants who died was significantly different among years ($X^2 = 14.1$, $p = 0.001$), there was no significant trend across years ($X^2 = 2.9$, $p = 0.09$). The greatest change was in the percentage of infants lost before outpatient retesting, which declined significantly across years of program operation; 36.3% for Y1, 24.3% for Y2, and 11.1% for Y3 ($X^2 = 204.0$, $p < 0.0005$). The conclusion that can be drawn is that the increasing percentage of infants returning for retesting with program year is because fewer were lost to follow-up with each successive year.

Figure 3 illustrates the comparison of the percentages of inpatient misses and fails returning as outpatients for rescreening. The open bars represent the percentage of inpatient misses and the black bars represent the percentage of inpatient fails returning for outpatient retesting, respectively. At every site, the percentage of inpatient fails returning for retesting was higher than the percentage of inpatient misses returning for retesting. As seen in Table 1, the percentage of inpatient fails returning for retesting (72%) was significantly higher than that for inpatient misses (31%) ($X^2 = 687$, $p < 0.0005$).

Investigation of whether outpatient outcome statistics were different between nursery types is shown in Table 2. The number of infants who failed inpatient screening and were referred for outpatient retesting and the percentage that returned for outpatient retesting are shown in rows 1 and 2, respectively. The return rate for NICU infants was 80%, and that for WN infants was 70%. Likewise, the percentage of misses (rows 3 and 4) who returned for outpatient retesting was higher for infants born into the NICU (34%) than for those born into the WBN (27%). Both of these differences were found to be statistically significant ($X^2 = 25.0$, $p < 0.0005$ for the former, $X^2 = 8.7$, $p < 0.003$ for the latter). The total percentage of infants returning for retesting (misses plus fails, Table 2, line 5) shows that the situation is reversed. That is, the total percentage of infants from the NICU who returned for retesting (52.6%) was lower than the percentage of infants from the WBN who returned for retesting (58.6%). This difference, too, was statistically significant ($X^2 = 15.5$, $p < 0.0005$). The reason that the total percentage of infants returning for retesting reverses between nursery types is that it is based on actual numbers, not the average of the percentages of misses and fails. Because the number of fails far exeeds the number of misses in the WBN, the number of fails dominates the percentage when the two categories are combined. Because of this, it may be more appropriate to look at the return rate in the categories of fails and misses. In these cases, the percentage of NICU infants returning is greater than that for the WBN infants, but only slightly so. One must remember that because of the large sample size, small differences will be statistically significant.

Figure 4 illustrates this concept well. This figure shows the percentage of infants from the NICU and WBN who failed inpatient testing and returned for outpatient retesting for each site (misses and fails combined). The open bars represent data for infants from the WBN, and the black bars represent data for infants from the NICU. First, Figure 4 illustrates that return of infant fails from both the WBN and NICU were high and fairly constant across hospitals. Five hospitals had more than 80% of infants from the WBN return for outpatient retesting (numbers 2, 4, 5, 6, and 7), and six sites had more than 80% of infants from the NICU

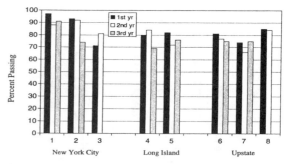

Figure 5. Percentage of infants passing the outpatient rescreening for individual hospitals with year of program operation. Bar color is the same as that used for Figure 1. There were similar percentages of infants passing the outpatient screening with successive years of program operation.

return for retesting (numbers 2, 4, 5, 6, 7, and 8). Secondly, for most hospitals, the percentage of infants from the WBN and NICU who returned for outpatient testing was only slightly different. One site had considerably more NICU infants return for outpatient testing (number 8), and four others had slightly more NICU than WBN infants return for retesting. The conclusion is that there are slight differences in the percentages of infants from the NICU and WBN returning for retesting. This slight difference actually may be clinically significant. Because the prevalence of hearing loss is greater in the NICU, it is important to get as many NICU infants as possible back for outpatient retesting.

The reasons for not returning for outpatient re-testing for the two nursery types are shown at the bottom of Table 2 (misses and fails are combined). The percentage of refusals for outpatient retesting was similar for infants cared for in the WBN (14.6%) and the NICU (11.9%) ($X^2 = 6.5$, $p = 0.13$). There were more NICU infants lost before outpatient retesting (30.8%) than WBN infants (25.9%) ($X^2 = 12.7$, $p < 0.0005$). The percentage of infants who died before outpatient retesting was significantly higher for NICU infants (4.1%) than for WBN infants (0.9%) ($X^2 = 124.0$, $p < 0.0005$).

There were differences noted across geographic region for outpatient outcome measures, as shown in Table 3. The percentage of inpatient fails who returned for outpatient retesting (row 2) was significantly different among regions ($X^2 = 130.0$, $p < 0.0005$). The percentage returning was substantially lower for hospitals

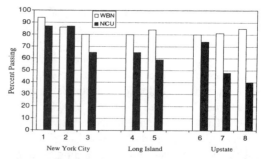

Figure 6. Percentage of infants passing the outpatient rescreening for individual hospitals in terms of nursery type. Bar color is the same as that used for Figure 4. A greater percentage of well-baby nursery (WBN) infants passed the outpatient rescreening than did neonatal intensive care unit (NICU) infants.

TABLE 3. Outpatient outcome measures—differences across geographic region.

	City			Long Island			Upstate		
	NICU	WBN	Total	NICU	WBN	Total	NICU	WBN	Total
Number of fails needing outpatient testing	112	394	506	179	456	635	306	1266	1572
Percentage of fails returning	57%	53%	54%	84%	84%	84%	86%	70%	73%
Number of misses needing outpatient testing	479	391	870	73	173	246	228	215	443
Percentage misses returning	32%	20%	27%	60%	47%	51%	32%	25%	28%
Percentage total returning	38%	42%	40%	77%	74%	75%	63%	63%	63%
Percentage refusing outpatient screen	14.6%	3.2%	8.2%	9.1%	16.5%	14.4%	9.6%	21.2%	18%
Percentage lost before outpatient screen	42%	55%	48.9%	9.9%	8.9%	9.2%	23.6%	13.9%	16.5%
Percentage died before outpatient screen	5.6%	0.2%	2.6%	1.6%	0%	0.45%	3%	0%	0.79%
Percentage in process	0%	0.1%	0.06%	2%	0.6%	1%	0.6%	1.5%	1.2%
Percentage pass re-screen	83%	86%	85%	63%	81%	76%	59%	83%	78%
Percentage referred DxABR	1.4%	0.3%	0.4%	2.3%	0.4%	0.7%	4.1%	0.8%	1.4%

NICU = neonatal intensive care unit; WBN = well-baby nursery; DxABR = diagnostic auditory brain stem response.

in New York City thant it was for hospitals in other regions of the state. The percentage of inpatient misses returning for outpatient screening was also significantly different among regions ($X^2 = 55.0$, $p < 0.0005$). It was highest in the Long Island region of the state, whereas the percentages for New York City and Upstate regions were similar (row 4). The percentage of infants refusing outpatient retesting was lowest in New York City (8.2%), with percentages of 14.4% and 18.0% for the Long Island and Upstate regions, respectively. These percentages were significantly different across sites ($X^2 = 50.0$, $p < 0.0005$). The percentage of infants lost before outpatient retesting was also significantly different among regions ($X^2 = 685.0$, $p < 0.0005$). It was substantially higher in New York City (48.9%) compared with Long Island (9.2%) and Upstate regions (16.5%). The percentage of infants who died was similar among regions ($X^2 = 8.0$, $p = 0.018$). Across geographic regions, infants from both the NICU and WBN returned for retesting in approximately the same percentages.

Figure 5 shows the percentage of infants passing the outpatient screening at each site for the 3 yr of program operation. Bar color is the same as that used in Figures 1 and 2. Almost every year at every site, more than 70% of the infants passed the outpatient screening. There was no apparent pattern among the years at each hospital. However, the pooled data (Table 1, row 9)

indicate that the percentage of infants passing outpatient screening decreased over the 3 yr ($X^2 = 15.6$, $p < 0.0005$). Because this does not seem to be a trend for individual hospitals, the significant decrease with year may reflect the large number of subjects rather than a clinically significant change. There were differences between the percentages of infants passing the outpatient screening among regions ($X^2 = 33.6$, $p < 0.0005$). In New York City, the percentage of infants passing the outpatient screening was slightly higher than for the other regions (Table 3).

The percentage of infants from the NICU and WBN who passed outpatient screening was 70% and 84%, respectively (Table 2). This difference was significant ($X^2 = 87.2$, $p < 0.0005$). To view this trend across hospitals, the percentage of infants passing outpatient screening based on nursery type is plotted in Figure 6. For seven out of eight hospitals, the percentage of infants from the WBN passing the outpatient screening was higher than the percentage from the NICU. The data shown in this figure suggest that inpatient test accuracy is better for infants from the NICU than for those from the WBN.

The percentages of infants passing the outpatient screening based on whether they were an inpatient fail or miss are plotted in Figure 7. At every hospital, the percentage of misses passing the outpatient screening was higher than the percentage of fails passing the outpatient screening. The percentage of inpatient misses and inpatient fails passing the outpatient screening was 80% and 77%, respectively, which was significantly different ($X^2 = 17.8$, $p < 0.0005$). The result of having a greater percentage of passes for inpatient misses is expected, given that the prevalence of hearing loss in the inpatient fails will be higher than that in the inpatient misses.

Another important outpatient outcome measure is the analysis of DxABR. These data are based in calendar years 1995 and 1996, rather than year of program operation. At the time of compilation of these data (September 1, 1998), 28% of infants born in 1997 still had not received or completed DxABRs. This large percentage could significantly affect calculations of prevalence of hearing loss; therefore, only those infants born in 1995 and 1996 were included in the reporting of

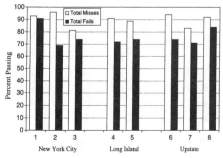

Figure 7. The percentage of inpatient misses and inpatient fails passing the outpatient rescreening. Bar color is the same as that used in Figure 3. For every site, the percentage of inpatient misses passing the outpatient rescreening was higher than that for inpatient fails.

TABLE 4. Summary of inpatient and outpatient data for calendar years 1995 and 1996.

Inpatient Data	NICU	WBN	Total
Number of live births/admissions	7059	37,566	44,625
Number/percentage refused inpatient screen	17/0.24	212/0.56	229/0.51
Number/percentage missed inpatient screen	714/10.11	678/1.80	1392/3.12
Number/percentage tested	6328/89.6	36,676/97.6	43,004/96.4
Number/percentage failed	392/6.19	1428/3.89	1820/4.23
Number/percentage referred for outpatient testing	1106/15.67	2106/5.61	3212/7.2
Outpatient Data			
Number of fails referred[a]	388	1324	1712
Number/percentage fails returning	296/76.3	949/71.9	1245/72.7
Number of misses referred[a]	501	572	1073
Number/percentage misses returning	168/33.5	139/24.3	307/28.6
Number/percentage total returning[b]	556/50.3	1217/57.8	1773/55.6
Percentage pass rescreen[c]	70.7	85.7	81.3
Number/percentage referred for DxABR[d]	201/3.1	184/0.5	385/0.9
Number/percentage refused, lost or died before outpatient rescreen	550/49.7	889/42.2	1439/44.4

[a] Data from hospital 2 not included because data were not reported in terms of misses/fails.
[b] Data from hospital 2 are included.
[c] This number reflects the percentage rescreened and excludes those infants who were not screened as outpatients but were referred directly for DxABR.
[d] Denominator for total tested is the number tested as inpatients plus the number of misses tested as outpatients. This total is slightly low because hospital 2 misses were not included in the misses for 1995 but is the best approximation for the number of infants tested.
NICU = neonatal intensive care unit; WBN = well-baby nursery; DxABR = diagnostic auditory brain stem response.

diagnostic data. Because the inpatient and outpatient data for calendar years 1995 and 1996 have not been reported as an aggregate in previous discussions, a summary is given in Table 4. The total number of infants screened in calendar years 1995 to 1996 was 43,311. A total of 6496 infants from the NICU and 36,815 from the WBN were screened. This number includes infants screened as inpatients and inpatient misses screened as outpatients. In these 2 yr, the percentage of infants referred for DxABR was low, approximately 0.5% and 3% for infants from the WBN and NICU, respectively.

Table 5 provides detailed data for the infants who were referred for DxABRs. Of those referred for DxABR, 83.6% of infants from the NICU and 70.7% from the WBN completed testing. Approximately the same percentages of infants from both nurseries were lost before diagnostic testing. The percentage of infants who refused DxABR testing was much higher for infants from the WBN (20%) than from the NICU nursery (9%). Two children died before completion of ABR testing, and they were both from the NICU.

A total of 85 infants were identified with PHL, either unilateral or bilateral; 75 of these had sen

sorineural hearing loss, six had mixed hearing loss, and four had permanent conductive hearing loss requiring surgery or amplification. Sixty-one percent of these infants were from the NICU nursery. A total of 75 infants were identified with TCHL. At the time of data compilation, two infants fro the WBN were identified with hearing loss, but type could not be determined. Because type was unknown, these two infants were left out of any further calculations. Combining both PHL and TCHL, a total of 160 infants were identified with hearing loss by the screening program. Fifty-six percent of the infants from the NICU and 51% of infants from the WBN who underwent diagnostic testing were identified with hearing loss.

The prevalence of hearing loss was calculated and is shown in Table 6. Based on the actual screening, the prevalence of PHL was 1.96/1000. The prevalence in the NICU was 8.0/1000, and that in the WBN was 0.9/1000. The prevalence of unilateral hearing loss was 0.83/1000, and that for bilateral hearing loss was 1.13/1000. The prevalence for TCHL was the same as that for PHL for the WBN and slightly less than that for PHL in the NICU. The prevalence for both types of hearing loss combined was 3.69/1000.

TABLE 5. Data for infants referred for diagnostic auditory brain stem response (DxABR).

	NICU	WBN
Number referred for DxABR	201	184
Percentage referred for DxABR	3.1	0.5
Number/percentage ABR completed	168/83.6	130/70.7
Number SNHL	45	30
Number mixed HL	5	1
Number perm. cond. HL	2	2
Total PHL	52	33
Number TCHL	42	33
Grand total with HL	94	66
Number normal-hearing	74	62
Number unknown type	0	2
Number/percentage lost before ABR	13/6.5	17/9.2
Number died before ABR	2	0
Number/percentage refused ABR	18/9	37/20

NICU = neonatal intensive care unit; WBN = well-baby nursery; SNHL = sensorineural hearing loss; HL = hearing loss; PHL = permanent hearing loss; TCHL = transient conductive hearing loss.

TABLE 6. Prevalence of hearing loss per 100 births.

	NICU	WBN	Total
PHL[a]	8.00	0.90	1.96
Unilateral	3.20	0.41	0.83
Bilateral	4.80	0.49	1.13
TCHL[a]	6.47	0.90	1.73
Total Combined[a]	14.47	1.80	3.69
Estimated PHL[b]	11.24	1.20	2.80
Estimated TCHL[b]	9.00	1.70	2.86
Estimated Total Combined[b]	20.24	2.90	6.74

[a] The denominator is the total number of infants tested.
[b] The denominator is the total number of live births/admissions.
NICU = neonatal intensive care unit; WBN = well-baby nursery; PHL = permanent hearing loss; TCHL = transient conductive hearing loss.

TABLE 7. Positive predictive values (PPVs).

	Inpatient Fail	Outpatient Fail
PPV for PHL		
NICU	12.5%	25.9%
WBN	2.2%	17.9%
Combined	4.5%	22.1%
PPV for TCHL		
NICU	10.0%	20.9%
WBN	2.2%	17.9%
Combined	3.9%	19.5%
PPV for PHL and TCHL		
NICU	22.5%	46.8%
WBN	4.4%	35.9%
Combined	8.3%	41.6%

PHL = permanent hearing loss; NICU = neonatal intensive care unit; WBN = well-baby nursery; TCHL = transient conductive hearing loss.

As explained in the Methods, the prevalence of hearing loss based on infants who were referred for DxABR tsting and did not complete it and for those not returning for outpatient retesting was calculated. The results also are shown in Table 6. As expected, these estimated prevalences were higher than the calculations based on the actual number who were identified. The estimated prevalence for PHL was 2.8/1000, and that for TCHL was 2.86/1000. The estimated total combined was 6.74/1000.

The positive predictive values (PPV), or the probability that given a positive test, an infant had a hearing impairment, were calculated. The PPVs are given in Table 7. The equation used to calculate PPV is given in Appendix A. The left column of the table provides estimates of PPV based on a positive inpatient fail for PHL, TCHL, and the two types of hearing loss combined. Inpatient misses were not included in this calculation. The PPV based on an inpatient fail was similar for PHL and TCHL, both being approximately 4%. For the two types of hearing loss combined, the PPV was approximately 8%. There were large differences in the PPV between NICU and WBN. The PPV for PHL was 12.5% in the NICU, whereas the PPV in the WBN was 2.2%. The PPV for TCHL in the NICU was approximately 10%, which was slightly lower than that for PHL in the NICU. In the WBN, PPV for TCHL was 2.2%, the same as that for PHL.

The right column indicates the PPV for hearing loss based on failing the outpatient retesting. For these calculations, both inpatient misses and fails were included. The PPV for PHL was 25.9% for NICU infants and 17.9% for WBN infants, substantial increases from predicting hearing loss based on only the inpatient screening. For TCHL, PPV for NICU infants is 20.9% and that for WBN infants is 17.9%. The PPV for detecting either type of hearing loss is 46.8% for infants from the NICU and 35.9% for infants from the WBN. Another finding is that the PPV based on failing an outpatient screen is more similar between nursery types than that based on failing an inpatient screen.

Discussion

Across the 3 yr of program operation, 72% of infants failing inpatient screening returned for outpa-

tient retesting. This percentage is considerably higher than the 48% reported by one group (Mehl & Thompson, 1998) and compares favorably with other published reports indicating that 68.5% (Finitzo et al., 1998) and 85% (Vohr et al., 1998) of infants returned for outpatient retesting. In one study, 91% of infants returned for outpatient testing (Mason & Herrmann, 1998); however, this program was designed to detect only bilateral hearing loss. The percentage of infants passing the rescreening was 79%, similar to other reports of 85% (Vohr et al., 1998; Watkin, 1996). The percentage of infants referred for a DxABR was 0.89%, within the range of published figures ranging from 0.4% (Finitzo et al., 1998) to 2.9% (Watkin, 1996). The prevalence of hearing loss was calculated to be 1.96/1000, also within the range of published reports from other universal newborn hearing screening programs for which unilateral and bilateral hearing loss were screened (Barsky-Firsker & Sun, 1997; Finitzo et al., 1998; Vohr et al., 1998).

Data by Year

One important aspect of the data analysis was to determine whether outpatient statistics improved with year of program operation. Similar to inpatient outcome measures (Spivak et al., 2000), some outpatient outcome measures improved with year of program operation. As an aggregate, the percentage of inpatient fails and misses returning for outpatient retesting increased with each successive year. The increase in the number of infants returning can be attributed to fewer numbers of infants lost to retesting, which declined from 36% to 11% between Y1 and Y3 of program operation because there were essentially no changes in the percentage of refusals or infant deaths among the 3 yr. For individual hospitals, increases were generally noted between at least 2, if not 3, yr of program operation; however, some individual hospitals showed little change or slight decreases in percentages of infants returning for retesting across years. Finitzo et al. (1998) also found this to be true among a group of 11 hospitals for which data were analyzed by chronological year. There could be several reasons for the improvements in percentages of infants returning for retesting with year of program operation. First, personnel may have gotten better at finding ways to track down infants through county public health programs and pediatricians. Second, the programs may have gained more acceptance in the second and third years from local medical personnel and the community, so parents were urged to have their children return for retesting.

One outcome measure that did not increase with program year was the percentage of infants passing the outpatient screening. The pooled data indicated that the percentage of infants passing outpatient screening decreased with program year, although this trend was not necessarily observed in individual hospital data. Vohr et al. (1998) found an increase in the percentage of infants passing the outpatient screening between the first and second years of data collection, then showed little change with subsequent years. In the current study, it is possible that percentage of passes decreasing with year is tied to the decreasing percentage of inpatient fails referred for outpatient testing with year (Spivak et al., 2000). With fewer infants referred for outpatient testing, the probability is greater that an infant may have hearing loss, so the percentage passing the outpatient retesting would be lower. The overall percentage of infants passing the rescreening was 79%, which is lower than that reported by Vohr et al. (1998). This also may be a reflection of the lower rates of referral for outpatient testing.

Data by Nursery Type

Another important area to explore was whether there were any differences in outpatient data between the two nursery types. The infants cared for in each nursery were quite different, and, therefore, it was possible that screening outcomes also would be different. The inpatient data indicated that there was a greater percentage of NICU misses than WBN misses and that fail rate was higher for NICU infants than for WBN infants (Spivak et al., 2000). Most of the outpatient outcome measures were slightly different for infants from the WBN and the NICU. The percentage of inpatient fails and misses returning for retesting was slightly higher for infants from the NICU than for infants from the WBN. The percentages of infants lost before retesting were within 5% of each other. Not surprisingly, the percentage of infants dying before retesting was higher among infants from the NICU than from the WBN. The biggest difference in outpatient outcome measures between the two nurseries was in the pass rate of the outpatient rescreening. Eighty-four percent of infants from the WBN, as compared with 70% of infants from the NICU, passed the outpatient screening. These differences would imply that the accuracy of inpatient testing is better for infants in the NICU than it is for infants in the WBN. There are may reasons that this may be the case. The most obvious difference is that infants in the WBN typically are discharged within 48 hr of birth, whereas NICU infants stay in the hospital much longer. It is likely that the infants from the WBN still have debris or vernix in the ear canal at the time of testing, which precludes them from passing the screen (Chang, Vohr, Norton, & Lekas, 1993; Doyle, Burggraph, Fujikawa, Kim, & MacArthur, 1997). At the time of rescreening, the debris is gone, and the infants meet passing criteria.

Another difference in outpatient outcome measures is the percentage of infants referred for DxABR testing. It is higher for NICU infants (3.1%) than for WBN infants (0.5%). These results are not surprising given that high risk factors for hearing loss are found more often among NICU infants.

Data by Region

Similar to the inpatient data for this project (Spivak, et al., 2000), there were some differences in the outpatient outcome data among the three regions of New York. The New York City region was much less successful at getting the infants who failed the inpatient screening back for retesting. This is true for both nursery types. The low percentage of return can be attributed mostly to the greater percentage of infants considered "lost to follow-up," which was considerably higher in New York City than in other regions. There are many possibilities for why this difference exists. It is possible that the infant tracking system was different or that the demographics of the population were different. As not all hospitals had the same protocols, it is also possible that this difference reflects a protocol rather than a geographic difference. For example, another difference among regions is that the Long Island region was able to get back 57% of their in-hospital misses for rescreening, whereas in the New York City and Upstate regions, the return rate for in-hospital misses was approximately 28%. These pooled data do not reflect every site, as one hospital in the Upstate region was able to get more than 60% of their missed infants to return for retesting. This finding may provide evidence that the procedures for getting missed infants to return is more of a protocol issue (e.g., the manner in which infants are tracked) rather than a regional issue. More research is needed to determine whether these differences are truly regional as opposed to procedural.

Misses versus Fails

Only one other study has attempted to screen as outpatients those infants who were "missed" as inpatients. Mason and Herrmann (1998), reporting data from a single hospital, found that 53% of infants missed in the hospital returned for retesting. In Y3, the New York State project approached a 50% return rate for in-hospital misses, but averaged across all years, the percentage was 31%. Figure 3 shows the dramatic differences in the percentages of inpatient misses and fails returning for retesting. These data suggest that it is better to screen the infants in the hospital before discharge. If infants are missed, it is difficult to locate them and have them return for retesting. All sites enlisted a statewide child tracking system to assist them in finding infants who needed to return for retesting. Additionally, all sites contacted the primary care physicians of the infants, urging them to advise their patients to obtain this free screening.

Even with this considerable effort, the percentages of misses returning for retesting was low. This finding is daunting given that all hospitals were funded for this project. The funding allowed hiring of personnel to track infants. It is uncertain how the statistics would change with fewer or no dollars available to fund these extreme measures. If a state did have universal newborn hearing screening, many of the infants from the NICU who were missed because they were too ill to screen before being transferred out of the hospital could be screened at another hospital. However, if a state tracking system were used would it be known that the infant had been screened. Because a high percentage of inpatient misses do not return for rescreening, and tracking efforts are expensive and time-consuming, the data suggest that as many infants as possible need to be tested before hospital discharge.

Prevalence of Hearing Loss

The prevalence of PHL from the current data set is 1.96/1000, which is within the range reported by other programs. Direct comparisons must be made carefully because some programs were designed to detect only bilateral hearing losses (Mason & Herrmann, 1998; Watkin, 1996). Some programs report prevalence based on actual screening numbers (Barsky-Firsker & Sun, 1997; Mehl & Thompson, 1998), and some programs report only adjusted prevalence (Finitzo et al., 1998). Overall prevalence rates are particularly difficult to compare across studies because prevalence of hearing loss in the NICU is approximately 10 times higher than in the WBN. Therefore, the percentage of NICU infants in the population from which the prevalence is calculated will heavily affect the overall prevalence rates.

The overall prevalence of 1.96/1000 found in the current data can be compared with other programs that screened for both unilateral and bilateral hearing loss. The prevalence is close to that of Vohr et al. (1998) and Mehl and Thompson (1998), who reported prevalences of 2.12/1000, respectively. It is slightly less than the 3.3./1000 reported by Barsky-Firsker and Sun (1997). It is interesting that the prevalence from the New York State project is slightly lower than that reported by others, when the percentage of NICU infants in the population is higher than that reported in the other studies. The estimated prevalence (adjusted for those infants not returning for rescreening or DxABR) is 2.80/1000, similar to the estimated prevalence reported by Finitzo et al. (1998) of 3.14/1000.

The prevalence of bilateral PHL in the New York State project was 1.13/1000, which is lower than other reports of bilateral PHL ranging from 1.4/1000 to 2.9/1000 (Barsky-Firsker & Sun, 1997; Mason & Herrmann, 1998; Mehl & Thompson, 1998; Vohr et al., 1998; Watkin, 1996). The prevalence of unilateral hearing loss from the New York State project (0.83/1000) was higher than other published reports of 0.38/1000 to 0.6/1000 (Barsky-Firsker & Sun, 1997; Mehl & Thompson, 1998; Vohr et al., 1998).

The prevalence of hearing loss varies with nursery type. The prevalence of hearing loss in the NICU, including both bilateral and unilateral PHL, was 8.00/1000, slightly less than the 9.75/1000 reported by Vohr et al. (1998) and less than the 13/1000 reported by Barsky-Firsker and Sun (1997). The estimated PHL in the NICU was 11.2/1000, still slightly less than that found by Barsky-Firsker and Sun (1997). Considering only bilateral PHL in the NICU, the prevalence of 4.8/1000 compares favorably with that reported by Mason and Herrmann (1998) of 5.0/1000. In the WBN, the prevalence from the New York State project was 0.9/1000, compared with that of Vohr et al. (1998) at 1.27/1000 and Barsky-Firsker and Sun (1997) at 2.0/1000. The estimated PHL in the WBN from the New York State project was 1.2/1000. The prevalence of a bilateral PHL in the WBN was 0.49/1000, less than that reported by Mason and Herrmann (1998) at 0.89/1000.

It is difficult to know what weight to place on differences in prevalence reported among the studies. There could be at least two reasons for the differences. The first is that the definition for hearing loss may be different among studies. A second possible explanation is that, because the prevalence of hearing loss is not high, the differences among the reported prevalence

rates may reflect sampling errors surrounding a true prevalence. Only large-scale studies or combined analysis across studies may help sort out these differences.

The prevalence of TCHL was calculated for this project; however, the detection of TCHL in a screening program, and calculation of its prevalence, are controversial for several reasons. First, some believe diagnostic testing should not be conducted on a disorder that is transient. Still, middle ear dysfunciton does produce hearing loss, and screening programs are designed to identify hearing loss, regardless of the type. It would be extremely difficult to accurately assess the type of hearing loss at birth given the current technologies (e.g., Thornton, Kimm, & Cafarelli-Dees, 1993). Secondly, because the disorder is transient, it is uncertain whether the retesting done at 4 wk of age and the subsequent diagnosis are due to the same transient disorder that may have occurred in the hospital. For example, it is possible that an infant failed the inpatient screening because of ear-canal blockage but failed the outpatient test because he or she has acquired middle ear dysfunction. Finally, it is possible that infants passed the in-hospital screening but developed transient middle ear dysfunction by 4 wk of age. Because these children were not retested at 4 wk of age, they are not identified with hearing loss.

The prevalence of TCHL was 3.9%, slightly lower than that for PHL. The prevalence of hearing loss including both PHL and TCHL was 3.69/1000, with 14.47/1000 in the NICU nursery and 1.80/1000 in the WBN.

Positive Predictive Value

PPV for PHL based on failing an inpatient screen was 12.5% in the NICU and 2.2% in the WBN, with a combined rate of 4.5%. This PPV was slightly higher than that reported by Vohr et al. (1998), who estimated a combined PPV of 2%. The reason for this is the difference in false alarm rates (false positives) between the two studies. In the current data set, the percentage failing the inpatient screening was approximately 4%, whereas in the program by Vohr et al. (1998), the inpatient fail rate was 10%. These rates are similar to PPVs of other infant screens for hypothyroidism (3%), cystic fibrosis (4%), and hemoglobinopathy (1%) (Mehl & Thompson, 1998). The PPV for WBN is within the range of these other established screenings, whereas the PPV for the NICU is considerably higher. The PPV for TCHL is similar to that for PHL. When the two types of hearing loss were combined, the PPV for NICU infants was 22.5%, that for WBN infants was 4.4%, and the combined PPV for all types of hearing loss in all nurseries was 8.7%. Again, the PPV for NICU infants was much higher than that for WBN infants.

The PPV based on outpatient fails is considerably higher than that for inpatient fails. The combined PPV for PHL based on a failed outpatient screen was 22.1%, with the PPV for NICU infants 25.9% and that for WBN infants at 17.9%. This PPV is higher than the 16% calculated by Vohr et al. (1998) but lower than the 27% calculated by Mason and Herrmann (1998). PPV for TCHL is similar to that of PHL. When combined together, the PPV for failing an outpatient screening was 46.8% for NICU infants, 35.9% for WBN infants, with a combined total of 41.6% for all infants. The PPVs based on outpatient screening between the two nurseries were similar, unlike the PPVs based on inpatient screenings. Perhaps one of the reasons for the lower PPV for WBN infants at inpatient screening was because of debris in the ear canal. Cleaning of debris in the ear canal has been shown to improve the pass rate (Chang et al., 1993; Doyle et al., 1997). It is more likely to be seen in infants from the WBN rather than the NICU because they typically are screened within 48 hr of birth.

These PPVs support two ideas about hearing screening programs. The first is that PPVs, even at the inpatient screening, compare favorably with other infant screening tests. Given the current technologies, and emerging new technologies, hearing screening should be considered worthwhile. The second point is that newborn hearing screening must be viewed in its entirety and that the screening process includes two separate screenings for those infants who fail an inpatient screen. This affects how we think about newborn hearing screening and how patients are counseled. If an infant fails an in patient screening, the parents should be told that the child did not pass, that children do not pass for a variety of reasons, and that most children pass the outpatient screening. If the infant fails the outpatient rescreening, it is more likely that the infant will have a hearing loss, especially if the infant was cared for in the NICU nursery.

Conclusions

1. More than 70% of infants who failed the in-hospital screening returned for outpatient retesting. This is significantly higher than the 31% of infants who were missed in the hospital who returned for outpatient screening. This outcome suggests that universal newborn hearing screening programs should minimize the number of infants missed in the hospital. Return rates for inpatient misses and fails varied among hospitals.

2. State-wide, the percentage of infants who returned for outpatient retesting increased with year of program operation. However, not every hospital showed this trend. The increased percentage of infants returning can be attributed to fewer infants being lost to retesting.

3. The percentages of infants failed and missed as inpatients who returned for outpatient testing from the NICU were slightly higher thatn those for infants from the WBN. The most dramatic difference in outpatient outcome measures between the two nursery types is the percentage of infants who passed the outpatient rescreen: 84% for WBN versus 70% for NICU.

4. Prevalence of hearing loss in the NICU (8.0/1000) was approximately 10 times higher than tat in the WBN (0.9/1000). The combined prevalence was 1.96/1000.

5. PPV was considerably higher in the NICU than in the WBN. It was also substantially higher for the outpatient screen than for the inpatient screen.

6. PPV for the in-hospital screen, even for the WBN, was similar to PPV for metabolic tests given at birth.

Acknowledgments

The majority of this project was funded by a grant from the New York State Department of Health. Individual hospitals contributed funding to some extent as well. The authors acknowledge the audiologists and personnel who tracked the infants, whose diligence and attention to detail made this project possible. In addition, thanks are given to the nurses, physicians, and hospital personnel for their cooperation. Gratitude is expressed to Drs. Michael Gorga, Deborah Hayes, and one anonymous reviewer for comments on an earlier version of this manuscript.

Address for correspondence and reprints: Beth A. Prieve, Ph.D., Communication Sciences and Disorders, 805 S. Crouse Avenue, Syracuse, NY 13244-2280.

Received August 20, 1999; accepted December 15, 1999.

References

Barsky-Firsker, L., & Sun, S. (1997). Universal newborn hearing screenings: A three-year experience. *Pediatrics, 6,* e4.

Chang, K.W., Vohr, B., Norton, S.J., & Lekas, M.D. (1993). External and middle ear status to evoked otoacoustic emission in neonates. *Archives of Otolaryngology, Head and Neck Surgery, 119,* 276-282.

Doyle, K.J., Burggraph, B., Fujikawa, S., Kim, J., & MacArthur, C.J. (1997). Neonatal hearing screening with otoscopy, auditory brainstem response and otoacoustic emissions. *Otolaryngology-Head and Neck Surgery, 116,* 597-603.

Finitzo, T., Albright, K., & O'Neal, J. (1998). The newborn with hearing loss: Detection in the nursery. *Pediatrics, 102,* 1452-1460.

Fowler, C.G., & Durrant, J.D. (1994). The effects of peripheral hearing loss on the auditory brainstem response. In J. Jacobson (Ed.), *Principles & applications in auditory evoked potentials* (pp. 237-250). Needham Heights, MA: Allyn and Bacon.

Joint Committee on Infant Hearing (1994). Position statement. *ASHA, 36,* 38-41.

Margolis, R.H., & Hunter, L.L. (1999). Tympanometry: Basic principles and clinical applications. In F. Musiek, W. Rintelman (Eds.), *Contemporary perspectives in hearing assessment* (pp. 89-130). Needham Heights, MA: Allyn and Bacon.

Mason, J.A., & Herrmann, K.R. (1998). Universal infant hearing screening by automated auditory brainstem response measurement. *Pediatrics, 101,* 221-228.

Mehl, A.L., & Thomson, V. (1998). Newborn hearing screening: The great ommission. *Pediatrics, 101,* e4.

Prieve, B., & Stevens, F. (2000). The New York State universal newborn hearing screening demonstration project: Introduction and overview. *Ear and Hearing, 21,* 85-91.

Spivak, L., Dalzell, L., Berg, A., Bradley, M., Cacace, A., Campbell, D., DeCristofaro, J., Gravel, J., Greenberg, E., Gross, S., Orlando, M., Pinheiro, J., Regan, J., Stevens, F., & Prieve, B. (2000). The New York State universal newborn hearing screening demonstration project: Inpatient outcome measures. *Ear and Hearing, 21,* 92-103.

Thornton, A.R.D., Kimm, L., & Cafarelli-Dees, D. (1993). External- and middle-ear factors affecting evoked otoacoustic emission in neonates. *British Journal of Audiology, 27,* 319-327.

Turner, R., Robinette, M., & Bauch, C. (1999). Clinical Decisions. In F. Musiek, W. Rintelman (Eds). *Contemporary perspectives in hearing assessment* (pp. 437-464). Needham Heights, MA: Allyn and Bacon.

Vohr, B.R., Carty, L.M., Moore, P.E., & Letourneau, K. (1998). The Rhode Island hearing assessment program: Experience with statewide hearing screening (1993-1996). *Journal of Pediatrics, 133,* 353-357.

Watkin, P. (1996). Neonatal ototacoustic emission screening and the identification of deafness. *Archives of Disease in Childhood, 74,* F16-F25.

Appendix A

PPV was calculated by the equation:
number of hits/number of hits + number of false alarms (Turner, Robinette, & Bauch, 1999).

This equation was chosen because it can be used when the percentage of hits and false alarms is not exactly known. This is the case with the current data set because the hearing of infants passing the inpatient and outpatient screening was not tested at a later date.

Universal Screening for Infant Hearing Impairment: Not Simple, Not Risk-Free, Not Necessarily Beneficial, and Not Presently Justified

Fred H. Bess
Division of Hearing and Speech Sciences, Vanderbilt University School of Medicine,
Bill Wilkerson Center, Nashville, TN

Jack L. Paradise
Dept of Pediatrics, University of Pittsburgh School of Medicine,
Children's Hospital of Pittsburgh, Pittsburgh, PA

Abbreviations. EOAE, evoked otoacoustic emissions; ABR, auditory brainstem response.

Screening for hearing impairment of all infants within the first 3 months of life, and preferably before discharge from the hospital newborn nursery, recently has been recommended in a National Institutes of Health Consensus Statement.[1] We agree with the desirability of identifying infants with congenital hearing impairment promptly, but we believe that the recommendation of universal screening is ill-considered and at this time ill-advised, and that its implementation might result in more harm than good. We also consider the Consensus Statement's discussions of the implications of acquired hearing loss during infancy and early childhood to be insufficiently balanced and qualified, and potentially encouraging of overly aggressive management.

The National Institutes of Health Consensus Statement was prepared by an independent 15-member panel representing audiology, otolaryngology, pediatrics, speech and hearing sciences, epidemiology, health care administration, various other child care areas, and the general public. The panel considered presentations and discussions at a 1fi day Consensus Development Conference on the Early Identification of Hearing Impairment in Infants and Young Children convened jointly by the National Institute on Deafness and Other Communication Disorders and the NIH Office of Medical Applications of Research, and cosponsored by the National Institute of Child Health and Human Development and the National Institute of Neurological Disorders and Stroke. The Consensus Statement has not, to our knowledge, been reprinted in any pediatric or general medical journal, but its recommendation of universal screening for hearing impairment by 3 months of age has been reported in pediatric news publications,[2,3] and free single copies of the Statement are available on request from NIH (1-800-644-6627).

Four main concerns seemed to underly the panel's recommendation of early screening. First, the prevalence of hearing impairment in infants and young children: "approximately 1 of every 1000 . . . born deaf, many more . . . born with less severe degrees of hearing impairment . . . [still] others develop[ing] hearing impairment during childhood." Second, the concern that "reduced hearing acuity [during the first three years of life] interferes with the development of speech and verbal language skills," and that "significantly reduced auditory input . . . adversely affects the developing auditory nervous system and can have harmful effects on social, emotional, cognitive, and academic development, as well as on . . . vocational and economic potential." Third, the concern that, despite persistent efforts to achieve early identification of children with hearing impairment, "the average age of identification in the United States remains close to three years [while] lesser degrees of hearing loss may go undetected even longer, [with] the result . . . that . . . for many hearing-impaired infants and young children, much of the crucial period for language and speech learning is lost." And fourth, the concern that the current practice of limiting hearing screening to infants who meet criteria for inclusion in a high-risk register[4] "misses 50 percent of children who are eventually diagnosed with severe to profound hearing impairment."

Reproduced with permission from *Pediatrics*, 93:330-334. Copyright 1994 by the AAP.

Received for publication Oct. 15, 1993; accepted Oct. 19, 1993.

Reprint requests to (F.H.B.) Division of Hearing and Speech Sciences, Vanderbilt University School of Medicine, Bill Wilkerson Center, 1114 19th Ave S, Nashville, TN 37212.

PEDIATRICS (ISSN 0031 4005). Copyright © 1994 by the American Academy of Pediatrics.

The consensus panel recommended a two-stage screening protocol. All infants would be screened with a test that measures evoked otoacoustic emissions (EOAEs), acoustic responses produced in the inner ear by physiologic activity of the outer hair cells of the cochlea, and measured with a sensitive microphone placed in the ear canal.[5] Infants who failed the EOAE test would receive an auditory brainstem response (ABR) screen at 40 dB nHL.* Failure at this second stage would call for a comprehensive diagnostic hearing assessment within 6 months.

Objections to the Consensus Statement

What are our objections to the Consensus Statement? Mainly, we are concerned that the consensus panel's recommendation of universal infant screening falls short of being justified on grounds of practicability, effectiveness, cost, and harm-benefit ratio. In addition, we are concerned that the Consensus Statement's dire and sweeping admonitions concerning the long-term developmental effects of early-life "hearing impairment" do not discriminate sufficiently between the acknowledged adverse effects of moderate to severe, persistent hearing loss, and the entirely speculative and perhaps nonexistent effects of mild or moderate temporary hearing loss. The reader is thus encouraged implicitly by the Consensus Statement to take an activist approach in screening for, and in managing, the conductive hearing losses that occur commonly throughout infancy and early childhood in association with episodes of otitis media—an approach that may involve various medical and surgical interventions, yet that remains largely unsubstantiated. Because the latter issue has been discussed in detail previously,[6-9] we confine our remaining comments to a consideration of the Consensus Statement's main recommendation of universal screening of young infants for hearing impairment.

When is Screening Appropriate?

For a disorder to warrant being screened for, several criteria must be met concerning, respectively, the disorder, the screening procedure, and the circumstances of eventual treatment.[10-14] The disorder must be important, i.e., it must cause substantial mortality, morbidity, or suffering. The screening procedure must be safe, acceptable, simple, reliable, valid, reasonably low in cost, and practicable. Finally, when the disorder is

found to be present, the treatment that follows must be efficacious, available, accessible, and readily complied with, and, crucially, early treatment must be more effective than later treatment.

Importance of Early Sensorineural Hearing Loss

No dispute exists as to whether early childhood hearing loss can impose burdens on the affected child, on the child's family, and on society. Early onset of persistent congenital or acquired hearing loss in the moderate to profound range (41 to 100 dB) affects speech perception adversely. This, in turn, may result in impairment of both receptive and expressive speech and language development, reduction in academic achievement, and disturbances in social and emotional development.[15-18] Further, difficulties in communication and frequently associated poor academic performance may lead to lowered self-esteem and to social isolation.[15] Even children with unilateral sensorineural hearing loss or mild (26 to 40 dB) bilateral sensorineural hearing loss may experience difficulties in speech or language development,[15,19,20] speech recognition under adverse listening conditions (e.g., classroom noise),[21-23] educational achievement,[21,24-27] and psychosocial behavior.[20]

Hearing impairment also imposes a significant economic burden; relatively few deaf persons are employed in professional, technical, and managerial positions.[28] The lifetime economic cost of congenital deafness is estimated currently to exceed 1 million dollars.[29] Other, less tangible costs borne by affected individuals and by their families derive from emotional stress, breakdowns in family communication, and isolation from peers and educational systems.[20,30]

Screening Tests for Hearing Loss in Young Infants

Because the screening procedure recommended in the Consensus Statement consists of two stages, the EOAE test first, followed by the ABR for those who fail the EOAE, we will consider the attributes of both tests as screening instruments. Because the ABR is the more familiar of the two tests and is widely accepted for use in both screening and diagnosis, it may serve to some extent as a standard against which to compare the EOAE.

Safety

Safety is not an issue with either test.

---

*nHL(normal Hearing Level)—click stimulus is referred to in terms of dB above the behavioral threshold of a group of normal listeners.

Acceptability and Simplicity

Acceptability to patients is not an issue with either test because the patients are newborns or young infants and neither test is invasive or traumatic. However, acceptability to the clinicians performing the tests, an often overlooked issue, is another matter. Using the diagnostic ABR equipment available in hospitals often is difficult and time-consuming, and test results are often difficult to interpret, even by professionals. In contrast, using EOAE equipment and automated ABR equipment appears to be easier and less time-consuming, and probably can be accomplished satisfactorily by trained nonprofessionals.

Reliability

The reliability of a test refers to the extent to which the test gives consistent results on repeated trials, by either the same or different observers, in the same individual. One might expect the reliability of both the ABR and the EOAE as screening tests to be high, but the issue warrants additional study.

Validity and Predictive Value

Validity consists of two components: sensitivity, the proportion of individuals with a disorder who have a positive test for the disorder, and specificity, the proportion of individuals without the disorder who have a negative test. Additional test characteristics of key importance in screening for a disorder are positive predictive value, the probability of an individual having the disorder when the test is positive, and negative predictive value, the probability of not having the disorder when the test is negative. The sensitivity and specificity of a test for a disorder tend to remain relatively stable, but the predictive value of the test for the disorder is highly dependent on the prevalence of the disorder in the population being tested. For a disorder of very low prevalence, even a highly specific test is likely to have a low positive predictive value. For example, a test that has a sensitivity of 90% and a specificity of 90% in detecting a disorder will have a positive predictive value of 79.4%, and thus a false-positive rate of 20.6%, if the prevalence of the disorder is 30%. However, the positive predictive value decreases to 50% if the prevalence is only 10%, to 8.3% if the prevalence is only 1%, and to 0.9%, with a false-positive rate of 99.1%, if the prevalence is only 0.1%.

In general, the ABR is highly sensitive in screening for moderate to severe hearing impairment in newborns and young infants. However, because the ABR uses a click stimulus it is primarily able to detect high-frequency hearing loss; the rare infant with low-frequency loss may be missed.[31] The specificity and positive predictive value of the ABR, when used as a screening test in well-baby nurseries, appear problematic. Thus, in keeping with the values we have cited above, the Consensus Statement notes the problem of over-referral as a consequence of ABR screening: "In the well-baby nursery . . . for every child with significant hearing impairment, more than 100 babies are referred." The same concerns necessarily apply to a recently devised, automated ABR instrument that is simpler to use and less expensive than conventional ABR equipment.[32]

EOAE testing also seems to offer high sensitivity, but its specificity in screening is even lower than that of ABR testing, so that, as pointed out in the Consensus Statement, ". . . newborn EOAE testing tends to have more false-positives when compared to ABR, especially during the first 48 hours of life." Further, most studies of EOAE testing in newborns have been conducted under "laboratory" conditions, i.e., by skilled professionals in sound-treated rooms. Use of the test by nonprofessionals in newborn nurseries, as would be required in the interest of practicability for mass screening, has not been evaluated but obviously risks being more problematic. Finally, additional problems reside in the facts that protocols using commercially available instrumentation for measuring EOAEs are based on normative data derived from adults rather than infants, that no consensus exists regarding pass/fail criteria, and that follow-up behavioral data on newborns who have passed the EOAE screen remain scant.

As for the two-stage, EOAE-ABR screening sequence recommended in the Consensus Statement, no data on actual use are available, to our knowledge. However, it is possible to gain some notion of the results to be anticipated, at best, from full implementation of this two-stage screen by using, in part, estimates cited in the Consensus Statement and by generously assuming that the EOAE and the ABR tests each have a sensitivity of 100%. Under these circumstances, of the approximately 4 million infants born in the United States each year and receiving the EOAE screen, 403,600 would fail it. Of these, 399,600 would be false positives and 4000 would be true positives. All 403,600 would then receive the ABR screen, of whom 359,640 would pass and 43,960 would fail. The 359,640 who passed would be discharged, but flagged for rescreening at age 3 to 6 months. The 43,960 who failed would be referred for comprehensive evaluation to differentiate the 4000 true positives from the 39,960 false positives.

Cost

Calculation of the cost of the proposed screening program must take into account not only the direct cost of the screening procedures themselves but also the cost of the assessment, monitoring, and intervention that would be undertaken as a consequence of the screening. Especially important are the costs deriving from false-positive tests: both the monetary costs of parents' lost time from work, transportation to care facilities, otherwise unnecessary tests, and unnecessary treatments; and the human and probably more consequential costs of attendant parental anxiety, distraction, and potential misunderstanding, of disturbance of family function, and of unnecessary or harmful procedures or treatments carried out on children. We estimate that the direct monetary costs alone of the proposed program, assuming ideal conditions, would approximate $200,000,000 annually.

Practicability

Currently, newborns in the United States are often discharged from hospital nurseries within 24 hours and usually within 48 hours. As noted previously, it is within that period that the specificity of EOAE testing is at its lowest level. Therefore, to undertake EOAE testing on newborns before hospital discharge is to invite even larger numbers than otherwise of false-positive tests, or to delay hospital discharge, or both, as well as to add to the burden of change, heightened activity, and emotion often borne by parents at that time. Further, an estimated 25% of births in this country occur in rural or remote areas, many of which lack qualified audiological professionals and sophisticated audiometric equipment; the second-stage screening and follow-up evaluation of infants from such areas would pose formidable problems of logistics and cost.

Treatment of Hearing Loss in Young Infants

Efficacy

Once hearing impairment has been accurately diagnosed, is treatment efficacious? Much theoretical understanding, intuitive belief, and clinical experience argue in favor of efficacy. Nonetheless, no direct evidence demonstrates conclusively that intervention appropriate by current standards results in more good than harm to the child and the family. Several case-control and cohort studies have suggested that intervention improves children's use of residual hearing and their speech-language skills, social and emotional status, and academic performance,[33-40] but other studies have failed to show such benefits.[41,42]

Critical review of all of the studies reveals important limitations in design or methodology that render interpretation of their findings difficult. These limitations include inadequate description of the population studied; selection bias; weighting of the study population with children who have severe or profound, as opposed to mild or moderate, sensorineural hearing loss; small sample size; questionable matching of cases and controls; failure to adjust for potentially confounding variables; failure to document the degree of compliance with recommended treatment; questionable validity and preciseness of outcome measures; failure to use blind examiners; and failure to differentiate maturation effects from treatment effects.

Availability and Accessibility

It is improper to screen for a disorder without certainty that facilities for suitable follow-up care of individuals who fail the screen are both available and accessible. Previously we expressed concern about the availability of qualified professionals in rural or remote areas to undertake the volume of follow-up diagnostic testing that a universal screening program would generate; the concern applies equally to the availability of such professionals for treatment. Moreover, families in such areas often lack health insurance or are underinsured, so that even if suitable professional services were available, they might not be affordable for such families until such time as a national health insurance program had come into being.

Compliance

The issue of compliance was not addressed in the Consensus Statement, but noncompliance has been one of the principal limitations of existing hearing screening programs for newborns. In some studies, proportions ranging from 25% to 80% of infants who failed newborn screening have been lost to follow-up despite aggressive recruiting efforts and the offering of cost-saving incentives to parents.[43,44] In other studies, after early identification of hearing loss, lag times of 8 to 9 months have transpired before infants returned for interventive services.[45-47] To our knowledge, no data have been reported on compliance in hearing screening programs for infants beyond the newborn period. It seems reasonable to anticipate that noncompliance would constitute a problem of substantial magnitude in any universal screening program, and that substantial effort and resources would be required to minimize its effects.

Early versus Later Treatment

Screening for hearing impairment can be justified only if treatment initiated before the impairment has become apparent is more effective than treatment initiated afterward. Although supported by theory and belief, no empirical evidence, to our knowledge, supports the proposition that outcomes in children with congenital hearing loss are more favorable if treatment is begun early in infancy rather than later in childhood (e.g., 6 months vs 18 months).

Conclusions

In our judgment, before any societal decision is made as to whether to institute a universal screening program for hearing impairment in young infants, many questions for which answers are not now available must be answered. To answer those questions will require extensive research. Clearly, the authors of the Consensus Statement were not unmindful of the scope of the problem, for they included in the Statement a listing of proposed future studies they considered important. Among these were: "controlled trials of screening by audiologists versus trained nonprofessionals or volunteers; controlled trials of the influence of different settings . . . on the effectiveness of screening procedures; comparison of early intervention with later intervention . . .; evaluate the validity and reliability of screening instruments . . .; test the feasibility of screening methods . . . in infant populations . . . in remote satellite clinics . . .; determine whether a two-tier screening system. . .works better than [a single screen] . . . study the cost-effectiveness of universal screening for infant hearing impairment." We heartily agree that these studies, and other studies, are important—indeed, crucial. So crucial, in fact, that, until they have been conducted and their results tabulated, no rational decision on undertaking universal screening for infant hearing loss is possible. We, too, believe that early identification is important; however, the precipitate launching of mass screening could work to deter the eventual development of an effective early identification program. In the meantime, to identify infants at risk for hearing impairment, continued reliance on the high-risk register as recommended by the Joint Committee on Infant Hearing,[4] but in combination with an automated rather than conventional ABR screen, seems to be a more practical, cost-effective approach.

Fred H. Bess, Ph.D.
Division of Hearing and Speech Sciences
Vanderbilt University School of Medicine
Bill Wilkerson Center
Nashville, TN

Jack L. Paradise, M.D.
Dept of Pediatrics
University of Pittsburgh School of Medicine
Children's Hospital of Pittsburgh
Pittsburgh, PA

References

1. NIH Consensus Statement. *Early Identification of Hearing Impairment in Infants and Young Children.* March 1-3,1993;11:1-24.
2. NIH Consensus panel report. *Newsletter.* Ambulatory Pediatric Association; 1993;29:18-19.
3. Hearing impairment screening. *AAP News.* July 1993;9:2.
4. Joint Committee on Infant Hearing. 1990 Position Statement. *AAP News.* April 1991;7:6,14. Reprinted in *Policy Reference Guide*, 6th ed. Elk Grove Village, IL: American Academy of Pediatrics; 1993:343-346.
5. Kemp, D.T. Stimulated acoustic emissions from within the human auditory system. *J Acoust Soc Am.* 1978;64:1386-1391.
6. Paradise, J.L. On tympanostomy tubes: rationale, results, reservations, and recommendations. *Pediatrics.* 1977;60:86-90.
7. Paradise, J.L., Smith, C.G. Impedance screening for preschool children: state of the art. In: Harford, E.R., Bess, F.H., Bluestone, C.D., Klein, J.O., eds. *Impedance Screening for Middle Ear Disease in Children.* New York: Grune & Stratton; 1978:113-123.
8. Paradise, J.L. Otitis media during early life: how hazardous to development? a critical review of the evidence. *Pediatrics.* 1981;68:869-873.
9. Paradise, J.L., Rogers, K.D. On otitis media, child development, and tympanostomy tubes: new answers or old questions? *Pediatrics.* 1986; 77:88-92.
10. Frankenburg, W.K. Selection of diseases and tests in pediatric screening. *Pediatrics.* 1974;54: 612-616.
11. Cadman, D., Chambers, L., Feldman, W., Sackett, D. Assessing the effectiveness of community screening programs. *JAMA.* 1984;251:1580-1585.
12. Sackett, D.L., Haynes, R.B., Tugwell, P. *Clinical Epidemiology—A Basic Science for Clinical Medicine.* Boston: Little, Brown & Co; 1985:139-155.
13. Fletcher, R.H., Fletcher, S.W., Wagner, E.H. *Clinical Epidemiology: The Essentials.* 2nd ed. Baltimore, MD: Williams & Wilkins; 1988:159-171.

14. Feightner, J.W. Screening in the 1990's: some principles and guidelines. In: Bess, F.H., Hall, J.W., eds. *Screening Children for Auditory Function*. Nashville, TN: Bill Wilkerson Center Press; 1991:1-16.

15. Davis, J., ed. *Our Forgotten Children: Hard of Hearing Pupils in the Schools*. Washington, DC: US Dept of Education; 1990:1-2.

16. Karchmer, M.A. *1990 Stanford Achievement Test Norms for Hearing Impaired Students*. Washington: Gallaudet University, Office of Demographic Studies; 1991.

17. de Villiers, P.A. Educational implications of deafness: language and literacy. In: Eavey, R.D., Klein, J.O., eds. *Hearing Loss in Childhood: A Primer*. Report of the 102nd Ross Conference on Pediatric Research. Columbus, OH: Ross Laboratories; 1992:127-135.

18. Holt, J.A. Stanford Achievement Test—8th Edition. [Reading Comprehension Subgroup Results]. *Am Ann Deaf*. 1993;138:172-175.

19. Goetzinger, C.P. Effects of small perceptive losses on language and on speech discrimination. *Volta Rev*. 1962;64:408-414.

20. Davis, J.M., Elfenbein, J., Schum, D., Bentler, R.A. Effects of mild and moderate hearing impairment on language, educational, and psychosocial behavior of children. *J Speech Hear Disord*. 1986;51:53-62.

21. Ross, M., Giolas, T.G. Effects of three classroom listening conditions on speech intelligibility. *Am Ann Deaf*. 1971 Dec; 580-584.

22. Bess, F.H., Tharpe, A.M., Gibler, A. Auditory performance of children with unilateral sensorineural hearing impairment. *Ear Hear*. 1986;7: 20-26.

23. Crandell, C.C. Speech recognition in noise by children with minimal degrees of sensorineural hearing loss. *Ear Hear*. 1993;14:210-216.

24. Quigley, S.P., Thomure, F.E. *Some Effects of Hearing Impairment on School Performance*. Springfield, IL: Illinois Office of Education; 1968.

25. Bess, F.H., Tharpe, A.M. Unilateral hearing impairment in children. *Pediatrics*. 1984;15:206-216.

26. Bess, F.H. The minimally hearing impaired child. *Ear Hear*. 1985;6:43-47.

27. Bess, F.H., editor. Unilateral sensorineural hearing loss in children. *Ear Hear*. 1986;7:1-54.

28. Downs, M.P. The rationale for neonatal hearing screening. In: Swigart, E.T., ed. *Neonatal Hearing Screening*. San Diego, CA: College-Hill Press; 1986.

29. Northern, J.L., Downs, M.P. *Hearing in Children*. 4th ed. Baltimore: Williams and Wilkins; 1991:1-31.

30. Maliszewski, S.J. The impact of a child's hearing impairment on the family: a parent's perspective. In: Bess, F.H., ed. *Hearing Impairment in Children*. Parkton MD: York Press; 1988;417-429.

31. Bess, F.H. Early identification of hearing loss: a review of the whys, hows, and whens. *Hear J*. 1993;46:22-25.

32. Hall, J.W. *Handbook of Auditory Evoked Responses*. Needham Heights, MA: Allyn and Bacon; 1992;475-508.

33. McConnell, F., Liff, S. The rationale for early identification and intervention. In: Glasscock, M.E., ed. Sensorineural hearing loss in children: early detection and intervention. *Otolaryngol Clin North Am*. 1975;8:77-87.

34. Greenstein, J. *Methods of Fostering Language Development in Deaf Infants: Final Report*. Washington, DC: Bureau of Education for the Handicapped (DHEW/OE); 1975. BBB00581.

35. Hanners, B.A. *A Study of Language Skills in Thirty-four Hearing Impaired Children for Whom Remediation Began before Age Three*. Nashville, TN: Vanderbilt University; 1977. Dissertation.

36. Clark, T.C. *Language Development Through Home Intervention for Infant Hearing Impaired Children*. University of North Carolina; 1979. Dissertation.

37. Greenberg, M., Calderon, R., Kusche, C. Early intervention using simultaneous communication with deaf infants: the effect on communication development. *Child Dev*. 1984;55:607-616.

38. Watkins, S. Long-term effects of home intervention with hearing-impaired children. *AAD*. 1988; 132:267-271.

39. Levitt, H., McGarr, N. Speech and language development in hearing-impaired children. In: Bess, F.H., ed. *Hearing Impairment in Children*. Parkton, MD: York Press; 1988:375-388.

40. Ramkalawan, T.W., Davis, A.C. The effects of hearing loss and age of intervention on some language metrics in young hearing-impaired children. *Br J Audiol*. 1992;26:97-107.

41. Musselman, C., Wilson, A., Lindsay, P. Effects of early intervention on hearing impaired children. *Exceptional Child*. 1988;55:222-228.

42. Weisel, A. Early intervention programs for hearing impaired children—evaluation of outcomes. *Early Child Dev Care*. 1990,41:77-87.

43. Shimizu, H., Walters, R.J., Proctor, L.R., Kennedy, D.W., Allen, M.C., Markowitz, R.K. Identification of hearing impairment in the neonatal intensive care unit population: outcome of a five-year project at the Johns Hopkins Hospital. *Semin Hearing*. 1990;11:150-160.

44. Diefendorf, A.O., Weber, B.A. Identification of hearing loss: programmatic and procedural considerations. In: Roush, J., Matkin, N., eds. *Infants and Toddlers with Hearing Loss: Family- Centered Identification, Assessment and Intervention*. Baltimore, MD: York Press; 1994.

45. Elssmann, S.F., Matkin, N.D., Sabo, M.P. Early identification of congenital sensorineural hearing impairment. *Hear J.* 1987;9:13-17.

46. Stein, L.K. Follow-up of infants in a neonatal hearing screening program. In: Swigert, E.T., ed. *Neonatal Hearing Screening.* San Diego, CA: College-Hill Press; 1986:99-106.

47. Stein, L.K., Jalsaley, T., Spitz, R., Stoakely, D., McGee, T. The hearing-impaired infant: patterns of identification and habilitation revisited. *Ear Hear* 1990:11:201-205.

Universal Screening for Infant Hearing Impairment: Replies to Bess and Paradise Selected Letters to the Editor

Statements appearing here are those of the writers and do not represent the official position of the American Academy of Pediatrics, Inc. or its Committees. Comments on any topic, including the contents of *Pediatrics*, are invited from all members of the profession: those accepted for publication will not be subject to major editorial revision but generally must be no more than 400 words in length. The editors reserve the right to publish replies and may solicit responses from authors and others.

To the Editor.—

I appreciate the opportunity to respond to the article by Drs Bess and Paradise[1] in the February 1994 issue of *Pediatrics* in which they debate the justification of the National Institutes of Health Consensus Statement recommendations for universal hearing screening using transient evoked otoacoustic emissions (TEOAE) and brainstem auditory-evoked response (BAER).[2]

One of the components of screening with which the authors take issue is the specificity and positive predictive value of the TEOAE/ BAER screen, a two-stage screen approach. Although the perfect screening tool for hearing impairment would have a positive predictive value of 100%, the seriousness of hearing impairment and its impact on the infant and the family would far outweigh the financial cost of performing a diagnostic audiologic assessment on a relatively small number of false positive infants. The most recent universal hearing screen data using a two-stage TEOAE/ABR system from our statewide program for the time period of July 1, 1993 to December 31, 1993 reveals a stage 2 fail rate of 1% (59 of 5760) (unpublished data). This stage 2 fail rate results in ten infants per thousand being referred for a diagnostic audiologic assessment by 6 months of age. This is lower than previously reported[3,4] as a result of software changes on the ILO88 apparatus, which produced an improved signal to noise ratio, and an improved probe-fitting technique.[3-5]

We demonstrated that the TEOAE technique can be easily administered in a nursery setting by paraprofessionals, supervised by an audiologist.[3,4] Costs of screening are therefore minimized, not only because the test can be easily administered by a paraprofessional, but because the test can be administered quickly.

It is surprising that Bess and Paradise question whether treatment for hearing impairment is efficacious. Although it is agreed that there are studies that have not demonstrated a positive effect of intervention on hearing-impaired children, the literature overwhelmingly reports the negative effects of mild, moderate, severe and profound hearing loss on child communicative development and the positive effects of medical, audiologic, and education intervention.[6-10]

In terms of availability and accessibility of services, it would appear critical that we as professionals in health care, audiology, and education develop strategies to provide cost-effective services for these infants and their families. I agree that poor compliance for follow-up and intervention is a societal problem that we must aggressively address. Families who are noncompliant tend to be poor, non-English speaking, single parent, and lack transportation. A newborn predischarge screen is one mechanism for beginning to address access barriers to this health care problem.

The issue of early versus late treatment for hearing impairment is supported by theory, i.e., the negative impact on the natural course of language development imposed by a hearing loss and published reports.[8-11] Studies that have documented speech and language delays secondary to mild hearing loss associated with otitis media during infancy also support the concept that early hearing impairments, if not addressed, will result in significant negative effects on speech and language.[12,13]

Finally, the overall issue of whether health care professionals should support universal hearing screening is in my opinion self-evident. Newborn metabolic screening for disorders such as phenylketonuria, hypothyroidism, and sickle cell disease are well accepted, despite the fact that they have lower prevalence rates than hearing impairment, and there are similar issues regarding follow-up for diagnostic tests, compliance for treatment, and efficacy of treatment.

In conclusion, it is imperative for health care professionals to advocate for infants and children with hearing impairment and to strive to provide the best possible care through universal hearing, screening, habilitation, and intervention services.

Betty R. Vohr, M.D.
Rhode Island Hearing Assessment Program
Department of Pediatrics
Women and Infants' Hospital
Providence, RI 02905

References

1. Bess, F.H., Paradise, J.L. Universal screening for infant hearing impairment: not simple, not risk-free, not necessarily beneficial, and not presently justified. *Pediatrics*. 1994;93:330-334

2. National Institutes of Health Consensus Development Conference on Early Identification of Hearing Impairments in Infants and Young Children. March 1-3, 1993

3. White, K.R., Vohr, B.R., Behrens, T.R. Universal newborn hearing screening using transient evoked otoacoustic emissions: results of the Rhode Island Hearing Assessment Project. *Semin Hear*. 1993;14:18-29

4. White, K.R., Vohr, B.R., Maxon, A.B., Behrens, T., Mauk, G. Screening all newborns for hearing loss transient evoked otoacoustic emissions. *Int J Pediatr Otorhinolaryngol*. In press

5. Chang, K.W., Vohr, B.R., Norton, S.J., Lekas, M.D. External and middle ear status related to evoked otoacoustic emission in neonates. *Arch Otolaryngol Head Neck Surg*. 1993;119:276-282

6. Davis, J.M., Elfenbein, J., Schum, D., Bentler, R.A. Effects of mild and moderate hearing impairment on language, educational, and psychosocial behavior of children. *J Speech Hear Disorder*. 1986;51:53-62

7. Bess, F.H., Tharpe, A.M., Gibler, A. Auditory performance of children with unilateral sensorineural hearing impairment. *Ear Hear*. 1986;7: 20-26

8. Ross, M. Implications of delay in detection and management of deafness. *Volta Rev*. 1990;92:69-79

9. Markides, A. Age at fitting of hearing aids and speech intelligibility. *Br J Audiol*. 1986;20:165-168

10. Bess, F.H., Klee, T., Culbertson, J.L. Identification, assessment and management of children with unilateral sensorineural hearing loss. *Ear Hear*. 1986,7:43-51

11. Madell, J.R. Identification and treatment of very young children with hearing loss. *Infants Young Child*. 1988;1:20-30

12. Teele, D.W., Klein, J.O., Rosner, B.A. Otitis media with effusion during the first three years of life and development of speech and language. *Pediatrics*. 1984;74:282

13. Friel-Patti, S., Finitzo-Heber, T., Conti, G.,Brown, C.K. Language delay in infants associated with middle ear disease and mild, fluctuating hearing impairment. *Pediatr Infect Dis J*. 1982;1:104

To the Editor—

The importance of early identification of hearing loss is summarized in the report issued by the United States (US) Department of Health and Human Services,[1] entitled "Healthy People 2000." The goal is to reduce the average age at which children with significant hearing impairment are identified to no more than 12 months. The report states:

> The future of a child born with significant hearing impairment depends to a very large degree on early identification (i.e., audiological diagnosis before 12 months of age) followed by immediate and appropriate intervention. If hearing-impaired children are not identified early, it is difficult, if not impossible, for many of them to acquire the fundamental language, social, and cognitive skills that provide the foundation for later schooling and success in society. When early identification and intervention occur, hearing-impaired children make dramatic progress, are more successful in school, and become more productive members of society. The earlier intervention and habilitation begins, the more dramatic the benefits (p. 460).

On the average, children in the US with severe to profound hearing impairment are not identified until 24 to 30 months of age, while children with milder, yet nonetheless, significantly detrimental hearing losses frequently are not identified until they are 5 to 6 years of age.[1,2] It is also alarming that only about 3% of all children born in the US participate in any type of newborn hearing-screening program.[3] The Joint Committee on Infant Hearing is in the process of revising their position on infant screening. Their 1990 Position Statement recommended hearing screening only for infants who exhibit one or more of ten risk factors for hearing loss.[4] However, recent research has revealed that as many of half of all children with bilateral severe-to-profound hearing losses have not exhibited any of the high-risk factors.[5,6]

The September 28, 1993 draft of the Joint Committee on Infant Hearing Position Statement recognizes these findings and states:[7]

> Because normal hearing is critical for speech and oral language development as early as the first six months of life, hearing loss in infants must be identified before three months of age. To acquire access to most infants, the Joint Committee on Infant Hearing recommends screening infants prior to hospital discharge from the newborn nursery.
>
> . . . a method of hearing screening must be able to identify infants with hearing losses of 30 dB HL and greater in one or both ears, in the frequency region important for speech

recognition (approximately 500 through 4000 Hz). Of the various approaches to newborn hearing screening currently available, two physiologic measures [auditory brainstem response (ABR) and otoacoustic emissions (OAE)] most nearly achieve this goal.

In addition to the National Institutes of Health Consensus Statement in support of universal hearing screening,[8] it is clear that many professionals from different disciplines now believe the time has come to support universal hearing screening. Much of the recent support has come as a result of studies showing that OAEs are capable of identifying infants with hearing loss of approximately 30 dB HL and greater.[9-13]

I have personal admiration for Doctors Bess and Paradise and their long-standing contributions to our understanding of effects of hearing disorders on children. However, I must express concern with their conclusions about the validity, predictive value, cost, practicability, and efficacy of using evoked otoacoustic emissions (EOAEs) for mass screening for infant hearing impairment, which led them to write the article entitled "Universal Screening for Infant Hearing Impairment: Not Simple, Not Risk-Free, Not Necessarily Beneficial, and Not Presently Justified."[14]

Doctors Bess and Paradise make some assumptions regarding prevalence of hearing loss, sensitivity, and specificity of TEOAE measures, use of the ABR for the second screen, and data taken from "laboratory" conditions for testing newborns under the heading of "Validity and Predictive Value." I respectfully disagree with their assumptions.

Although prevalence of bilateral profound hearing loss in children has historically been reported as 1 to 1.3/1000, our population of interest is unilateral/bilateral mild to profound sensorineural hearing loss where the prevalence is estimated to be 1.5 to 6/1000.[13,15,16] For mathematical examples I will use the prevalence of 5.95/1000 reported by White and Behrens (1993).[13] They also reported that sensitivity of TEOAEs approaches 100%, based on behavioral audiological evaluations as the "gold standard."[13]

Recent data on specificity is much better than reported in early studies.[17] The Rhode Island Hearing Assessment Project utilizes EOAE as the initial infant screen and has now screened over 23,000 newborns since February 1990. With their experience, software and hardware modifications, and improved clinical techniques, specificity has improved to above 90% for the initial screen. Their latest technique includes an immediate recheck for collapsed canals or ears occluded with vernix caseosa for the initial EOAE screen.

When the initial screening result is "fail" the recheck includes replacing the disposable tip on the probe and rescreening immediately. This procedure yielded a fail rate of only 4.9% for 1223 infants tested at Women's and Infants Hospital (November through December 1993, K.R. White and B.R. Vohr, personal communication, 1993-1994).[17] The average fail rate for other hospitals in the Rhode Island Project varies, depending on the length of screening experience, but averages 8.4%. These fail rates cover all births regardless of when they were discharged from the hospital and includes the categories of both "fail" and "partial pass." Their screening procedures are accomplished in nurseries with background noise levels of 45 to 60 dBA, not unrealistic "laboratory" type sound treated rooms. Usually it is the infants own noise (breathing, etc) that prolongs the test time beyond 1 minute. However, if other sounds are problematic, a quiet isolette with a lid reduces the ambient noise levels to 45 to 50 dBA. In addition, the "fail" rate for the second EOAE screens accomplished 2 to 6 weeks later is only 9% of those failing the initial screen. Hospital nursery employees such as trained assistants or clerks perform the screening before discharge. Audiologists interpret test results from computer files and schedule rechecks and follow-up.

As an example of a three-step screening program to meet the goals of the Joint Committee, consider the following cost estimates using fail rates and prevalence of hearing loss from the Rhode Island project (based on 1000 live births).

In their article Bess and Paradise calculated the cost to screen 4 million live births at approximately 200 million dollars. The yield would be 4000 hearing-impaired children at a cost of $50,000 per identified child. We would estimate the cost to be 144 million to identify 23,800 hearing-impaired children at a cost of $6,045 per identified child (only 12% of the Bess and Paradise estimate).

The comments of Bess and Paradise about efficacy are surprising. First they admit that "Much theoretical understanding, intuitive belief, and clinical experience argue in favor of efficacy."(p. 332) Then they conclude that, "Nonetheless no direct evidence demonstrates conclusively that intervention appropriate by current standards results in more good than harm to the child and the family." If they truly believe that current evidence is not sufficiently "conclusive" for universal newborn screening, why then, is it "conclusive" enough for screening at risk infants? Are we less concerned about "harm" to families of at risk children than to families of children not at risk? Interested readers may wish to review the article by Kuhl et al[17] in addition to the eight publications supporting early intervention cited by Bess and Paradise.

If one accepts the premise that early identification of hearing loss and appropriate amplification and language stimulation is valuable, one way to measure its value would be in educational savings. If efficacy is measured in terms of statistical outcomes, then indeed, it may be difficult to show that student "X" will score better than student "Y" later on in life on some standard test. However, placement of students in the educational system is based on their performance, and if even a small percentage of children born with hearing loss can reach standard classroom placement, then the overall savings to society will be sufficient to pay for the program.

The following example is offered to show how educational cost savings might offset the costs of universal screening. The cost to educate one child K-12 in a regular classroom is about $44,000 in Rhode Island. The cost for a hearing- impaired child in a self-contained class is $126,000 and $429,000 in a residential school. By dividing the cost to identify each hearing-impaired child by the cost difference between education in a regular versus self-contained classroom and multiplying the quotient by 100, one can estimate the percent of early identified hearing-impaired children that would need to be educated in regular classrooms in place of self-contained classrooms for the universal screening/diagnostic program to pay for itself in educational savings. For example, $6,045 ÷ [$126,000 − $44,000] ˜ 100 = 7.4%. As a second example, if only

Procedure	Number	Charge ($)	Total ($)
First OAE screen (Fail rate 8%)	1000	30.00	30,000.00
Second OAE screen80 (Fail rate 10%)		30.00	2,400.00

Test battery on eight infants per 1000 who fail both OAE screens:

• Threshold ABR including sedation	$270.00
• Audiologic pediatric evaluation	54.00
• High frequency tympanometry	21.00
• ENT consult	101.00
Total Charge	$446.00

Total newborn screens = $32,400 + 8 diagnostics (3,568)	= $35,968.00
Cost per newborn for screens and diagnostic: $35,968/1000	= $36.00
Cost per infant with sensorineural hearing loss: $35,968/5.95	= $6,045.00

2% of children identified early could be educated in self-contained classes rather than residential schools, the identification program would pay for itself.

The views expressed here, I believe, are in concert with clinicians who have extensive hands-on experience with testing infants, children, and adults with EOAEs. We have found EOAE measures to yield frequency-specific data and to be simple, quick, noninvasive, objective, sensitive, and cost-efficient. Accurate measurements do not require highly-skilled personnel. Results of mass screening have demonstrated success in identifying large numbers of infants with impaired hearing.

Clearly we have reached the point where the usefulness of OAEs as a universal newborn hearing screening tool should be considered. The questions that remain pertain to refining the method, optimizing the procedures, expanding the availability of services, and the development of models of service delivery to match national demographics.

Martin S. Robinette, Ph.D.
Mayo Clinic
Rochester, NY 55905

References

1. US Department of Health and Human Services *Healthy People 2000: National Health Promotion and Disease Prevention Objectives*. Washington, DC: Public Health Service; 1990
2. Commission on Education of the Deaf. *Towards Equality: Education of the Deaf*. Washington, DC: US Government Printing Office;1988
3. Bess, F.H., Hall, J.W. *Screening Children for Auditory Function*. Nashville, TN: Bill Wilkerson Center Press; 1992
4. Joint Committee on Infant Hearing (1990). Position statement. *ASHA*. 1991;33(suppl 5):3-6
5. Elssmann, S.F., Matkin, N.D., Sabo, M.P. Early identification of congenital sensorineural hearing impairment. *Hear J*. 1987;40:13-17
6. Mauk, G.W., White, K.R., Mortensen, L.B., Behrens, T.R. The effectiveness of screening programs based on high-risk characteristics in early identification of hearing impairment. *Ear Hear*. 1991;12:312-319
7. Draft: Tuesday, September 28, 1993. Joint Committee on Infant Hearing 1993 Position Statement, pp. 1-11
8. NIH Consensus Statement. *Early Identification of Hearing Impairment in Infants and Young Children*. March 1-3, 1993;11:1-24
9. Bonfils, P., Uziel, A., Pujol, R. Screening for auditory dysfunction in infants by evoked otoacoustic emissions. *Arch Otolaryngol Head Neck Surg*. 1988;114:887-890
10. Stevens, J., Webb, H., Hutchinson, J., Connell, J., Smith, M., Buffin, J. Click evoked otoacoustic emis-

sions compared to brainstem electric response. *Arch Dis Child*. 1989;64:1105-1111

11. Stevens, J., Webb, H., Hutchinson, J., Connell, J., Smith, M., Buffin, J. Click evoked otoacoustic emissions in neonatal screening. *Ear Hear*. 1990; 11:128-133

12. Kennedy, C., Kimm, L., Dees, D., Evans, P., Hunter, M., Lenton, S., Thornton, A. Otoacoustic emissions and auditory brainstem responses in the newborn. *Arch Dis Child*. 1991;66:1124-1129

13. White, K.R., Behrens, T.R., eds. The Rhode Island Hearing Assessment Project: Implications for Universal Newborn Hearing Screening. *Seminars in Hearing*. 1993;14:1-119

14. Bess, F.H., Paradise, J.L. Universal screening for infant hearing impairment: not simple, not risk-free, not necessarily beneficial, and not presently justified. *Pediatrics*. 1994;93:330-334

15. Watkin, P., Baldwin, M., McEnery, G. Neonatal at risk screening and the identification of deafness. *Arch Dis Child*. 1991;66:1130-1135

16. Parving, A. Congenital hearing disability-epidemiology and identification: a comparison between two health authority districts. *Int J Pediatr Otolaryngol*. 1993;27:29-46

17. Kuhl, P.K., Williams, K.A., Lacerda, F., Stephens, K.N., Lindbloom, B. Linguistic experience alters phonetics perception in infants by six months of age. *Science*. 1992;255:606-608

To the Editor.—

Neonatal hearing screening has come to the forefront of interest within our professional communities and among the general public, particularly over the last year. Identifying children with hearing loss at the earliest age possible, however, has been a long-standing tenet of audiologists, pediatricians, otolaryngologists, and early childhood specialists, based both on knowledge of developmental processes and abundant clinical experiences. Indeed, the identification of conditions present in early childhood that can result in long-term disabilities are critical components of current legislative (Individuals with Disabilities Education Act [IDEA], Part H Public Law 102-119 [formerly 99-457])[1] and public health initiatives (Healthy People 2000).[2] Subsequent intervention has been shown to positively influence outcome when such programs are initiated in early life.[3] Moreover, congenital or early-onset, sensory or neurologic disorders that result in long-term developmental disabilities are known to be more costly to society when such deficits are first detected at older ages. Thus, the concept of hearing screening programs designed to identify debilitating hearing loss in early childhood is well founded. Both the National Institutes of Health (NIH) Consensus Statement[4] and the Joint Committee on Infant Hearing (JCIH) Position Statement[5] (currently in revision) reflect this challenge of the identification of hearing loss as early in life as possible.

Recently, in their commentary in *Pediatrics* entitled "Universal Screening for Infant Hearing Impairment: Not Simple, Not Risk-Free, Not Necessarily Beneficial, and Not Presently Justified," Bess and Paradise[6] raised important and relevant questions regarding the concept of mass screening for hearing loss in the neonatal period. Their letter was motivated by the Consensus Panel Statement that resulted from the NIH Conference of March 1 through 3, 1993. Among other recommendations, the Panel advised that universal hearing screening of all newborns be implemented; preferably before hospital discharge, but no later than 3 months of age. Specifically, the Panel recommended that evoked otoacoustic emissions (EOAE) be used as the first-level screening procedure, followed by auditory brainstem response (ABR) screening of all infants who failed the EOAE screen.

Bess and Paradise articulated numerous practical and fiscal concerns about these recommendations. Moreover, Bess and Paradise argued that insufficient empirical evidence exists to support the sweeping recommendations for universal neonatal hearing screening and a two-stage screening protocol. They further argued that neither the instrumentation currently available, nor the testing and follow-up protocols suggested met the rigorous prerequisites necessary for instituting any screening initiative. Bess and Paradise specifically questioned: 1) the simplicity, efficiency, reliability and predictive value of the screening devices/ protocols recommended; 2) the availability, accessibility, and efficacy of treatment options; 3) the provisions for ensuring compliance with follow-up for infants who failed screening; 4) whether thorough cost analyses of the recommendations had been completed *a priori*; and most importantly, 5) whether neonatal hearing screening was "risk-free" when measured in human terms (the unnecessary worrying of parents/caregivers in cases of false-positive outcomes).

As the three pediatric audiologists who served as members of the Planning Committee for the NIH Consensus Development Conference, we deem it important to address the comments of Bess and Paradise in light of our participation in, and perceptions of, the NIH Conference and the subsequent Consensus Statement. The body of evidence presented by numerous respected scientists and clinicians over the 2-day period that led to the development of the NIH Position Statement was clear. The following facts appear, then and now, irrefutable: 1) our current models for the identification of potentially-disabling hearing loss in infancy and early childhood are inadequate. For example, the use of the High-Risk Register[5] for the identification of infants and young children at risk for hearing loss followed by the direct auditory screening of those so designated[7] identifies only about 50% of young children who have congenital or early-onset permanent hearing loss;[8-11] 2) except for the neonatal period, our current health-care delivery system provides us no other opportunity to pursue an organized, direct screen of hearing until children enter the public school system—for most, at about 5 to 6 years of age; 3) although delayed language and speech development are the primary indicators of a hearing disability, most parents and primary care providers do not suspect hearing loss as a possible etiology. Most primary care providers lack sufficient information regarding normal communication development and early-onset hearing loss, neither do the majority of providers systematically evaluate speech, language or hearing during routine well-baby visits;[12-14] 4) in the United States, the average age when permanent hearing disabilities are identified remains at about 18 months for severe to profound bilateral impairments and as late as 60 months for unilateral impairments or bilateral losses of lesser degree.[11] Although the prevalence of bilateral profound hearing loss has been historically reported as 1:1000 live births, the target population also includes mild to moderate losses/unilateral losses. For these degrees of permanent impairment, prevalence estimates are higher (1.5 to 6 per 1000 births[15,16]). Thus, our goal remains to identify these children before school age and the onset of costly academic failure and/or the need for special service provision; 5) instrumentation (e.g., EOAE and automated ABR) is available and currently undergoing rapid technological improvement, thereby affording simple, relatively risk-free, and cost-effective screening device options for clinicians pursuing the initiation of neonatal hearing screening programs.

We agree with Bess and Paradise that experience and research with well-devised and implemented mass neonatal hearing screening programs is needed before many important questions can be thoroughly addressed. Some of these authors' concerns, such as treatment efficacy, however, will likely not be amenable to empirical study because of ethical and moral concerns. We cannot imagine knowingly withholding intervention from a group of young children with hearing loss as part of a planned, prospective, case-control investigation designed to determine the age and audiometric variables that significantly influ-

ence communicative/ developmental outcome. It would seem unlikely that an Institutional Review Board or more importantly, an informed parent, would agree to deny intervention (amplification, aural habilitation, medical monitoring and parent counseling) to a young child identified as having a permanent hearing loss. The risk-benefit ratio for such a protocol would preclude such a circumstance. The exact "formula" for determining *which* children may suffer significant, long-standing consequences will likely be determined by the synergistic interaction of the specific degree, configuration, type and age of onset of the hearing loss, as well as the specific set of intrinsic and extrinsic factors each *individual* child brings to this unique developmental equation.

Simply viewed, the NIH Consensus Panel had two choices: maintain the status quo or set a vision for the future. The Panel, composed of both professionals and the lay public, opted for the latter. Further, the Consensus Panel determined from the data presented that current technology would allow the direct and accurate screening of hearing in very young children. One could argue that the cause might have been better served if the Panel had been less specific about the test protocol and time lines, for example, while placing more emphasis on the development of site-specific innovative alternative approaches to the early identification of hearing loss. Hindsight not withstanding, the NIH Consensus Panel took an important, decisive and knowingly controversial position on newborn hearing screening.

The importance of Bess and Paradise's critical commentary on this important topic is appreciated. Their article has challenged professionals to re-examine positions, long-held beliefs, and current screening initiatives. We also believe, however, that such commentary should not dissuade professionals from aggressively pursuing the vision of universal early identification and amelioration of hearing loss. This goal must be maintained as one of our most important clinical challenges. To suggest otherwise would be to deny that optimal child development is facilitated by the rich and abundant input provided through hearing.

Judith S. Gravel, Ph.D.
Albert Einstein College of Medicine and the Montefiore Medical Center Bronx, NY

Allan O. Diefendorf, Ph.D.
Indiana University School of Medicine Indianapolis, IN

Noel D. Matkin, Ph.D.
Children's Hearing Clinic University of Arizona Tucson, AZ

References

1. Early intervention programs for infants and toddlers with handicaps: final regulations. *Fed Reg*. 1989;54:(#119)26306-26348

2. Healthy People 2000. United States Department of Health and Human Services, Public Health Service. *Healthy People 2000: National Health Promotion and Disease Prevention Objectives*. Washington, DC: US Government Printing Office; 1990

3. Infant Health and Development Program. Enhancing the outcomes of low-birth-weight, premature infants. A multisite, randomized trial. *JAMA*. 1990;263:3035-3042

4. NIH Consensus Panel Report. Newsletter. *Ambulatory Pediatr Assoc*. 1993;29:18-28

5. Joint Committee on Infant Hearing. 1990 Position Statement. *AAP News*. April 1991;7:6,14. Reprinted in *Policy Reference Guide*, 6th edition. Elk Grove Village, IL: American Academy of Pediatrics; 1993:343-346

6. Bess, F.H., Paradise, J. Universal screening for infant hearing impairment: not simple, not risk-free, not necessarily beneficial, and not presently justified. *Pediatrics*. 1994;93:330-334

7. American Speech-Language-Hearing Association. Guidelines for audiologic screening of newborn infants who are at-risk for hearing impairment. *ASHA* 1989;31:89-92

8. Mahoney, T.M., Eichwald, J.G. The ups and "Downs" of high-risk hearing screening: The Utah statewide program. *Semin Hear*. 1987;8: 155-163

9. Epstein, S., Reilly, J.S. Sensorineural hearing loss. *Pediatr Clin North Am*. 1989;36:1501-1520

10. Stein, L., Clark, S., Kraus, N. The hearing-impaired infant: patterns of identification and habilitation. *Ear Hear*. 1983;4:232-236

11. Elssmann, S., Matkin, N., Sabo, M. Early identification of congenital sensorineural hearing impairment. *Hear J*. 1987;9:13-17

12. Shah, C., Chandler, D., Dale, R. Delay in referral of children with impaired hearing. *Volta Rev*. 1978;80:207

13. Kenworthy, O.T., Triggs, E., Perrin, J., Bess, F. Current-screening practices of primary care physicians. Paper presented at the Conference on Otitis Media and Development: Screening, Referral and Treatment. 1987; Vanderbilt University, Nashville, TN

14. Diefendorf, A.O., Weber, B.A. Identification of hearing loss: programmatic and procedural considerations. In: Roush, J., Matkin, N., eds. *Infants and Toddlers with Hearing Loss: Family- Centered Identification, Assessment and Intervention*. Baltimore, MD: York Press; 1994:43-64

15. White, K.R., Behrens, T.R., eds. The Rhode Island Hearing Assessment Project: implications for universal newborn hearing screening. *Semin Hear*. 1993;14:1-119

16. Watkin, P., Baldwin, M., McEnery, G. Neonatal at risk screening and the identification of deafness. *Arch Dis Child*. 1991;66:1130-1135

To the Editor—

In their recent commentary Bess and Paradise[1] impugn the recommendations of the National Institutes of Health (NIH) Consensus Development Conference on Early Identification of Hearing Impairment in Infants and Young Children (March 1-3, 1993) for universal infant hearing screening. Bess and Paradise challenge the validity and predictive value of the recommended two-sequence screening procedure, evoked otoacoustic emissions (EOAE), and auditory brainstem response (ABR). Although they confirm that EOAE and ABR testing is highly sensitive, they contend that the specificity and positive predictive value of these procedures are problematic. To illustrate their concern, Bess and Paradise report a hypothetical outcome of hearing screening all 4 million infants born annually in the United States per the recommended NIH procedure. Bess and Paradise apparently base their calculations on test sensitivity of 100%, test specificity of 90%, and prevalence of 1:1000 births. They calculate that 43,960 infants will be referred for comprehensive evaluation to detect 4000 infants who are truly hearing-impaired (39,960 false-positives), an over-referral of almost 10 normally-hearing infants for every infant with hearing loss.

This calculation exaggerates the problem of over-referral. First, Bess and Paradise cite an inaccurate prevalence estimate. Prevalence of hearing impairment in infants is considerably >1:1000 births. This prevalence rate refers only to well-babies who are profoundly deaf and fails to account for prevalence of hearing-impairment in infants at-risk for developmental disabilities and well-babies with moderate-to-severe sensorineural hearing loss. Based on results from infant hearing screening studies, 5.5 to 6 per 1000 is a more accurate estimate of prevalence of moderate, severe, and profound sensorineural hearing loss in infants.[2-5] Second, specificity of both traditional and automated ABR screening exceeds 95%.[6,7] Recalculation of the Bess/Paradise example using more accurate prevalence data (5.7 per 1000) and ABR test specificity (95%) predicts referral of 19,886 normally hearing infants to detect 22,800 infants who are truly hearing-impaired, an over-referral of fewer than one normally-hearing infant for every infant who is truly hearing-impaired.

Implementation of a national universal program for infant hearing screening will undoubtedly require ongoing and substantial professional commitment. Future research on the efficacy of early identification and early intervention strategies will depend on large-scale universal screening programs. Whether or not one agrees with all the NIH Consensus Panel recommendations, the suggested screening protocol is a worthwhile effort to move us in the direction of better and improved methods for early detection of hearing loss.

It is premature and detrimental to conclude that universal hearing screening of infants is not simple, not risk-free, not necessarily beneficial and not presently justified. Screening for sensorineural hearing loss in infants is justified because 1) the disorder of childhood hearing loss is important; 2) currently available screening procedures are safe, effective, simple, reliable, valid, reasonably low cost, and practicable; and 3) treatment is effective.

Jerry L. Northern, Ph.D.
University of Colorado Health Sciences Center
Department of Otolaryngology
Denver, CO 80262

References

1. Bess, F.H., Paradise, J.L. Universal screening for infant hearing: not simple, not risk-free, not necessarily beneficial, and not presently justified. *Pediatrics.* 1994,93:330-334

2. Simmons, F.B. Automated hearing screening test for newborns: the Crib-o-gram. In: Mencher, G., ed. *Early Identification of Hearing Loss.* Basel: Karger; 1976:171-180

3. Galambos, R., Hicks, G., Wilson, M. Hearings loss in graduates of a tertiary intensive care nursery. *Ear Hear.* 1982;3:87-90

4. Hosford-Dunn, H., Johnson, S., Simmons, F.B., Malachowski, N., Low, K. Infant hearing screening: program implementation and validation. *Ear Hear.* 1987;8:12-20

5. White, K.R., Behrens, T.R., eds. The Rhode Island hearing assessment project: implications for universal newborn hearing screening. *Semin Hear.* 1993;14:1-122

6. Hyde, M.L., Riko, K., Malizia, K. Audiometric accuracy of the click ABR in infants and risk for hearing loss. *J Am Acad Audiol.* 1990;1:59-66

7. Jacobson, J., Jacobson, C., Spahr, R.C. Automated and conventional ABR screening techniques in high-risk infants. *J Am Acad Audiol.* 1990;1:187-195

To the Editor.—

In March 1993, the Consensus Panel of the National Institutes of Health (NIH) Consensus Development Conference on Early Identification of Hearing Impairment in Infants and Young Children recommended universal infant hearing screening and reinforced the goal of early intervention for infants with hearing loss. In an editorial commentary, Bess and Paradise opposed the recommendation for universal infant hearing screening and disparaged the benefit and effectiveness of early intervention.[1] I am concerned that pediatricians will underestimate the importance of childhood hearing loss and the effectiveness of early intervention.

Bess and Paradise contend that ". . . no direct evidence demonstrates conclusively that intervention appropriate by current standards results in more good than harm to the child and the family. . . ." Early intervention for infants with hearing loss is delivered in a family-centered approach and includes substantial family support and counseling by a multidisciplinary team, selection, evaluation, fitting and monitoring of appropriate amplification, and auditory and language stimulation. When correctly applied, none of these components results in physical, emotional, or psychological harm to the child or family. On the contrary, establishment of a supportive environment fostered by early intervention promotes child development even in the face of difficult challenges such as deafness.[2]

Bess and Paradise further contend that ". . . no empirical evidence . . . supports the proposition that outcomes in children with congenital hearing loss are more favorable if treatment is begun early in infancy rather than later in childhood. . . ." For ethical reasons, it is not possible to implement a prospective study comparing intervention versus nonintervention in infants with hearing loss. Furthermore, because the average age of identification of infants with hearing loss continues to exceed 12 months,[3-5] a large population of children who benefitted from early (e.g., before 6 months of age) identification is difficult to obtain. Nevertheless, the benefit of early intervention is well-documented. In a thorough longitudinal study of language and communication skills in children with hearing loss, Levitt, McGarr, and Geffner report that, of the many variables examined, the age at which special education began showed the largest effect on the development of language and communication skills.[6] Those children who received early intervention sustained significantly higher speech and language scores than those children for whom intervention was delayed.

Early, appropriate, beneficial, and effective intervention can only occur in the presence of early identification. Current high-risk registry techniques fail to identify at least 50% of babies with hearing loss.[4,7,8] Implementation of universal infant hearing screening is an important first step toward improving outcomes for infants with hearing loss.

Deborah Hayes, Ph.D.
University of Colorado Health Sciences Center
Department of Pediatrics
The Children's Hospital
Denver, CO 80218

References

1. Bess, F.H., Paradise, J.L. Universal screening for infant hearing impairment: not simple, not risk-free, not necessarily beneficial, and not presently justified. *Pediatrics.* 1994;93:330-334

2. First, L.R., Palfrey, J.S. The infant or young child with developmental delay. *N Engl J Med.* 1994;330:478-483

3. Stein, L., Clark, S., Kraus, N. The hearing-impaired infant: patterns of identification and habilitation. *Ear Hear.* 1983;4:232-236

4. Elssmann, S., Matkin, N., Sabo, M. Early identification of congenital sensorineural hearing impairment. *Hear J.* 1987;40:13-17

5. Stein, L., Jabaley, T., Spitz, R., Stoakley, D., McGee, T. The hearing-impaired infant: patterns of identification and habilitation revisited. *Ear Hear.* 1990;11:201-205

6. Levitt, H., McGarr, N.S., Geffner, D. Development of language and communication skills in hearing-impaired children. *ASHA Monographs Number 26.* Rockville, MD: American Speech-Language-Hearing Association; 1987

7. Pappas D. A study of the high-risk registry for sensorineural hearing impairment. *Arch Otolaryngol Head Neck Surg.* 1983;91:41-44

8. Mauk, G., White, K., Mortensen, I., Behrens, T. The effectiveness of screening programs based on high-risk characteristics in early identification of hearing impairment. *Ear Hear.* 1991;12: 312-319

To the Editor.—

Drs Bess and Paradise are to be commended on their timely, intelligent, and well-informed response[1] to the National Institutes of Health (NIH) Consensus Statement[2] that advocates universal screening for infant hearing impairment. I share their concerns and have been arguing along similar lines since the release of the statement.

It is lamentable that so many of the recommendations we make as clinicians involved in the care and habilitation of children with permanently impaired hearing are based on theoretical assumptions, anecdotal evidence, and impressions informed by "clinical experience." Although I advocate strongly for early intervention in the course of patient care, it is disquieting to realize at the same time how little the literature provides in the way of solid empirical support for its effectiveness. In addition, there is a tendency in this literature to overstate the dimensions of the evidence that does exist. For example, Markides[3] reported that children with severe congenital hearing loss who were fit with hearing aids before 6 months of age received higher teacher ratings of speech intelligibility than those fit after this time. This study has, however, been variously cited as showing how early fitting of hearing aids "alleviates or avoids . . . many of the disabling and handicapping consequences of deafness,"[4] or the benefit of such intervention for both "linguistic and cognitive development."[5]

There are certainly formidable obstacles to designing and conducting methodologically rigorous studies in this area. Such studies should nevertheless be supported and undertaken, if for no other reason than that they may provide evidence that will strengthen the case of those who seek to help hearing-impaired children through earlier diagnosis and intervention. The effectiveness of a newborn or infant hearing screening program in enhancing communicational, cognitive, and social competence could be investigated in a large scale randomized clinical trial. Newborns would be assigned at birth to one of three conditions: screening using evoked otoacoustic emissions followed by auditory brainstem response testing, screening by application of high-risk criteria,[6] or no screening, and would then be followed prospectively to at least the mid-elementary school level. Such a study would address directly the potential value of the NIH proposal, and would also provide invaluable data on the development of hearing-impaired infants born to hearing parents. Generally accepted notions of the disadvantages these children face in terms of language development, literacy, and educational attainment could potentially be altered dramatically if their hearing losses were routinely identified in the first months of life.

As the screening debate goes on, we should heed the caution that "widespread implementation of untested methods of early diagnosis make later rigorous evaluation more difficult and less decisive, while discouraging research into alternative strategies in the interim."[7] For the present, there are short- and medium-term goals to be met, including first, to define what the target of screening should be—severe hearing loss? Any degree of loss? Second, we need some idea of the compliance with recommendations for follow-up and intervention that may be expected from parents of an apparently healthy newborn when first informed of the possibility or presence of a severe sensorineural hearing loss. Third, it would be highly desirable to assemble a coherent intervention plan consisting of those measures known to be most efficacious. Apart from amplification, however, it might prove difficult to agree on the components of such a plan due to differences in opinion between various factions in deaf and hard- of-hearing habilitation.

In my opinion, collaborative efforts in the form of research and consultation on the part of those serving children with hearing loss may be more important than getting submerged in a flurry of action related to the implementation of newborn hearing screening programs.

Anton R. Miller, MBCHB, FRCPC
Dept of Pediatrics, University of British Columbia and the Hearing Disorders Program British Columbia's Children's Hospital Vancouver British Columbia V6H 3V4 Canada

References

1. Bess, F.H., Paradise, J.L. Universal screening for infant hearing impairment: not simple, not risk-free, not necessarily beneficial, and not presently justified. *Pediatrics.* 1994,93:330-334

2. NIH Consensus Statement. Early Identification of Hearing Impairment in Infants and Young Children. March 1-3, 1993;11:1-24

3. Markides, A. Age at fitting of hearing aids and speech intelligibility. *Br J Audiol.* 1986;20:165-167

4. Sancho, J., Hughes, E., Davis, A., Haggard, M. Epidemiological basis for screening hearing. In: McCormick, B., ed. *Pediatric Audiology 0-5 years.* London Taylor and Francis; 1988:4

5. Haggard, M.P. Hearing screening in children-state of the art(s). *Arch Dis Child.* 1990;65:1193-1195

6. Joint Committee on Infant Hearing 1990 Position Statement. AAO-HNS Bulletin. March 1991: 15-18

7. Sackett, D.L., Haynes, R.B., Guyatt, G.H., Tugwell, P. *Clinical Epidemiology: A Basic Science for Clinical Medicine.* 2nd ed. Boston: Little, Brown & Co; 1991:167

To the Editor.—

As is the case with the recommendation from the National Institutes of Health Consensus Meeting on Early Hearing Screening, the opinion of the European Concerted Action on Otoacoustic Emissions is to consider it necessary to test sensitivity, specificity, and predictive values of otoacoustic emissions as basis for early hearing screening and subsequent identification of hearing impairment in children in preparation for an earlier and thus optimal rehabilitation of the hearing-impaired. Like Bess and Paradise, we had no doubts about "the desirability of identifying infants with congenital hearing impairment promptly" based on the fact that an untreated hearing loss in "the crucial period for language and speech learning" permanently would reduce "verbal language skills," "the developing auditory nervous system" and in consequence "have harmful effects on social, emotional, cognitive, and academic developments."

The reservations of Bess and Paradise towards introducing a general screening at the moment seem primarily to reflect practical considerations highly conditioned by local circumstances. The United States is a vast country where great economic disparity often leads to a lack of health insurance or even to citizens who are uninsured, leaving many people in the lurch partly because they cannot afford to participate in the follow-up of a screening with identification, and partly because many people living in large, thinly populated areas cannot afford the cost of transportation. Lastly reduced availability of qualified personnel in rural and remote areas will render impossible the treatment necessary after identification. In Europe conditions are more favorable and the socioeconomic reservations are therefore less valid. Should the United States introduce conditions offering the handicapped the same opportunities as those available in Europe, on the whole, these reservations would often vanish.

In regard to the evidence of the value of early start to rehabilitation Bess and Paradise refer to many positive papers, but they claim that one cannot trust that "intervention improves (their) speech-language skills, social and emotional status, and academic performance" since other papers fail to demonstrate any advantage in early intervention. Bess and Paradise find that an uncertainty remains due to selection bias. However, throughout the world identification of congenital deaf children is late thus precluding a systematic evaluation of early intervention. However, morphological changes of the central neural pathways have been demonstrated as a result of an early experimental acoustic deprivation[1] in contrast to an impressive development of phonetic perception during the first 6 months of life.[2] When, as mentioned in the introduction, we as well as Bess and Paradise are convinced of the value of an early start, it stems from the general clinical experience that at least some children seem to profit most effectively from an early start of rehabilitation. In our view it is shameful, as well as unethical, (for economic reasons only) not to give even some of the hearing-impaired children the chance for an optimal rehabilitation and a lifelong improvement in communicative skills and quality of life. Moreover, as regards the projective economic considerations, we can reassure Bess and Paradise that the percentage of children failing the emission screening (the yield) appears to be far less than stated (personal examinations of 5000 newborns).[3] Incidentally, Bess and Paradise account only for the credit side and omit the debit (the retrenchment). For every child rehabilitated in Europe, we estimate that the social expenses in the interval 20 to 60 years is reduced with at least 300,000 United States dollars (in Northern Europe closer to 500,000 to

600,000 United States dollars) and this must be compared to the expenses of the screening effort. As a minimum, 10% of the children will experience an increased (usable) work capacity. Even if the savings in social expenses could not finance the screening, you have to ask firstly, who would refuse treatment of a patient with a 10% chance of healing, and secondly, how do you estimate the value of a better quality of life?

Finally, it would have been valuable if Bess and Paradise would have put forward alternative constructive suggestions to improve early identification and thereby diminish the uncertainty of the statistical effect of early intervention. An example of an alternative approach would be to compare two health authority districts as suggested by Parving.[4]

THE EUROPEAN CONCERTED ACTION ON OTO-ACOUSTIC EMISSIONS

F. Grandori (Italy)
L. Collet (France)
D. Kemp (Great Britain)
G. Salomon (Denmark)
K. Schorn (Germany)
A.R.D. Thornton (Great Britain)

References

1. Eggermont, Bock. *Acta Otolaryngol.* 1986;(suppl 429)
2. Kuhl et al. *Science.* 1992;255:606-608
3. Kok et al. *Audiology.* 1993;32:213-224
4. Parving, A. *Int J Pediat Otolaryngol.* 1993;27:29-46

Universal Screening for Infant Hearing Impairment: A Reply

Fred H. Bess

Division of Hearing and Speech Sciences, Vanderbilt University School of Medicine,
Bill Wilkerson Center, Nashville, TN

Jack L. Paradise

Department of Pediatrics, University of Pittsburgh School of Medicine,
Children's Hospital of Pittsburgh, Pittsburgh, PA

Abbreviations. EOAE, evoked otoacoustic emissions; ABR, auditory brainstem response.

In Reply.—

We are pleased that our challenge[1] of the National Institutes of Health Consensus Conference recommendation[2] that all infants be screened for hearing impairment within the first 3 months of life, and preferably before discharge from the newborn nursery, has generated so much response. We thank Dr Miller for his approving comments and particularly for his suggestions concerning screening-related research. We also welcome the provocative rejoinders from the proposed screening program's advocates, first, because in answering their various criticisms we hope to shed further light on key component issues, and second, because heightened attention in these pages to the problem of hearing loss in young infants can only lead to heightened general vigilance and therefore earlier case detection.

Overview of the Issues

Unarguably, all infants with handicapping degrees of hearing impairment should ideally be identified as early as possible. However, it is important to emphasize at the outset that universal screening within the first 3 months of life will identify relatively few infants with hearing impairment who would not have been identified by screening all newborns who meet high-risk-register criteria[3] and/or are admitted to an intensive-care nursery (HRR/ICN infants). On the other hand, the added cost of universal screening—in monetary terms and, more importantly, in harm done—could be immense.

Collectively, the respondents advocating an early infant screening program have underrated the problems it would pose in implementation and follow-through,

overstated its potential benefits, and virtually ignored its indirect costs and risks.

Regarding *implementation and follow-through,* the advocates have glossed over complex issues involving in-hospital personnel requirements and logistics, particularly in the face of the rapidly growing, if not virtually universal practice of discharging newborns within 24 to 48 hours of birth. They have also largely failed to address procedures for fulfilling standard screening-program requirements, particularly 1) assuring in advance the availability of adequate resources—facilities, personnel, and financing—for accomplishing recommended interventions; 2) establishing and maintaining mechanisms for maximizing and monitoring compliance; and 3) educating and counseling parents of infants with false-positive test results and evaluating the near- and long-term impact of those results.

In projecting *benefits,* the advocates have, variously, 1) broadened the definition of handicapping hearing loss to include children with milder degrees of sensorineural loss (in whom untoward developmental effects, and the effectiveness of early intervention, are uncertain) thereby arriving at higher estimates of prevalence than the 0.1% (1:1000) rate we used in calculating expected outcomes of the recommended screening protocol; 2) neglected to distinguish between cases in which hearing loss is present at birth and therefore would be potentially detectable by the screening program proposed, and cases in which hearing loss develops only later and therefore would not be detectable by screening early in infancy; 3) failed to note that relatively early identification is already being accomplished in many locales; 4) projected more optimistic estimates of the validity of the proposed screening protocol than are justified by a comprehensive overview of experience to date, 5) failed to make clear the differences to be expected in cost-yield relationships between screening HRR/ICN infants and screening healthy, non-HRR/ICN infants; and 6) assumed a greater degree of certainty about the efficacy of early intervention for infants with hearing impairment than is justified by available evidence.

Regarding *costs and risks*, the respondents advocating universal screening have failed to confront the fact that, of the hundreds of thousands of initial test failures by infants each year that would result from the proposed screening program, over 95% would be false-positives by even the most optimistic estimates of test validity. Thus, few of the advocates mentioned, and none acknowledged as substantial concerns, the quantum of needless parental anxiety, potentially harmful labeling, and other psychological disturbance that the proposed program might generate among families of normally-hearing infants. Finally, none of the advocates adverted to another, more consequential risk of universal infant screening that we cited in our commentary[1], namely, the risk of unnecessary or harmful diagnostic procedures or treatments carried out on children.

Individual Issues

Here we address, summarizing for brevity, the various arguments advanced by the respondents advocating universal screening. Parentheses indicate by whom the respective arguments were advanced.

Prevalence of Hearing Loss

Respondent argument: If one includes mild to moderate unilateral and bilateral sensorineural hearing loss, the overall prevalence may be as high as 0.6%, rather than the 0.1% rate that we used (Gravel et al; Hall; Northern; Robinette). Including mild to moderate loss is justified by studies showing speech and language delays secondary to the mild conductive loss that accompanies otitis media (Vohr).

Reply: True prevalence is poorly understood. Prevalence rates will vary depending on the population tested, the type and degree of hearing loss, the tests used to measure hearing, and the ages at which the hearing tests were administered. As noted previously, the higher estimates of prevalence cited include cases in which sensorineural loss would not yet have developed or been detectable during early infancy.

Regarding mild to moderate hearing loss, studies attributing speech and language delays to mild conductive loss secondary to otitis media have had major limitations and cannot be considered conclusive.[4-6] For that reason, and because the developmental effects of

milder degrees of sensorineural loss also are uncertain, it seems inappropriate at present to include infants with such loss in the target population of any screening program.

Regarding moderate to profound unilateral and bilateral sensorineural loss—for which we agree screening would be justified if the screening protocol gave satisfactory outcomes—prevalence in the ICN is around 2 to 4%,[7-9] whereas estimates of prevalence in the well-baby nursery range from 0.05 to 0.1%,[8-11] i.e., about 1/40 , the prevalence in the ICN.

Identification of Hearing Loss

Respondent argument: Half or more of the children with significant hearing impairment are not identified by the HRR (Dennis et al; Gravel et al; Hayes; Robinette).

Reply: There is no assurance that a universal screening program would identify many or most of such children not identified by the HHR. Many cases of significant hearing impairment are not present at birth. Some that develop later—e.g., as a consequence of genetic abnormality, congenital or postnatal infection, exposure to ototoxic drugs, or persistent pulmonary hypertension—would ordinarily not be detectable by any type of newborn screening.[12-15] Further, some of the cases not identified by the HRR would be identified by routinely screening all babies in the ICN. For example, in the Rhode Island project, to be discussed in greater detail later, eight of the 11 cases identified as having sensorineural hearing loss were HRR/ ICN infants.[18]

Respondent argument: On average, children in the United States with severe to profound hearing impairment are not identified until approximately 2fi years of age (Koop, Robinette).

Reply: That statistic was also cited in the NIH Consensus Statement.[2] However, indications exist that the average age of identification of such children is decreasing in many locales, probably due to increased screening of HRR/ ICN infants and to enhanced awareness of hearing loss on the part of families, pediatricians, and other primary-care providers. Recently the reported average age of identification has been less than 11 months in Utah,[17] 14 months in the Chicago area,[18] and 16 to 17 months at Boys Town Institute.[19] Currently, the average age is 14 to 16 months at the Bill Wilkerson Center in Nashville. Thus it appears that, even without universal screening, we may be closing in on Dr Koop's goal of 12 months by the year 2000.

Advantages of Screening Newborns

Respondent argument: Our current health care system provides no opportunity for systematic screening of children's hearing until the children enter the public school system; most primary-care providers do not routinely evaluate hearing at well-baby visits (Gravel et al). Universal hearing screening before discharge from the newborn nursery would relieve physicians of the obligation to arrange systematic screening subsequently (Stewart and Davis-Freeman).

Reply: As noted previously, many cases of sensorineural hearing loss are not present or detectable in the newborn period. Therefore, passing the newborn screen may, in some cases, impart a false sense of security, and testing will of necessity be required at later ages to achieve optimal identification. Clearly, far greater efforts than have been applied heretofore need to be applied toward educating both primary health care providers and parents to be on the alert for hearing loss in infants. The monetary costs of such efforts should be far less than the costs of a universal newborn screening program. Physicians' offices, hospital clinics, public health well-baby clinics, and day-care centers constitute settings in which such educational efforts could logically take place. That the average age of identification has been reduced in some locales speaks to the possibility that such efforts can be successful.

Test Performance of the Proposed 2-Stage Screening Protocol

Respondent argument: The evoked otoacoustic emissions (EOAE) test, the first stage of the proposed 2-stage test protocol, is a better screening test than we indicated in our commentary.[1] We failed to reference the appropriate supporting research (Koop). The percentage of infants failing EOAE screening is far lower than the 10% value we projected[1] (European Concerted Action Group). Moreover, newer data from the Rhode Island project—the pilot project on whose results the NIH Consensus Statement recommendations were largely based—show better results than the 27% first-stage failure rate reported originally;[16] the rate is currently down to 8.6% statewide (Vohr) and 5% at Women and Infants Hospital of Rhode Island (Robinette and personal communication, Betty R. Vohr, MD).

Reply: Other than those from the Rhode Island project, the studies of EOAE testing cited by Dr Koop[11,20-22] were carried out under controlled conditions by skilled examiners; one cannot assume that comparable results would be obtained under standard nursery conditions by paraprofessionals. These studies indeed documented high levels of test sensitivity, but the test failure rates averaged about 20%. Other investigators[23-25] have reported failure rates of 22 to 43% if testing is conducted during the first 24 hours of life; one group concluded that newborns should not be screened before 4 days of age.[25] Even after the first few days of life, other centers have reported findings far different from those now being cited from Rhode Island; EOAE failure rates at these centers have ranged from 33 to 78%.[26-29] Because increasingly in the United States most normal newborns are discharged by 2 days, or even 1 day of age, it seems unlikely that EOAE failure rates nationwide would be much lower than the range of values just cited. Finally, one must note that a test failure rate even as low as 5%, combined with a prevalence even as high as 2:1000, would result in 96% of the test failures being false-positives.

Respondent argument: Contrary to our admonition that auditory brain stem response (ABR) testing is problematic, ABR techniques, both conventional and automated, are readily accepted by most clinicians (Dennis et al; Hall; Northern). The specificity of ABR screening, the second stage of the proposed 2-stage protocol, is not 90%, as both the NIH Consensus Statement[2] and we had cited,[1] but, rather, at least 95% (Northern; Raffin and Matz; Stewart and Davis-Freeman).

Reply: To be acceptable, a screening tool should be simple and easily and quickly operated, and its findings should be easy to interpret. Conventional ABR testing does not meet those criteria, although automated ABR testing probably does. The data suggesting that the specificity of ABR testing is as high as 95% were collected in university-based hospital programs on small and biased samples—i.e., mostly high-risk infants—by skilled audiologists whose clinical and academic interests have centered on auditory electrodiagnosis.[30-34] Specificity values are likely to be substantially lower when ABR testing is carried out on large numbers of normal infants in community hospitals by paraprofessional personnel.[35] Here even the estimate of 90% may be overly optimistic. Beyond specificity values, it is well known that the proportion of children eventually shown to have sensorineural hearing loss is lower than early life ABR failure rates would indicate.[10,21,36]

Respondent argument: Failure rates for automated ABR testing in the well-baby population are 5% or less, resulting in substantially lower over-referral rates than the 99% value cited both in the NIH Consensus Statement[2] and in our commentary[1] (Dennis et al; Hall).

Reply: Failure rates as low as 5% have been reported in two papers recently at seminars.[37-38] Whether these values can be replicated on a larger-scale basis with nonprofessional staff has not yet been determined. Typically, more errors can be expected with routine screening.[39]

Practicability of the Screening Protocol

Respondent argument: EOAE testing can be easily and quickly performed in a nursery setting by paraprofessionals, supervised by an audiologist (Vohr).

Reply: That paraprofessionals in the Rhode Island project are supervised by audiologists is but one indicator that an EOAE screening program in a hospital nursery is not to be undertaken lightly or without substantial commitment. The following excerpts from a description of the Rhode Island program by its developers[40] provide further insight into what may be called for:

". . . regular monitoring of all screeners . . . (was) critical. . . . Screeners who worked fewer than 10 hours per week . . . produced a comparatively high percentage of invalid results. . . . Testing could be accomplished more rapidly if low-frequency background noise was reduced. . . . It was also important to attempt to reduce the infant physiological noise that occurs because of mucus, loud sucking, whimpering, respiratory distress, or crying. . . . Infants were. . . snugly swaddled with a blanket and patted and caressed until an appropriate state was achieved. . . . If the infant remained restless, a pacifier was offered and the lights were dimmed. If none of these maneuvers produced the desired results, the infant was rescheduled for later in the day or the following day. Recognizing the key factors in the infant's behavior that indicated a probability of completing a valid screen in a reasonable time was an ongoing challenge for the scheduling and screening staff. . . . Screening every live birth for hearing loss . . . involves all aspects of existing hospital procedures, staffing arrangements, and facilities. . . . It is absolutely essential to have systematic training and certification of screeners as well as regular monitoring (by an audiologist) thereafter. If these steps are not taken, there will be an unnecessarily high rate of invalid results. . . ."

Costs and Risks

Respondent argument: The costs of newborn hearing screening are relatively low. We accept as necessary the costs of screening for phenylketonuria (PKU) hypothyroidism, and sickle-cell disease; why not also for hearing loss? (Dennis et al, Vohr).

Reply: The consequences of delay in the detection of hearing loss, serious though they may be, cannot be fairly equated with the disastrous consequences of failure to detect PKU or hypothyroidism in the neonatal period, or of undiagnosed sepsis in the infant with sickle-cell disease. Moreover, the current combined cost of metabolic and sickle-cell screening is less than $10, compared with $30 or more for only the first-stage EOAE screen. Finally, the false-positive rates in screening for PKU and hypothyroidism are substantially lower than in infant hearing screening.

Respondent argument: Newborn hearing screening programs have been successfully implemented in many hospitals without the adverse consequences we projected in our commentary.[1] The risk consists only of unnecessary worrying by parents and caregivers in the cases of infants who prove to be false-positives (Gravel et al).

Reply: No newborn hearing screening program, to our knowledge, has actually investigated adverse consequences among false-positive infants or their families. Two types of adverse outcome warrant concern. First, it seems likely that, of the large numbers of false-positive infants identified by screening, many will be subjected to discomfort, costs, and risks as a consequence of additional diagnostic and inappropriate therapeutic procedures. In particular, we would be concerned that many will show evidence of conductive hearing loss that will be ascribed (rightly or wrongly) to otitis media with effusion, and that some of these infants will be subjected inappropriately to tympanostomy-tube placement. That this risk is real is supported both by our own observations and by a recent report[41] documenting, in a large, insured population of children, that the operation is frequently recommended for inappropriate indications.

Second, it seems likely that in many cases the false-positive identification itself will harm parents and children. A number of reports[42,43] and reviews[44-46] document the extent to which parental misunderstanding and anxiety concerning the false-positive state may persist as important problems long after the diagnosis in question has been dismissed. The newborn period, in particular, appears to be a sensitive time when identifying the infant as abnormal, even if only temporarily, may result in the infant's being "labeled" unfavorably or in other long-term adverse effects on the parent-child relationship and/or the child's psychological development.[45]

Follow-up, Access, and Compliance

Respondent argument: Before initiating screening, each program should be encouraged to resolve issues concerning accessibility and availability of facilities for suitable follow-up and compliance (Stewart and Davis-Freeman). On the other hand, a newborn predischarge screen is one mechanism for beginning to address both access barriers and poor compliance (Vohr).

Reply: "Encouraged" is not sufficient. Accessibility and availability of both diagnostic and treatment facilities, as well as the likelihood of reasonable compliance, are key *prerequisites* for initiating a screening program.[47] To undertake a program without these elements reasonably assured in advance not only will undercut the objective of the program—to benefit children—and waste its efforts, but will result inevitably in much parental confusion, frustration, and anxiety. Access barriers and poor compliance are societal and health-system problems that screening programs cannot solve.

Respondent argument: Because of differing health-system, socioeconomic, and geographic circumstances between European countries and the United States, there should be fewer reservations about newborn hearing screening in Europe (European Concerted Action Group).

Reply: Fewer, perhaps, but reservations nonetheless, because the adverse effects of false-positive identification would likely constitute risks as substantial in Europe as in the United States.

Neuropsychological Considerations

Respondent argument: Morphological changes in central neural pathways have been shown to result from early experimental acoustic deprivation (European Concerted Action Group).

Reply: The studies referred to are interesting, but they have been carried out only on birds and rats; extrapolating the findings to humans would be problematic.

Respondent argument: Phonetic perception in infants undergoes impressive development during the first 6 months of life, constituting a reason for detecting hearing loss early (European Concerted Action Group; Robinette).

Reply: The evidence cited is credible and important. However, no parallel evidence exists that the first 6 months constitute a critical period, and that satisfactory phonetic perception cannot develop later.

Efficacy of Intervention

Respondent argument: Our commentary[1] did not sufficiently acknowledge the effectiveness and benefits of early intervention, once children with hearing impairment have been identified. The educational (regular versus special classrooms) and quality-of-life savings would more than compensate for the costs of screening (European Concerted Action Group; Hayes; Robinette; Stewart and Davis-Freenman; Vohr).

Reply: The possibility of optimizing habilitation, communication skills, and quality of life for even a few individuals constitutes a strong argument for early identification. Early identification, followed by intervention that at present is deemed appropriate, makes intuitive sense, and surely all health professionals, we included, support it. Nonetheless it must be acknowledged that, for the reasons outlined in our commentary,[1] available empirical evidence to support the effectiveness of early intervention is far from conclusive.

Respondent argument: If evidence of the effectiveness of early intervention is not conclusive enough to justify universal screening, why is it conclusive enough to justify screening at-risk newborns (Robinette)?

Reply: Our objection to universal screening is not based on the weakness of evidence supporting intervention; we simply call attention to that weakness while agreeing that, for infants with confirmed hearing impairment, one *must* intervene in whatever manner seems best at the moment. Rather, our objection to universal screening is based on 1) lack of evidence, and skepticism, that it will result in more effective identification and better eventual outcomes than targeted HHR/ICN screening; and 2) concern about the harm that could result from universal screening, as discussed previously.

It is important to appreciate that among normal newborns, as compared with high-risk newborns, the proportion likely to be benefited by screening is much lower and the proportion likely to be harmed is much higher. Another factor favoring the screening of high-risk newborns but not normal newborns is that high-risk newborns have substantially longer hospital stays, so that they can be tested at times when test results are substantially more valid than during the first day or two of life, by which time normal newborns are generally discharged.

Feasibility and Ethics of Research on Screening

Respondent argument: The questions and concerns about screening that we raised in our commentary[1] are not amenable to study because of ethical and moral constraints. One cannot withhold intervention from young children with known hearing loss in a planned, prospective investigation. The NIH Consensus panel was obliged to choose between maintaining the status quo and setting a vision for the future. If we have any alternative, constructive suggestions, what are they? (European Concerted Action Group; Gravel et al; Hayes; Raffin and Matz).

Reply: As suggested in Dr Miller's response, the effectiveness of an early infant hearing screening program certainly *can* be subjected to experimental study—without resort to withholding intervention from young children with known hearing loss—and *should* be subjected to experimental study before deciding whether to launch such a program nationwide. The underlying principles and essential features of randomized trials of screening programs have been well delineated by Sackett, Haynes, and Tugwell.[47]

A randomized trial of hearing screening would require a large population of newborns. Eligibility would be limited to those who were apparently normal and risk-free, with those who met HRR criteria and/or who were admitted to an ICN having been excluded and screened because of their at-risk status. The normal newborns would be randomly assigned to be offered (experimental group) or not offered (control group) the screening protocol. Control infants would receive clinical care in the conventional, pre-trial manner, but the parents of all infants in both study groups would receive, at baseline and periodically, standardized educational materials about the importance of remaining alert to possible signs of hearing loss in their infants. The outcomes of all infants randomized to be screened—including those whose parents either declined the offer, dropped out later, or failed to comply with recommended interventions—would be compared with the outcomes of all control infants. Screened infants would be subcategorized according to their designated status on completing the screening protocol—i.e., true-positive, false-positive, or negative. The outcomes analyzed over the course of follow-up would include, at minimum, the proportions of infants correctly and incorrectly identified as having hearing loss, and the ages of the identifications; the numbers of diagnostic and therapeutic procedures; measures of children's functional status, behavior, and psychosocial adjustment; measures of parental stress and anxiety; and monetary costs.

The cost of a study such as this would be high, but far less than the first-year costs alone of a nationwide screening program and the diagnostic and therapeutic procedures it would generate. If the study showed that screening had resulted in favorable benefits overall in relation to risks and costs, one could then proceed to implement a nationwide program with confidence. If, on the other hand, the results showed no clear advantage of screening, immense effort and cost for years to come could properly be avoided. As pointed out by Sackett et al,[47] "the widespread implementation of untested methods of early diagnosis renders their subsequent rigorous evaluation much more difficult and less decisive; indeed it may even become impossible to correct the original error."

Current Recommendations

Because of the potential benefits of early detection of hearing loss and the potential risks of delayed detection, and because the prevalence of sensorineural hearing loss is far higher in infants who meet HRR criteria than in normal newborns, we recommended in our commentary[1] and continue to recommend that screening, using automated ABR methods, be performed on all HRR infants. Importantly, although most newborns admitted to an ICN also will meet HRR criteria, in our recommendation we neglected to make specific reference to ICN infants who do not meet HRR criteria; such infants should have been included and also should be screened.

In contrast to HRR/ICN infants, apparently normal newborns ought not be subjected to hearing screening (except as subjects in a properly designed study). Some of the difficulties and pitfalls inherent in attempting to screen and follow-up such infants have recently been underscored by Galambos, a pioneer in the study and use of ABR testing in newborns, and his co-workers.[48] In expressing skepticism about universal screening, based on their extensive experience with ICN infants, they wrote, "After the ICN infants have been taken away, few of the infants left behind in the normal nursery will be deaf, because normal infants almost always have normal hearing." To detect those rare deaf infants in the normal nursery, a vigorous campaign directed at educating primary-care providers and parents to be continually alert to the possibility of hearing loss makes far more sense and would cost far less than a program of universal screening.

Fred H. Bess, Ph.D.
Division of Hearing and Speech Sciences
Vanderbilt University School of Medicine and
the Bill Wilkerson Center
Nashville, TN

Jack L. Paradise, M.D.
Department of Pediatrics
University of Pittsburgh School of Medicine
and the Children's Hospital of Pittsburgh
Pittsburgh, PA

References

1. Bess, F.H., Paradise, J.L. Universal screening for infant hearing impairment: not simple, not risk-free, not necessarily beneficial and not presently justified. *Pediatrics.* 1994,93:330-334

2. NIH Consensus Statement. *Early Identification of Hearing Impairment in Infants and Young Children.* March 1-3,1993;11:1-24

3. Joint Committee on Infant Hearing. 1990 Position statement. *AAP News.* April 1991;7:6-14 Reprinted in *Policy Reference Guide,* 6th ed. Elk Grove Village, IL: American Academy of Pediatrics; 1993:343-346

4. Ventry, I.M. Effects of conductive hearing loss: fact or fiction. *J Speech Hear Dis.* 1980;45:143-156

5. Paradise, J.L. Otitis media during early life: how hazardous to development? A critical review of the evidence. *Pediatrics.* 1981;68:869-873

6. Paradise, J.L., Rogers, K.D. On otitis media, child development, and tympanostomy tubes: new answers or old questions? *Pediatrics.* 1986; 77:88-92

7. American Speech-Language-Hearing Association. Guidelines for audiologic screening of newborn infants who are at-risk for hearing impairment. *ASHA.* 1989;31:89-92

8. Turner, R.G. Modeling the cost and performance of early identification protocols. *J Am Acad Audiol.* 1991;2:195-205

9. Turner, R.G., Cone-Wesson, B.K. Prevalence rates and cost-effectiveness of risk factors. In Bess, F.H., Hall, III J.W., eds. *Screening Children for Auditory Function.* Nashville, TN: Bill Wilkerson Center Press; 1992:79-104

10. Newton, V.E. Aetiology of bilateral sensorineural hearing loss in young children. *J Laryngol Otol.* 1985;10(suppl):40-41

11. Plinkert, P.K., Sesterhenn, G., Arold, R., Zenner, H.P. Evaluation of otoacoustic emissions in high-risk infants by using an easy and rapid objective auditory screening method. *Eur Arch Otorhinolaryngol.* 1990;247:356-360

12. Nield, T.A., Schrier, S., Ramos, A.D., Platzker, A.C.G., Warburton, D. Unexpected hearing loss in high-risk infants. *Pediatrics.* 1986;78:417-422

13. Salamy, A., Eldredge, L., Tooley, W.H. Neonatal status and hearing loss in high risk infants. *J Pediatr.* 1989;114:847-852

14. Walton, J.P., Hendricks-Munoz, K. Profile and stability of sensorineural hearing loss in persistent pulmonary hypertension of the newborn. *Speech Hear Res.* 1991;34:1362-1370

15. Fowler, K.B., Dahle, A., Boppana, S.B., Stagno, S., Britt, W.J., Pass, R.F. The importance of congenital cytomegalovirus infection in identifying childhood hearing impairment. Abstract. *Pediatr Res.* 1994;34(4, Part 2):296A

16. White, K.R., Vohr, B.R., Behrens, T.R. Universal newborn hearing screening using transient evoked otoacoustic emissions: results of the Rhode Island Hearing Assessment Project. *Semin Hear.* 1993;14:18-29

17. Mahoney ,T.M., Eichwald, J.G. The ups and "DOWNS" of high-risk hearing screening: the Utah statewide program. *Semin Hear.* 1987;8: 155-163

18. Stein, L.K., Jabaley, T., Spitz, R., Stoakley, D., McGee, T. The hearing-impaired infant: patterns of identification and habilitation revisited. *Ear Hear.* 1990;11:201-205

19. Mace, A.L., Wallace, K.L., Whan, M.A., Stelmachowicz, P.G. Relevant factors in the identification of hearing loss. *Ear Hear.* 1991;12:287- 293

20. Bonfils, P., Uziel, A., Pujol, R. Screening for auditory dysfunction in infants by evoked otoacoustic emissions. *Arch Otolaryngol Head Neck Surg.* 1988;114:887-890

21. Stevens, J.C., Webb, H.D., Hutchinson, J., Connell, J., Smith, M.F., Buffin, J.T. Click evoked otoacoustic emissions compared with brain stem electric response. *Arch Dis Child.* 1989;64:1105-1111

22. Kennedy, C.R., Kimm, L., Cafarelli Dees, D., et al. Otoacoustic emissions and auditory brainstem responses in the newborn. *Arch Dis Child.* 1991;66:1124-1129

23. Saloman, G., Anthonisen, B., Groth, J., Thomsen, P.P. Otoacoustic hearing screening in newborns: optimization. In: Bess, F.H., Hall, III J.W., eds. *Screening Children for Auditory Function.* Nashville, TN: Bill Wilkerson Center Press; 1992:191-206

24. Chang, K.W., Vohr, B.R., Norton, S.J., Lekas, M.D. External and middle ear status related to evoked otoacoustic emission in neonates. *Arch Otolaryngol Head Neck Surg.* 1993;119:276-282

25. Kok, M.R., van Zanten, G.A., Brocaar, M.P., Wallenburg, H.C.S. Click-evoked otoacoustic emissions in 1036 ears of healthy newborns. *Audiol.* 1993; 32:213-224

26. Uppenkamps, S., Jakel, M., Talartschick, B., Buschel, J., Kollmeister, B. Evozierte otoakustische emissionen als screening test fur die horprufung bei neu-und fruhgeborenen? *Laryngoorhinootologie.* 1992;71:575-529

27. Jacobson, J.T., Jacobson, C.A. The effects of noise in transient EOAE newborn hearing screening. *Int J Pediatr Otorhinolaryngol.* 1994; 29:235-248

28. Hall, J.W., Baer, J.E., Chase, P.A., Rupp, K.A. Transient and distortion product otoacoustic emissions in infant hearing screening. Paper presented at annual meeting of the American Academy of Audiology; April 1994; Richmond, VA

29. Taff, J.H., Cox, E.L. TEOAE hearing screenings in the special care nursery. Paper presented at annual meeting of the American Academy of Audiology; April 1994; Richmond, VA

30. Jacobson, J.T., Morehouse, C.R., Johnson, M.J. Strategies for infant auditory brainstem response assessment. *Ear Hear.* 1982;3:263-270

31. Dennis, J.M., Sheldon, R., Toubas, P., McCaffee, M.A. Identification of hearing loss in the neonatal intensive care unit population. *Am J Otol.* 1984;5:201-205

32. Ruth, R.A., Dey-Sigman, S., Mills, J.A. Neonatal ABR hearing screening. *Hearing J.* 1985;38:39-45

33. Jacobson, J.T., Jacobson, C.A., Spahr, R.C. Automated and conventional ABR screening techniques in high-risk infants. J *Am Acad Audiol.* 1990;1:187-195

34. Kileny, P.R. ALGO-1 automated infant hearing screener: preliminary results. *Sermin Hear.* 1987;8:125-131

35. Ransohoff, D.F., Feinstein, A.R. Problems of spectrum and bias in evaluating the efficacy of diagnostic tests. *N Engl J Med.* 1978;299:926-930

36. Durieux-Smith, A., Picton, T.W., Edwards, C.G., MacMurray, B., Goodman, J.T. Brainstem electric-response audiometry in infants of a neonatal intensive care unit. *Audiol.* 1987;26:284-297

37. Davis, S. Hearing screening at Baptist Memorial Hospital, Memphis, TN. Paper presented at Universal Infant Hearing Screening National Seminar; November 1993, Nashville, TN

38. Joseph, J.M., Herrmann, B.S., Thornton, A.R., Pye, R.K. Well-baby hearing screening using automated ABR. Paper presented at the American Speech-Language-Hearing Association Annual Convention; November 1993; Anaheim, CA

39. Holtzman, N.A. What drives neonatal screening programs? *N Engl J Med.* 1991;325:802-804

40. Johnson, M.I., Maxon, A.B., White, K.R., Vohr, B.R. Operating a hospital-based universal newborn hearing screening program using transient evoked otoacoustic emissions. *Semin Hear.* 1993; 14:46-56

41. Kleinman, L.C., Kosecoff, J., Dubois, R.W., Brook, R.H. The medical appropriateness of tympanostomy tubes proposed for children younger than 16 years in the United States. *JAMA.* 1994; 271:1250-1255

42. Sorenson, J.R., Levy, H.L., Mangione, T.W., Sepe, S.J. Parental response to repeat testing of infants with "false-positive" results in a newborn screening program. *Pediatrics.* 1984;73:183-187

43. Tluczek, A., Mischler, E.H., Farrell, P.M., et al. Parents' knowledge of neonatal screening and response to false-positive cystic fibrosis testing. J *Dev Behav Pediatr.* 1992;13:181-186

44. Feldman, W. How serious are the adverse effects of screening? J *Gen Intern Med.* 1990;5(suppl): S50-S53

45. Clayton, E.W. Issues in state newborn screening programs. *Pediatrics.* 1992,90:641-646

46. Clayton, E.W. Screening and the treatment of newborns. *Houston Law Review.* 1992;29:85-148

47. Sackett, D.L., Haynes, R.B., Tugwell, P. *Clinical Epidemiology: A Basic Science for Clinical Medicine.* Boston: Little, Brown & Co; 1985:302-310

48. Galambos, R., Wilson, M.J., Silva, P.D. Identifying hearing loss in the intensive care nursery: a 20-year summary. J *Am Acad Audiol.* 1994;5: 151-l62

V. Minimal Hearing Loss

In this section, we present a collection of articles that deal with three groups of children frequently thought not to be at risk for auditory disabilities. These are not easily categorized into other sections of this book, yet they are considered essential for the study of pediatric audiology.

For many years it was believed that children with significant unilateral sensorineural hearing loss experienced few, if any, communicative or psychoeducational difficulties. The typical management strategy for this population was to identify the loss, inform the parents that the hearing loss existed, but assure them that there was no problem and, occasionally, experiment with a CROS-type hearing aid. Educators, audiologists, speech-language pathologists, and otolaryngologists held the time-honored belief that one good ear was sufficient for normal auditory, linguistic, cognitive, and educational development. The article by Bess and Tharpe challenged the long-standing premise that unilaterally hearing impaired children did not present with problems and, in fact, demonstrated that many of these children experience a number of auditory and psychoeducational difficulties. Most important was the finding that almost one-half of these children had either failed a grade or needed resource assistance in the schools.

Since the early 1950s, there has been a multitude of studies exploring the possible developmental consequences of early childhood otitis media with effusion. Many of these earlier studies were fraught with design limitations that confounded the interpretation of the data. Some of the limitations of this research included the retrospective nature of the studies, small sample size, questionable matching of cases and controls, questionable validity of test measures, and inadequate documentation of the disease process and hearing loss. An excellent critique of many of the earlier studies on the developmental effects of otitis media is presented next by Ventry. Ventry stated that insufficient evidence existed to allow one to conclude that otitis media causes speech, language, cognitive, or educational problems. This article offered valuable insight into the need for audiologists to consider carefully design issues and methodology before accepting carte blanche the results and conclusions of studies in otitis media.

Hearing loss is considered the most common sequelae of otitis media with effusion (OME); however, few controlled studies have examined the natural history of hearing loss associated with this disease. Fria, Cantekin, and Eichler offer one of the few data-based studies that documents the degree and variability of hearing loss associated with otitis media. This study, which showed that hearing impairment averaged about 30 dB and ranged from 10 to 55 dB, provided impetus for the premise that OME and subsequent hearing loss may have deleterious effects on speech and language development.

Whether early otitis media with effusion and subsequent fluctuating hearing loss lead to later life developmental problems remains unclear. Holm and Kunze (1969) were the first investigators to suggest that early otitis media could lead to later developmental problems. Numerous studies followed the Holm and Kunze article—many of these studies implied an association between otitis media and developmental complications; others did not. Again, design limitations precluded interpretation of many of these investigations. The first prospective studies to demonstrate an effect of mild hearing loss associated with OME in early life and emerging language were the studies of Friel-Patti and Finitzo (1990) and Wallace et al. (1988).

Two studies are included here to demonstrate the possible effects of persistent, early otitis media with effusion. Jerger and coworkers demonstrated that otitis media can temporarily arrest the development of word recognition ability, under adverse listening conditions. Similarly, Gravel and Wallace reported that young infants with a history of early otitis media required a more favorable signal-to-noise ratio for speech understanding than did children with no history of otitis media. Whether the speech recognition problems observed by Jerger et al. and Gravel and Wallace persist into the school-age years has not yet been determined, although a more current investigation by Schilder and colleagues (1994) suggests this may be the case. This question still requires further investigation. Nevertheless, these two articles signal the need for audiologists to monitor carefully those children with a history of early middle ear disease.

Finally, we include two investigations on school-age children with minimal sensorineural hearing loss--minimal hearing loss typically refers to three different types of hearing loss: unilateral hearing loss, bilateral hearing loss, and high-frequency hearing loss. These mild hearing losses usually average 20 to 40 dB HL through the frequency range 1, 2, and 4 kHz, in one or both ears or exhibit losses greater than 25 dB HL above 2 kHz in one or both ears. These children are considered to be within the normal range for hearing. In fact, many of these children will pass the school hearing screening program. These two studies, by Crandell and Bess and colleagues, offer evidence that children with minimal hearing loss are at risk for academic failure and psychosocial dysfunction. The findings suggest that improved efforts to manage these children could well result in meaningful improvement in educational progress and psychosocial well being.

References

Friel-Patti, S., and Finitzo, T. 1990. Language learning in a prospective study of otitis media with effusion in the first two years of life. *Journal of Speech and Hearing Research* 33:188-194.

Holm, V.A., and Kunze, L.H. 1969. Effects of chronic otitis media on language and speech development. *Pediatrics* 43:833-839.

Schilder, A., Snik, A., Straatman, H., and van den Broek, P. 1994. The effect of otitis media with effusion at preschool age on some aspects of auditory perception at school age. *Ear and Hearing* 15(3):224-231.

Wallace, I.F., Gravel, J.S., Ruben, R.J., McCarton, C.M., Stapells, D., and Bernstein, R.S. 1988. Otitis media, language outcome and auditory sensitivity. *Laryngoscope* 98:64-70.

Additional Readings

Bess, F.H. 1985. The minimally hearing-impaired child. *Ear & Hearing* 6:43-47.

Bess, F.H. 1986. Unilateral sensorineural hearing loss in children. *Ear & Hearing* 7:1-54.

Paradise, J.L. 1981. Otitis media during early life: How hazardous to development? A critical review of the evidence. *Pediatrics* 68:869-873.

Roberts, J.E., Burchinal, M.R., Davis, B.P., Collier, A.M., and Henderson, F.W. 1991. Otitis media in early childhood and later language. *Journal of Speech and Hearing Research* 34:1158-1168.

Unilateral Hearing Impairment in Children

Fred H. Bess, Ph.D., and Anne Marie Tharpe, M.S.

Division of Hearing and Speech Sciences, Vanderbilt University School of Medicine, and The Bill Wilkerson Hearing and Speech Center, Nashville, Tennessee 1984

Abstract

An overview and update are offered on difficulties experienced by children with monaural sensorineural deafness. It is the general consensus that children with unilateral hearing loss experience few, if any, communication and/or educational problems. The medical and educational status of a group (N = 60) of children with unilateral, hearing impairment are described. In addition, the auditory, linguistic, and behavioral manifestations of unilateral hearing impairment were studied in considerable detail for a subsample of these 60 children. The results revealed that approximately one third of the children with unilateral hearing loss had failed at least one grade. Nearly 50% of the group had either failed a grade and/or needed resource assistance in the schools. The small subsample of children with unilateral hearing loss performed much poorer than a matched group of children with normal hearing on both a localization and a syllable recognition task. Finally, the data on behavioral and linguistic manifestations of monaural hearing loss indicate that children with unilateral hearing impairment are experiencing more problems than previously supposed. *Pediatrics* 1984;74:206-216; *monaural sensorineural deafness, language, behavior, hearing impairment.*

A unilateral hearing impairment has never been viewed as a handicapping condition for children. Parents are characteristically advised that preferential classroom seating will afford sufficient auditory input for educational purposes and that the hearing loss will not cause any undue communicative problems. A recent statement by Northern and Downs[1] best illustrates the current thinking regarding this population: ". . . audiologists and otolaryngologists are not usually concerned over such deafness, other than to identify its etiology and assure the parents that there will be no handicap." It is of interest to note that experimental evidence supporting this widespread clinical impression is almost nonexistent. To the contrary, studies on adults with monaural deafness suggest that this type of hearing loss can produce a variety of communication difficulties.[2,3] Furthermore, there is indirect evidence to suggest that longstanding unilateral hearing losses in children can present some educational problems.[4,5] The emergence of recent research on monaural deafness, however, demonstrates more conclusively that some children with this type of hearing condition exhibit deficits in auditory and psycholinguistic skills as well as experience considerable difficulty in the schools.[6-9]

Because the primary care physician, especially the pediatrician, is usually the first to encounter children with unilateral hearing loss, it is important that they have an understanding of the various communicative and educational problems that can occur in this population. Hence, it is the purpose of this report to review the present status of unilateral hearing impairment in children.

Demography

It is estimated that there are close to 6.5 million Americans with some degree of unilateral hearing loss. The prevalence rate for school-aged children with unilateral hearing losses of 45 dB or more is 3:1,000 and, if the milder losses (26 to 45 dB) are included, the rate increases to 13:1,000.[10] Presently, there are no prevalence figures available for children less than 3 years of age.

In a sample of 122 patients with unilateral hearing loss, Everberg[11] noted a greater prevalence of affected males (62.3%) than females (37.7%); 52.5% of these subjects had impaired left ears whereas 47.5% exhibited impaired right ears. The cause of monaural deafness is not clearly understood. Depending on the study, etiology is reported as unknown in 42% to 66% of the subjects examined.[7,11-14] Heredity is considered the most common congenital factor, whereas the most frequently acquired forms of unilateral hearing loss originate from viral complications and meningitis.

Unilateral hearing loss is generally discovered much later in life than the bilateral hearing impairment. It is not unusual for the hearing loss to go undetected until the child is screened in the school system, proba-

Reproduced with permission from *Pediatrics*, 74:206-216. Copyright 1984 by the AAP.

Received for publication Jan 3, 1983; accepted Oct 28, 1983.

Reprint requests to (F.H.B.) Division of Hearing and Speech Sciences, Vanderbilt University School of Medicine, Nashville, TN 37212

PEDIATRICS (ISSN 0031 4005). Copyright □ 1984 by the American Academy of Pediatrics.

bly because language appears to develop normally, and thus does not attract attention to the handicap. Studies have shown that the hearing loss is usually detected when the children enter the first year of school, although many unilateral impairments are not discovered until the children are 7 years of age or older.[7,8]

Background

To appreciate fully the potential problems that can be encountered by a child with unilateral hearing impairment, it is helpful to review three specific areas that are most pertinent to this topic: the importance of binaural hearing, the effects of noise on children, and educational considerations.

Importance of Binaural Hearing

It has long been recognized that two ears provide a listening advantage over one ear alone. Several factors are known to contribute to this binaural advantage. First is the concept of binaural summation which can be defined as an improvement in auditory thresholds for pure tones and speech (approximately 2 to 3 dB) when presented binaurally as opposed to a monaural presentation.[15-23] Although an advantage of only 3 dB may not seem consequential, its favorable effect on speech understanding and ease of listening is well documented.[24,25]

Another factor contributing to the binaural advantage is the head shadow effect. The head serves to attenuate sounds before reaching the ear farthest from the source. In fact, the head attenuates speech intensity by as much as 6.4 dB as a signal progresses from one ear to the other.[26-28] The degree of the shadowing effect varies according to the type and origin of the acoustic signal.[24] For a person with unilateral deafness, the shadowing effect can result in favorable and unfavorable listening conditions. A favorable listening condition exists if the primary signal is directed to the normal ear and a competing message or noise is transmitted to the impaired ear. In this situation, the intensity of the competing signal is attenuated by as much as 6.4 dB at the good ear, thus minimizing its distractiveness. Conversely, if the primary signal is directed to the impaired ear and the competing signal is transmitted to the normal ear, a more unfavorable listening condition is experienced. Not only is the noise reaching the normal ear with full impact, but the primary signal is reduced in intensity as it crosses from one side of the head to the other. Consequently, it is often difficult for the listener with unilateral hearing impairment to detect the primary signal embedded in the

noise. Head shadow effects are always present in normal listening conditions; thus a binaural listener has an advantage over a monaural listener. A binaural listener typically has one ear in a favorable listening position unless both the speech and noise sources located directly in front or in back of the head.

The "squelch effect" also contributes to the binaural advantage. The squelch effect refers to the ability of the two ears to suppress background noise to the advantage of the primary signal. In 1950, Koenig[29] first observed that listeners with binaural hearing could disregard interfering background noises, such as automobiles or voices, and attend to wanted auditory stimuli. Studies have shown that this phenomenon results in improved speech perception ability in the presence of noise when listening in a binaural as opposed to a monaural mode. This effect holds true even if the monaural condition is such that the ear is favorably positioned with regard to the primary signal.[28,30-34] Hence, the far ear seems to play an important role in contributing to the listening advantage resulting from the squelch effect.

Finally, an important consideration in the discussion of binaural hearing is localization of sound in the horizontal plane. The ability to localize a sound source in space is clearly a binaural phenomenon; therefore, it is not surprising that people with unilateral hearing loss experience difficulty with directionality. In general, as the threshold difference between ears increases, errors in localization also increase. Bergman,[25] however, has noted that localization can occur in persons with marked disparities between ears, provided the sound in the poorer ear is audible.

Auditory Effects of Noise

Another important factor relative to the possible effects of unilateral hearing loss in young children is the high noise level found in the classroom. Although in most school systems there are certain architectural goals set for classroom acoustics, sound levels in kindergarten and elementary classrooms often exceed these standards, especially in classrooms for hearing-impaired children.[35-42] For example, the average noise intensity of an occupied classroom ranges from 50 to 70 db(C) depending on the type of room. (Sound level meters have three weighting networks: A, B, and C, which are designed to respond differently to the frequencies of noise. The A network weights (filters) the low frequencies and approximates the response characteristics of the human ear. The B network also weights the low frequencies but not as much as the A network.

The C scale provides a fairly flat response, whereas there is no weighting on the linear scale. The federal government recommends the use of the A network for measuring noise.) Such noise levels result in signal-to-noise ratios (S/N) that range from –6 to +6 dB. The S/N ratio (often referred to as primary-to-secondary, P:S) expresses (in decibels) the relationship between speech and the ambient noise reaching a person's ear. A positive S/N ratio indicates that the speech is louder than the noise, whereas a negative S/N ratio denotes that the noise is louder than the speech. For hearing-impaired children to function maximally for speech understanding, a S/N ratio of +20 to +30 dB is required.[37]

In addition to high noise levels, classrooms are often too reverberant. That is, there is present a considerable amount of reflected sound, resulting in a more uniform distribution of noise within the room. When reverberation is high, the binaural listener has a definite advantage over the unilaterally impaired listener, especially when the normal ear is farthest from the primary signal.[33-42]

If such noise and reverberant conditions are sufficient to interfere with verbal communication in adults, they may also be sufficient to interfere with the acquisition of important language and listening skills in young children. In fact, even children with normal hearing yield significantly more speech recognition errors with classroom noise present than in quiet conditions.[43] Furthermore, it is recognized that noise and reverberation in combination produce significant problems in speech understanding for children with binaural hearing loss. When one considers the probable adverse effects of noise on the speech recognition of persons with unilateral hearing loss, it is reasonable to assume that the acoustic environment could interfere with the learning skills of these children. It is believed that the ability to perceive speech in the presence of noise is important to the normal development of auditory function in children.[44] When the ability to separate the desired signal from a background of noise is impaired, disintegration of perception occurs. This inability to differentiate auditory figure from ground may be a factor in the difficulties faced in some learning-disabled or language-delayed children. There is evidence to suggest that weakness in the auditory discrimination of speech sounds is one of the most frequent causes of poor reading skills.[45,46] Hence, one can speculate that the difficulties that children with unilateral hearing impairment experience in noise might interfere with normal language development, necessary auditory figure-ground identity, and auditory discrimination skills.

Educational Considerations

Although there is almost no clinical or experimental information on the communicative and educational skills of children with monaural deafness, there is some indirect evidence to suggest that at least some of these children could be scholastically handicapped. For example, one study that demonstrated language delay in school-aged children with slight hearing losses (15 to 26 dB) reported that "a number of students had unilateral impairment."[4] Unfortunately, information on the number of subjects with unilateral hearing impairment, degree of hearing loss, and type of hearing loss (conductive v sensorineural) was not available. Further support for the assumption that children with unilateral hearing impairment[6] may demonstrate auditory and/or language deficits was reported by Boyd.[5] Boyd noted lags in academic achievement among a small group of children with unilateral hearing loss. Specifically, 38% of the children exhibited reading problems, 31% had spelling problems, and 23% had problems with arithmetic. In addition to the small sample size, however, limitations to this study included a retrospective design as well as a failure to provide normative data.

In summary, children with unilateral hearing impairment constitute a population currently ignored in our educational system. Yet, there is reason to believe that a unilateral hearing impairment can impose a handicapping condition. An abundance of available research affirms that binaural listening is superior to monaural listening. Moreover, it is well documented that high noise levels present in most classrooms make speech understanding more difficult for a hearing-impaired child. Finally, there are indirect data that suggest that some children with monaural deafness have difficulty learning in school. Although these factors lead one to suspect that a child with unilateral hearing impairment can experience scholastic difficulty, systematic research designed to examine this premise is almost nonexistent.

Report of a Recent Study

A recent study conducted at Vanderbilt University School of Medicine and The Bill Wilkerson Hearing and Speech Center revealed that some children with unilateral hearing loss do indeed demonstrate considerable difficulty in the classroom. Although described in detail elsewhere,[6-8] a brief review of the methods and procedures will be included here.

Methods and Procedures

The study was divided into two basic components. In the first portion, 60 children with unilateral hearing loss were selected on the basis of convenience from the patient files of The Bill Wilkerson Hearing and Speech Center, the files of the Nashville Metropolitan School System, and those of other local educational agencies in the mid-Tennessee region. The only criteria used in the selection of this group was a sensorineural loss of 45 dB or greater (500, 1,000, 2,000 Hz) in the impaired ear and thresholds no poorer than 15 dB (500, 1,000, 2,000 Hz) in the good ear. The children ranged in age from 6 to 18 years with a mean age of 13 years. Forty-five percent of the subjects were boys; 55% of the subjects were girls. Medical and educational case history data were then obtained via parental interview and/school records.

The second portion of the study involved selection of 25 of the 60 children with unilateral hearing impairment; these 25 children received a more comprehensive examination of their auditory and linguistic skills. A matched group of 25 children with normal hearing was also selected for this part of the investigation. The following criteria were used in the selection of the group with monaural hearing loss: (1) age range between 6 and 13 years; (2) hearing thresholds in the good ear no poorer than 15 dB hearing level (HL) (re: American National Standards Institute, [ANSI], 1969) through the speech frequency range (500 to 2,000 Hz) with a monaural word-recognition score greater than 90%; (3) hearing thresholds in the sensorineural impaired ear no better than 45 dB (re: ANSI, 1969) through the speech frequency range (500 to 2,000 Hz); (4) presence of the hearing impairment for at least 3 years as reported by the parent; (5) a negative case history of recurring episodes of middle ear effusion in the good ear; (6) normal intelligence as determined by a licensed psychological examiner; (7) no evidence of central auditory dysfunction; and (8) normal growth and development and freedom from other significant medical problems.

Criteria for the control group included hearing thresholds no poorer than 15 dB HL bilaterally at octave intervals 250 to 8,000 Hz, normal tympanometry in both ears, normal intelligence as determined by a licensed psychological examiner, and a negative history of otitis media. These two groups of children were then matched for age (±6 months), sex, intelligence (±1 SD), race, and socioeconomic status.[47] There were some subject pairs that did not meet all of the matching criteria. Three of the matched pairs exceeded the ±6 month criteria for age, in two pairs by 3 months and in another pair by 4 months. Four of the matched pairs exceeded the ±1 SD criteria on the Wechsler Intelligence Scale for Children (WISC-R). The average point difference in total IQ for the 25 matched pairs was 10. The mean total IQ for those with normal hearing was 107, whereas the mean total IQ for those with unilateral hearing impairment was 102.

Behavioral Manifestations

A Behavioral Rating Scale (BRS) was distributed to the teachers of the 50 children. The scale was constructed by the psychological examiner for this study, and the test items were piloted in the local schools. The scale included behavioral descriptors in five main areas: attention to academic tasks, peer relations and social confidence, dependence-independence, emotional lability, and organization. In each area, both positive and negative descriptors were included. The scores were based on the percentage of negative responses for each category and for the total test. The BRS also includes a three-point rating scale in which teachers can rate a child's academic achievements as average, above average, or below average.

Auditory Skills

The test battery used to assess auditory skills included measures of localization and syllable recognition. Localization was assessed in an anechoic chamber (6 m × 6 m × 6 m). The apparatus used for sound localization has been detailed in an earlier report.[48] Briefly, the stimuli consisted of pure tones (500 Hz, 3,000 Hz) that were delivered to a series of 13 loudspeakers. The speakers were mounted on a light framework, separated by 15-degree intervals, and placed on an arc of 180 degrees in a horizontal plane at ear level. The signals were presented at a sound pressure level of 60 dB.

Prior to each presentation, a warning light flashed to ready the subject for the listening task. The subject was instructed to maintain head fixation until the termination of the trial. The subject then reported verbally which of the various loudspeakers (clearly numbered) was activated. This procedure was repeated four times for each experimental condition (500 Hz and 3,000 Hz). For the analysis, the initial trial was discarded, and only the final three trials were considered in the computation of the error indices.

The localization score was obtained by determining the number of speakers from the sound source the subject was in error. This error score was then divided by the error score due to guessing, thus yielding an error index value. An error index of 1.0 depicts random guessing whereas an index value of 0.0 would mean perfect localization performance.

Syllable recognition ability was assessed using the Nonsense Syllable Test.[49] A preliminary study with these materials revealed that performance of children between the ages of 6 and 13 years was similar to that of an adult population. Furthermore, the test has been shown to be a valued and reliable index of syllable recognition in children.[6] The Nonsense Syllable Test is comprised of consonant-vowel and vowel-consonant syllables categorized into seven subtests of seven to nine syllables each. The composite score obtained on this test is expressed in percent correct, similar to other standard monosyllabic speech recognition tests. The format is a closed-set, forced-choice test. The carrier phrase "you will mark _____ please" is used with each stimulus item.

Each subject was placed in the center of an acoustically treated room. Two speakers were located at 45 degrees from midline at a distance of 1.83 m from the subject's head. The signal from the primary speaker was presented at a level of 65 dB sound pressure level. A cafeteria noise was used to achieve the desired primary-to-secondary (P:S) ratios (+20, +10, 0, −20). A quiet condition was also employed.

The children with unilateral hearing impairment were evaluated in a monaural direct condition (speech to the good ear and noise to the impaired ear) and a monaural indirect condition (speech to the poor ear and noise to the good ear). The children with normal hearing were assessed with speech to the right ear and noise to the left ear.

Language

The language abilities of the matched pairs were assessed using a number of standard tests. The battery consisted of the following: (1) The Token Test for Children[50]; (2) Wiig-Semel Test of Linguistic Concepts[51] (1976 version); (3) Illinois Test of Psycholinguistic Abilities (ITPA)[52]: (a) Auditory Association subtest, (b) Visual Association subtest, (c) Grammatic Closure subtest; (4) Auditory Verbal Learning Test[53]; (5) Detroit Test of Learning Aptitudes (DTLA)[54]: (a) Verbal Opposites subtest, (b) Auditory Attention Span subtest, (c) Oral Directions subtest; and (6) Sample of Spontaneous Language: (a) Mean Length of Utterance in Morphemes, (b) Mean Length of Utterance in Words, (c) Complex Sentence Analysis. A detailed description of these language measures can be found elsewhere.[7] In addition to the language tests, a measure of cognitive development was administered

to each child in the sample. The test used was the WISC-R, both performance and verbal scales.

For the auditory skills and language measures, a one-way analysis of covariance taking the WISC-Performance IQ as the covariate was used. Although the difference in performance IQ between groups was not statistically significant, it was believed that the point spread was sufficient (seven points) to warrant an analysis of covariance design. Hence, group differences were viewed having partialled out the contribution of nonverbal intelligence to the difference.

Results

Educational and Behavioral Manifestations

Examination of the case histories obtained on the total group of 60 children with hearing impairment revealed that 35% had failed one or more grades. This percentage value is in contrast to only 3.5% of the Nashville public school population that fail a grade between kindergarten through sixth grade. It is also significant to note that many children, although not required to repeat a grade, were in need of resource help in the schools. Hence, if one considers the number of students who had sufficient difficulty in the classroom to warrant either resource assistance or a grade repetition, it encompasses 48.3% of the hearing-impaired children in our test population. A distribution of the grades failed by these children can be seen in Fig 1. Most of the children who failed did so at the first grade level, although approximately half of the subjects failed grades above the first grade.

Examination of the subsample of 25 children with unilateral hearing impairment presented data similar to that for the total group of 60 children. That is, 32% of these children failed a grade (predominantly kindergarten and first grade) whereas none of their matched counterparts repeated a grade. Furthermore, when asked to rate their students' academic performance as being above average, average, or below average, of 37 teachers who responded (19 teachers of students with normal hearing and 18 teachers of hearing-impaired students), only 22.2% considered their hearing-impaired students above average academically. In contrast, 47.3% of the students with normal hearing were rated as above average.

In addition to the academic problems encountered by the hearing-impaired subjects, it appears that they also exhibited behavioral difficulties in the classroom. On four of the five categories of the BRS, the hearing-impaired children had a higher percentage of negative ratings from their classroom teachers than did their peers with normal hearing. The only category in which no difference between groups was observed was organizational skills. On the total BRS, the mean percentage of negative ratings was 10.83% for the group with unilateral hearing impairment and 4.42% for the children with normal hearing. Thus, the BRS responses suggest that the children with unilateral hearing impairment have more difficulty in the classroom than do children with normal hearing across a variety of behavioral and academic dimensions.

These findings were indeed surprising because, as mentioned previously, it has long been assumed that children with unilateral hearing loss have few, if any, problems in school. It thus appears that the listening difficulties imposed by a unilateral hearing impairment might have an effect on the individual's classroom performance. Because all of the hearing-impaired children in this study were receiving preferential classroom seating, it can be concluded that greater efforts are needed to help them overcome the apparent listening difficulties they encounter in the educational setting.

Auditory Skills

A composite audiogram for the normal and hearing-impaired ears of the 25 children in the subsample is shown in Fig 2. The data points represent mean hearing threshold levels, and the associated numbers in parentheses represent those ears that exhibited no responses at that particular frequency.

The findings obtained for sound localization are shown in Fig 3, which shows the mean error indices and SD ($\pm$1 SD) at each experimental condition for the hearing-impaired children and their matched counterparts. Mean error index values taken from another study conducted at our facility are also provided for comparison.[48] Several interesting points are shown: First, the hearing-impaired children exhibited significantly higher error indices than did their counterparts with normal hearing at both experimental conditions ($P < .001$). Second, both the children with normal hearing and those with hearing impairment showed greater difficulty localizing a high-frequency signal than a low-frequency sound. Third, there is considerable variability for localization skills among the hearing-impaired children as exhibited by the large SDs. The wide variability may have been due to differences in the hearing threshold levels of the impaired ears. Both Viehweg and Campbell[55] and Humes et al,[48] suggested that there was a relationship between the degree of hearing impairment and localization skills. That is, the more severe the hearing loss the poorer the localization performance. An analysis of our data supports a relationship between the degree of hearing level in the impaired ear and the error index score. For the pure tone at 500 Hz, a positive correlation (Pearson product-moment coefficient) of .78 ($P < .001$) was obtained, whereas at 3,000 Hz (correlated with average hearing loss at 2,000 and 4,000 Hz), the correlation was .51 ($P < .05$).

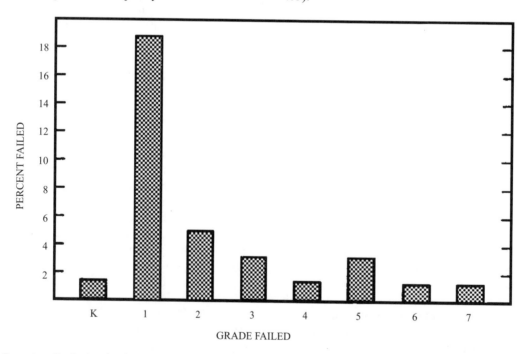

Figure 1. Percentage distribution showing grades failed by children with unilateral sensorineural hearing loss. One child failed two grades.

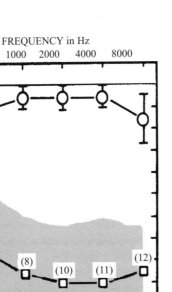

Figure 2. Audiogram depicting mean hearing threshold levels for normal ears (circles) and impaired ears (squares) on 25 children with unilateral hearing loss. Vertical bars represent SD (±1 SD) for normal ears and shaded area represents SD (±1 SD) for impaired ears. Values in parentheses at each test frequency depict number of ears that failed to yield response at maximum output of audiometer.

The mean syllable recognition scores in percent correct for both the children with normal hearing and those with hearing impairment at several different P:S ratios and in quiet are depicted in Fig 4. These scores show that the children with unilateral hearing impairment exhibited considerably greater difficulty than did the children with normal hearing under all listening conditions. A somewhat unexpected finding was that the children with unilateral hearing impairment performed poorer than the children with normal hearing under all monaural direct (signal directed to good ear) conditions. That is, even when the primary signal was directed to the good ear with noise striking the poor ear with full impact, subjects with unilateral hearing impairment did not perform as well as their peers with normal hearing. These differences were significant (*P* < .05) at two of the four listening conditions (Q [quiet] and 0 dB P:S). It is also apparent from this figure that the child with unilateral hearing impairment exhibits considerable difficulty coping with an adverse listening condition. The more adverse the listening condition, the greater the discrepancy between the listeners with normal hearing and those with unilateral hearing impairment. In the monaural indirect condition (signal to poor ear, noise to good ear), the children with unilateral hearing loss showed a rather marked breakdown in

syllable identification even under the more favorable S/N ratios.

Language Manifestations

Recall that no significant differences were found on the WICS-R between groups. Within the hearing-impaired population, however, there was a significantly lower verbal IQ (*P* < .007) for those children who failed a grade, suggesting that verbal ability may be partially responsible for teachers holding these children back a grade. Finally, WISC-Full Scale IQ was shown to be significantly lower in children with the more severe (∅ 60 dB HL) unilateral hearing losses (*P* < .03). This finding suggests that the more severe the unilateral loss, the more devastating the effect on verbal abilities, as measured by this test.

For the language measures, no significant differences were found between those with normal hearing and those with hearing impairment. However, we have not yet completed the analysis of the spontaneous language data. Within the hearing-impaired children, no significant differences were noted when the data were analyzed for academic failure *v* academic success and right ear impairment *v* left ear impairment. Once again, however, the subjects with the more severe losses (∅60 dB HL) performed significantly poorer (P < .05) than the children with the milder losses for several language

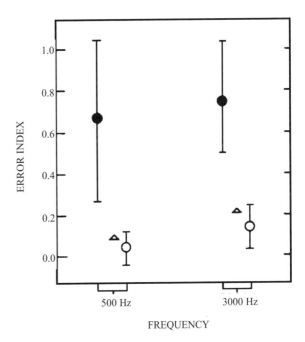

Figure 3. Mean error index values and SDs for hearing-impaired children (solid circles; N = 20) and those with normal hearing (open circles; N = 20) at two experimental conditions. Data for adult population[61] are also provided (triangles).

measures including the Detroit Test of Learning Aptitudes (Verbal Opposites subtest and Auditory Attention Span subtest) and the Token Test (part 4).

Discussion and Conclusions

It is generally believed that a unilateral hearing impairment does not produce a handicapping condition for children. The findings from this study, however, suggest that children with unilateral hearing impairments do experience a variety of difficult listening complications that may be compromising their educational progress. In a survey of 60 children with monaural hearing impairment, 35% were found to have failed at least one grade in the schools. If one also considers those children who are in need of resource help, the total number experiencing difficulty increases to almost 50%. In support of these findings, the teachers' responses on the BRS revealed that the children with unilateral hearing loss were judged by their teachers to have greater difficulty in school than their matched counterparts.

In view of previous assumptions regarding children with unilateral hearing loss, it is only natural to

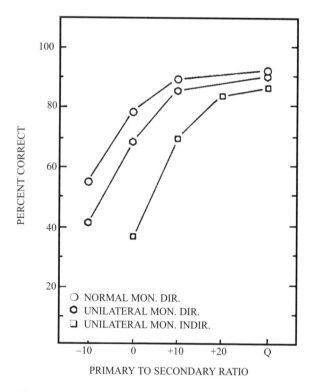

Figure 4. Mean sound field composite scores (in percent) on nonsense syllable test (NST) across several primary-to-secondary (P:S) ratios for normal children (n = 25) and children with unilateral hearing loss (n = 25). The hearing-impaired children were assessed in monaural direct and monaural indirect conditions whereas children with normal hearing were tested in monaural direct condition only.

pose the question, "Why do these children experience educational problems?" The data presented on auditory skills may help, in part, to answer that question. The localization of sound in space is recognized as a very basic and fundamental auditory skill, yet in our study children with unilateral hearing impairment performed significantly poorer on these tasks than did those with normal hearing. These findings are consistent with some of the previous work on sound localization in subjects with unilateral hearing impairment.[48,55,56]

This study also demonstrated clearly that children with unilateral hearing loss experience considerable difficulty understanding speech in the presence of a competing message. Perhaps the most significant finding was that some children with unilateral hearing impairment performed poorer than those with normal hearing even when the primary signal was presented to the good ear. In considering these data, one cannot help but question the value of classroom seating preference. These findings also suggest that children with unilateral hearing impairment will experience difficulty communicating efficiently in a classroom environment.

The language data may also help to explain some of the problems experienced by the children with unilateral hearing impairment. Recall that we were unable to find any overall group differences between the children with normal hearing and the hearing-impaired children and that there were no obvious differences between children within the hearing-impaired group due to either side of loss or success in school. However, one factor contributing to lower language performance may be the severity of the unilateral hearing loss. Those children with losses greater than 60 dB HL performed more poorly on at least several language measures. The language findings need to be tempered, however, with the following remarks. First, many of the children included in this study may have acquired a unilateral loss past the critical period for language learning. It is possible that if a loss was acquired past this period, it would not result in a significant decrement in language abilities. Second, if a unilateral hearing loss has an effect on language development in childhood, these particular language tests may not have been sensitive to registering the deficit. Indeed, further test development is needed in estimating language abilities of school-age children. Needless to say, we are anxiously awaiting the results of the spontaneous language sample.

Certainly, there are other factors that may be contributing in some unknown and complicated way to the problems of these children. For instance, there are a number of animal studies that have reported subtle degenerative changes in the CNS following auditory deprivation.[57-62] Whether, in fact, such subtle changes could affect learning and, even more pertinent, whether such changes actually occur in humans have not been established. Indeed, the effects of auditory deprivation on humans is a research area that deserves further inquiry. Other causative factors that may be operating are the complications that produced the hearing impairment. Certain prenatal and perinatal conditions are known to produce damage not only to the cochlea and eighth nerve but also to the central auditory pathways.[63-67] Whatever the reason or reasons for the problems exhibited by these children with monaural deafness, there is no doubt they do exist and their prevalence is greater than originally suspected.

The results from our study also prompt the need for a reexamination of present management strategies for this population. To date, the only course of management has been to assure the parents that no significant problem exists, recommend classroom seating preference, and occasionally experiment with a hearing aid (CROS-type) on a trial basis. CROS amplification is a special device designed to give directional assistance to the listener with unilateral hearing loss. It is now apparent that there is a need to determine the hearing loss earlier than the first grade, preferably before 2 years of age, so that appropriate intervention can be implemented. If we hope to detect these children with hearing loss earlier, however, there will need to be more emphasis on neonatal and infant screening. Once determined as having unilateral hearing loss, the child should be monitored carefully by the physician, a speech-language pathologist and/or audiologist, the local education agency, and the parents. If the child exhibits some communication and/or educational difficulty, a program of management may be recommended. For preschool-aged children, such a program might involve the enhancement of listening skills through auditory training, facilitating parent-child interaction patterns that foster the growth of linguistic skills, and, if necessary, enhancing infant vocalization patterns that are the precursors of speech training. For school-aged children, special tutoring in specific topic areas may be indicated. The feasibility of amplification might also be explored for those children who experience trouble in the schools. Toward this end, we have found that frequency modulation (FM) amplification systems can be used successfully with some children with unilateral hearing impairment. It has already been shown that children with unilateral hearing loss experience considerable difficulty understanding speech in the presence of a competing background. The advantage of the FM system is that it affords an acceptable S/N ratio for speech understanding. Traditionally, a transmitter/microphone is worn around the teacher's neck and a frequency modulated signal is broadcast to an FM student receiver unit worn by the child. External receivers coupled to personal earmolds can be used with the student units or it is possible to couple a personal hearing aid to the student receiver. We have found good success with using on the good ear a very mild gain hearing aid (open earmold) that is coupled to the student FM receiver. In contrast, we have not experienced much success with directly amplifying the impaired ear or using a CROS-type hearing aid.

Finally, we would be remiss not to point out the limitations in the design of this study and subsequently to caution the reader in the interpretation of the findings. The subject samples were relatively small, and there is a need to examine the potential problems of these children using a much larger population. Further, several reports have outlined the limitations in using a between-subject design along with a paired-matching technique.[68-74] The difficulty in controlling for all variables (i.e., number of siblings, parent stimulation, etc) that can affect linguistic skills is well recognized. Another shortcoming in the design was our failure to maintain a blind technique with all aspects of the study. For example, because the psychologist and audiologist determined whether a child satisfied the criteria for subject selection with respect to intelligence and hearing, they usually knew whether the subject had normal hearing or was hearing impaired. Finally, the problems with selecting appropriate and valid language measures for school-aged children have long been recognized.

Nevertheless, even when one considers the confinements of this study, it seems quite certain that children with unilateral hearing loss experience considerably more difficulty in education and in communication than was previously supposed. Obviously, there is a significant need for reexamination of our basic assumptions underlying the detection and management of this population.

Acknowledgments

This research was supported in part by grant No. MCR-470428-02-0, Maternal and Child Health Services, Bureau of Community Health, US Public Health Service, Department of Health, Education and Welfare.

The authors thank Thomas Klee for assistance on the language section, Barb Coulson for typing the manuscript, and Don Riggs for preparing the figures.

References

1. Northern, J., Downs, M.: *Hearing in Children,* ed 2. Baltimore, Williams & Wilkins, 1978, p. 143

2. Giolas, T.G., Wark, D.J.: Communication problems associated with unilateral hearing loss. *J Speech Hear Disord* 1967;41:336-343

3. Rosenbaum, S.: *Evaluation of the Hearing Handicap Scale for Individuals with Monaural Mild, and Moderate Sensorineural Hearing Impairment,* Doctoral dissertation. Columbia University, New York, 1976

4. Quigley, S.P., Thomure, F.E.: *Some Effects of Hearing Impairment on School Performance.* Springfield, IL, Illinois Office of Education, 1968

5. Boyd, S.F.: *Hearing Loss: Its Educationally Measurable Effects on Achievement,* Masters degree research requirement. Department of Education, Southern Illinois University. Springfield, IL, 1974

6. Bess, F.H., Gibler, A.M.: Syllable recognition skills of unilaterally hearing-impaired children. Paper presented at the American Speech-Language-Hearing Association Convention, Los Angeles, November 1981

7. Bess, F.H., Culbertson, J., Davis, E., et al.: Children with unilateral hearing loss. *Ear and Hearing*, Special Supplement, in press, 1984

8. Bess, F.H.: Children with unilateral hearing loss. *J Acad Rehad Aud* 1982;15:131-144

9. Binhero, R.: A *Study of the Relationship Between Unilateral Hearing Impairment and Academic Achievement,* doctoral dissertation. Gallaudet College, Washington, DC, 1982

10. Berg, F.S.: *Educational Audiology: Hearing and Speech Management.* New York, Grune & Stratton, 1972, p. 2

11. Everberg, G.: Etiology of unilateral total deafness. *Ann Otol Rhinol Laryngol* 1960;69:711-730

12. Kinney, C.: Hearing impairments in children. *Laryngoscope* 1953;63:220

13. Tarkkanen, J., Aho, J.: Unilateral deafness in children. *Arch Otolaryngol* 1966;61:270-278

14. Lehnhardt, E.: Zur einseitigen Taubheit in Kindesalter. *Arch Ohren Nasen Kehlkopfheilkd* 1962;180:230

15. Keys, J.W.: Binaural versus monaural hearing. *J Acoust Soc Am* 1974;19:629-631

16. Shaw, W.A., Newman, E.B., Hirsh, I.J.: The difference between monaural and binaural thresholds. J *Excep Psych* 1947;37:229-242

17. Pollack, I.: Monaural and binaural threshold sensitivity for tones and white noise. *J Acoust Soc Am* 1948;20:52-58

18. Breaky, M.R., Davis, H.: Comparisons for thresholds of speech. *Laryngoscope* 1949;59:236-250

19. Bocca, E.: Binaural hearing: Another approach. *Laryngoscope* 1955;65:572-578

20. Pollack, I., Pickett, J.M.: Stereophonic listening and speech intelligibility against voice babble. *J Acoust Soc Am* 1958;30:131-133

21. Reynolds, G.S., Stevens, S.S.: Binaural summation of loudness. *J Acoust Soc Am* 1960;32:1337-1343.

22. Lochner, J.P., Burger, J.F.: The binaural summation of speech signals. *Acustica* 1961;9:313-317.

23. Coles, R.R.A., cited by Markides, A.: *Binaural Hearing Aids.* New York, Academic Press, 1977, p. 2

24. Konkle, D., Schwartz, D.: Binaural amplification: A paradox, in Bess, F.H., Freeman, B.A., Sinclair, S. (eds): *Amplification in Education.* Washington DC. Alexander Graham Bell Assoc for the Deaf, 1981, pp. 342-357

25. Bergman, M.: Binaural hearing. *Arch Otolaryngol* 1957;66:572-578

26. Tillman, T.W., Kasten, R.N., Horner, J.S.: Effect of head shadow on reception of speech. *ASHA* 1963;5:778-779

27. Olsen, W.O.: The effect of head movement on speech reception under monaural and binaural listening condition. *ASHA* 1965;7:405

28. Olsen, W.O., Carhart, R.: Development of test procedures for evaluation of binaural hearing aids. *Bull Prosthet Res* 1967;10:22-49

29. Koenig, W.: Subjective effects in binaural hearing. *J Acoust Soc Am* 1950;22:61-62

30. Norlund, B., Fritzell, N.: The influence of azimuth on speech signals. *Acta Otolaryngol* 1963; 56:1-11

31. Harris, J.D.: Monaural and binaural speech intelligibility and the stereophonic effect based on temporal cues. *Laryngoscope* 1965;75:428-446

32. Carhart, R.: Monaural and binaural discrimination against competing sentences. *Int Audiol* 1965,4:5-10

33. Moncur, J., Dirks, D.: Binaural and monaural speech intelligibility in reverberation. *J Acoust Soc Am* 1967;10:186-195

34. MacKeith, N.W., Coles, R.R.A.: Binaural advantages in hearing of speech. *J Laryngol Otol* 1971; 85:213-232

35. Sanders, D.: Noise conditions in normal school classrooms. *Except Child* 1965;31:344-353

36. Mills, J.H.: Noise and children: A review of literature. *J Acoust Soc Am* 1975;58:767-779

37. Bess, F.H., McConnell, F.E.: *Audiology Education and the Hearing Impaired Child.* St Louis, CV Mosby, 1981, pp. 188-200

38. Finitzo-Hieber, T.: Classroom acoustics, in Roeser, R., Downs, M.P. (eds): *Auditory Disorders in Children.* New York, Thieme-Stratton Inc., 1982, pp. 250-262

39. Olsen, W.O.: Acoustics and amplification in classrooms for the hearing impaired, in Bess, F.H. (ed): *Childhood Deafness: Causation Assessment and Management.* New York, Grune & Stratton, 1977, pp. 251-266

40. Bess, F.H., Gravel, J.S.: Recent trends in educational amplification. *Hear Instrum* 1981;32:24-29

41. Olsen, W.O.: The effects of noise and reverberation on speech intelligibility, in Bess, F.H., Freeman, B.A., Sinclair, J.S. (eds): *Amplification in Education.* Washington, DC, Alexander Graham Bell Assoc for the Deaf, 1981, pp. 151-163

42. Nabalek, A.K.: Temporal distortions and noise considerations, in Studebaker, G.A., Bess, F.H. (eds): *The Vanderbilt Hearing Aid Report* (Monographs in Contemporary Audiology). Upper Darby, PA, 1982, pp. 51-59

43. Finitzo-Hieber, T., Tillman, T.W.: Room acoustic effects on monosyllabic word discrimination ability for normal and hearing impaired children. *J Speech Hear Res* 1978;21:440-448

44. Siegenthaler, B.M., Barr, C.A.: Auditory figure-ground perception in normal children. *Child Dev* 1967;38:1163-1167

45. Goetzinger, C.P., Dirks, D.D., Baer, C.J.: Auditory discrimination and visual perception in good and poor readers. *Ann Otol Rhinol Laryngol* 1960;69:121-136

46. Clark, A.D., Richards, C.J.: Auditory discrimination among economically disadvantaged and nondisadvantaged preschool children. *Except Child* 1966;33:259-262

47. Stahlman, M., Hedvall, G., Dolanski, E., et al.: A six-year follow-up of clinical hyaline membrane disease. *Pediatr Clin North Am* 1973;20:433-446

48. Humes, L.E., Allen, S.K., Bess, F.H.: Horizontal sound localization skills of unilaterally hearing-impaired children. *Audiology* 1980;19:508-518

49. Levitt, H., Resnick, S.B.: Speech reception by the hearing impaired: Methods of testing and the development of new tests. *Scand Audiol* 1978;6: 107-130

50. DiSimoni, F.G.: *The Token Test for Children.* Hingham, MA, Teaching Resources Corp, 1978

51. Wiig, E.H., Semel, E.M.: *Language Disabilities in Children and Adolescents.* Columbus, OH Charles E Merrill, 1976

52. Kirk, S.A., McCarthy, J.J., Kirk, W.D.: *The Illinois Test of Psycholinguistic Abilities.* Urbana, IL, University of Illinois Press, 1968

53. Rey, A.: Auditory Verbal Learning Test, in Taylor, E.M. (ed): *Psychological Appraisal of Children with Cerebral Defects.* Cambridge, MA, Harvard University Press, 1961

54. Baker, H.J., Leland, B.: *Detroit Tests of Learning Aptitude.* Indianapolis, Bobbs-Merrill Co, 1958

55. Viehweg, R., Campbell, R.A.: Localization difficulty in monaurally impaired listeners. *Trans Am Otolaryngol Soc* 1960;48:339-350

56. Nordlund, B.: Directional audiometry. *Acta Otolaryngol,* 1964;57:12-17

57. Webster, D.B., Webster, M.: Neonatal sound deprivation affects brain stem auditory nuclei. *Arch Otolaryngol* 1977;103:392-396

58. Webster, D.B., Webster, M.: Effects of neonatal conductive hearing loss on brainstem auditory nuclei. *Ann Otol Rhinol Laryngol* 1979;88:684-688

59. Coleman, J., O'Connor, P.: Development of neurons of the ventral cochlear nucleus following monaural sound deprivation, abstracted. *Anat Rec* 1978;190:366

60. Batkin, S., Groth, H., Watson, J.R., et al.: Effects of auditory deprivation on the development of auditory sensitivity in albino rats. *Electroencephalogr Clin Neurophysiol* 1970;28:351-359

61. Clopton, B.M., Silverman, M.S.: Plasticity of binaural interaction: II. Clinical period and changes in midline response. *J Neurol* 1977;40:6

62. Ochs, M., Tharpe, A.M.: Auditory deprivation: A review. Paper presented at Workshop on the Problem of Children with Very Mild Hearing Loss: A Closer Look. The Bill Wilkerson Hearing and Speech Center, Nashville, TN, Sept 16-17, 1982

63. Johnston, W.H., Angara, V., Baumal, R., et al.: Erythroblastosis fetalis and hyperbilirubinemia: Five-year follow-up with neurologic, psychologic, and audiologic evaluation. *Pediatrics* 1967;39:88-92

64. Overall, J.C.: Neonatal bacterial meningitis. *J Pediatr* 1970;76:499-511

65. Carhart, R.: Probable mechanisms underlying kernicterus hearing loss. *Acta Otolaryngol Suppl* 1967;221:6-41

66. Sells, C.J., Carpenter, R.L., Ray, C.G.: Sequelae of central nervous system enterovirus infections. *N Engl J Med* 1975;293:1-4

67. Ferry, P.C., Cooper, J., Sitton, A.B., et al.: Sequelae of hemophilus influenzae meningitis: Preliminary report of a long-term follow-up study. Paper presented at the Conference of the Biology of Hemophilus influenzae, Pinehurst, NC, April 24, 1981

68. Ventry, I.M.: Research design issues in studies of effects of middle ear effusion, in Workshop on effects of otitis media on the child. *Pediatrics* 1983;71:639-652

69. Paradise, J.L.: Long-term effects of short-term hearing loss—Menace or myth?, in Workshop on effects of otitis media on the child. *Pediatrics* 1983;71:639-652

70. Bess, F.H.: Impedance screening for children—A need for more research. *Ann Otol Rhinol Laryngol* 1980;89:(68):228-232

71. Rapin, I.: Conductive hearing loss: Effects on children's language and scholastic skills. *Ann Otol Rhinol Laryngol* 1979;88:(60):3-12

72. Menyuk, P.: Design factors in the assessment of language development in children with otitis media. *Ann Otol Rhinol Laryngol* 1979;88:(60): 78-87

73. Ventry, I.M.: Effects of conductive hearing loss: Fact or fiction. *J Speech Hear Disord* 1980;45: 143-156

74. Paradise, J.L.: Otitis media during early life: How hazardous to development?: A critical review of the evidence. *Pediatrics* 1981;68:869-873

Effects of Conductive Hearing Loss: Fact or Fiction

Ira M. Ventry
Teachers College, Columbia University, New York, New York

This paper reviews the empirical evidence implicating conductive hearing impairment as a causal agent in learning disability, language dysfunction, and central auditory problems. From this review one can conclude that there are few, if any, valid data linking conductive hearing impairment to any of these problems. Suggestions for improving research in this area conclude the article.

Many authors recently have expressed concern about the deleterious effects of conductive hearing loss, especially mild and fluctuating conductive loss, on auditory and language function and on educational achievement. This concern is most apparent in a recent article by Katz (1978), in which he reviews a variety of studies and concludes that conductive hearing impairment can indeed cause auditory and language dysfunction. The concern about the educational effects of conductive hearing impairment also serves as a major rationale for ASHA's 1979 guidelines for acoustic immittance screening of school children. This article presents a critical evaluation of the research evidence cited by Katz and others. The evaluation shows that few valid data support a causal link between conductive hearing impairment (including mild and fluctuating losses) and language, learning, or nonperipheral auditory deficits. This article also offers some suggestions for improving the quality of research in this area.

Katz (1978) views conductive hearing loss as a "long standing form of sensory deprivation" (p. 885) which can interfere with the acquisition of good auditory perceptual skills, can adversely influence language development, can increase the likelihood of having a significant learning disability, and can lead to aberrant results on auditory tests, such results being mistaken as signs of gross retrocochlear lesions or brain lesions. Katz concludes, in part, that "the effects of deprivation [conductive hearing loss] may be far-reaching and no doubt involve the retrocochlear system and the brain" (p. 885); that "the greater the hearing loss and the longer the period of deprivation, the more extreme the retrocochlear signs" (p. 885); that "disruption in auditory perception and language (presumably cerebral functions) are associated with fluctuating hearing loss, especially unilateral problems and with early age of onset" (p. 885); and that "even after the mechanical blockage has been removed, abnormal auditory function may persist" (p. 885). While not subscribing to all of Katz's conclusions, other writers have expressed similar views (ASHA Committee on Audiometric Evaluation, 1979; Brooks, 1978; Downs, 1978; Needleman, 1977; Webster and Downs, 1978; Zinkus, Gottleib, and Schapiro, 1978).

The Evidence

Effects of Conductive Hearing Loss on Auditory Function

Katz cites a variety of studies purportedly demonstrating that there is more to a conductive hearing loss than simply a mechanical disruption of the middle ear transmission system. An important shortcoming of Katz's review is his heavy reliance on unpublished studies. Because these studies are unpublished, identifying methodological shortcomings, problems with data analysis, or faulty interpretation of the results is impossible. Most important is that unpublished studies have not been subject to peer review, that is, a review conducted by objective and knowledgeable readers whose purpose is to evaluate the quality of a given research study and to determine if the research should be published. An occasional reference to an unpublished work is acceptable; overuse of unpublished sources is not.

Katz cites a series of studies conducted in the early and mid-1960s that sought to determine if temporary threshold shift (TTS) data could differentiate aural pathologies. These studies generally demonstrated "bizarre" (Katz and Epstein, 1962) results for subjects with middle ear disorders because there was greater TTS and slower recovery for people who presumably had normal sensory mechanisms. The results of these studies are difficult to explain especially when considering that few other studies have demonstrated "bizarre" results for people with conductive hearing loss. For individuals with conductive impairments, test results on a peripheral test battery are not unlike those obtained for normal hearing subjects except, of course, when the conductive pathology itself affects the test results (for example, an abnormal tympanogram). For the most part, however, people with conductive hearing impairment do not demonstrate "bizarre" results on Bekesy audiometry, on word identification tests, on tone decay tests, or on SISI tests (Konkle and Rintlemann, 1979; Olsen and Matkin, 1978). In addition, the "bizarre" TTS results have not been replicated by investigators other than Katz, his students, and his associates. Finally, the use of TTS data to differentiate aural pathologies has not received recent attention.

Perhaps the major methodological flaw of these early studies lies in subject selection. In Epstein and Bower (1962), four groups of subjects were employed: normal-hearing subjects, conductive subjects, subjects with cochlear hearing loss, and subjects with presbycusis. The conductive group differed from the other three groups not only with respect to type of pathology but also in the severity of the hearing impairment. The same was true for the three subject groups employed by Epstein, Katz, and Dickenson (1962). In fact, in the latter study, the authors' statistical analysis demonstrated that if threshold sensitivity loss is taken into account, subjects with conductive impairment did not demonstrate significantly greater TTS than normal subjects. Although an attempt was made to compensate for threshold differences by presenting a stimulating tone at the same sensation level for all subjects, the more meaningful procedure would have been to study subjects with different pathologies but who were matched on severity of threshold loss (for example, a subject with cochlear lesion and a threshold impairment of 40 dB vs. a subject with a conductive lesion and a threshold impairment of 40 dB). As long as there are important threshold differences among subjects, the effect of pathology per se is difficult to parcel out.

There were other problems with these early studies. The test frequency that was used by Katz (1965) was 6000 Hz, a frequency that nearly always has the largest intersubject variability of any audiometric frequency (Corso, 1958). This variability combined with a small sample, and relatively small TTS differences between conditions makes interpretation difficult. In the Epstein and Bower (1962) study as well as the Epstein, Katz, and Dickenson (1962) study, the order of frequency presentation was such that 4000 Hz was always the first frequency tested. As a result, order effects were not controlled by either counterbalanced or random presentations. This result is especially important because the TTS data were most unusual at 4000 Hz. That the results at 4000 Hz were contaminated by short-term maturation effects (that is, practice or learning) is entirely possible. In short, methodological problems plus the absence of published replicative studies plus the "bizarre" findings raise serious questions about the adequacy of these early studies of TTS in conductive hearing impairment.

Animal Studies

Three studies were cited by Katz (1978) to support the effects of auditory deprivation. One study is unpublished and therefore cannot be analyzed. However, the most recent study by Webster and Webster (1977) is available. Three groups of mice were studied: one normal group, one group whose auditory experiences were restricted, and one group that had external ear canal atresia. Webster and Webster found abnormalities in the dorsal cochlear nuclei and trapezoid bodies of the sensory-restricted animals and concluded that even incomplete conductive lesions can lead to abnormal central structures. What is noteworthy here is that the Websters had nine measures of neuron lengths and nine measures of neuron packing densities. Thus, there was a possible total of 54 differences (3 groups ˇ 2 neuron conditions ˇ 9 measures in each neuron condition). Webster and Webster found that the experimental mice differed significantly from the controls for two neuron length measures (four differences out of a possible 27) and under only one neuron density condition (two differences out of a possible 27). Thus, conductive mice differed from normal mice on six (11%) of 54 measures. On the basis of the actual data, Webster and Webster's conclusion seems premature at best and unwarranted at worst. At the very least, Webster and Webster's study bears replication. In this regard, recent research on auditory brain-stem-evoked responses (BER) has demonstrated nothing unusual about the responses of individuals with conductive impairment other than a shift in the latency of wave V. The shift in latency, however, is attributed to the different spectra of air- and bone-conducted signals and not to the conductive hearing impairment per se (Mauldin and Jerger, 1979).

Finally, the data of Batkin, Groth, Watson, and Ansberry (1970) showing poorer responses to puretone stimuli by sound-isolated rats are not supported by Liberman's (1978) recent study of auditory-nerve responses from cats raised in a low-noise chamber.

Once again, the studies and data cited by Katz are subject to different or contrary interpretations. Although a review of these studies suggests an obvious need for further research, considerable caution still needs to be exercised in generalizing from laboratory studies of mice and cats to the effects of conductive hearing loss on children and adults.

Effects on Auditory Perception

The last body of research reviewed by Katz deals with the possible effects of conductive hearing loss on auditory perception. Nowhere is Katz's bias more evident than in his treatment of two delayed auditory feedback (DAF) studies performed in the late 1950s. On the basis of these two studies, Katz (1978) makes the following statement: "The results of the delayed speech feedback studies implicate brain dysfunction" (p. 883). In one study cited by Katz, Butler and Galloway (1959) tested three groups of subjects—normal hearing, sensorineural, and conductive—under two levels (50 and 80 dB) of DAF. Katz reports that the conductive group had more interference than the sensorineural group, and he expressed interest in the fact "that such a faint level . . . caused so much disruption to speech production . . ." (p. 883). Butler and Galloway's actual data showed that at the faint level (50 dB), the mean number of errors for the sensorineural subjects was 2.2, while for the conductive subjects it was 3.2, a mean difference of one error. In addition, Katz failed to point out that at the 80 dB level, conductive subjects had fewer mean errors than the other two groups although between-group differences continued to remain small. Butler and Galloway's actual data simply do not support Katz's conclusion.

In a second study cited by Katz, Harford and Jerger (1959) found conductive subjects to be more affected by DAF than four other groups, including a group of "plugged" normal subjects. The data, however, must be interpreted cautiously because of the small sample size ($N = 10$ in each group), the small differences in median error scores between the three most affected groups, the large intersubject variability, and the absence of any statistical analysis. Also, the three groups most affected by DAF had poorer hearing thresholds than the two groups least affected, once again implicating hearing threshold level differences as a possible contaminant of the data. In a more recent study, Grönäs, Quist-Hanssen, and Bjelde (1968) found no difference between conductive subjects and "plugged" normal subjects in their performance under DAF, and they found that both of these groups had significantly more errors than normal hearing subjects or operated otosclerotic subjects. These data are contrary to those reported by Harford and Jerger and fail to lend support to Katz's argument. A careful analysis of the DAF studies cited by Katz yields equivocal findings at best and offers little support for the statement that DAF studies implicate brain dysfunction.

The last portion of Katz's paper cites a number of studies purporting to show brain dysfunction differences between subjects with and without conductive hearing loss. Again, the use of unpublished material or unrefereed reports is striking.[1] Two published studies cited by Katz are notable because they bear on the issue of the possible effects of conductive hearing loss on language dysfunction in children. Holm and Kunze (1969), in perhaps the most widely cited study, found that children with long-standing conductive hearing loss had generally poorer language performance on a variety of measures than did a group of matched subjects with no history of conductive hearing loss. Although the study was reasonably well done, several important methodological problems may have confounded the results. One problem that Holm and Kunze recognized was that the subjects ($N = 16$ in each group) were not matched on intelligence, environmental stimulation, motivation, and language experience in the home and that these factors could have accounted for the group differences. Careful matching of subjects in research of this sort is an extremely important methodological issue. Other procedural factors that might have confounded the results of the study were the extent of the hearing impairment at the time of the language evaluation (not measured), lack of control over experimenter expectancies or attributes (there is no indication that subjects were seen "blind," thus the experimenter may have known into which group a child was placed and this knowledge may have introduced experimenter bias), and the test instrument employed (the experimental version of the Illinois Test of Psycholinguistic Abilities [ITPA]).

Recently, Kirk and Kirk (1978) noted that there was some question about the equivalence of the experimental and revised editions of the ITPA. In addition, they also cited three major limitations of research using the ITPA. The first limitation is the difficulty obtaining comparable control and experimental groups. We have already identified this as an important limitation of the Holm and Kunze (1969) study. Second, Kirk and Kirk indicate that children must be age-appropriate for the ITPA. They specifically caution against the use of the ITPA with nine- and ten-year-old children. The age range of the children studied by Holm and Kunze was from 5fi-9 yrs, with a mean age of 7.4 years. Determining how many of the Holm and Kunze subjects were nine years of age or slightly older is not possible. Since control subjects were matched within six months of the age of their experimental counterparts, the control group may have had more children who were nine years of age or older, thus compromising the test data. Finally, Kirk and Kirk (1978) strongly emphasize that the ITPA must be administered by people adequately trained and pre-

---

[1]It is discouraging to note that in the ASHA guidelines on Acoustic Immittance Screening (1979), five of seven references dealing with the educational implications of middle-ear disease are to unrefereed sources.

pared to use the instrument. Holm and Kunze do not identify the one or more individuals who administered the test, and thus there is no way to assess their qualifications. The Holm and Kunze study was a first step in the right direction. That it was a first step, and not the definitive study, was recognized by Holm and Kunze (1969) with the following statement: "This was a pilot study with all the problems inherent in a retrospective design. Further prospective studies . . . are obviously needed" (p. 839).

The second published study cited by Katz is another reasonably well-controlled study conducted by Lewis (1976). In this study, two groups of Australian aborigine children were compared; one group ($N = 14$) had chronic ear disease while the other group ($N = 18$) was free of such disease. A group of 18 European children without ear disease was also tested. Lewis evaluated the children on seven measures: the Wepman Auditory Discrimination Test; a speech discrimination test in quiet and in noise; an investigator-developed phonemic synthesis test; a dichotic listening test; and tests of verbal and of nonverbal intelligence. Language performance was not assessed directly. Although Katz (1978) suggests that conductively impaired children had "considerably poorer auditory perceptual performance" (p. 885), Lewis's actual data reveal only three statistically significant findings, those being on the Wepman Test, on the phonemic synthesis test (on which no validity or reliability data were reported by Lewis), and on the verbal intelligence test. On the speech discrimination-in-quiet task, there was less than a one-word difference between the aborigine groups. Although there are other problems with the Lewis study, suffice it to say that Lewis's data do not offer unequivocal support for the hypothesis that conductive hearing impairment in children causes cerebral dysfunction.

Other studies of the effects of conductive hearing loss on children have been published, but many have flaws similar to those mentioned. Needleman (1977) studied two groups of 20 children each, one group with a history of otitis media and one without such a history. In the former group, there were 13 males and in the latter group there were only 8 males. Could the sex difference account for the fact that children with otitis media had significantly poorer articulation? Despite the fact that there was only one other significant difference between groups (there were four nonsignificant differences), Needleman focuses her discussion on the differences and ignores the implications of the nonsignificant findings.

Needleman's study had additional flaws that sorely compromised the data. Some of these flaws include vague subject selection criteria especially with respect to the identification of incidents of otitis media, the absence of any reliability or validity data on an experimenter-designed test instrument, the failure to control for experimenter expectancies, the inappropriate use of some standardized tests (for example, the Peabody Picture Vocabulary Test as the sole measure of mental age), the failure to randomize or counterbalance the seven tests employed, the use of overall rather than pair matching, and the absence of audiologic or impedance measurements. These shortcomings are typical of those that might be found in published but unrefereed sources.

At first glance, a study by Zinkus, Gottlieb, and Schapiro (1978) seems well done. They studied the developmental and psychoeducational sequelae of chronic otitis media in two groups of children. One group contained 18 subjects with long-standing histories of severe chronic otitis, while the other ($N = 22$) included subjects with relatively mild otitis media during the first three years of life. One positive feature of this investigation was that all evaluations were done without the examiner's knowledge of subject classification (that is, severe vs. mild). Unfortunately, though, the study is flawed in several important respects. For example, a major shortcoming was that speech and language development was assessed by asking parents at what age subjects had acquired a four- to ten-word vocabulary and formulated and utilized three-word sentences. The accuracy of the parental reports notwithstanding, defining speech and language development in this fashion is naive and superficial. The study, in fact, says nothing about speech and language development despite the authors' assertion that children with severe chronic otitis media "were delayed in the major areas of speech and language development" (p. 1102) and "suffered profound delays in language development"(p.1103). Additionally, the mean data reported for the severe group could easily be interpreted as falling within normal developmental expectations (Words = 18 months, S.D. = 2.2 months; Sentences = 34 months, S.D. = 4.1 months). Secondly, the Wechsler Intelligence Scale for Children (WISC) was the sole measure used to evaluate verbal and nonverbal abilities. The problem lies not with the use of the WISC but with the interpretation of the WISC results. The authors state that "the results suggest a general intellectual deficit among the children with severe otitis media" (p. 1102), when, in fact, the mean full scale WISC score was 100.6 for this group and the Verbal IQ was within 3 points of the Performance IQ. In the treatment of subtest performance, Zinkus et al. ignored the fact that the severe group scored at normal or above normal levels on six of 11 subtests including analytical reasoning and expressive vocabulary (for some reason, data for five additional WISC subtests were not reported).

Although 20 statistical comparisons are reported in the article, the authors fail to identify the type of statistical test used, the values found, the degrees of freedom, or whether the tests were one-tailed or two-tailed. These are important omissions because all of the authors' conclusions are based on statistically significant differences between the severe and the mild groups. Because of the lack of detail, there is no way to assess the adequacy of the statistical treatment of the data. Finally, although the authors did a reasonably good job in matching the two groups of subjects on extraneous variables such as socioeconomic status, sex, and race, they failed to consider health problems other than otitis media occurring during or after the first three years of life. For instance, children with severe otitis media could have had other chronic illnesses that required significant periods of hospitalization during their first three years or that resulted in frequent absences from school. Health history differences between groups were not controlled. Despite the above-noted flaws and despite the small N, the Zinkus, et al study received extensive coverage in a *New York Times* article (December 26, 1978) titled "Middle-Ear Disease Is Linked to Learning."

Masters and Marsh (1978) found in their study a 12% higher prevalence of Type B and Type C tympanograms among children with learning disabilities (25% prevalence) than was found among normal children (13% prevalence). Unfortunately, the authors incorrectly interpret their significant Chi Square value as "indicating a reliable relationship between learning disabilities and middle ear pathology" (p. 105). The Chi Square test says nothing about reliability and in this application simply demonstrates a difference between groups. The Utah Test of Language Development failed to demonstrate significant differences between normal children with and without abnormal tympanograms or between learning-disabled children with and without middle ear problems. Probably because 75% of the learning disabled children did not have abnormal tympanograms, Masters and Marsh correctly suggest that a cause and effect relationship cannot be assumed and that there is an obvious need for further research.

Finally, there is an early study by Kaplan, Fleshman, Bender, Baum, and Clark (1973) that reports data on the long-term effects of otitis media on Alaskan Eskimo children. This study, too, has significant shortcomings, not the least of which are inade-

quate audiologic data (for example, bone conduction measurements made in a quiet schoolhouse or community room using a portable audiometer, classification of hearing loss on the basis of poorer ear results, and absence of impedance measures), unexplained differences in sample sizes (for example, 489 children with ear disease histories but audiometric results only on 361; verbal and performance intelligence scores on 380 children but data reported for only 283 subjects), lack of description of the statistical tests employed, a nearly incomprehensible presentation and treatment of the data, and attention given to only those aspects of the data that lend support to the hypothesis that otitis media has a deleterious effect on intelligence and scholastic achievement.

A careful evaluation of published research on the relation between conductive hearing impairment and language and learning difficulties suggests that the relationship has been poorly documented, that methodological flaws in the published research have contaminated the data and confounded the reported results, and that there is a continuing need, as so many investigators have emphasized, for ongoing research in this area.

Some Comments and Suggestions for Researchers and Consumers of Research

Merely identifying the methodological or interpretive shortcomings of previous research is not sufficient—the topic is too important. While I take issue with the way previous research has been conducted and with the uncritical acceptance of the interpretations drawn from the research, I do not take issue with the hypothesis that there may be a link between conductive hearing impairment and language, learning, and auditory dysfunction. If such a link can be demonstrated, it could have profound implications for audiologists, speech-language pathologists, physicians, and above all, parents and children. Because of these implications, we must conduct the most rigorous and exacting kind of research possible. Also, the reader of research has the responsibility for critical evaluation of the published research and for not succumbing to the intuitively appealing notion that there must be a cause and effect relationship between conductive hearing impairment and language, learning, and auditory dysfunction.

Research on the effects of conductive hearing impairment is no simple matter.[2] At the heart of the difficulty is that true experimental research is nearly impossible. That is, researchers simply cannot manipulate (that is, induce) hearing impairment on human subjects and then study the effects of that manipulation on behavior or function. This type of cause-and-effect study might be done with laboratory animals, but generalizations to humans would be sorely limited.[3]

As a result, most of the research on conductive hearing impairment has to be descriptive; either two or more groups are compared (comparative research), or relationships are studied (correlational research), or changes in subjects are observed over time (longitudinal research), or there is a comparative-experimental design (mixed design). The vast majority of research on the effects of conductive hearing loss has utilized the comparative design rather than the much stronger mixed design in which there can be experimental manipulation of variables that might differentiate conductive subjects and nonconductive subjects. Young (1976) has also proposed a way of strengthening comparative research by focusing on predictive potential rather than on differences between group means.

Threats to Internal Validity[4]

Whatever the type of research, there are several overriding considerations for the researcher and the reader. First, in between- subject comparative research (for example, a group of children with conductive hearing loss vs. a group of children without conductive hearing loss compared on a variety of measures such as the Wepman or the ITPA), the major threat to internal validity lies in subject selection. The two (or more) groups being compared should be similar on all subject variables except for the classification variable that differentiates the groups (for example, presence or absence of conductive hearing loss). These important subject variables include age, intelligence, sex, socioeconomic status, race, grade level, and the like. Without this comparability which, by the way, is best achieved by a pair-matching technique such as that employed by Holm and Kunze (1969), one or more of the subject variables (for example, intelligence) could account for any group differences as well as or instead of the hearing status of the subjects. The requirement for group comparability applies equally to mixed designs, that is, to designs that have both an experimental and a comparative component. When groups are compared, the groups should be as similar as possible on those variables that might mimic the effect of the classification variable. Obtaining group comparability is no simple matter but is worth the effort because it reduces or eliminates the subject selection threat to internal validity.

This type of comparative research has another pitfall. Because one group of subjects has had conductive pathology and one group has not, the former group will probably have a hearing impairment while the latter group will not. Any difference in hearing sensitivity

must be considered in choosing presentation levels of all test stimuli. For example, the examiner must be certain that the subject is hearing the instructions during administration of an intelligence test. Researchers need to measure the hearing levels of all subjects prior to the administration of the research tasks; since hearing levels in conductive impairments can fluctuate, there should be as short an interval as possible between hearing measurements and the research task. The obtained hearing threshold data should be reported by the researcher.

One issue that needs to be clarified is whether it is fluctuating conductive hearing loss per se that may cause dysfunctions or whether it is hearing loss, irrespective of type, that is the culprit. The argument seems to be that it is the effects of fluctuating conductive hearing loss that are of most consequence and, in fact, these effects underlie the major rationale for acoustic immittance screening of school children. But, as we have seen, the evidence here is scanty. Two other important questions remain: Does chronic middle-ear pathology that results in significant hearing impairment produce language and learning problems? and Are these problems similar to those that are produced by longstanding sensorineural hearing impairment? Brooks (1978) cites a study by Hamilton suggesting a positive answer to both questions. Unfortunately, Hamilton's study was published in a rather obscure source, *Occasional Paper No. 6, North Regional Association for the Deaf*, and it is not available to me for evaluation purposes. Nonetheless, this type of comparative research with normal subjects, conductive subjects, and sensorineural subjects should be replicated because it may demonstrate that the severity of the hearing impairment, and not necessarily the type, has the most important consequences for language development, learning, and educational achievement.

In addition to the subject selection threat to internal validity, another major threat needs to be controlled by researchers.[5] It is the threat posed by instrumentation. The instrumentation threat is important because it transcends the type of research conducted. Faulty, inappropriate, or inadequate instrumentation can be as

---

[2]Hanson and Ulvestad (1979) present an extensive discussion of design consideration in research dealings with the effects of conductive hearing impairment. Ventry and Schiavetti (1980) provide a detailed description of the research evaluation process.

[3]Merely labeling one group of subjects as an experimental group (for example, conductive subjects) and another group as a control group (for example, nonconductive subjects) does not mean that the study is experimental. There may or may not be an experimental component; there will certainly be a comparative component, and for this reason, subject selection criteria are of utmost importance.

much of a problem in experimental as in descriptive research and thus deserves the careful attention of both the researcher and reader alike.

Most of us are aware of the importance of carefully calibrated instrumentation in the conduct of research. What may be less apparent, however, is that instrumentation includes paper and pencil tests, standardized and nonstandardized materials, and questionnaires. Instrumentation also includes the human experimenter. With respect to research on the effects of conductive hearing loss, valid and reliable instruments must be used to collect the data. This rule is relatively easy to apply to those test instruments that have undergone extensive standardization (for example, the ITPA). Even here, however, the researcher and the reader must be certain that the standardized test is the most appropriate instrument for the purposes of the research, that it is appropriate for the subjects studied, and that it is the best instrument of the many available.

The tasks of doing and evaluating research become more complicated when nonstandardized instruments are employed. These are instruments developed by the researcher for the specific purposes of a given research study. In this case, the researcher has an obligation to provide, at the very least, data attesting to the reliability of the instrument. Ideally, the researcher should also address the issue of the validity of the test instrument employed. There should be examples of the test items, a description of the rationale underlying the selection of the items, and details of how the test is scored. An unreliable or invalid nonstandardized test instrument makes suspect any data reported by the investigator.

The human observer as an instrument also needs careful consideration by researcher and evaluator. Much has been written about the effects of experimenter attributes and expectancies as instrumentation threats to internal validity (Rosenthal, 1966; and Barber, 1976). In an area in which investigators may be inclined to see what they wish to see, control of experimenter expectancies is especially important. A variety of methods is available to the investigator to control this threat to internal validity. Perhaps the best method is to use a blind technique whereby the individual who collects the data does not know into which group or treatment condition a subject belongs. This approach is exemplified in the study by Zinkus, Gottlieb, and Schapiro (1978). This is the only study of

the many reviewed that employed a blind technique. Another method for controlling experimenter bias is to record and analyze responses through the use of mechanical or electrical devices. Still another method is to differentiate the experimenter from the investigator. The former merely collects the data with or without knowledge of the hypothesis under investigation while the latter designs the study, analyzes the data, and writes the research report. Finally, strict experimental and research protocols need to be used, with frequent checks by the investigator that the experimenter is adhering to the protocol. Whatever method is used, investigator biases must be controlled so that they do not pose a threat to internal validity. The researcher, of course, has the responsibility to describe the methods employed to control experimenter bias.

A Threat to External Validity

In addition to threats to internal validity, the researcher needs to be concerned about threats to the ability to generalize the data, that is, about threats to external validity (Campbell and Stanley, 1966). External validity, in both experimental and descriptive research, asks the question: "To what populations, settings, treatment variables, and measurement variables can the effect be generalized?" (p. 5). Although Campbell and Stanley discuss four such threats, I will treat the one that appears to pose the major threat to the external validity of studies evaluating the effects of conductive hearing loss. Previously, I discussed subject selection as a threat to internal validity. That discussion centered essentially around who the subjects were and whether, in fact, they were comparable on important dimensions other than the classification variable. The threat to external validity arises from how subjects are selected. Random selection of subjects is generally considered one of the best methods for increasing external validity. For a variety of reasons, random selection of subjects from the total population of interest is usually not feasible. As a result, the studies of the effects of conductive hearing impairment have not employed random samples of subjects. To overcome this problem, investigators in other fields have relied on replicative studies, on using fairly large samples of subjects, and on cautious and prudent generalizations. This has not been the case in studies of the effects of conductive hearing loss. There have been no published replications, sample sizes have been small, and investi-

---

[4]A study has internal validity when the researcher has minimized or controlled those nuisance or extraneous variables that can mimic the effect of experimental treatment or can serve as alternative explanations of the results. See Campbell and Stanley (1966) and Ventry and Schiavetti (1980) for a complete discussion of internal validity in experimental and descriptive research.

---

[5]Campbell and Stanley (1966) describe eight threats to internal validity. For the sake of brevity, I have limited my discussion to the two most pervasive threats: subject selection and instrumentation.

gators have, for the most part, been imprudent in their generalizations. In addition, experimenter expectancies have led researchers to generalize from a few statistically significant findings while ignoring a large number of findings that were not consistent with their basic hypothesis. Drawing meaningful generalizations from a single study is rarely possible. Rather, the accumulation of valid empirical evidence from research with different subjects, different experimenters, different settings, and different tasks will allow us to answer the question: What are the effects of conductive hearing loss on children? At present, we cannot answer the question. The search must continue, albeit at a higher and more rigorous level than in the past.

Acknowledgment

My thanks goes to Margaret Lahey for convincing me that the importance of the subject demanded a constructive article rather than an angry letter to the Editor. My appreciation is also extended to Honor O'Malley for her helpful comments on portions of the article. Requests for reprints should be directed to Ira M. Ventry, Department of Speech Pathology and Audiology, Teachers College, Columbia University, 525 West 120th Street, New York, New York 10027.

References

ASHA Committee Audiometric Evaluation, Guidelines for acoustic immittance screening of middle-ear function. *Asha*, 21, 283-288 (1979).

Barber, T.X., *Pitfalls in Human Research: Ten Pivotal Points*. New York: Pergamon Press (1976).

Batkin, S., Groth, H., Watson, J.R., and Ansberry, M., Effects of auditory deprivation on the development of auditory sensitivity in albino rats. *Electroenceph. Clin. Neurophysiol.*, 28, 351-359 (1970).

Brooks, D.N., Acoustic impedance testing for screening auditory function in schoolchildren. *Maico Audio. Libr. Ser.*, 15, Report 8 (1978).

Butler, R.A., and Galloway, F.T., Performance of normal hearing and hard-of-hearing persons on the delayed feedback task. *J. Speech Hear. Res.*, 2, 84-90 (1959).

Campbell, D.T., and Stanley, J.C., *Experimental and Quasi-Experimental Designs for Research*. Chicago: Rand McNally (1966).

Corso, J.F., Proposed laboratory standard for normal hearing. *J. Acoust. Soc. Amer.*, 30, 14-23 (1958).

Downs, M.P., Auditory screening. *Otolar. Clin. N. Amer.*, 11, 611-629 (1978).

Epstein, A., and Bower, D.R., Auditory fatigue in differentiating aural pathology. *Ann. Otol. Rhinol. Lar.*, 71, 970-989 (1962).

Epstein, A., Katz, J., and Dickenson, D.T., Low level stimulation in the differentiation of middle ear pathology. *Acta Otolar.*, 55, 81-96 (1962).

Grönäs, H.E., Quist-Hanssen, S., and Bjelde, A., Conductive hearing loss with and without a functioning stapedius muscle. *Acta Otolar.*, 66, 13-19 (1968).

Hanson, D.G., and Ulvestad, R.F., (Eds.), Otitis media and child development. *Ann. Otol. Rhinol. Otolar.*, Suppl. 60, part 2 (1979).

Harford, E., and Jerger, J., Effect of loudness recruitment on delayed feedback. *J. Speech Hear. Res.*, 2, 361-368 (1959).

Holm, V.A., and Kunze, L.H., Effect of chronic otitis media on language and speech development. *Pediatrics*, 43, 833-839 (1969).

Kaplan, G.J., Fleshman, J.K., Bender, T.R., Baum, C., and Clark, P.S., Long term effects of otitis media: A ten-year cohort study of Alaskan Eskimo children. *Pediatrics*, 52, 577-585 (1973).

Katz, J., Temporary threshold shift, auditory sensory deprivation, and conductive hearing loss. *J. Acoust. Soc. Amer.*, 37, 923-924 (1965).

Katz, J., The effects of conductive hearing loss on auditory function. *Asha*, 20, 879-886 (1978).

Katz, J., and Epstein, A., A hypothesis considering non-mechanical aspects of conductive hearing loss. *Acta Otolar.*, 55, 145-150 (1962).

Kirk, S.A., and Kirk, W.D. Uses and abuses of the ITPA. *J. Speech Hear. Dis.*, 43, 58-75 (1978).

Konkle, D.F., and Rintlemann, W.F., Peripheral and central auditory systems: Test battery interpretation. In W.F. Rintlemann (Ed.), *Hearing Assessment*. Baltimore, Md.: University Park Press (1979).

Lewis, N., Otitis media and linguistic incompetence. *Archs Otolar.*, 102, 387-390 (1976).

Liberman, M.C., Auditory-nerve response from cats raised in a low-noise chamber. *J. Acoust. Soc. Amer.*, 63, 442-455 (1978).

Masters, L., and Marsh, G.E., II, Middle ear pathology as a factor in learning disabilities. *J. Learning Disabilities*, 11, 103-106 (1978).

Mauldin, L., and Jerger, J., Auditory brain stem evoked responses to bone-conducted signals. *Archs Otolar.*, 105, 656-661 (1979).

Needleman, H., Effects of hearing loss from early recurrent otitis media on speech and language development. In B. Jaffe (Ed.), *Hearing loss in children*. Baltimore, Md.: University Park Press (1977).

Olsen, W.O., and Matkin, N.D., Differential Audiology. In D.E. Rose (Ed.), *Audiological Assessment* (2nd ea.) Englewood Cliffs, N.J.: Prentice-Hall (1978).

Rosenthal, R., *Experimenter effects in behavioral research*. New York: Appleton-Century-Crofts (1966).

Ventry, I.M., and Schiavetti, N., *Evaluating research in speech pathology and audiology: A guide for clinicians and students.* Reading, Mass.: Addison Wesley (1980).

Webster, D., and Downs, M.P., Conductive hearing loss and critical periods in mice and men. Presented to the Annual Convention of the American Speech and Hearing Association, San Francisco, California (November, 1978).

Webster, D.B., and Webster, M., Neonatal sound deprivation affects brain stem auditory nuclei. *Archs Otolar.*, 103, 392-396 (1977).

Young, M.A., Application of regression analysis concepts to retrospective research in speech pathology. *J. Speech Hearing Res.*, 19, 15-18 (1976) .

Zinkus, P.W., Gottlieb, M.L., and Schapiro, M., Developmental and psychoeducational sequelae of chronic otitis media. *Am. J. Dis. Child*, 132, 1100-1104 (1978).

Received October 4, 1979
Accepted December 20, 1979

Hearing Acuity of Children with Otitis Media with Effusion

Thomas J. Fria, Ph.D., Erdem I. Cantekin, Ph.D., and John A. Eichler

*Department of Otolaryngology, University of Pittsburgh School of Medicine
and Children's Hospital of Pittsburgh*

Hearing levels are reported for a cohort of 222 infants (aged 7 to 24 months) and 540 older children (aged 2 to 12 years) with otitis media with effusion (OME). The infants had an average speech awareness threshold of 24.6 dB hearing level (HL). The older group had mean bone conduction thresholds less than 10 dB HL, and air conduction thresholds averaged 27 dB HL; however, acuity was 7 dB less impaired at 2,000 Hz. The mean three-frequency pure tone average and speech reception threshold were 24.5 and 22.7 dB, respectively. Hearing acuity was not significantly related to age or previous duration of OME. The otoscopic observation of an air-fluid level or bubbles was associated with less hearing impairment; however, a predictive relationship between hearing levels and tympanogram characteristics could not be demonstrated. (*Arch Otolaryngol* 1985;111:10-16)

Otitis media manifests itself in various ways, and these manifestations collectively represent a ubiquitous disease in early childhood. A particularly common manifestation involves the effusion of liquid into the middle ear space without the signs and symptoms of an acute infection, and is known as otitis media with effusion (OME), commonly named "secretory" otitis media. Despite the frequent occurrence of OME in early childhood and its reputed association with impaired language and development, several issues remain unresolved. For example, there is no universally accepted scheme for classifying the forms of the disease, the pathogenetic factors continue to be studied, and the efficacy of various methods of treatment has not been determined. In addition, our knowledge of the various sequelae associated with the disease remains incomplete. One of these sequelae, hearing loss, is closely related to the function of the child and is, therefore, especially important to understand.

Several descriptions of the hearing loss associated with OME have appeared in the literature.[1-8] For a variety of reasons, these reports have not provided a complete profile of what the clinician might expect of the disease's effect on hearing acuity. Two of the six studies were retrospective reviews of patient charts, with no assurance that the disease was uniformly diagnosed or that the diagnostic tools employed were validated. The larger series of patients represent more severe, chronic forms of the disease; for example, Cohen and Sade[2] described only the "worse" audiograms observed in each case, and Kokko[4] studied only children having chronic OME. Selected studies—namely, those of Harbert and colleagues[7] and Bergman[5]—gave either no description of the subjects or an incomplete description.

The profile given herein represents the largest series of patients with an accurate diagnosis of OME of varying durations. Moreover, the data represent an age continuum from 7 months to 12 years.

Subjects and Methods

Subjects

A total of 977 children were participants in two clinical trials evaluating the medical treatment of OME. Of these, 663 were subjects in a trial investigating the efficacy of an oral decongestant-antihistamine combination,[9] and the remaining 314 were enrolled in an efficacy study of oral antibiotics. Children with symptoms of acute suppurative otitis media, purulent or chronic rhinitis, sinusitis, adhesive otitis media, tympanic membrane perforation or retraction pockets, history of middle ear surgery other than tympanocentesis, or a clear indication of sensorineural hearing loss were excluded from the studies. All subjects were seen in the Otolaryngology Ambulatory Care Center of Children's Hospital of Pittsburgh, and informed consent was obtained for each child before participation.

The audiometric data of each patient were examined for completeness. Any child not having air conduction thresholds at all frequencies and a speech reception threshold (SRT) for both ears was excluded from the analysis, as was any infant without a speech awareness threshold (SAT). There were 215 such children with

Reprinted by permission of authors and American Medical Association. Copyright 1985. *Archives of Otolaryngology*, 111, pp. 10-16.

Accepted for publication Aug. 22, 1984.

Reprint requests to Audiology Division, Children's Hospital of Pittsburgh, 125 DeSoto St., Pittsburgh, PA 15213 (Dr. Fria).

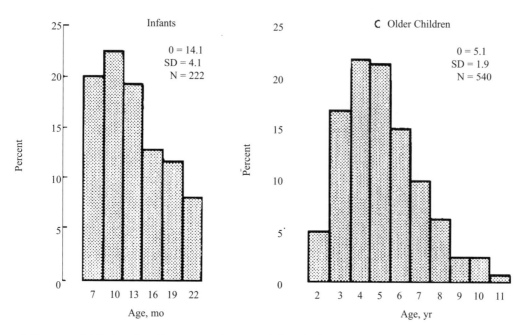

Figure 1. Frequency distribution of age for younger patient group (left) and older patient group (right). Months shown for younger group represent lower limit of interval. Associated descriptive statistics are displayed in this and all subsequent figures.

incomplete audiometric data. The remaining 762 children were divided into two groups—222 infants and 540 older children—for analysis purposes. The abundance ratio of the SRT and the SAT scores according to the subject's age was determined; it was established that the SRT was the predominant datum by 25 months of age. Consequently, children with SAT scores (aged 7 to 24 months) constituted the infant group, and children with SRT measures (aged 2 to 12 years) constituted the older children group. Figure 1 shows the age distribution of subjects in each group. More than 60% of the infants were 7 to 15 months old, and the largest proportion of the older children were 4 and 5 years old. Certain selected patient characteristic are shown in Table l: bilateral disease was more frequent than unilateral; 71% of the subjects were white; and about 30% of the children had OME of less than eight weeks' duration.

Diagnosis of OME

Before audiologic testing, the presence or absence of OME was determined with a diagnostic algorithm that incorporated otoscopy, tympanometry, and the acoustic middle ear muscle reflex. Pneumatic otoscopy was performed by clinicians who previously had been validated against myringotomy[10] and were blinded to the tympanogram when examining the children. Tympanograms were recorded by an electroacoustic impedance bridge (Madsen model Z073) coupled to an

XY plotter (Hewlett-Packard). Tympanometry was always performed by changing the external canal air pressure from 200 to –600 mm H_2O with a constant pressure rate of 35 to 38 mm H_2O/s. The ipsilateral and contralateral acoustic reflex were measured for an eliciting stimulus of 1,000 Hz at 105 dB sound pressure level (SPL). Tympanometry was performed by certified audiologists who classified the tympanometric patterns according to a schema proposed by Paradise et al.[11] Tympanometry findings were combined with the findings of acoustic reflex and otoscopy in accordance with the algorithm described by Cantekin.[12]

Audiologic Assessments

The audiometric technique was varied to suit the functional age of the child. Behavioral observation audiometry, incorporating a conditioned response to an animated toy, was used for the infants. The target response was the SAT to monitored live voice presented through a loudspeaker. Air and bone conduction thresholds for pure tone stimuli (500 through, 4,000 Hz) were determined with conventional audiometric procedures for children 4 to 12 years of age, and monitored live-voice presentation of "spondaic" words was used to determine the SRT. Conditioned, "play" audiometry was employed to obtain pure tone thresholds for children 2 to 4 years of age, and picture identification was used for the SRT.

Table 1. Selected Patient Characteristics of Study Population

	No. of Patients		
	Infants (N = 222)	Older Children (N = 540)	Total (N = 762)
Trial			
Decongestant-antihistamine	111	359	470
Antibiotic	111	181	292
Sex			
M	144	322	466
F	78	218	296
Race			
White	121	421	542
Nonwhite	101	119	220
Laterality of OME*			
Unilateral	59	155	214
Bilateral	163	385	548
Duration of OME, wk			
0-3	46	72	118
4-8	43	76	119
>8	72	189	261
unknown	61	203	264

*OME indicates otitis media with effusion.

Hearing tests were conducted in an acoustically shielded test booth (IAC model 401). Loudspeakers were positioned at 45° azimuth approximately 90 cm from the child. The audiometer (Grason-Stadler model 1704) and impedance meter (Madsen model Z073) were biologically calibrated each day, and electroacoustic calibrations were performed at six-week intervals. The study audiologists were clinically certified by the American Speech-Language-Hearing Association.

In the analysis of data, the 222 children in the infant group were treated separately, since their hearing sensitivity was defined by the SAT scores and since each child had only one measure of hearing irrespective of the disease laterality. The 540 children in the older group, however, had ear-specific measures for pure tone thresholds and for SRT scores. In these subjects, we randomly chose the data from one ear in children with bilateral OME, and only included the hearing measures of the involved ear in the unilateral cases to describe the hearing sensitivity of the cohort. This selection process was thought to be necessary for the unbiased representation of the data, i.e., each child with OME, regardless of the disease laterality, contributed only one ear to the data set.

Results

The distributions of air conduction thresholds for pure tone stimuli are shown in Fig 2. The air conduction thresholds showed that OME was associated with an average hearing level of approximately 27 dB HL at 500, 1,000, and 4,000 Hz. The disease had less of an effect on the sensitivity at 2,000 Hz, where the average threshold was approximately 20 dB HL. For simplicity, pure tone sensitivity via bone conduction is not shown in this figure, but the mean values for these test frequencies were 4.8, 5.8, 6.9, and 7.9 dB HL (and the associated SDs 5.3, 5.4, 6.5, and 7.7 dB HL), respectively.

The distribution of air conduction thresholds was qualitatively different across the test frequencies. Hearing levels were distributed in apparently normal fashion around the mean value at 500 Hz, but the degree of skewing toward less impairment increased at 1,000 Hz and was quite noticeable at 2,000 Hz. The Poisson-like distribution at 2,000 Hz was unique to this frequency, however; the 4,000-Hz distribution showed a transition from a Poisson to a Gaussian shape. The simplest observation from these four distributions is that the threshold distribution at 2,000 Hz was highly skewed and was different from the other three frequencies. The consequences of this 2,000-Hz advantage is reflected in the average of pure tone thresholds (PTA) at 500, 1,000, and 2,000 Hz. The apparent skewing of the PTA distribution probably reflects a biasing of the average due to less impairment at 2,000 Hz.

Figure 3 illustrates the distribution of the SRT and SAT scores associated with OME. The average levels were 22.7 and 24.6 dB HL, respectively. The SRT was in close agreement with the PTA, but it was about 5 dB better than the thresholds at 500, 1,000, and 4,000 Hz.

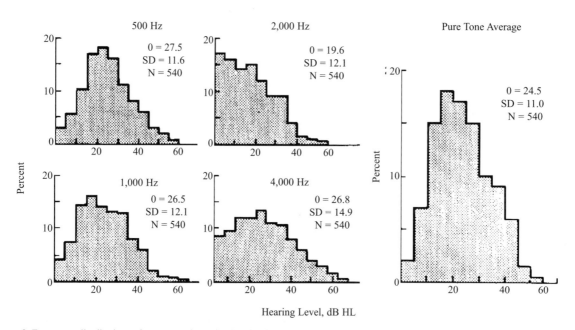

Figure 2. Frequency distributions of pure tone air conduction thresholds associated with otitis media with effusion. Shown are individual test frequencies and average of pure tone thresholds at 500, 1,000, and 2,000 Hz. HL indicates hearing level.

Therefore, it would appear that the better acuity at 2,200 Hz was also reflected in the SRT.

Further exposition of the data for older children is provided by Table 2, which shows percentile rankings of air conduction thresholds as well as the PTA and the SRT. These rankings were generally similar for pure tone sensitivity with the exception of thresholds at 2,000 Hz. One way to interpret these data is to note the level that describes the majority (i.e., 60%) of scores. For 500, 1,000, and 4,000 Hz, this level was 30 dB HL, but it was 20 dB HL at 2,000 Hz. The majority of SRT scores was described by 25 dB HL; this level approximated the majority of PTA scores. If the majority cutoff is moved to 70%, the corresponding level

was 35 dB HL for 500, 1,000, and 4,000 Hz, 25 dB HL for 2,000 Hz, and 30 dB HL for the SRT and PTA. In the context of hearing acuity for speech, thresholds associated with OME were elevated by 25 dB or more in 40% of cases and by 30 dB or more in 30% of cases.

The distribution of SAT scores shown in Fig 3 represents infants from 7 to 24 months of age with unilateral and bilateral disease. Consequently, these data reflect the average minimum response level for speech stimuli for the infants regardless of age and laterality of disease. Both of these factors are considered in Table 3, which gives a breakdown of the SAT in five age categories according to disease laterality. For

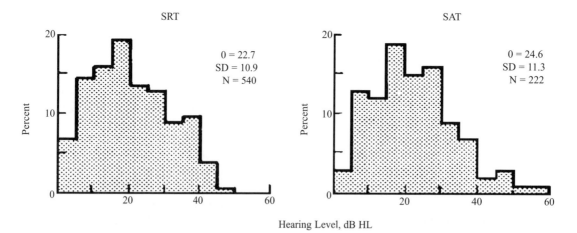

Figure 3. Frequency distribution of thresholds for speech stimuli associated with otitis media with effusion. Left, Speech reception threshold (SRT) of older children; right, speech awareness threshold (SAT) of infants. HL indicates hearing level.

Table 2. Percentile Rankings of Hearing Thresholds for Air Conduction Thresholds by Frequency, Pure Tone Average, and Speech Reception Threshold (N = 540)

Percentile	Test Frequency, Hz				Pure Tone Average	Speech Reception Threshold
	500	1,000	2,000	4,000		
10	15	10	5	10	12	10
20	20	15	10	15	15	14
30	20	20	10	20	20	20
40	25	20	15	20	20	20
50	25	25	20	25	23	20
60	30	30	20	30	27	25
70	35	35	25	35	30	30
80	35	35	30	40	35	34
90	45	45	35	45	40	38

comparison, the expected SAT scores suggested by Wilber[13] for each of these categories are also shown. As might be expected, overall, infants with unilateral disease responded at lower levels than infants with bilateral OME ($P < .05$). Also notable was the surprising similarity of SAT scores across age categories. In other words, the anticipated decrease in the SAT with increasing age was neither evident nor statitistically significant for these infants, regardless of the laterality of disease.

To determine the optimal hearing sensitivity of a given child, the PTA of the better ear of each child was evaluated with respect to the laterality of disease. Figure 4, left, shows that children with unilateral OME averaged 10 dB better hearing than children with bilateral OME. This can be attributed to the better hearing levels of the uninvolved ear. The overlap of the frequency distributions was less than 50%, emphasizing

the hearing acuity differences between the children with unilateral and those with bilateral OME.

Figure 4, right, shows the distribution of the PTA for the worse ear of children with unilateral and bilateral OME. Although there was considerable overlap between the distributions for the two groups, their mean levels were separated by 8 dB; the respective means were 22.8 and 31.3 dB HL. Consequently, a continuum of hearing levels emerged from this analysis. The best levels were represented by the better ears of children with unilateral disease, followed by the worse ears of unilaterally impaired children and the better ears of children with bilateral OME; the poorest levels were observed for the worse ears of children with bilateral disease.

To determine the possible influence of selected patient characteristics on pure tone hearing sensitivity, we examined the cumulative distribution of the PTA according to the patient's age and the previous duration

Table 3. Speech Awareness Thresholds for Infant Group in Relation to Age and Laterality of Otitis Media with Effusion (OME) (N = 222)

	Speech Awareness Threshold, dB HL,* by Age				
	7-9 mo	10-12 mo	13-15 mo	16-20 mo	21-24 mo
Total group					
Mean 26.3	23.8	25.0	24.4	22.8	
SD	11.5	11.0	9.7	13.1	10.8
N	45	51	46	55	25
Unilateral OME					
Mean 27.0	19.4	24.5	21.8	16.7	
SD	12.3	6.8	13.0	12.5	10.3
N	10	16	10	17	6
Bilateral OME					
Mean 26.1	25.9	25.1	25.5	24.7	
SD	35	5	36	38	19
Expected levels[†]					
Mean 20.0	10.0	5.0	5.0	5.0	
SD	10.0	10.0	10.0	10.0	10.0

*HL indicates hearing level. †From Wilber.[13]

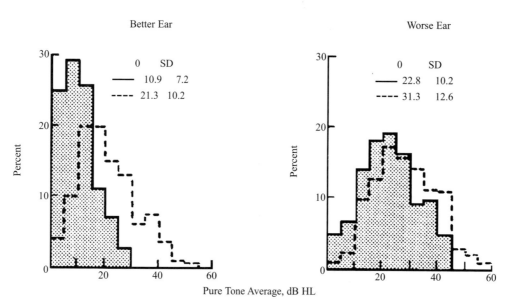

Figure 4. Distribution of pure tone averages for better ear (left) and worse ear (right) of 155 children with unilateral otitis media with effusion (OME) (solid line) and 385 children with bilateral OME (broken line). HL indicates hearing level.

of OME (Fig 5). The effect of age was examined according to four groupings (25 to 30 months, 31 to 36 months, 37 to 40 months, and older than 40 months) based on the premise that the children younger than 40 months might yield thresholds that were different from those of the older children. The results are shown in Fig 5, left; no consistent difference in the PTA could be attributed to these age groupings. Figure 5, right, shows that the duration of OME had no differential effect on the PTA.

The relationship between hearing sensitivity and clinical measures used in the diagnosis of OME, namely otoscopy and tympanometry, was also examined. Figure 6 illustrates the distribution of air conduction thresholds at the individual test frequencies and the PTA according to the presence or absence of otoscopic evidence of an air-fluid level or bubbles behind the tympanic membrane. Such evidence was present in 114 ears and absent in 421 ears. As shown in Fig 6, a significant advantage of approximately 8 dB (*P* < .001) was associated with the presence of air-fluid level or bubbles. The advantage was more apparent for 2,000 and 4,000 Hz than for 500 and 1,000 Hz. The greatest advantage appeared to be at 2,000 Hz, where approximately 90% of 114 ears with this otoscopic observation had thresholds better than 25 dB HL. The hearing acuity advantage associated with this condition was reflected in the PTA: 70% of ears with air-fluid level or bubbles had scores better than 25 dB HL, whereas only 34% of ears without this observation had a PTA better than 25 dB HL.

To determine the relationship between hearing sensitivity and tympanometric features, we performed a correlation analysis. The three major characteristics of the tympanogram (location of the peak in relationship to atmospheric pressure, height of the peak, and the gradient of the peak)[11] were compared with air conduction thresholds, PTA, and SRT. Table 4 shows the correlation coefficients (*r*) generated for this comparison. Also shown are the square of the coefficient (*r*≈), which indicates the percent variance that could be explained by the variability in the tympanometric feature, and the statistical significance of the coefficient (*P*). The correlation between hearing sensitivity and middle ear pressure was not significant, and essentially none of the variance in hearing level could be explained by the variance in pressure. All measures of hearing sensitivity were significantly correlated with the height and gradient of the tympanogram. The variations in peak compliance or tympanogram slope, however, could only explain 4% of the variance associated with the audiometric indexes. Consequently, hearing sensitivity could not be reasonably predicted on the basis of tympanometric features.

Comment

It is not unreasonable to expect hearing to be affected by an inflammation of the middle ear, especially when this is accompanied by an effusion of liquid into the middle ear space. The ensuing increase in stiffness and mass components of the middle ear

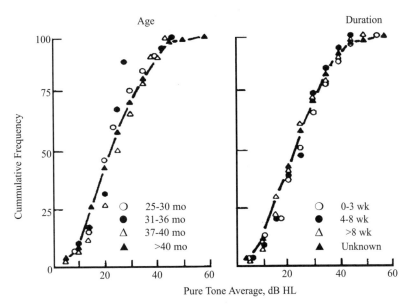

Figure 5. Cumulative frequency distributions of pure tone averages according to patient"s age (left) and duration of disease (right). Respective numbers of patients in four age groups were 13, 19, 46, and 462; in the four duration groups, 72, 76, 189, and 179. HL indicates hearing level.

impedance can have an impact on the threshold acuity.[14]

Our findings demonstrate that OME was not always associated with a mild to moderate conductive hearing loss. The PTA scores were distributed around a mean of 24.5 dB HL; this score also approximated the 50th percentile for the group. The findings, however, do not support a contention that the disease rarely has

a substantial effect on hearing acuity; 50% of ears had a PTA poorer than 23 dB HL, and 20% were poorer than 35 dB HL. These proportions approximately correspond to those reported by Kokko[4] and Cohen and Sade.[2] Bergman[5] did not indicate the distribution of thresholds, but the mean levels were approximately 10 dB poorer than our data and those reported by Kokko. These differences might be attributed to the various

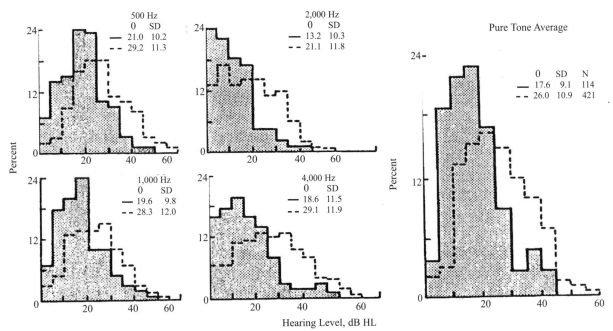

Figure 6. Frequency distributions of air conduction thresholds for individual test frequencies and pure tone averages according to presence (solid line) and absence (broken line) of air-fluid line or bubbles behind tympanic membrane. Numbers of patients shown for pure tone averages also applies to each of individual test frequencies. HL indicates hearing level.

Table 4. Correlation Statistics for Relationship Between Audiometric Indexes and Tympanometrically Determined Middle Ear Pressure (N = 538), Height of Tympanogram (N = 535), and Slope of Tympanogram (N = 533)

	Test Frequency, Hz				Pure Tone Average	Speech Reception Threshold
	500	1,000	2,000	4,000		
Pressure						
r	−.06	−.05	.00	.00	−.04	−.06
r^2	.00	.00	.00	.00	.00	.00
P	.10	.14	.48	.47	.21	.09
Height						
r	−.18	−.15	−.11	−.15	−.16	−.14
r^2	.03	.02	.01	.02	.02	.02
P	<.001	<.001	.006	<.001	<.001	.001
Slope						
r	−.20	−.17	−.13	−.11	−.18	−.20
r^2	.04	.03	.02	.01	.03	.04
P	<.001	<.001	.001	.005	<.001	<.001

stages of the disease in subjects in different studies, but the present data do not support the influence of duration of OME on hearing on a short-term basis. Chronic OME, however, may manifest other effects on hearing that may explain those differences.

The peak in hearing sensitivity at 2,000 Hz is distinctive, but this pattern has been reported by others in the context of OME.[4,5,7] It was observed as early as 1948 by Johansen,[14] who suggested that this was caused by the increase in the mass component of impedance (due to the fluid load on the tympanic membrane) in combination with a related increase in stiffness (due to an accompanying relative fixation of the ossicular chain). In other words, the interaction of mass and stiffness secondary to OME would serve to raise the resonant frequency of the middle ear system, which, combined with the changes in the acoustics of the external auditory canal due to a more reflecting tympanic membrane, may explain this observation.

The present findings also demonstrate a tendency for hearing to be less impaired for simple speech material (spondaic words) than for pure tone stimuli in the speech frequencies (500, 1,000, and 2,000 Hz). This is not surprising when the 2,000-Hz advantage is considered. Better hearing at 2,000 Hz would permit slightly better reception of simple, familiar words, such as spondees, while the PTA would be elevated by the inclusion of 500 and 1,000 Hz, where hearing was more impaired. This observation influences the interpretation of the effect of OME on hearing. Previous profiles have almost exclusively reported the effect on pure tone sensitivity. The PTA represents the purest summary index of air conduction acuity for the frequencies traditionally associated with everyday speech, but our findings demonstrate that the PTA can overesti-

mate the true impairment for speech material in the context of OME.

The significantly better SAT scores of unilaterally v bilaterally impaired infants would be anticipated on the basis of the non-ear-specific nature of the procedure and the consequent contribution of the better hearing of the uninvolved ear. Although there was a trend for older infants to respond to speech stimuli at lower levels, the SAT did not significantly vary with age. Wilber's[13] compilation of published auditory response levels in infants portends an average difference of 20 dB HL between the SAT scores of 7- and 24-month-old infants. In the present study, the average decrease in the SAT of unilaterally impaired infants was only 10 dB HL for the same age range. The apparent discrepancy is probably due to procedural differences. The responses of infants in the present study were reinforced with an animated toy located above the stimulus speaker. This tends to decrease age-dependent differences.[15] The expected SAT levels compiled by Wilber were based on behavioral observation audiometry, which historically yields more variable age-dependent auditory response levels.

It might prove interesting to equate the infant SAT findings to the SRT scores of the older children. To do so, however, would require assumptions for which supporting data are lacking. One approach might be to adjust the SAT scores by subtracting the levels suggested by Wilber. This would provide a baseline awareness level independent of age, but, as shown in Table 3, such a manipulation would overadjust for the younger infants and produce a misleading profile of the hearing levels associated with OME. Even if such an adjustment was possible, there is no evidence that the 10-dB difference between SAT and SRT scores in older children and adults also applies to infants. Extrapolating from existing data in preschool children,[16] it is feasible that the articulation function for speech material in infants has a more gradual slope. Consequently, infants probably require larger stimulus-intensity increments to achieve a given level of speech discrimination. This makes it difficult to compare the SAT data with the SRT values of older children. Therefore, the SAT data serve as reasonable indexes of detection levels associated with OME, but further investigation is needed to assess the reception and processing of speech sounds in infants in the context of the disease.

The response advantage stemming from the uninvolved ears of unilaterally impaired infants was also apparent in the older children. Children with unilateral disease had PTA scores in their better ear that were significantly better than those in the better ear of children with OME in both ears. Consequently, it would appear that the laterality of disease affects the optimal hearing acuity of the child. Children with bilateral OME were more impaired than children with the disease in only one ear. Unilaterally impaired children with the same hearing level in their better ears may not function equally, however, since the acuity in their poorer ears could be widely disparate. These issues are now beginning to emerge and have been investigated on a preliminary basis by Bess and Tharpe.[17]

The potential relationship between hearing sensitivity and the results of other clinical tests is of practical importance. Hearing levels were significantly better when otoscopy demonstrated an air-fluid level or bubbles behind the tympanic membrane. The effect of OME on hearing was believed to be related to the viscosity of the effusion; i.e., mucoid effusion would have more of an impact than would serous liquid. This was disproved by Bluestone and his colleagues,[3] and subsequently Wiederhold and associates[18] demonstrated in cats that thresholds were related to the volume of the effusion, but not the viscosity. The present findings add further support to this concept since the observation of an air-fluid level or bubbles would imply quantitatively less fluid in the middle ear space.

Unlike other investigators,[19,20] we were unable to uncover a meaningful association between hearing and middle ear pressure. In addition, the data did not support the prediction of hearing level on the basis of the slope (or gradient) of the tympanogram. This possibility was suggested by Fiellau-Nikolajsen,[19] who found this tympanometric feature to have "high predictive value" in 79 ears. The apparent discrepancy between our findings and those of Fiellau-Nikolajsen is puzzling, especially in view of the fact that the equipment and method used in determining the slope of the tympanogram were identical between the studies. The most plausible explanation relates to a difference in the number and nature of the subjects involved in the two studies. The previous study was conducted on an unselected group of 79 ears of 3-year-old children, whereas the present study population (the older group) comprised 540 children aged 2 to 12 years who were referred for recurrent or persistent middle ear disease.

Several key questions remain unanswered and represent challenges for future studies. For example, the natural history of hearing loss accompanying the disease is of paramount importance, and our findings demonstrate only the point prevalence of elevated hearing levels. Viable methods for describing longitudinal variations in hearing over longer periods of time have yet to be devised. Finally, the effect of the hearing impairment portrayed in this report should be investigated further to delineate the association between the sequelae of OME and speech and language dysfunction.

Conclusions

The following represent our conclusions, based on the foregoing data:

The hearing acuity of children with OME was characterized by the average air conduction thresholds of 27 dB HL at 500, 1,000, and 4,000 Hz and 20 dB HL at 2,000 Hz with the bone conduction thresholds not being affected.

The child's hearing acuity was dependent on the laterality of OME; the children with bilateral disease had 10 dB more impairment than the children with unilateral disease.

Hearing sensitivity was related to the presence or the absence of air-fluid level or bubbles in the middle ear.

Features of the tympanogram were not predictive of the hearing sensitivity.

Acknowledgment

This investigation was supported in part by grant NS-16337 from the National Institutes of Health.

Cheryl Palfrey, MA, Cynthia Dellecker, MA, Victoria Ashoff, MA, and Lori Griffith, MA, conducted the audiometric and acoustic impedance tests. Marie Mazza helped prepare the manuscript.

References

1. Carter, B.S.: Secretory otitis media as a cause of conduction deafness in children. *Proc R Soc Med* 1963;56:699-702.

2. Cohen, D., Sade, J.: Hearing in secretory otitis media. *Can J Otolaryngol* 1972;1:27-29.

3. Bluestone, C.D., Beery, Q.E., Paradise, J.L.: Audiometry and tympanometry in relation to middle ear effusions in children. *Laryngoscope* 1973;83:594-604.

4. Kokko, E.: Chronic secretory otitis media in children. *Acta Otolaryngol*, 1974, suppl 327, pp 7-44.

5. Bergman, M.: Audiology in secretory otitis media in children, in Sade, J. (ed): *Secretory Otitis Media and Its Sequelae.* New York, Churchill Livingstone, 1979, pp. 102-124.

6. Thelin, J.W., Thelin, S.J., Kieth, R.W., et al.: Effect of middle ear dysfunction and disease on hearing and language in high risk infants. *Int J Pediatr Otorhinolaryngol* 1979;1:125-136.

7. Harbert, F., Young, I.M., Menduke, H.: Audiologic findings in serous otitis media. *EENT Monthly* 1970;49:36-41.

8. Bluestone, C.D., Klein, J.O., Paradise, J., et al.: Workshop on effects of otitis media on the child. *Pediatrics* 1983;71:639-652.

9. Cantekin, E.I., Mandel, E.M., Bluestone, C.D., et al.: Lack of efficacy of a decongestant-antihistamine combination for otitis media with effusion ('secretory' otitis media) in children. *N Engl J Med* 1983;308:297-301.

10. Bluestone, C.D., Cantekin, E.I.: Design factors in the characterization and identification of otitis media and certain related conditions. *Ann Otol Rhinol Laryngol* 1979;88(suppl 60):13-28.

11. Paradise, J.L., Smith, C.G., Bluestone, C.D.: Tympanometric detection of middle ear effusion in infants and children. *Pediatrics* 1976;58:198-210.

12. Cantekin, E.I.: Algorithm for the diagnosis of otitis media with effusion. *Ann Otol Rhinol Laryngol* 1983;92(suppl 107):6.

13. Wilber, L.A.: Threshold measurement methods and special considerations, in Rintelmann, W.F. (ed): *Hearing Assessment.* Baltimore, University Park Press, 1979, p. 20.

14. Johansen, H.: Relation of audiograms to the impedance formula. *Acta Otolaryngol,* 1948, suppl. 74, pp. 64-75.

15. Matkin, N.D.: Assessment of hearing sensitivity during the preschool years, in Bess, F.H. (ed): *Childhood Deafness: Causation, Assessment, and Management.* New York, Grune & Stratton Inc, 1977, pp. 127-134.

16. Sanderson-Leepa, M.E., Rintelmann, W.F.: Articulation functions and test-retest performance of normal-hearing children on three speech discrimination tests: WIPI, PBK-50, and NU auditory test No. 6. *J Speech Hearing Dis* 1976;41: 503-519.

17. Bess, F.H., Tharpe, A.M.: Unilateral hearing impairment in children. *Pediatrics* 1984;74:206-216.

18. Wiederhold, M.L., Zajtchuk, J.T., Vap, J.G., et al.: Hearing loss in relation to physical properties of middle ear effusions. *Ann Otol Rhinol Laryngol* 1980;89(suppl. 68):185-189.

19. Fiellau-Nikolajsen, M.: Tympanometry and middle ear effusion: A cohort study in 3 year old children. *Int J Pediatr Otolaryngol* 1980;2:39-49.

20. Lildholdt, T., Courtois, J., Kortholm, B., et al.: The correlation between negative middle ear pressure and the corresponding conductive hearing loss in children. *Scand Audiol* 1979;8:117-120.

Development of Speech Intelligibility in Children with Recurrent Otitis Media*

Susan Jerger, James Jerger, Bobby R. Alford, and Sue Abrams

Department of Otorhinolaryngology and Communicative Sciences,
Baylor College of Medicine, Houston, Texas

Abstract

This study defined developmental functions for Pediatric Speech Intelligibility word and sentence materials presented in quiet and in competition for 25 normal children and 25 children with recurrent otitis media. Ages ranged from 24 to 56 mos. In normal children, developmental functions for Pediatric Speech Intelligibility speech materials showed earlier development of performance (1) in quiet than in competition and (2) for words than for sentences (competing condition). In children with otitis media, developmental functions were normal for both words and sentences in quiet and for sentences in competition. However, developmental functions were grossly abnormal for words in competition.

The effect of recurrent otitis media on the development of speech processing abilities remains unresolved. Animal-deprivation and cross-language studies[6,11,47-49,56,57] have consistently suggested that the nature of environmental sounds experienced by a developing animal or human influences the development of anatomical, physiological, and behavioral auditory mechanisms. These findings encouraged many attempts[3,7,12,25,26,32,36,41,50,58] to study the effect of conductive hearing loss due to otitis media on the development of speech processing skills. Almost without exception, results documented depressed linguistic and auditory processing abilities in children with a history of otitis media. However, the validity of most previous studies (before 1981) on the effects of otitis media on development has been challenged.[39,43,45,50,55] Criticisms primarily allege faulty methodology and/or experimental design. In particular, the value of studies limited to older children with a history of otitis media has been questioned because results do not reveal probable developmental mechanism(s) underlying the abnormal behavior.

In short, developmental abnormalities that may lead to eventual speech processing disorders in children with otitis media have been suggested, but not definitively isolated, by previous investigations. The purpose of the present study was to examine the influence of recurrent conductive hearing loss due to otitis media on the development of speech intelligibility.

Reprinted by permission of authors and Williams & Wilkins. Copyright 1983. *Ear & Hearing*, 4, No. 3, pp. 138-145.

*This study was supported by Public Health Service Research Grant NS-10940 from the National Institute of Neurological and Communicative Disorders and Stroke.

Method

Subjects

Subjects were 50 Caucasian children, 25 girls and 25 boys, between 24 and 56 mos of age. Nine children were 24 to 26 mos old, 10 children were 27 to 29 mos old, 7 children were 30 to 32 mos old, 9 children were 33 to 35 mos old, 7 children were 36 to 38 mos old, 4 children were 39 to 47 mos old, and 4 children were 48 to 56 mos old. All 50 children had normal sensitivity [less than or equal to 20 dB HL (re: ANSI 1969)] on both ears for pure-tone signals between 250 and 4000 Hz. All children passed a neurologic screening test for developmental normalcy.

The normal (control) group contained 25 children, 14 girls and 11 boys, with no known episodes of otitis media. Ages ranged from 24 to 38 mos. Children had received regular otoscopic examinations at well-baby pediatric evaluations. By parental report, no child had a history of otitis media, frequent upper respiratory infections, or allergy.

The otitis media (experimental) group contained 25 children, 14 boys and 11 girls, with medically documented recurrent episodes of otitis media. Ages ranged from 24 to 56 mos. Age of onset of documented otitis media ranged from 2 weeks to 36 mos. The average age of documented onset was 15 mos. Documented onset was before 12 mos of age in 60% of children. The average number of documented otitis media episodes per year was 7 and ranged from 1 to 24 per year. Seventeen of the 25 children had a history of ventilating (PE) tubes inserted into at least one tympanic membrane. One child had undergone a tympanoplasty.

At the time of the present study, the PE tubes were still present in nine children and had fallen out or been surgically removed in eight children.

Subjects in both the normal and otitis media groups represented diverse socioeconomic and cultural levels. Categorization of parental occupations in each group was distributed approximately as follows: professional (42%), managerial or administrative (19%), clerical or sales (19%), technical (10%), and semi-skilled or unemployed (10%).

Materials and Instrumentation

Children were evaluated with a battery of tests designed to assess speech intelligibility performance, middle ear immittance, hearing sensitivity, neurologic status, verbal ability, nonverbal skills, social maturity, environmental factors, and physical growth. The reason for including neurologic, psychologic, physical, and social scales in the test battery was (1) to describe characteristics of the two subject groups and (2) to allow us to evaluate factors, other than otitis media, that might be related to differences in the development of speech intelligibility performance.

Speech intelligibility performance was assessed with the Pediatric Speech Intelligibility (PSI) test.[30,31] The PSI test consists of word and sentence messages composed by normal children. The sentence messages are formed into two different syntactic constructions, referred to as format I and format II sentences. Format I sentences are appropriate test materials for children with relatively low receptive language (RL) ability; format II sentences are appropriate test materials for children with relatively high RL skills.[30] Performance for PSI word materials does not differ as a function of RL skill.[30]

PSI speech messages were recorded on a dual track magnetic tape recorder (Ampex 351). Channel 1 contained PSI word and sentence test items. Channel 2 contained PSI competing sentence messages. The test items and the competing sentences were recorded by different male talkers with general American dialect. The interitem interval was 10 sec for the sentence test and 7.5 sec for the word test. Speech level was defined as the SPL of a 1000 Hz sinusoid recorded at the average level of frequent peaks of the speech as monitored on a VU meter. The tape playback system consisted of a multichannel tape recorder (Sony TC-788-4) fed through amplifying, attenuating, and mixing circuits (Broadcast Electronics, Series Audio Console 8S150) to a loudspeaker (Phillips, type 22RH544/64R).

Immittance measures were obtained with an electroacoustic bridge (American Electromedics, model 83). Hearing sensitivity measures were obtained with a portable pure-tone audiometer (Beltone, model 10D). Neurologic status was assessed with the Denver Prescreening Developmental Questionnaire (PDQ).[18] Verbal ability was defined with the Peabody Picture Vocabulary test (PPVT)[16] and the Verbal Language Developmental Scale (VLDS).[38] Nonverbal skill was measured with the Southern California Figure Ground Visual Perceptual test (VPT).[2] Social maturity was assessed with the Vineland Scale.[14] Environmental factors were quantified by three subtests of the Home Observation for Measurement of the Environment (Home).[8] The subtests assessed (1) the emotional responsivity of the mother, (2) the provision of appropriate play materials, and (3) the opportunity for a variety of daily stimulation. Information for the Home questionnaire was obtained by parental report and observation of mother-child interaction in the test environment, rather than by a visit to the home site. Physical growth was defined by height measurements with a standard medical scale (Continental Scale Works).

Procedure

Children were tested inside a sound-treated booth in a single session of approximately 1.5 hr. Individual test procedures were administered in the following order: the PSI test, pure-tone audiometry, the VPT, the PPVT, height, immittance measures, and parental questionnaires—the Vineland, the VLDS, the PDQ, and the Home.

For the PSI test, word and sentence test items were presented as lists of five items each. Each list had a corresponding picture identification response card. The child was seated at a table with a response card. After each sentence or word had been presented, the child responded by pointing to the picture corresponding to the sentence or word that he heard. PSI results were obtained in the sound field. A loudspeaker was placed opposite the test ear at a distance of 20 cm.

All children were tested with the same four word lists. Successive trials progressed through each word list (with one replication in a different random order) until all four lists (20 word items) had been presented. At that time, if necessary, the five words of a list(s) were presented again in a different random order. For sentence materials, all children were tested with format I sentence messages. Successive trials represented the same five sentences presented in different random orders. One-half of children were tested with list A sentences and one-half with list B sentences. The equivalence of sentence and word lists has been previously established in a group of normal children.[30] The order of administration of word and sentence materials was counterbalanced.

Performance-intensity (PI) functions for PSI speech materials were constructed by presenting blocks of words or sentences at several suprathreshold intensity levels. The initial test intensity was 50 to 60 dB SPL. Intensity was then reduced in 10 dB steps until one point below the "knee" of the PI function (i.e., the point of inflection below which performance decreases rapidly with further decrease in intensity) was obtained (see Fig. 1). Finally, intensity was raised to 70 to 80 dB SPL to define the high-intensity region of the PI function. Performance was not obtained at SPLs greater than 80 dB because the young children of this study would not tolerate higher speech intensity levels.

PI functions were obtained in quiet and in the presence of a competing speech message. The message-to-competition ratio (MCR) was constant across intensity levels: 0 dB for sentences and +4 dB for words. The two standard competing message conditions are the MCRs yielding 95 to 100% correct performance in normal children between 3 and 6 yrs of age.[30] Different MCR test conditions for sentences and words were selected in an attempt to equate performance for the two different types of speech materials in normal children.

At any given intensity level, a listening trial consisted of the presentation of each of the five sentences or words of a list. If performance on this trial was 80 to 100% or 0 to 20%, only one trial (five items) was presented at that test condition. If performance on the first trial was between 21 and 79%, then a second trial was presented at that test condition. In other words, PI function data are based on five items for performance levels between 80 and 100% and 0 and 20%, and on 10 items for performance levels between 21 and 79%.

Hearing sensitivity was screened on both ears at 20 dB HL at all octave frequencies between 250 and 4000 Hz. In addition, absolute threshold hearing sensitivity was obtained at 1000 Hz on the right ear. A threshold level was defined by the traditional descending-ascending staircase procedure. Administration of the remaining procedures in the test battery was carried out according to standardized technique.

All 50 children successfully completed the PSI test and the neurologic screening test (PDQ). However, other procedures in the battery were not successfully completed by every child due to fatigue, the presence of PE tubes, etc. Table 1 summarizes the number of children in each group successfully completing each of the 10 test procedures. With the exception of immittance measures, the number of children completing

each test in each group ranged from 18 to 25 (72 to 100%).

Results

Subject Characteristics

Comparison of the normal group and an age-matched otitis media group on eight behavioral indices is shown in Table 2. To equate chronological age in the two subject groups for this comparison, the eight children in the otitis media group above 38 mos of age were temporarily eliminated from consideration. In other words, data in Table 2 for the otitis media group were confined to children between the ages of 24 and 38 mos. Performance scores for the eight indices were characterized by markedly skewed distributions. For this reason, results in each group are described with distribution-free, nonparametric statistical measures.

Table 2 summarizes median chronological age and median results for verbal skill, social maturity, nonverbal ability, hearing sensitivity, physical height, and home environment. The median chronological age was equal, 30 mos, in the two groups (Mann-Whitney U test, $p > 0.10$).[†]

Verbal skills (PPVT and VLDS) and social maturity (Vineland) were significantly different between the two groups. Performance for children in the normal group was 5 to 8 mos advanced compared to results in the otitis media subgroup. On the PPVT, the median vocabulary age was 36 mos in the normal group, but only 31 mos in the otitis media subgroup. On the VLDS, the median language age was 41 mos in the normal group, but only 33 mos in the otitis media subgroup. On the Vineland, the median "social" age was 39 mos in the normal group, but only 34 mos in the otitis media subgroup. The difference between groups

Table 1. Number of children in each group ($N = 25$) successfully completing each of the 10 test procedures.

Test Procedure	Group	
	Normal	Otitis media
PSI test	25	25
Neurologic screen (PDQ)	25	25
Pure-tone audiometry	25	25
Immittance measures	20	14
Vision (VPT)	20	23
Vocabulary (PPVT)	21	23
Language (VLDS)	19	22
Vineland	19	22
Height	18	21
Home	19	22

Table 2. Comparison of median scores of normal group and age-matched otitis media subgroup on eight indices.[a]

Indices	Group	
	Normal (N = 25)	Otitis media (N = 17)
Age	30 mos	30 mos
Verbal skills		
Vocabulary (PPVT)[b]	36 mos	31 mos
Language (VLDS)[b]	41 mos	33 mos
Social maturity		
Vineland[b]	39 mos	34 mos
Nonverbal skill		
Vision (VPT)	5 items	4 items
Hearing sensitivity		
1000 Hz	14 dB HL	18 dB HL
Height	36 inches	36 inches
Home environment	100%	100%

[a]For this comparison, age ranged from 24 to 38 mos in both groups.
[b]$p < 0.05$.

was significant for the PPVT (U test, $p < 0.05$), the VLDS (U test, $p < 0.05$), and the Vineland (U test, $p = 0.05$). A difference between children with otitis media and normal controls on vocabulary and language tests is a prevalent finding of most previous investigations.[3,12,25,26,32,36,41,50,58]

In contrast to verbal skills, nonverbal (visual perception) ability in the two groups of children was statistically equivalent (U test, $p > 0.10$). Mental age equivalency scores for median visual perceptual (VPT) performance[28] were about 32 mos (five items) in the normal group and about 27 mos (four items) in the otitis media subgroup. This finding is consistent with Brandes and Ehinger's[7] results on visual perceptual ability in 7- to 9-yr-old children with and without a history of middle ear pathology. However, Sak and Ruben[50] observed relatively advanced visual sequential memory in 8- to 11-yr-old children with a history of otitis media.

Hearing sensitivity, physical height, and the quality of the home environment were equivalent in the two groups (U test, $p > 0.10$). Median pure-tone (1000 Hz) sensitivity was 14 dB HL in the normal group and 18 dB HL in the otitis media subgroup. Median height measures, 36 inches, corresponded to a mental age equivalency score (weighted for sex)[53] of approximately 32 mos in each group. The median quality of the home environment was 100% in both groups.

[†]Mann-Whitney U values are not specified within the text because data were frequently characterized by either a large sample size or a large proportion of ties involving both groups. If either of these circumstances occurred, observed U values were transformed into z scores to determine the probability. Tables of critical values are not available when $n_2 > 20$. For a discussion of the Mann-Whitney test, see Siegel.[51]

In overview, age-matched children in the normal group and otitis media subgroup did not differ significantly in nonverbal skills, hearing sensitivity, physical height, or quality of the home environment. However, the two subject groups did differ significantly in verbal abilities and social maturity. The reciprocal relation between verbal skills and social development was recently discussed by Rediehs.[46]

Immittance measures (not shown in Table 2) may be compared in the normal and otitis media groups without the necessity of controlling for age effects. Not unexpectedly, the pattern of results differed in the two groups. In the normal group, tympanometry showed normal, type A, shapes in 18 children and type C shapes (more than −200 deca Pascals) in 2 children. Acoustic reflex thresholds at 500 to 4000 Hz were present at normal HLs (70 to 100 dB) in all 20 children. In the otitis media group, tympanometry and acoustic reflex thresholds were normal in three children. In contrast, tympanograms were an abnormal type B ($N = 8$) or C ($N = 3$) shape in 11 children. In these latter children, acoustic reflex thresholds were elevated (greater than 100 dB HL) in one child and absent (greater than 110 dB HL) in 10 children. Immittance measures could not be successfully carried out in five children in the normal group and in 11 children in the otitis media group.

Illustrative PI Functions

Figure 1 presents PI functions for two children from the present study. One child was a girl, 26 mos old, from the normal group; the other child was a girl, 27 mos old, from the otitis media group. Results in these two children are representative of median results in both subject groups.

In the normal child, maximum intelligibility scores for both words and sentences were 100% in quiet and 60 to 80% in competition. For the competing condition, performance was relatively better for words (80%) than for sentences (60%). In the child with otitis media, maximum intelligibility scores for words and sentences were 80 to 100% in quiet and 20 to 60% in competition. In the two children, performance for words and sentences in quiet and for sentences in competition was relatively equivalent. However, performance for words in competition showed a striking discrepancy. In the normal child, the function plateaued at 80%, but in the otitis media child, the function peaked at only 20%.

Normal Control Group

Figure 2 shows the developmental function for PSI word and sentence materials in quiet and in competition for the normal group. Individual data were obtained from maximum scores of PI functions for each of the four conditions. Results are grouped into five age subgroups between 24 and 38 mos of age. Each age subgroup contained four to seven children. Due to the skewed distributions of results, data in Figure 2 are medians. Due to the small number of children in some cells, quartile deviations for each median are not reported.

Figure 2 highlights two important findings: (1) a difference between performance in quiet versus in competition; and (2) a difference between performance for words in competition versus sentences in competition. First, notice that children between 24 and 26 mos of age show a large performance difference between quiet and competing conditions. In this age subgroup, median performance for both words and sentences was 100% correct in quiet, but only about 45% correct in competition. This initial performance difference between quiet and competing conditions systematically resolved, however, by 36 mos of age. The difference between performance in quiet versus in competition was approximately 55% in the 24- to 26-mo-olds, but was 0% (no difference) in the 36- to 38-mo-olds. In the total group of 25 children, the difference between quiet and competing conditions was statistically significant for words (Wilcoxon matched pairs signed ranks test, $t = 0$, $p < 0.005$, one-tailed test) and for sentences (Wilcoxon $t = 0$, $p < 0.005$, one-tailed test). These results are consistent with data on the effect of experience on visual perception.[19,44]

The second observation in Figure 2 concerns the relative performance difference for words and sentences in competition. For the quiet condition, perfor-

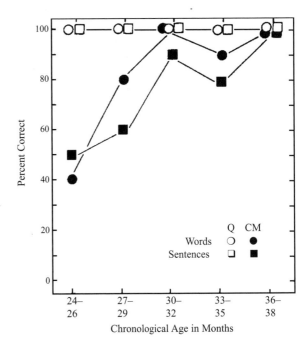

Figure 2. Developmental function for PSI word and sentence materials in quiet (Q) and in competition (CM) in 25 normal children between 24 and 38 mos old.

mance for word and sentence materials was equivalent. For the competing condition, however, the rate of developmental change was greater for word materials than for sentence materials. With the exception of results in the 24- to 26-mo-old and 36- to 38-mo-old subgroups, performance for words was approximately 10 to 20% better than sentence performance. In children between 27 and 35 mos of age, performance for words versus sentences in competition was significantly different (Wilcoxon $t = 6$, $p < 0.05$).

In short, normal developmental functions for PSI speech materials show earlier development of performance (1) in quiet than in competition and (2) for words than for sentences (competing condition). These two features of PSI developmental functions are reminiscent of results of diagnostic speech audiometry in adults with central nervous system auditory disorders. Previous investigators[27,29] have emphasized that central auditory dysfunction is more apparent on auditory tests administered in the presence of a competing message rather than in quiet and on tests consisting of sentence materials rather than word items.

The observed developmental changes in PSI performance with increasing age may reflect normal development of central auditory function and/or may be associated with the maturation of many different auditory and nonauditory skills. Increasing performance with age may be related to developmental change in (1) the central nervous system,[54] (2) basic cognitive skills and the ability to adopt more appropriate task-processing strategies,[22,23,33,34] (3) specific lan-

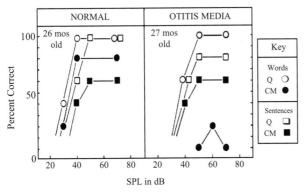

Figure 1. Illustrative PI functions for PSI words and sentences in quiet (Q) and in competition (CM) in a 26-mo-old girl from the normal control group and a 27-mo-old girl from the otitis media experimental group.

guage-processing skills,[17,37,40,42] (4) the amount and organization of information in the child's knowledge base and his overall information-processing capacity,[4,33,40] (5) the ability to attend selectively to relevant information,[1,15,21,59] and (6) the discrimination of acoustic cues and the linguistic organization of acoustic patterns.[5,9,52]

Otitis Media Experimental Group

Figure 3 shows the developmental function for PSI speech materials in quiet versus in competition for the otitis media group. Results are grouped into seven age intervals between 24 and 56 mos of age. Each age subgroup contained three to four children.

Two results in Figure 3 merit attention. The first concerns the delay in the growth of PSI performance in competition versus in quiet. In the 24- to 26-mo age subgroup, median performance was 100% correct in quiet, but only about 45% correct in competition. The performance difference between quiet and competing conditions resolved with increasing age, however. In the 39- to 56-mo-olds, the difference between performance in quiet versus in competition was 0% (no difference). In the total group of children between 24 and 38 mos, performance in quiet versus in competition was significantly different for both words (Wilcoxon t = 0, $p < 0.005$, one-tailed test) and sentences (Wilcoxon $t = 0$, $p < 0.005$, one-tailed test).

The second result in Figure 3 concerns the relatively better performance for sentences in competition than for words in competition. In the normal control group (Figure 2), the growth of performance was more rapid for words in competition than for sentences. In the otitis media group, the reverse was true. Growth of performance was more rapid for sentences in competition than for words. With the exception of results in the 24- to 26-mo-olds and the 39- to 56-mo-olds, sentence performance in competition was approximately 15 to 20% better than word performance. In children between 27 and 38 mos of age, performance for sentences and words in competition was significantly different (Wilcoxon $t = 5$, $p < 0.01$).

Intergroup Comparisons

Comparison of developmental functions for PSI speech materials in the normal and otitis media groups (Figs. 2 and 3) shows that performance in quiet was the same, 100%, in both groups. Children in both the normal and otitis media groups had the vocabulary skills and cognitive abilities to perform the PSI task. In

the presence of speech competition, however, there were significant intergroup differences.

Developmental functions for PSI words in competition (Fig. 4) showed striking differences between the two subject groups. In the normal group, performance for words in competition increased approximately 60% in the 6-mo period between 24 to 30 mos of age. In the otitis media group, however, performance for words in competition increased only about 10% during the entire 12-mo interval between 24 and 36 mos of age. The growth of word performance in competition between 24 and 38 mos was significantly different in the two groups (U test, $p < 0.05$). In children between 24 and 38 mos old, the correlation between age and word intelligibility performance in competition was significant for the normal group (Spearman rank order $r = 0.70$, $p < 0.005$, one-tailed test), but was not significant in the otitis media group ($r = 0.27$, $p > 0.05$; maximum tabled critical probability value is 0.05, one-tailed test).

In contrast to word results, PSI performance for sentences in competition (Fig. 4) was comparable in the two groups. The growth of performance between 24 and 38 mos of age was statistically equivalent between groups (U test, $p > 0.50$). Median performance in both groups was approximately 45% in the 24- to 26-mo-olds and 80 to 100% in the 36- to 38-mo-olds. In children between 24 and 38 mos, the correlation between age and sentence intelligibility performance in competition was significant for the nor-

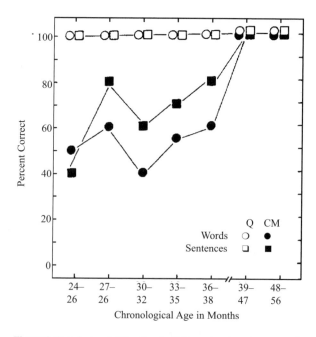

Figure 3. Developmental function for PSI word and sentence materials in quiet (Q) and in competition (CM) in 25 children between 24 and 56 mos old with recurrent otitis media.

mal group ($r = 0.65$, $p < 0.005$, one-tailed test) and for the otitis media group ($r = 0.52$, $p < 0.025$, one-tailed test).

The difference between groups for PSI words in competition may be highlighted by comparing the percentage of children in the normal and otitis media groups achieving an arbitrarily defined criterion score of at least 80% correct performance. For this analysis, data were confined to children in the age subgroups between 24 and 38 mos of age. Performance for PSI sentence materials in competition reached the criterion score in 52% of the normal group and in 53% of the otitis media subgroup. In contrast, performance for PSI word materials in competition met the criterion score in 72% of the normal group, but in only 29% of the otitis media subgroup. Previous investigators have noted both normal[24] and abnormal[17] performance for word materials in older children with a history of otitis media (for summary of references before 1981, see Ref. 26).

In short, developmental functions for PSI words in competition are grossly abnormal in children with recurrent otitis media. The abnormality is in contrast to normal performance for both words and sentences in quiet and sentences in competition.

Generality of Effect

To what extent was the "word abnormality" effect common to all children in the otitis media group? To answer this question, we compared the distributions of sentence-word difference scores in the normal and oti-

tis media groups. Subjects were the children in the age subgroups from 27 to 35 mos in the normal group and 27 to 38 mos in the otitis media group. These age ranges represent the portions of the developmental functions that showed the characteristic sentence-word relation (Figs. 2 and 3). Children in both the youngest age subgroup (24 to 26 mos) and the oldest age subgroups (36 to 38 mos, normal group; 39 to 56 mos, otitis media group) were excluded.

Figure 5 shows the distributions of sentence-word difference scores (sentence score minus word score) for the competing condition in the normal subgroup and in the otitis media subgroup. The difference score on the abscissa represents the midpoint of an interval encompassing a range of 12.5%, e.g., –4% is the midpoint of an interval ranging from –10 to +2.5%. A negative difference score indicates better performance for words than for sentences; a positive difference score indicates better performance for sentences than for words.

The two distributions in Figure 5 show only slight overlap between subgroups. For example, 14 of 15 children in the normal subgroup had negative sentence-word difference scores. In contrast, 11 of 13 children in the otitis media subgroup had positive sentence-word difference scores. Sentence-word difference scores ranged from –60 to +30% in the normal subgroup and from –20 to +40% in the otitis media subgroup. One child in the normal subgroup showed a positive sentence-word difference score and two children from the otitis media subgroup showed negative difference scores.

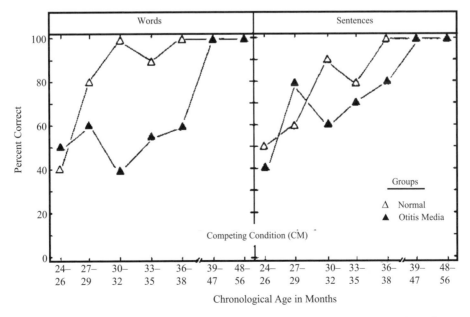

Figure 4. Comparison of developmental functions for PSI speech materials in competition in the normal and otitis media groups.

Subject Characteristics

To what extent was the magnitude of the sentence-word difference scores related to specific subject characteristics? To answer this question, we carried out a retrospective analysis of subject factors in relation to the magnitude of the difference score. Results failed to reveal any uniquely explanatory subject characteristic. The magnitude of the difference score was not related to vocabulary skill (PPVT), language ability (VLDS), social maturity (Vineland), sex, age of onset of documented otitis media, number of documented episodes per year, or presence or absence of ventilating (PE) tubes. Furthermore, the incorrect word responses of children in the otitis media subgroup with positive difference scores (better performance for sentences than for words) did not cluster around any particular phonemes (or distinctive features) and did not differ from the incorrect word responses of children in the normal subgroup with negative difference scores.‡ In short, abnormal development of PSI word performance in competition in children with otitis media did not appear to be related to any discernable subject characteristic.

Discussion

The literature suggests that the isolated word abnormality observed in the present study is not unexpected. In fact, Menyuk[40] and Dobie and Berlin[13] anticipated these results. In a theoretical discussion of aspects of language processing that might be affected by otitis media, Menyuk theorized abnormality of ". . . phonological (speech-sound) categorization and rules and lexical (word) retrieval" (p. 257).

Dobie and Berlin, in an experimental investigation of the possible patterns of imperception consequent on otitis media, analyzed speech waveforms filtered to simulate the typical hearing loss of children with otitis media. Spectral analysis suggested degradation of brief utterances and high-frequency information, but preservation of vocalic and temporal information. In other words, their results suggested degradation of the acoustic-phonetic information important to word understanding, but preservation of the global information important to sentence comprehension. Lenneberg[35] has previously stressed the importance of suprasegmental information to a child's initial processing of speech messages. Various mechanisms underlying discrimination of words versus sentences have been discussed in depth by Walk and Pick[56] and Garrett.[20]

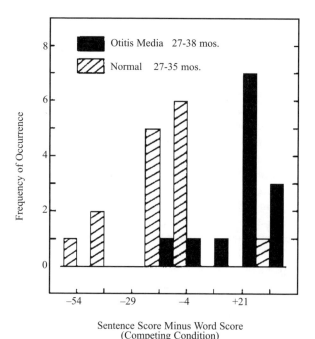

Figure 5. Distributions of sentence-word difference scores for the competing condition in subgroup of normal children ($N = 15$) ranging in age from 27 to 35 mos and a subgroup of children with otitis media ($N = 13$) ranging in age from 27 to 38 mos.

In adults with normal pure-tone sensitivity, but a history of previous conductive hearing loss, performance on diagnostic speech audiometry is usually within normal limits. Recently, however, Chadwell and Greenberg[10] reported abnormal intelligibility scores for nonsense syllables in low-pass filtered noise. Their subjects were adults with previous unilateral stapedectomies. Hearing sensitivity was normal bilaterally in all subjects. Results in the operated ear were significantly poorer than results in the unoperated ear. These authors related difficulty in speech intelligibility to absence of the acoustic reflex in the operated ear. In contrast to Chadwell and Greenberg's conclusions, results in the present study do not implicate absence of acoustic reflexes as a contributory factor for two reasons. First, speech levels in the present study were relatively low (less than or equal to 80 dB SPL or 60 dB HL) compared to threshold levels for the acoustic reflex. Second, the magnitude of the sentence-word difference scores was not related to presence or absence of the acoustic reflex in individual children.

Finally, one important limitation concerning the patterns of development in Figures 2, 3, and 4 is that results were obtained from a cross-sectional, rather than a longitudinal, experimental design. Consequently, data of the present investigation do not allow us to infer characteristics of development for individual children.

Summary and Conclusions

1. In normal children, developmental functions for PSI speech materials showed earlier development of performance (1) in quiet than in competition and (2) for words than for sentences (competing condition).

2. In children with recurrent otitis media, developmental functions were normal for both PSI words and PSI sentences in quiet and PSI sentences in competition. However, developmental functions for PSI words in competition were grossly abnormal.

3. Recurrent conductive hearing loss appears to be associated with temporarily arrested development of word understanding in competition in some children.

References

1. Anooshian, L., and L. Prilop. 1980. Developmental trends for auditory selective attention: dependence on central-incidental word relations. *Child Dev.* 51, 45-54.

2. Ayres, J. 1978. Southern California Figure Ground Visual Perception Test. Sixth printing. Western Psychological Services, Los Angeles, CA.

3. Bergstrom, L. 1980. Continuing management of conductive hearing loss during language development. *Int. J. Pediatr. Otorhinolaryngol.* 2, 3-9.

4. Berlin, C., L. Hughes, S. Lowe-Bell, and H. Berlin. 1973. Dichotic right ear advantage in children 5 to 13. *Cortex* 9, 393-401.

5. Boothroyd, A. 1970. Developmental factors in speech recognition. *Audiology* 9, 30-38.

6. Bornstein, M. 1979. Perceptual development: stability and change in feature perception. pp. 37-81. In M. Bornstein and W. Kessen, eds. *Psychological Development from Infancy: Image to Intention.* Lawrence Erlbaum Assoc., Hillsdale, NJ.

7. Brandes, P., and D. Ehinger. 1981. The effects of early middle ear pathology on auditory perception and academic achievement. *J. Speech Hear. Disord.* 46, 250-257.

8. Caldwell, B., and R. Bradley. 1970. Home observation for measurement of the environment. University of Arkansas, Center for Child Development and Education, Little Rock, AR.

9. Carpenter, R. 1976. Development of acoustic cue discrimination in children. *J. Commun. Disord.*, 9, 7-17.

10. Chadwell, D., and H. Greenberg. 1979. Speech intelligibility in stapedectomized individuals. *Am. J. Otol.* 1, 103-108.

11. Coleman, J., and P. O'Connor. 1978. Development of neurons of the ventral cochlear nucleus following monaural sound deprivation. *Anat. Rec.* 190, 366-367.

12. Dalzell, J., and H. Owrid. 1976. Children with conductive deafness: a follow-up study. *Br. J. Audiol.* 10, 87-90.

13. Dobie, R., and C. Berlin. 1979. Influence of otitis media on hearing and development. *Ann. Otol. Rhinol. Laryngol.* Suppl. 60, 48-53.

14. Doll, E. 1965. Vineland Social Maturity Scale. Ed. 2. American Guidance Service, Inc., Circle Pines, MN.

15. Doyle, A. 1973. Listening to distraction: a developmental study of selective attention. *J. Exp. Child Psychol.* 15, 100-115.

16. Dunn, L., and L. Dunn. 1981. Peabody Picture Vocabulary Test. Revised edition. American Guidance Service, Circle Pines, MN.

17. Entwisle, D., and N. Frasure. 1974. A contradiction resolved: children's processing of syntactic cues. *Dev. Psychol.* 10, 852-857.

18. Frankenburg, W., W. van Doorninck, T. Liddell, and N. Dick. 1976. Denver Prescreening Developmental Questionnaire. Ladoca Publishing Foundation, Denver, CO.

19. Ganz, L. 1978. Innate and environmental factors in the development of visual form perception. pp. 437-488. in R. Held, H. Leibowitz, and H. Teuber, eds. *Handbook of Sensory Physiology, III. Perception.* Springer-Verlag, Berlin.

20. Garrett, M. 1978. Word and sentence perception. pp. 611-625. in R. Held, H. Leibowitz, and H. Teuber, eds. *Handbook of Sensory Physiology, III. Perception.* Springer-Verlag, Berlin.

21. Geffen, G., and M. Sexton. 1978. The development of auditory strategies attention. *Dev. Psychol.* 14, 11-17.

22. Hagen, J. 1972. Strategies for remembering. pp. 65-79. in Farnham-Diggory, ed. *Information Processing in Children.* Academic Press, New York.

23. Halford. G., and W. Wilson. 1980. A category theory approach to cognitive development. *Cognit. Psychol.* 12, 356-411.

24. Hoffman-Lawless, K., R. Keith, and R. Cotton. 1981. Auditory processing abilities in children with previous middle ear effusion. *Ann. Otol. Rhinol. Laryngol.* 90, 543-545.

25. Holm, V., and L. Kunze. 1969. Effect of chronic otitis media on language and speech development. *Pediatrics* 43, 833-839.

26. Howie, V. 1980. Developmental sequelae of chronic otitis media: a review. Development and behavior. *Pediatrics* 1, 34-38.

27. Jerger, J., and D. Hayes. 1977. Diagnostic speech audiometry. *Arch. Otolaryngol.* 103, 216-222.

---

‡The PSI word test consists of different message sets of five highcontrast words (e.g., hat, fork, sun, train, bird).

28. Jerger, S., and S. Abrams. 1980. Unpublished data. Baylor College of Medicine, Houston, Texas.

29. Jerger, S., and J. Jerger. 1981. *Auditory Disorders. A Manual for Clinical Evaluation.* Little, Brown & Co., Boston.

30. Jerger, S., J. Jerger, and S. Lewis. 1981. Pediatric Speech Intelligibility test. II. Effect of receptive language and chronological age. *Int. J. Pediatr. Otorhinolaryngol.* 3, 101-118.

31. Jerger, S., S. Lewis, J. Hawkins, and J. Jerger. 1980. Pediatric Speech Intelligibility test. I. Generation of test materials. *Int. J. Pediatr. Otorhinolaryngol.* 2, 217-230.

32. Kaplan, G., J. Fleshman, T. Bender, C. Baum, and P. Clark. 1973. Long-term effects of otitis media. A ten-year cohort study of Alaskan Eskimo children. *Pediatrics* 52, 577-585.

33. Keating, D., A. Keniston, F. Manis, and B. Bobbitt. 1980. Development of the search-processing parameter. *Child Dev.* 51, 39-44.

34. Kramer, P., E. Koff, and B. Fowles. 1980. Enactment vs picture-choice tasks in studies of early language comprehension: when a picture is not worth 10,000 words. *Psychol. Rep.* 46, 803-806.

35. Lenneberg, E. 1969. On explaining language. *Science* (Wash. DC) 164, 635-643.

36. Lewis, N. 1976. Otitis media and linguistic incompetence. *Arch. Otolaryngol.* 102, 387-390.

37. Marshall, L., J. Brandt, L. Marston, and K. Ruder. 1979. Changes in number and type of errors on repetition of acoustically distorted sentences as a function of age in normal children. *J. Am. Aud. Soc.* 4, 218-226.

38. Mecham, M. 1971. Verbal Language Development Scale. Ed. 2. American Guidance Service, Inc., Circle Pines, MN.

39. Menyuk, P. 1979. Design factors in the assessment of language development in children with otitis media. *Ann. Otol. Rhinol. Laryngol.* Suppl. 60, 78-87.

40. Menyuk, P. 1980. Effect of persistent otitis media on language development. *Ann. Otol. Rhinol. Laryngol.* Suppl. 68, 257-263.

41. Needleman, H. 1977. Effects of hearing loss from early recurrent otitis media on speech and language development. pp. 640-649. in B. Jaffe, ed. *Hearing Loss in Children.* University Park Press, Baltimore.

42. Nelson, N. 1976. Comprehension of spoken language by normal children as a function of speaking rate, sentence difficulty, and listener age and sex. *Child Dev.* 47, 299-303.

43. Paradise, J. 1981. Otitis media during early life: how hazardous to development? A critical review of the evidence. *Pediatrics* 68, 869-873.

44. Pettigrew, J. 1974. The effect of visual experience on the development of stimulus specificity by kitten cortical neurons. *J. Physiol.* (Lond.) 237, 49-74.

45. Rapin, I. 1979. Conductive hearing loss: Effects on children's language and scholastic skills. A review of the literature. *Ann. Otol. Rhinol. Laryngol.* Suppl. 60, 3-12.

46. Rediehs, G. 1982. Social and cognitive development: the first three years. pp. 1-13. in J. Marlowe, ed. *Seminars in Speech, Language, and Hearing 3.* Brian C. Decker Division, Thieme-Stratton, Inc., New York.

47. Riesen, A. 1975. *The Developmental Neuropsychology of Sensory Deprivation.* Academic Press, New York.

48. Ruben, R. 1980. A review of transneuronal changes of the auditory central nervous system as a consequence of auditory defects. *Int. J. Pediatr. Otorhinolaryngol.* 89, 303-311.

49. Ruben, R., and I. Rapin. 1980. Plasticity of the developing auditory system. *Ann. Otol. Rhinol. Laryngol.* 89, 303-311.

50. Sak, R., and R. Ruben. 1981. Recurrent middle ear effusion in childhood: implications of temporary auditory deprivation for language and learning. *Ann Otol. Rhinol. Laryngol.* 90, 546-551.

51. Siegel, S. 1956. *Nonparametric Statistics for the Behavioral Sciences.* McGraw-Hill Book Co., New York.

52. Simon, C., and A. Fourcin. 1978. Cross-language study of speech-pattern learning. *J. Acoust. Soc. Am.* 63, 925-935.

53. Simon, F. 1979. Pediatric Clerkship Manual. The University of Texas Medical School, Houston.

54. Valenstein, E. 1981. Age-related changes in the human central nervous system. pp 87-106. in D. Beasley, and G. Davis, eds. *Aging. Communication Processes and Disorders.* Grune & Stratton, New York.

55. Ventry, I. 1980. Effects of conductive hearing loss: fact or fiction. *J. Speech Hear. Disord.* 45, 143-156.

56. Walk, R., and H. Pick. 1978. *Perception and Experience.* Plenum Press, New York.

57. Webster, D., and M. Webster. 1977. Neonatal sound deprivation affects brain stem auditory nuclei. *Arch. Otolaryngol.* 103, 392-396.

58. Zinkus, P., and M. Gottlieb. 1980. Patterns of perceptual and academic deficits related to early chronic otitis media. *Pediatrics* 66, 246-253.

59. Zukier, H., and J. Hagen. 1978. The development of selective attention under distracting conditions. *Child Dev.* 49, 870-873.

Acknowledgments

We thank Herman A. Jenkins, M.D.; Paul E. Johnson, M.D.; Robert H. Miller, M.D.; J. Gail Neely, M.D.; Robert B. Parke, M.D.; William J. Dichtel, M.D.; and Michael G. Forrester, M.D. for assistance on this project.

These data were obtained with a new PSI computer-aligned tape recording prepared by Dr. C. Berlin, Dr. M. Miller, and the staff of the Kresge Hearing Research Laboratory of the South.

Address reprint requests to Susan Jerger, M.S., 11922 Taylorcrest, Houston, TX 77024.

Received July 14, 1982
Accepted January 3, 1983

Listening and Language at 4 Years of Age: Effects of Early Otitis Media

Judith S. Gravel and Ina F. Wallace
Albert Einstein College of Medicine, Bronx, NY

The effect of early otitis media on preschoolers' listening and language abilities was examined in a cohort of prospectively followed children. At 4 years of age, children considered otitis negative and otitis positive during the first year of life were examined using a speech-in-competition task and several standardized measures of language and cognitive function. An adaptive test procedure was used, with sentence materials from the Pediatric Speech Intelligibility Test (PSI) (Jerger & Jerger, 1984). Results indicated that children with positive histories of otitis media during the first year required a more advantageous signal-to-competition ratio to perform at 50% sentence intelligibility than did their otitis-negative peers. There was no interaction between birth status (high-risk or full-term) and adaptive PSI listening task outcome. No differences between the groups were found in either receptive or expressive language abilities or in cognitive abilities. Further, there was no relationship between any language or cognitive measure and the adaptive PSI result.

Key Words: otitis media, pediatric hearing assessment, language development

Research examining the sequelae of otitis media (OM) has been equivocal, particularly with regard to the effects of middle ear disease on communication development. Some investigators who have retrospectively examined the impact of otitis media on communication and learning skills have suggested that a positive OM history may be associated with auditory processing deficits. Studies with school-age children have attributed poor selective attention, reduced sequential auditory memory, and attention deficits to early recurrent otitis media (Brandes & Ehinger, 1981; Gottlieb, Zinkus, & Thompson, 1979; Sak & Ruben, 1981; Zinkus & Gottlieb, 1980). In several of these studies, auditory deficits were further linked to learning disorders. One of the few retrospective studies that has examined higher auditory processing in preschoolers as a function of otitis media is that of Susan Jerger and her colleagues (Jerger, Jerger, Alford, & Abrams, 1983). They found that children with positive OM histories had more difficulty recognizing monosyllabic words in a fixed level of background competition than did their otitis-negative peers. However, because all of these studies were retrospective in design, their conclusions can be criticized for numerous methodological shortcomings (Paradise, 1981; Ventry, 1980).

Several recent investigations that used prospective designs have found associations between positive histories of otitis media and attentional problems in the absence of global language deficits. In two separate studies, Feagans and her colleagues (Feagans, McGhee, Kipp, & Blood, 1990; Feagans, Sanyal, Henderson, Collier, & Applebaum, 1987) found that higher order language processes and attention were associated with recurrent episodes of middle ear effusion. In the earlier study (Feagans et al., 1987), children who had many episodes of OM in the first 3 years of life were found to have impaired narrative skills and attentional behaviors at 5 and 7 years of age. In contrast, the same subjects did not have deficits in their mean length of utterance, a global measure of productive language. The later study (Feagans et al., 1990) examined toddlers' attention to language during a book-reading task. The results indicated that even when middle ear function was normal at the time of testing, toddlers with histories of frequent episodes of OM had poorer attention than toddlers with few episodes of otitis media. In addition, a recent study by Roberts and her colleagues (Roberts et al., 1989) reported similar findings: Total days with OM in the first 3 years of life were related to task orientation and the ability to work independently as rated by third-grade teachers. Moreover, these investigators also reported that no relationship was found between total days with OM and linguistic abilities in these same children at 4fi-6 years of age (Roberts, Burchinal, Davis, Collier, & Henderson, 1991).

The results of these retrospective and prospective investigations support models of the sequelae of otitis media that suggest that the effect of OM is more complex than previously believed. Menyuk (1986) suggested that OM might affect language skills as a result of the inconsistent auditory input children experience during recurrent episodes of otitis media when hearing sensitivity fluctuates. Building on Menyuk's model, Feagans (1986) and her colleagues (Feagans, Blood, & Tubman, 1988) proposed a model of the effects of OM in which the degraded auditory input leads to poorer attention to language. In other words, children with recurrent OM may not learn to attend to language input as consistently as their otitis-negative peers and thus may have an attention deficit for language-related tasks. We further hypothesize that when auditory deprivation occurs during critical periods of communication development, the foundation for higher order listening skills, in addition to attention, may not be firmly established. Poorly developed auditory abilities would be particularly problematic in the educational setting, when prolonged attention to language-related tasks (e.g., instruction, direction, content listening) is highly relevant to successful performance in school.

The purpose of the present investigation was to examine a cohort of preschoolers whose middle ear status during the first year of life was well documented (see Gravel, McCarton, & Ruben, 1988). These young children have been the subjects of previous reports on the effects of early recurrent otitis media on emerging language (Wallace, Gravel, & Ganon, 1991; Wallace, Gravel, McCarton, & Ruben, 1988a; Wallace et al., 1988b). Our earlier studies demonstrated significantly poorer expressive language abilities at 1 and 2 years of age for otitis-positive children in comparison to their otitis-negative peers (Wallace et al., 1991; Wallace et al., 1988a; Wallace et al., 1988b), though no differences were found in their receptive language or cognitive capacities. In addition, children considered otitis positive during the first year had, as a group, significantly poorer peripheral auditory sensitivity as estimated by the conventional click ABR (auditory brainstem response) (Wallace et al., 1988b).

In the present investigation, we examined the language and cognitive abilities of this prospectively followed sample of children at 4 years of age. In addition, we examined the higher level auditory abilities of these same subjects at 4 years of age using a modification of the Pediatric Speech Intelligibility Test (PSI) (Jerger & Jerger, 1984). The PSI is a closed-set, picture-pointing test for preschoolers that examines monosyllabic word and sentence recognition performance in a fixed level of background competition. Specifically, the ability of the children to listen in a competitive background (auditory figure-ground; Keith, 1988) was examined using the sentence materials of the PSI in an adaptive test procedure.

Method

Subjects

The children in this investigation are subjects of the Clinical Research Center for Communicative Disorders, which draws subjects from the longitudinal Infant Follow-up and Evaluation (LIFE) Program of the R.F. Kennedy Center, Albert Einstein College of Medicine, Bronx, New York. All children in the Clinical Research Center are enrolled at 40 weeks postconceptional age (corrected for prematurity) and receive all medical and neurobehavioral follow-up through the LIFE Program. The 23 children who were included in the present investigation were subjects of previous studies (Wallace et al., 1991; Wallace et al., 1988a; Wallace et al., 1988b) on the linguistic and cognitive sequelae of otitis media. These 23 subjects include all of those seen at 4 years of age for the measure of speech intelligibility in the presence of a competing message (the adaptive PSI task). Seven subjects from our original studies (Wallace et al., 1988a; Wallace et al., 1988b) were not included in the present investigation: One was not tested on the PSI at 4 years; 1 was unable to perform the listening task because of behavior problems; and 5 were lost to attrition at 4 years.

Subjects of this investigation were either high-risk (HR) infant graduates of a Neonatal Intensive Care Unit (NICU) (*n* = 14) or full-term (FT) graduates of the well-baby nursery (*n* = 9) of Jacobi Hospital (an affiliated Bronx Municipal Hospital Corporation facility). HR infants were cared for in the NICU because of very low birthweights (≤ 1500 grams, *n* = 11) or severe perinatal asphyxia (*n* = 3). All subjects were drawn from low socioeconomic urban neighborhoods and their mean socioeconomic status was classified using Hollingshead's (1975) index. Many families are of Hispanic background; however, subjects recruited for the Clinical Research Center come from homes in which English was reported to be the primary language spoken.

During the first year of life (corrected age), all infants in this study received frequent examinations of their middle ear status (see Gravel et al., 1988). Pediatric nurse practitioners completed pneumo-otoscopic examinations during each scheduled well-baby visit. On the basis of otoscopic histories during the first year, two groups of infants were identified for study purposes: One was considered otitis positive (OM+; *n* = 10), the other otitis negative (OM–; *n* = 13). An infant was considered otitis positive when bilateral otitis media was detected at 30% or more of the baby's

Table 1. Perinatal and demographic characteristics of subjects.

			Group										
	Otitis positive ($n = 10$)					Otitis negative ($n = 13$)							
Characteristic	n	%	M	SD	Range	n	%	M	SD	Range	t/x^2	df	p
High risk	7	70				7	54				.13	1	.72
Birthweight (g)			1868.5	944.3	1140-3320			2503.8	1018.1	820-3400	1.53	21	.141
Gestational age (weeks)			34.2	4.3	30-40			36.5	4.7	27-40	1.22	21	.236
Small for gestational age	1	10				1	8				.00	1	1.00
Apgar (5 min)[a]			8.3	1.0	7-9			7.0	2.5	3-10	−1.51	19	.147
Maternal age (years)			27.1	5.5	18-34			23.9	5.6	16-32	−1.36	21	.189
Sex													
Male	7	70				8	62				.00	1	1.00
Race													
Black	5	50				7	54				2.09	3	.554
Hispanic	4	40				5	38						
White	1	10				0							
Other	0					1	8						
SES (Hollingshead, 1975)			27.6	11.7	11-51			26.2	12.8	14-48	−.28	21	.783
% visits bilateral OM (1st yr.)			43.7	8.4	30-50			8.0	8.1	0-20	−10.34	21	.001
% visits bilateral normal (1st yr.)			42.9	13.7	20-63			90.3	7.3	80-100	9.92	12	.001
Average click-ABR threshold in dB nHL (1st yr.)[b]			33.5	11.7	18-48			22.3	7.8	8-38	−2.60	19	.018

[a]Apgar information was missing on 2 children; n's for the variable are 9 and 12. [b]ABR thresholds were not available for 2 otitis-negative children; n for this group is 11.

first year visits. An infant was considered otitis negative when middle ear status was rated as normal in both ears during 80% or more of the first-year visits. Electrophysiologic and behavioral measures completed on these infants revealed none to have sensorineural hearing loss. In addition, no infant considered neurologically compromised was included in the sample.

Demographic, perinatal, and 1-year middle ear and electrophysiologic findings for the 23 study children are presented in Table 1. As the table shows, the groups did not differ on any demographic or perinatal status variable. However, the groups did differ as to middle ear status and electrophysiologic outcome. During the first year, the group considered otitis positive had, on average, poorer auditory sensitivity as estimated by click ABR than those babies considered otitis negative (see Wallace et al., 1988b).

All 23 subjects were seen within 3 months of their 4th birthday (corrected age) for assessment of auditory abilities (M = 4 years, 1 month 6 days, SD = 1 month 5 days). There was no difference between the two groups in age of assessment (M_{OM+} = 49.1 months, SD = .99; M_{OM-} = 49.1 months, SD = 1.04). Numbers of subjects vary somewhat for cognitive and language measures.[1]

Children were generally seen on the same test day for all measures. However, when the entire battery could not be completed on one test day, children returned for completion of the measures.

Materials and Instrumentation

Auditory measures. A modification of the PSI was administered to each child. The primary sentence items of the PSI consist of 10 sentences that were generated by a large group of normal-language children aged 3-6 years (Jerger, Lewis, Hawkins, & Jerger, 1980). Each sentence is composed of eight syllables on average (range: six to nine syllables) (Jerger & Jerger, 1984). The PSI is a closed-set response task. The items are depicted pictorially with five sentence items per response card (A & B). The child responds by pointing to the picture that corresponds to the sentence heard. An example of the sentence-items is "A rabbit is painting an egg." For the present investigation, the Format II sentences (those without a carrier phrase), Response Card A, were used. The equivalence of Lists A and B has been previously established (Jerger & Jerger, 1984). The competing sentences of the PSI were selected from the sentence items rejected for use as primary sentences (Jerger & Jerger, 1984). Twenty sentences serve as competitive phrases. An example of a competing sentence is "A big bad wolf is catching some fish."

The commercially available (Auditec, Inc.) cassette-tape recordings of the PSI were used in this investigation. The message-to-competition ratio (MCR) function recording consists of blocks of the five randomized primary sentence-items (for a given response card) on one channel of the tape. A total of 140 presentations of the five stimulus items are available on each tape. The competing sentences are recorded on the second channel of the cassette. The onset of the primary sentences occurs simultaneously with the onset of the competing message (Jerger & Jerger, 1984).

The PSI primary sentence (S) items were delivered through one channel of a stereo cassette tape deck (Realistic SCT-35) and routed to the tape-input section of a two-channel clinical audiometer (Grason-Stadler GSI-16). The Competing Messages (CM) were led to the second tape input of the same audiometer. Inputs were mixed and delivered through TDH-50P earphones housed in MX41-AR cushions with standard headband assembly. A 1000-Hz calibration tone (approximating the level of the peaks of the speech materials) (Jerger & Jerger, 1984), recorded on each channel at the beginning of the MCR function tape, was adjusted to achieve 0 on the audiometer's VU meter for each channel. The overall levels of the primary and competing sentences could be varied independently. The mixed S and CM materials were delivered binaurally (a diotic listening condition).

All testing was carried out in a sound-treated test booth. The examiner, child, and all test equipment were located within the test suite. A visual reinforcement display unit was located directly in front of the child.

Initially, the child was acquainted with the five sentence items by the examiner. Eight randomizations of the 5 PSI sentences (40 items) served as practice. Jerger and Jerger (1984) suggest that presenting at least 20 items should eliminate the possibility of practice effects. The level of the sentences was held constant at 60 dB HL. Initially, 5 items were presented in quiet. Thereafter, the remaining 35 practice sentences were delivered in systematically increasing levels of background-message competition. Generally, 5 items were presented at a +40 dB S/CM, 5 at +30 dB S/CM, and 5 at +20 dB S/CM; thus, 20 practice items were presented in relatively easy listening conditions. The level of the competing message for the remaining 20 practice

[1]One subject who was able to perform the PSI was untestable on cognitive and language measures because of severe emotional disturbance. Another subject refused so many items on both scales of the SICD that her test was unscorable.

items was then varied in intensity, beginning at +10 dB S/CM, in 2-dB steps, until the child missed a sentence item. Thereafter, the CM was varied around that point to give the child experience with the competitive listening task.

At the end of the 40 practice sentences, an S/CM that reduced sentence intelligibility to approximately 50% was determined for each child using a modified adaptive test procedure (Levitt, 1978). That is, with the level of the primary sentence held constant (60 dB HL), the level of the CM was raised in 6-dB steps (beginning at 36 dB HL or +24 dB S/CM) until the child missed two out of the three primary sentences. The intensity level of the CM was then lowered and raised in 2-dB steps using the same two-out-of-three decision rule. A S/CM was computed on the average of the last four of six response reversals. During the test session, visual reinforcement for correct responding was used to maintain the child's attention and motivation. This consisted of randomly activating and illuminating one of three mechanical toys in a display. The examiner listened to the primary sentences via a monitoring earphone, scored the results manually, and adjusted the S/CM according to the procedure described above.

In addition to the PSI procedure, a pure-tone audiogram was obtained on each child. A conventional clinical staircase procedure (descending-ascending) was used. Thresholds for each ear of all subjects were obtained at octave frequencies from 500 through 4000 Hz (at a minimum) (ANSI, 1969). A tympanogram (probe frequency 220 Hz) was also obtained in each ear using a screening tympanometer (Grason-Stadler GSI-27A).

Cognitive and Language Measures. The cognitive measure administered was the Stanford-Binet 4th Edition (Thorndike, Hagen, & Sattler, 1986).[2] It is designed for individuals from the age of 2 to adulthood. The test yields a composite IQ score as well as area scores for verbal reasoning, abstract/visual reasoning, quantitative reasoning, and short-term memory. Because we were investigating relationships with language skills, only the verbal reasoning IQ score and the global IQ score were included in the present analysis.

The only language measure included in the following analyses was the Sequenced Inventory of Communication Development-Revised (SICD-R) (Hedrick, Prather, & Tobin, 1984). The SICD-R is a standardized measure of communicative functioning that combines parental report with direct assessment of the child. Separate scales are included to measure receptive and expressive skills. The skills measured on the receptive scale include orienting to auditory stim-

Table 2. Four-year outcome auditory, cognitive, and language results.

Measure	Otitis positive				Otitis negative				t	df	p
	n	M	SD	Range	n	M	SD	Range			
PSI S/CM (dB)	10	−6.8	2.8	−3 to −11	13	−9.7	2.6	−6 to −14	2.63	21	.016
Pure-tone average (dB)											
Right ear	10	15.8	4.1	10-21.6	13	14.9	3.2	6.6-20	.58	21	.570
Left ear	10	15.8	4.1	10-21.6	13	14.6	3.3	6.6-16.6	.76	21	.454
Stanford-Binet Global IQ	9	87.8	14.8	75-122	13	86.0	8.6	72-102	−.36	20	.725
Stanford-Binet Verbal Reasoning IQ	9	88.3	15.9	72-117	13	84.3	9.4	70-106	−.75	20	.463
SICD Expressive Language (in months)	8	36.0	5.2	32-44	12	39.0	6.2	28-48	1.13	18	.274
SICD Receptive Language (in months)	8	35.5	5.4	28-44	13	37.8	5.3	20-48	.97	19	.342

uli, comprehension of word meanings, discrimination between words, and understanding directions. The expressive scale includes items assessing the use of prelinguistic vocalizations and gestures, imitation of actions, production of sound sequences and words, use of words and sentences, and ability to respond orally to simple sentences. Communication ages are the standardized scores provided for each scale. Although the age range of the SICD-R is 4-48 months, all but 2 children had communication age scores that were less than 48 months (one child on each scale). Given that the children in our sample actually performed in the range of younger children, there appears to be no ceiling effect on the SICD-R; hence it seems to be an appropriate measure for these children. The individual who assessed the children's cognitive and language abilities was unaware of each child's middle ear status.

Results

Means and standard deviations for the 4-year outcome measures for the two groups of children are presented in Table 2. T Tests were performed between the two groups in order to examine group differences. As can be seen, the only significant difference between the groups was in their performance on the adaptive PSI competitive listening task. The otitis-negative group had a significantly lower mean S/CM (M_{OM-} = −9.7) than the otitis-positive group (M_{OM+} = −6.8). In other words, otitis-positive children as a group required a more advantageous signal-to-competing message ratio than did the otitis-negative children to maintain performance at 50% sentence understanding. Moreover, using omega squared, 20% of the variance in the children's performance was explained by otitis media status.[3]

In contrast, there were no group differences on the other outcome measures. First of all, pure-tone averages were similar in the two groups and indicated that all children had normal peripheral hearing sensitivity. Secondly, global intelligence, verbal reasoning, expressive language, and receptive language scores did not differ as a function of otitis media status during the first year of life.

Because both high-risk and full-term children were included in the study, it seemed important to examine whether risk status contributed to the results. An ANOVA was performed to examine the joint effect of risk status and early otitis media status on PSI scores. Figure 1 presents the results of the adaptive PSI competitive listening task by OM status and risk status. There was neither an interaction between risk status and OM status nor a significant main effect due to risk status. In fact, full-term and high-risk children were similar in their performance. The only significant finding was the main effect of early otitis media status ($F[1, 19]$ = 5.93, $p < 0.05$). These results suggest that the ability to perform on a task of sentence intelligibility in background competition is related more to early otitis media history than to risk status.

Finally, correlations were computed between the PSI scores and each of the other outcome measures. No significant relationships were detected between the

---

[2]It is recognized that the Stanford-Binet 4th Edition is not an ideal measure of cognitive ability for preschoolers, particularly those who function in the low-average range. However, given the measures that were available in 1988, it seemed to be the best choice in terms of multifactorial conception of IQ, length of administration time (45 min), and recency and adequacy of norms.

PSI and any of the other measures. Three of the correlations were close to zero (r = −.10, .05, .06), whereas the correlation between the PSI and receptive language was r = .31. The correlations obtained here suggest that performance on the PSI is largely independent of intellectual and language abilities.

Discussion

The results of this investigation demonstrate a relationship between a history of early recurrent otitis media and performance on a competitive listening task. Children who had numerous episodes of otitis media in the first year of life performed more poorly when listening to sentence material in the presence of background competition than did children who were considered otitis negative during the same period. The validity of this finding is bolstered by the fact that all children had normal peripheral hearing sensitivity (i.e., had normal pure-tone audiograms) and normal middle ear functioning on the day of testing. Moreover, all of the children were able to identify the stimuli with perfect accuracy in quiet. That is, children scored 100% sentence intelligibility when listening to only the primary sentence. However, when a competing sentence was introduced, the group of 4-year-olds who were otitis negative in infancy were found to tolerate significantly more competition (i.e., they required a less advantageous S/CM) than did the early otitis-positive group. Thus, early recurrent otitis media appears to affect children's higher level auditory abilities (selective listening) at later ages, even when peripheral sensitivity and middle ear function are normal.

We found that not only did the groups differ significantly in their ability to listen in competition, but also that 20% of the variance in listening performance was accounted for by early otitis media status. Although this still leaves 80% unexplained, we believe that 20% is a substantial amount in view of the length of time that elapsed between the early episodes of otitis media and the children's performance on the PSI at 4 years of age. Nevertheless, we recognize that there are many other factors that could affect children's auditory abilities, such as previous listening experience in linguistically complex environments, as well as the child's overall attentional and motivational capacities.

Our results support the findings of Jerger and her colleagues (1983), which demonstrated a relationship between otitis media history and performance on the PSI. In their study, intelligibility of both monosyllables

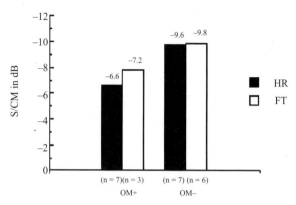

Figure 1. Results of the adaptive PSI competitive listening task for otitis-postive (OM+) and otitis-negative (OM−) groups as a function of birth status (HR = high-risk, FT = full-term).

and sentences was compared at various ages using the standard fixed message-to-competition ratios (+4 dB and 0 dB for words and sentences, respectively). Jerger et al. found that children with retrospectively documented histories of otitis media had significantly more difficulty than otitis-negative children with monosyllabic word recognition in competition. No differences were found between groups for sentence materials. Because Jerger and her colleagues (1983) examined sentences at a relatively advantageous message-to-competition ratio (0 dB), differences in performance on sentence materials between groups may not have been apparent. It is conceivable that a 0-dB message-to-competition ratio was a relatively easy listening condition for both groups on the sentence materials. The use of the PSI sentences in an adaptive test paradigm, however, imposes no fixed limitations on performance in the competitive-message condition. Indeed, the advantage of using the PSI in an adaptive test paradigm (Levitt, 1978) is that children's performance can be compared as to the S/CM that reduces intelligibility to 50%. Thus, performance differences between subject groups can be examined (see Dirks, Morgan, & Dubno, 1982).

In contrast to the group differences on the PSI, no significant differences were detected on cognitive or language measures as a function of early otitis media status.[4] We administered other standardized tests of more specific functions, but we did not detect differences between groups on these measures, either.[5] However, it is possible that if we had included measures that require the integration of higher order language abilities, such as paraphrase skills (as did Feagans and colleagues, 1987), we might have found differences between groups. Although the power of the statistical tests was low because of small sample sizes, our failure to find differences is in accord with the results of other investigators who have examined cog-

---

[3]Omega squared is defined by Hays (1973) as "the proportion of variance in Y accounted for by X" (p. 414). The formula he provides for estimating omega squared is: est $T^2 = (t^2 − 1)/(t^2 + N_1 + N_2 − 1)$.

nitive and language sequelae in lower social class children and have not detected differences as a function of early otitis media status (Roberts et al., 1991; Roberts, Burchinal, Koch, Footo, & Henderson, 1988; Teele, Klein, Rosner, & The Greater Boston Otitis Media Study Group, 1984).

However, it cannot be concluded that the children in our sample have done well. Both otitis-positive and otitis-negative groups performed well below age expectation on all standardized measures. The group differences in emerging expressive language skills reported previously (Wallace et al., 1991; Wallace et al., 1988a; Wallace et al., 1988b) were no longer apparent at 4 years, which we speculate may be due to socioenvironmental factors. In other words, the overwhelming impact of our children's social environment may have overshadowed any negative effects due to early otitis media.

We also failed to find any differences due to perinatal risk status. The current findings parallel the outcome of the larger cohort from which our sample was drawn. In two large cohorts (Cohort I: 65 HR, 19 FT; Cohort II: 102 HR, 25 FT) our Clinical Research Center is following, no differences between high-risk and full-term groups have been found in language or cognition in the preschool years. However, a substantial proportion of children in all groups (range: 8-67%, depending on age of assessment) were found to have language and cognitive deficits that we attribute to socioenvironmental factors. Furthermore, despite the many studies that have longitudinally followed high-risk children (Greenberg & Crnic, 1988; Hubatch, Johnson, Kistler, Burns, & Moneka, 1985; Menyuk, Liebergott, Schultz, Chesnick, & Ferrier, 1991; Siegel, 1982; Zarin-Ackerman, Lewis, & Driscoll, 1977), consensus has not been reached on the cognitive and language outcomes of children as a function of perinatal risk status.

Importantly, children's performance on the PSI is not dependent on learning, language level, or cultural experiences. Keith (1988) suggested that it is important that measures of auditory perceptual ability be clearly delineated from tasks that actually examine higher order language and cognitive capacities. This is critical because most of the children, regardless of otitis media or birth history, demonstrated impaired performance on the standardized measures of language and cognition. Furthermore, because no relationship was found between adaptive PSI outcome and language or cognitive ability, the result is likely attributable to a deficit in auditory processing ability. It is not surprising that performance on the competitive listening task was unrelated to performance on individually administered tests of language and cognitive abilities. In those measures,

messages may be maximized through repetition and visual cues. In contrast, the auditory task relied on only a single input channel and provided both distractions and restricted message redundancy.

A question could arise as to the importance of the finding of a 3-dB difference between groups on the PSI adaptive test procedure. Stated differently, is a 3-dB difference in S/CM *functionally* significant? Konkle and Schwartz (1981) and Bess and Tharpe (1986) have suggested that a 3-dB threshold advantage (such as is available in binaural versus monaural listening) can mean as much as a 30% improvement in speech intelligibility depending upon the slope of the performance-intensity (PI) function of a particular speech message set. Duquesnoy (1983) found that a 1-dB difference in signal-to-noise ratio could equal a 17-20% change in intelligibility of sentence materials for elderly adults. Because only five sentences were used in the present PSI task, the slope of the PI function for the PSI sentence materials is likely quite steep, suggesting that small differences in S/CM ratio could mean substantial performance differences in speech intelligibility.

It appears that children with histories of otitis media have more difficulty in recognizing familiar sentences in the presence of background competition. This task (speech in competition) is similar to the situation in classroom environments in which children must attend to a primary message and ignore a competing (potentially distracting) phrase. Our findings appear consistent with the model proposed by Feagans (1986; Feagans et al., 1988), as well as with the results of Roberts and her colleagues (1989; Roberts et al., 1991), suggesting that auditory attention is affected deleteriously by an early history of recurrent otitis media. Further, our results support earlier retrospective investigations that speculated that recurrent OM can affect higher level or "central" auditory abilities (such as selective auditory attention and discrimination of speech in noise) that could subsequently lead to verbal-

----

[4] In a related study (Wallace, Gravel, & Ganon, 1991) concerning language outcomes as a function of early otitis media, the findings and sample composition were somewhat different. First of all, the sample reported on at 4 years differed to some extent from the sample in this study because of some subjects' failure to return for the auditory procedures and, in one case, the inability to perform the PSI during training. Secondly, the differences reported pertained only to those children who had IQ scores in the normal range (IQ > 78). In brief, the OM+ (n = 10) had lower receptive and expressive SICD scores than the OM− group (n = 12).

[5] Although the only language measure included here is the SICD, children were administered other formal measures, including the Peabody Picture Vocabulary Test-Revised, Test of Early Language Development, and subtests of the Illinois Test of Psycholinguistic Abilities. In addition, an audiotaped language sample was obtained. Because there were many children in each group who were unable to complete these measures, the data were not included. However, preliminary analyses did not detect any significant differences between the two groups on these measures.

ly based learning disorders (Brandes & Ehinger, 1981; Gottlieb et al., 1979; Sak & Ruben, 1981; Zinkus & Gottlieb, 1980).

One limitation of our study is the reduction in available information concerning these children's middle ear status after the first year of life. During the second year, children were seen for regular follow-up less frequently, on average only four times.[6] Children considered otitis positive continued in the second year to have a higher percentage of visits that were characterized as bilaterally positive than did the group considered otitis negative, though the differences were not significant.[7] The subsequent regular follow-up of these children after the second year has been annual (in keeping with the present LIFE follow-up protocol). Thus, regular otoscopy was not completed during the third or fourth years postterm, and we are therefore unable to characterize adequately the groups' middle ear status for that time period. In consequence, it is possible that one reason for the failure to find differences in language abilities at age 4 was that there was a greater similarity between the groups in middle ear status during years 3 and 4. However, we feel this is unlikely for two reasons. First of all, most researchers have failed to find a relationship between early otitis media and performance on standardized measures of language abilities during the preschool years (Feagans et al., 1987; Roberts et al., 1991). Secondly, when researchers have found a relationship between otitis media and language, only middle ear disease occurring in the first year of life was related to outcome (Teele et al., 1984).

It remains to be seen whether these same children will demonstrate observable difficulties in the classroom environment. We intend to follow these children into the educational setting to determine whether these findings in the preschool period are functionally apparent at school age. It may be that we are able, through such early measures of listening ability, to pinpoint children who are at high risk for auditory processing problems in complex and acoustically challenging listening environments. Such auditory abilities go far beyond those examined by conventional audiometry and suggest the need to assess the auditory system at multiple levels in determinations of the long-term sequelae of early otitis media.

Acknowledgments

This work was supported by a NIH-NIDCD Program Project Grant #DC 00223 and Mental Retardation Center Grant #HD 01799. Thanks are due to Ellen Ganon for assistance in data collection, to two anonymous reviewers, and to Mark Haggard, who provided valuable comments on an earlier version of this manuscript.

References

American National Standards Institute. (1969). *Specifications for audiometers* (ANSI S3.6-1969). New York: ANSI.

Bess, F.H., & Tharpe, A.M. (1986). An introduction to unilateral sensorineural hearing loss in children. *Ear and Hearing, 7,* 3-13.

Brandes, P.J., & Ehinger, D.M. (1981). The effects of early middle ear pathology on auditory perception and academic achievement. *Journal of Speech and Hearing Disorders, 46,* 301-307.

Dirks, D.D., Morgan, D.E., & Dubno, J.R. (1982). A procedure for quantifying the effects of noise on speech recognition. *Journal of Speech and Hearing Disorders, 47,* 114-123.

Duquesnoy, A.J. (1983). The intelligibility of sentences in quiet and in noise in aged listeners. *Journal of the Acoustical Society of America, 74,* 1136-1144.

Feagans, L. (1986). Otitis media: A model for long-term effects with implications for intervention. In J.F. Kavanagh (Ed.), *Otitis media in child development* (pp. 192-208). Parkton, MD: York Press.

Feagans, L., Blood, I., & Tubman, J.G. (1988). Otitis media: Models of effects and implications for intervention. In F.H. Bess (Ed.), *Hearing impairment in children* (pp. 347-374). Parkton, MD: York Press.

Feagans, L.V., McGhee, S., Kipp, E., & Blood, I. (1990, April). *Attention to language in day-care attending children: A mediating factor in the developmental effects of otitis media.* Paper presented at the Meeting of the International Conference on Infancy Studies, Montreal, Canada.

Feagans, L., Sanyal, M., Henderson, F., Collier, A., & Applebaum, M. (1987). Relationship of middle ear disease in early childhood to later narrative and attentional skills. *Journal of Pediatric Psychology, 12,* 581-594.

Gottlieb, M.I., Zinkus, P.W., & Thompson, A. (1979). Chronic middle ear disease and auditory perceptual deficits. *Clinical Pediatrics, 18,* 725-732.

Gravel, J.S., McCarton, C.M., & Ruben, R.J. (1988). Otitis media in NICU graduates: A one-year prospective study. *Pediatrics, 82,* 44-49.

Greenberg, M.T., & Crnic, K.A. (1988). Longitudinal predictors of developmental status and social interaction in premature and full-term infants at age two. *Child Development, 59,* 554-570.

---

[6]The average number of visits for the otitis-positive group was $M = 4.3$, $SD = 1.5$, and for the otitis-negative group $M = 4.4$, SD = 1.2.

Hays, W.H. (1973). *Statistics for the social sciences* (2nd ed.). New York: Holt, Rinehart, & Winston.

Hedrick, D.L., Prather, E.M., & Tobin, A.R. (1984). *Sequenced Inventory of Communication Development—Revised.* Seattle, WA: University of Washington Press.

Hollingshead, A. (1975). *Four factor index of social status.* Working paper available from Department of Sociology, Yale University, New Haven, CT.

Hubatch, L.M., Johnson, C.J., Kistler, D.J., Burns, W.J., & Moneka, W. (1985). Early language abilities of high-risk infants. *Journal of Speech and Hearing Disorders, 50,* 195-207.

Jerger, S., & Jerger, J. (1984). *Pediatric Speech Intelligibility Test.* St. Louis, MO: Auditec.

Jerger, S., Jerger, J., Alford, B.R., & Abrams, S. (1983). Development of speech intelligibility in children with recurrent otitis media. *Ear and Hearing, 4,* 138-145.

Jerger, S., Lewis, S., Hawkins, J., & Jerger, J. (1980). Pediatric Speech Intelligibility Test: I. Generation of test materials. *International Journal of Pediatric Otorhinolaryngology, 2,* 217-230.

Keith, R.W. (1988). Tests of central auditory function. In R. Roeser & M. Downs (Eds.), *Auditory disorders in school children* (2nd ed., pp. 83-97). NY: Thieme.

Konkle, D.F., & Schwartz, D.M. (1981). Binaural amplification: A paradox. In F.H. Bess, B.A. Freeman, & J.S. Sinclair (Eds.), *Amplification in education,* (342-357). Washington, DC: A.G. Bell Association for the Deaf.

Levitt, H. (1978). Adaptive testing in audiology. *Scandinavian Audiology Supplement, 6,* 241-292.

Menyuk, P. (1986). Predicting speech and language problems with persistent otitis media. In J.F. Kavanagh (Ed.), *Otitis media in child development* (pp. 83-96). Parkton, MD: York Press.

Menyuk, P., Liebergott, J., Schultz, M., Chesnick, M., & Ferrier, L. (1991). Patterns of early lexical and cognitive development in premature and full-term infants. *Journal of Speech and Hearing Research, 38,* 88-94.

Paradise, J.L. (1981). Otitis media during early life: How hazardous to development? A critical review of the evidence. *Pediatrics, 68,* 869-873.

Roberts, J.E., Burchinal, M.R., Collier, A.M., Ramey, C.T., Koch, M.A., & Henderson, F.W. (1989). Otitis media in early childhood, and cognitive, academic, and classroom performance of the school-aged child. *Pediatrics, 83,* 477-485.

Roberts, J.E, Burchinal, M.R., Davis, B.P., Collier, A.M., & Henderson, F.W. (1991). Otitis media in early childhood and later language. *Journal of Speech and Hearing Research, 34,* 1158-1168.

Roberts, J.E., Burchinal, M.R., Koch, M.A., Footo, M.M., & Henderson, F.W. (1988). Otitis media in early childhood and its relationship to later phonological development. *Journal of Speech and Hearing Disorders, 53,* 416-424.

Sak, R., & Ruben, R.J. (1981). Recurrent middle ear effusion in childhood: Implications of temporary auditory deprivation for language and learning. *Annals of Otology, Rhinology, and Laryngol*ogy, 90, 546-551.

Siegel, L. (1982). Reproductive, perinatal and environmental factors in the cognitive and language development of pre-term and full-term infants. *Child Development, 53,* 963-973.

Teele, D., Klein, J., Rosner, B., & The Greater Boston Otitis Media Study Group. (1984). Otitis media with effusion during the first three years of life and development of speech and language. *Pediatrics, 74,* 282-287.

Thorndike, R.L., Hagen, E.P., & Sattler, J.M. (1986). *The Stanford-Binet Intelligence Scale: 4th Edition.* Chicago: Riverside.

Ventry, I.M. (1980). Effects of conductive hearing loss: Fact or fiction. *Journal of Speech and Hearing Disorders,* 45, 143-156.

Wallace, I.F., Gravel, J.S., & Ganon, E.C. (1991). Preschool language outcomes as a function of otitis media and parental linguistic styles. *Abstracts of the Fifth International Symposium Recent Advances in Otitis Media* (Abstract No. 211).

Wallace, I.F., Gravel, J.S., McCarton, C.M., & Ruben, R.J. (1988a). Otitis media and language development at 1 year of age. *Journal of Speech and Hearing Disorders,* 53, 245-251.

Wallace, I.F., Gravel, J.S., McCarton, C.M., Stapells, D.R., Bernstein, R.S., & Ruben, R.J. (1988b). Otitis media, auditory sensitivity, and language outcomes at one year. *Laryngoscope, 98,* 64-70.

Zarin-Ackerman, J., Lewis, M., & Driscoll, J.M. (1977). Language development in 2-year-old normal and risk infants. *Pediatrics, 59,* 982-986.

Zinkus, P.W., & Gottlieb, M.I. (1980). Patterns of perceptual and academic deficits related to early chronic otitis media. *Pediatrics, 66,* 246-253.

Received Jan 22, 1991; accepted Sept 5, 1991

---

[7]The mean percentage of visits in the 2nd year that were characterized as bilaterally positive for the otitis-positive group was 39.6 (SD = 36.2); for the otitis-negative group, the mean percentage was 17.3 (SD = 21.3). The difference was not significant, $t(21)$ = 1.85, n.s.

Contact author: Judith S. Gravel, Ph.D., R. F. Kennedy Center, Room 842, Albert Einstein College of Medicine, 1300 Morris Park Avenue, Bronx, NY 10461.

Speech Recognition in Noise by Children with Minimal Degrees of Sensorineural Hearing Loss

Carl C. Crandell

Callier Center for Communication Disorders, University of Texas at Dallas, Dallas, Texas

1993

Abstract

It is well recognized that the acoustical environment in a classroom is an important variable in the psychoeducational achievement of hearing-impaired children. To date, however, there remains a paucity of information concerning the importance of classroom acoustics for children with minimal degrees of sensorineural hearing loss (SNHL). The present investigation examined the effects of commonly reported classroom signal to noise ratios (+6, +3, 0, –3, and –6 dB) on the sentence recognition of 20 normal-hearing children and 20 children with minimal degrees of SNHL (i.e., pure-tone averages of 15- 30 dB HL through the speech frequency range). Results indicated that children with minimal degrees of SNHL obtained poorer recognition scores than normal-hearing children across most listening conditions. Moreover, the performance decrement between the two groups increased as the listening environment became more adverse. Educational implications of these data, such as acoustical modification of the classroom and/or the utilization of frequency modulation sound field amplification systems, are discussed.

Numerous investigators have stressed the importance of appropriate classroom acoustics in the educational management of hearing-impaired children (e.g., Bess, 1985; Bess, Sinclair, & Riggs, 1984; Blair, Peterson, & Veihweg, 1985; Crandell, 1991a; Crandell & Bess, 1987; Crum & Matkin, 1976; Davis, Elfenbein, Schum, & Bentler, 1986; Finitzo-Hieber, 1988; Finitzo-Hieber & Tillman, 1978; Ross, 1978; Ross & Giolas, 1971; Sanders, 1965). A review of such research has demonstrated that elevated levels of classroom noise and/or reverberation can deleteriously affect not only speech recognition ability, but also may compromise psychoeducational and psychosocial development in children with mild to profound degrees of sensorineural hearing loss (SNHL). Despite the important educational and therapeutic implications of these findings, there remains a paucity of data concerning the communicative efficiency of children with minimal, or "borderline," degrees of SNHL (i.e., pure-tone thresholds between 15 and 30 dB HL through the speech frequency range). Although the incidence of minimal hearing impairment in children is not known, it is well recognized that incidence rates increase as a function of decreasing hearing loss (Bess, 1985; Bess & McConnell, 1981; Davis et al, 1986; Gearheart & Weishahn, 1982; Northern & Downs, 1991; Ross, Brackett, & Maxon, 1982). Hence, it is reasonable to assume that a significant number of school-age children may exhibit minimal degrees of SNHL.

A review of the available evidence suggests that children with minimal degrees of SNHL experience greater speech recognition difficulties than normal-hearing children, particularly in the presence of environmental distortions such as noise and reverberation (Boney & Bess, 1984; Ross & Giolas, 1971). Ross and Giolas (1971), for example, assessed the speech recognition ability of six children with minimal to mild degrees of SNHL in a classroom setting. The children's hearing loss averaged 35 dB HL or less through the speech frequency region (500-2000 Hz). Stimuli consisted of phonetically balanced kindergarten monosyllabic words presented at a level of 65 dB SPL. Results indicated that the hearing-impaired group performed significantly poorer than the normal-hearing children. Specifically, recognition scores of 46% were obtained by the hearing-impaired children compared to 91% for the normal-hearing group. Unfortunately, it is difficult to generalize these findings exclusively to children with minimal degrees of SNHL, as the investigation only examined a small, heterogenous population of children with degrees of hearing loss ranging from minimal to mild levels. The trends noted in speech recognition performance, therefore, may not be applicable to children with only minimal degrees of SNHL.

To date, only the unpublished Boney and Bess (1984) investigation has specifically examined the effects of environmental distortions on the speech recognition of children with minimal degrees of SNHL. Minimally hearing-impaired children ($N = 6$) exhibited pure-tone thresholds between 15 and 30 dB HL for frequencies of 500, 1000, and 2000 Hz, with pure-tone thresholds no poorer than 40 dB HL at 4000 Hz. Monosyllabic word and sentence recognition were assessed in acoustical conditions often encountered in the classroom. Specifically, speech recognition was evaluated in noise [signal to noise ratio (SNR) = +6 dB], reverberation (T = 0.8 sec), and in noise and reverberation (SNR = +6 dB; T = 0.8 sec). The following results of this study are most pertinent to this investigation. First, the minimally hearing-impaired children performed significantly poorer than the normal-hearing children under most listening conditions. Second, in a listening condition commonly reported in the classroom setting (SNR = +6 dB; T = 0.8 sec), children with minimal degrees of hearing loss obtained sentence recognition scores of 54% compared to approximately 80% for the normal-hearing children. These data strongly suggest that noise and reverberation levels characteristic of many classroom environments can cause significant reductions in the speech recognition of minimally hearing-impaired children. However, it is again difficult to generalize these findings to children with minimal degrees of SNHL due to the small sample size. Certainly, if minimal hearing loss is an important educational variable in pediatric listeners, additional investigations are needed concerning the communicative efficiency of these children in everyday listening environments. Indeed, if it can be demonstrated that minimally hearing-impaired children do experience greater recognition difficulties in the learning environment, it is imperative that appropriate intervention strategies be developed to assist this population in the classroom setting.

With these considerations in mind, the purpose of the present investigation was to examine the effects of commonly reported classroom SNRs on the speech recognition abilities of children with minimal degrees of SNHL. Specifically, the sentence recognition of 20 children with pure-tone averages ranging from 15 to 30 dB HL through the speech frequency range were evaluated at SNRs of +6, +3, 0, –3, and –6 dB. All SNRs were chosen as representative of those values commonly found in classroom environments (e.g., Bess et al, 1984; Blair, 1977; Crandell, 1991a; Finitzo-Hieber, 1988; McCroskey & Devens, 1975; Paul, 1967; Pearsons, Bennett, & Fidell, 1977; Sanders, 1965).

Methodology

Subject Selection Criteria

Forty children, 20 with minimal degrees of SNHL and 20 with normal hearing, served as subjects for this investigation. Subjects ranged in age from 5 to 15 yr

with a mean age of 9 yr, 1 mo. All children were selected from the patient files at the Callier Center for Communication Disorders and the Dallas Independent School District.

The minimally hearing-impaired group met the following criteria:

1. pure-tone average (PTA) of 500, 1000, and 2000 Hz between 15 and 30 dB HL in at least one ear with no air conduction threshold poorer than 45 dB HL from 250 to 4000 Hz in octave intervals;
2. no air-bone gap greater than 10 dB HL at any frequency;
3. normal middle ear function (peak compliance between ±100 mm H_2O) as indicated by tympanometry;
4. sentence recognition scores of 90% or better in quiet as assessed by the Bamford-Kowal-Bench (BKB) Standard Sentence Test presented at a level of 65 dB SPL;
5. normal development and intelligence as reported by the parent; and
6. free from any significant medical problems.

The normal control group met the same criteria; however, all subjects in this group exhibited pure-tone air conduction thresholds no poorer than 15 dB HL from 250 to 8000 Hz in octave intervals. Subjects were matched for age (±1 yr). A composite audiogram for the normal and minimally hearing-impaired children is presented in Figure 1. The mean PTAs for the normal-hearing and minimally hearing-impaired groups were 4.5 and 19.5 dB HL, respectively. Only one of the minimally hearing-impaired children had any prior experience with amplification (personal hearing aid).

Speech Stimuli

The BKB Standard Sentence Test (Bench & Bamford, 1979; Bench, Koval, & Bamford, 1979) was used to assess sentence recognition. The BKB test consists of 21 syntactically and semantically equivalent sentence lists, each containing 16 sentences. Within each of these lists, 50 words have been designated as key words, which are scored for correctness (i.e., The *Clown* had a *Funny Face*). Percentage correct scores are calculated by dividing the number of correct responses by the total number of responses. Because the BKB lists were originally developed using British English vocabulary, an Americanized version of the test developed by Kenworthy, Klee, and Tharpe (1990), with permission from the original authors, was

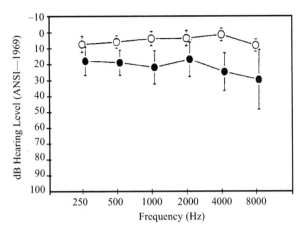

Figure 1. Mean audiograms for the normal and minimally hearing-impaired children. ○, Normal-hearing; ●, minimally hearing-impaired children. The vertical bars depict ±1 SD from the mean.

utilized in this investigation. In the Americanized version of the BKB stimuli, the British English words were converted to their equivalent standard American English forms. The Americanized BKB lists were recorded by an adult male who has both a General American English dialect and professional speaking experience. Master recordings were taped in a sound-treated room using a fi inch microphone (Bruel and Kjaer 4165) and a reel to reel tape recorder (Revox A-77). The sentences were then equalized for average intensity and re-recorded on tape. Recall that all subjects achieved recognition scores of 90% or better when listening to these sentences in quiet.

Competing Noise

Because a child in the classroom environment rarely listens to speech without the presence of noise, background noise was added simultaneously to the speech signal. The multibabble recording derived from the Speech Perception in Noise (SPIN) test (Bilger, 1984; Kalikow, Stevens, & Elliott, 1977) was used as the noise competition. The SPIN noise was generated by recording 6 adults (3 males/3 females) reading a passage in an anechoic room. The 6 recordings were then combined with a second recording of the same speakers, producing a 12 speaker babble. The SPIN noise has a long-term spectrum equivalent to the long-term spectrum of speech. The multibabble was chosen for the noise competition because its spectral shape is similar to the background noises commonly encountered in everyday listening situations (Aniansson, 1974). The BKB sentences and SPIN noise were dubbed onto two separate channels of high-quality recording tape.

Subject Listening Tasks

Speech recognition was assessed in a double-walled IAC sound-treated room under TDH-49 earphones mounted in MX-41/AR supra-aural cushions. The speech stimuli and the noise were separately attenuated, mixed, amplified, and presented monaurally to the subject. Only one ear of each subject was assessed. The speech stimulus was presented at a level of 65 dB SPL to simulate normal conversational levels. The noise was presented at levels of 59, 62, 65, 68, and 71 dB SPL, which resulted in SNRs of +6, +3, 0, –3, and –6 dB. As noted previously, all SNRs were chosen as representative of those values commonly reported in classroom environments (Bess et al, 1984; Blair, 1977; Crandell, 1991; Finitzo-Hieber, 1988; McCroskey & Devens, 1975; Paul, 1967; Pearsons et al, 1977; Sanders, 1965). In quiet listening conditions, the output of the channel producing the noise was disconnected.

The child's task was to repeat each sentence. Subjects were encouraged to guess when necessary. A silent period of approximately 8 sec followed each stimulus item to allow for the child's response. Each child listened to approximately two BKB lists per experimental condition. No child received any specific BKB list more than once to avoid possible learning effects. Furthermore, practice trials were given to each subject to familiarize the listener with the experimental task. Total test time for the investigation was approximately 2 hr per subject, which was completed in a single session. To ensure subject attentiveness, frequent breaks (approximately every 15 min) were permitted throughout the testing sequence.

Results

Mean sentence recognition scores and SDs (in percent correct) as a function of listening condition for the normal-hearing and minimally hearing-impaired children are presented in Table 1. These findings illustrate several trends. First, children with minimal degrees of SNHL obtained poorer recognition scores than the normal-hearing children across most listening conditions. A multifactor, repeated measures analysis of variance (ANOVA) indicated that these differences were statistically significant ($F = 9.25$; df = 1,5; $p < 0.0001$). Post hoc analyses, utilizing the Newman-Kuels test, indicated that these differences were significant at SNRs ranging from +3 to –6 dB at the $p = 0.01$ level. Second, note that the performance decrement between the two groups increased as the listening environment became more adverse. For example, at a SNR of +6 dB, the minimally hearing-impaired children obtained recognition scores of 83% compared to 96% for the normal-hearing children (a 13% difference). At a SNR of –6 dB, however, the performance discrepancy between the two groups increased to 33%, as the minimally hearing-impaired children obtained recognition scores of 38% compared to 71% for the normal-hearing controls. Finally, children with minimal degrees of SNHL exhibited marked variability in speech recognition performance, as demonstrated by the large SDs. This finding was not surprising, as it is well documented that hearing-impaired listeners tend to exhibit greater variability on speech recognition tasks, particularly in noise and/or reverberation (e.g., Cooper & Cutts, 1971; Crandell, 1991b; Dirks, Morgan, & Dubno, 1982; Keith & Talis, 1972; Nabelek & Pickett, 1974; Plomp, 1986; Suter, 1985).

Discussion

The results of this investigation revealed that children with minimal degrees of SNHL obtained significantly poorer recognition scores in commonly reported classroom SNRs than their normal-hearing counterparts. Moreover, the more adverse the listening condition, the greater the discrepancy between the two groups. The speech recognition difficulties experienced by these children may explain, in part, the psychoedu-

cational and psychosocial deficits often seen in this population (Boyd, 1974; Downs, 1988; Goetzinger, Harrison, & Baer, 1960; Quigley & Thomure, 1968; Waldman, Wade, & Aretz, 1930). Quigley and Thomure (1968), for example, reported that children with minimal hearing losses of 15 to 26 dB HL exhibited an average educational delay of approximately 1.1 grades.

The speech recognition deficits experienced by minimally hearing-impaired listeners emphasize the need to consider the acoustical environment of these children. Certainly, stringent acoustical requirements should be used for classrooms utilized by minimally hearing-impaired listeners to ensure that classroom noise levels are within recommended criteria. Acoustical standards suggest that unoccupied classroom noise levels should not exceed 30 to 35 dB(A) for maximum communication to occur in hearing-impaired listeners (Bess & McConnell, 1981; Crandell, 1991a; Crandell & Bess, 1987; Finitzo-Hieber, 1988; McCroskey & Devens, 1975; Olson, 1977, 1981, 1988; Ross, 1978). Unfortunately, a review of the literature indicates that this acoustical recommendation is rarely achieved (Bess et al, 1984; Blair, 1977; Crandell, 1991a; Finitzo-Hieber, 1988; Markides, 1986; McCroskey & Devens, 1975; Paul, 1967; Pearsons et al, 1977; Ross, 1978; Ross & Giolas, 1971; Sanders, 1965). Bess et al (1984) reported that the median noise level of 19 classrooms was 41 dB(A), with a range of 28 to 52 dB(A). Crandell (1991a) reported that the mean noise level in 32 classrooms was 51 dB(A), with a range of 34 to 61 dB(A). Discouragingly, only 1 of the 32 classrooms actually met recommended criteria.

Noise levels in a listening environment can be minimized in several ways. First, it is imperative that classrooms utilized for the rehabilitation or counseling of minimally hearing-impaired individuals be located away from external noise sources, such as traffic, construction, and furnace/air conditioning unit noise. Landscaping strategies such as the placement of shrubs or earthen banks can provide interference and absorption of outside environmental noise. An additional procedure to reduce external noise is to relocate the room and/or the noise source. That is, classrooms must be relocated away from high noise sources within the building such as areas adjacent to other rooms, cafeterias, or busy hallways. If relocation of the room or the noise source cannot be accomplished, then acoustical modifications of the room should be considered. Acoustical treatments such as thick or double-wall construction, carpeting of hallways, double-paned windows, and acoustically treated or well-fitting doorways can help to attenuate extraneous noise sources in the classroom.

Table 1. Means and SDs, in percent correct, of normal-hearing and minimally hearing-impaired children for the BKB sentences across six test conditions.

Test Condition	Normal Hearing	Minimal Hearing Loss
Quiet		
Mean	99.7	96.3
SD	(0.7)	(6.9)
+6 dB		
Mean	96.2	83.5
SD	(6.0)	(14.6)
+3 dB		
Mean	94.7	74.9
SD	(5.6)	(21.0)
+0 dB		
Mean	93.2	67.3
SD	(5.2)	(21.1)
–3 dB		
Mean	84.4	53.8
SD	(7.6)	(22.1)
–6 dB		
Mean	70.7	38.1
SD	(15.4)	(25.4)

A high degree of ambient noise originates from within the room itself. Obvious sources here include such activities as children talking, the sliding of chairs or tables, dropping of books, and the shuffling of feet. Heating and cooling systems may also contribute to the overall classroom noise level. Acoustical treatments such as the installation of thick carpeting, acoustical paneling on the walls and ceiling, acoustically treated furniture, and hanging of thick curtains can reduce ambient noise generated within the classroom. In addition, the rearrangement of listeners away from high noise sources, such as fans, air conditioners, or heating ducts, can also provide a more favorable listening environment for minimally hearing-impaired individuals.

Although the present investigation examined only the effects of noise on speech recognition, a further consideration in providing an appropriate listening environment for the minimally hearing-impaired child is the reduction of reverberation. Reverberation refers to the persistence or prolongation of sound within an enclosure as sound waves reflect off hard surfaces in a room. Reverberation time (T) refers to the amount of time it takes for a steady-state sound to decay 60 dB from its initial onset (Bolt & MacDonald, 1949; Kurtovic, 1975; Lochner & Burger, 1964; Nabelek & Pickett, 1974). Available research suggests that classroom environments are often far too reverberant for maximum communication to occur. Specifically, the range of reverberation in unoccupied classroom settings has been reported to be from 0.4 to 1.2 sec (Crandell, 1991a; Finitzo-Hieber, 1988; Kodaras, 1960; McCroskey & Devens, 1975; Nabelek & Pickett, 1974; Ross, 1978). Such high levels of reverberation in the classroom are alarming, as acoustical standards suggest that for optimum speech recognition to occur, levels of reverberation should not exceed 0.4 sec (Crandell & Bess, 1986, 1987; Crum, 1974; Finitzo-Hieber, 1988; Finitzo-Hieber & Tillman, 1978; McCroskey & Devens, 1975; Nabelek & Nabelek, 1985; Niemoeller, 1968; Olson, 1981, 1988; Ross, 1978). Reverberation can be reduced by covering the hard, reflective surfaces in a room (i.e., bare cement walls and ceilings, glass or mirrored areas, and uncarpeted floors) with absorptive materials. Acoustical paneling on the walls and ceiling, carpeting on the floors, the placement of cork bulletin boards on the walls, curtains on the windows, and the positioning of mobile bulletin boards at angles other than parallel to the walls can also decrease reverberation levels in an enclosure. For a more detailed description of acoustical treatments to reduce noise and reverberation levels in the classroom, the reader is directed to Finitzo-Hieber (1988), Nabelek and Nabelek (1985), Olson (1988), and Ross (1978).

Another consideration in reducing the damaging effects of noise and reverberation is to ensure that the child receives the teacher's voice at the most favorable speaker-to-listener distance possible. Specifically, the minimally hearing-impaired child needs to be in a face-to-face situation and in the direct sound field of the teacher, where the interaction of noise and reverberation are less detrimental to speech recognition skills. To achieve this recommendation, the restructuring of classroom activities must be considered. For example, small group instruction is recommended over more "traditional" classroom settings, where the teacher instructs in front of numerous rows of listeners. Close proximity to the teacher and face-to-face contact should also aid the minimally hearing-impaired listener in maximizing speech-reading skills. Such a recommendation has practical limitations, however, as in typical classrooms, the "critical distance"* for maximum speech recognition is present only at distances relatively close to the teacher (Peutz, 1971). Hence, the simple recommendation of preferential seating may not be adequate to ensure an appropriate listening environment for the child with minimal degrees of SNHL.

If further acoustic modifications in the room or restructuring of the enclosure are not possible due to room design or cost, another consideration for improving the acoustical environment for the minimally hearing-impaired child is the utilization of an assistive listening device. Unfortunately, recent research indicates that amplification systems are rarely recommended for children with minimal degrees of hearing loss (Crandell & Karasik-Rush, 1991; Davis et al, 1986; Shepard, Davis, Gorga, & Stelmachowicz, 1981). Several potentially beneficial amplification systems include: frequency modulation (FM) systems, personal hearing aids, and/or FM wireless sound field amplification systems. With the latter system, speech is picked up via a wireless microphone located near the speaker's mouth, where the voice is considerably stronger than the ambient noise in the room. The signal is then amplified and delivered to the listener via a room loudspeaker system. Several investigators have reported that the utilization of such systems in the classroom can significantly enhance speech recognition ability and, consequently, psychoeducational achievement for both normal-hearing and hearing-impaired children (e.g., Berg, 1987; Crandell & Bess, 1987; Flexer, 1989; Flexer, Millin, & Brown, 1990; Ray, Sarff, & Glassford, 1984; Sarff, 1981; Sarff, Ray, & Bagwell, 1981). For instance, Sarff (1981) utilized a sound field amplification system in a classroom with normal-hearing children and children with minimal degrees of SNHL. Results indicated that both groups of children, particularly the minimally hearing-impaired children, demonstrated significant improvements in academic achievement when receiving amplified instruction. Moreover, younger children demonstrated greater academic improvements than older children.

To summarize, the preceding discussion has highlighted several salient points concerning the speech recognition abilities of minimally hearing-impaired children in the classroom setting. First, commonly reported classroom acoustics have a deleterious effect on the speech recognition of children with minimal degrees of SNHL. Such findings are alarming, as it is well recognized that inappropriate classroom acoustics can adversely affect not only speech recognition ability, but also psychoeducational achievement. Hence, inadequate classroom acoustics may place minimally hearing-impaired children at risk for later language, literacy, social, and academic difficulties. Finally, this discussion has addressed several strategies to enhance speech recognition for minimally hearing-impaired children in the classroom setting. Specifically, the following areas were discussed: (1) acoustical modifications to reduce levels of noise and reverberation; (2) modifying classroom activities to achieve optimum speaker-listener distance; and (3) the utilization of amplification systems, such as FM sound field amplification systems.

This discussion indicates the need for further research in several areas. First and foremost, screening programs need to be developed that accurately identify those children with minimal degrees of hearing impairment. Current identification programs that screen pure-tone sensitivity at a level of 25 dB HL may fail to isolate many of these children. Clearly, research needs be conducted utilizing a 10 or 15 dB HL screening level in a sound-treated environment to provide precise incidence rates of minimal hearing loss in children. Second, ongoing collaboration and research among audiologists, psychoacousticians, acoustical/architectural engineers, and speech scientists is required in order to determine the most appropriate classroom acoustics (i.e., noise and reverberation levels) for maximizing speech recognition in minimally hearing-impaired children in the classroom setting. Third, the most appropriate classroom intervention strategies

(such as FM sound field amplification systems) for these populations will need to be isolated and developed. Fourth, the auditory and/or cognitive mechanisms responsible for diminished speech recognition in populations of minimally hearing-impaired children must be identified. Finally, if a relationship between auditory and/or cognitive deficits and speech recognition is substantiated in these populations, additional research will be required to develop assessment procedures for identifying specific processing difficulties in individual minimally hearing-impaired children. Assessment procedures will require the development of reliable, time-cost effective paradigms that do not require extensive instrumentation or subject training. Certainly, it is reasonable to assume that only through detailed analysis of how the individual hearing-impaired child processes various parameters of auditory information in difficult listening environments can we achieve maximum speech recognition and, consequently, academic achievement for minimally hearing-impaired children in the classroom setting.

References

Aniansson, G. Methods for assessing high frequency hearing loss in everyday listening situations. *Acta Otol Suppl* 1974;320:1-50.

Bench, J., and Bamford, J. Speech-Hearing Tests and the Spoken Language of Partially-Hearing Children. New York: Academic Press, 1979.

Bench, J., Koval, A., and Bamford, J. The BKB (Bamford-Koval-Bench) sentence lists for partially-hearing children. *Br J Audiol* 1979;13:108-112.

Berg, F. Facilitating Classroom Listening. Boston: College-Hill Press, Division of Little Brown, 1987.

Bess, F. The minimally hearing-impaired child. *Ear Hear* 1985;6(1):43-47.

Bess, F., and McConnell, F. Audiology, Education and the Hearing-Impaired Child. St. Louis: C.V. Mosby, 1981.

Bess, F.H., Sinclair, J.S., and Riggs, D. Amplification in schools for the hearing-impaired. *Ear Hear* 1984;5:138-144.

Bilger, R. Speech recognition test development. *Asha Rep* 1984;14:2-15.

Blair, J.C. Effects of amplification, speechreading, and classroom environment on reception of speech. *Volta Rev* 1977;79:443-449.

Blair, J.C., Peterson, M.E., and Veihwig, S.H. The effects of mild hearing loss on academic performance of young school-age children. *Volta Rev* 1985;87(2):87-93.

Bolt, R., and MacDonald, A. Theory of speech masking by reverberation. *J Acoust Soc Am* 1949;21: 577-580.

Boney, S.J., and Bess, F.H. Noise and reverberation effects in minimal bilateral sensorineural hearing loss. Paper pre-

---

*Critical distance (D$_c$) refers to the distance from a sound source at which the intensity of the direct sound field is equal to the intensity of the reverberant sound field. Operationally, D$_c$ can be defined by the following formula:

$$Dc = (0.20)(VQ/nT) - 1/2,$$

where V = volume of the room in m^3, Q = directivity factor of the source, n = number of sources, and T = reverberation time of the enclosure at 1400 Hz.

sented at the American Speech-Language and Hearing Association Convention, San Francisco, CA, 1984.

Boyd, S.F. Hearing loss: Its educationally measurable effects on achievement. Masters degree research requirement, Dept. of Education, Southern Illinois University, 1974.

Cooper, J., and Cutts, B. Speech discrimination in noise. *J Speech Hear Res* 1971;14:332-337.

Crandell, C. An update of classroom acoustics for hearing-impaired children. *Asha* 1991a;33:93.

Crandell, C. Individual differences in speech recognition ability: Implications for hearing aid selection. *Ear Hear* 1991b;12(6):100-108.

Crandell, C., and Bess, F. Speech recognition of children in a "typical" classroom setting. *Asha* 1986;28:82.

Crandell, C., and Bess, F. Sound-field amplification in the classroom setting. *Asha* 1987;29:87.

Crandell, C., and Karasik-Rush, S. Noise effects on the speech recognition of children with minimal hearing loss. *Asha* 1991;32:64.

Crum, D. The effects of noise, reverberation, and speaker-to-listener distance on speech understanding. Unpublished doctoral dissertation, Northwestern University, Evanston, IL, 1974.

Crum, M., and Matkin, N. Room acoustics: The forgotten variable? *Lang Speech Hear Serv Schools* 1976;7:106-110.

Davis, J.M., Elfenbein, J., Schum, R., and Bentler, R.A. Effects of mild and moderate hearing impairments on language, educational, and psychosocial behavior of children. *J Speech Hear Disord* 1986;51:53-62.

Dirks, D., Morgan, D., and Dubno, J. A procedure for quantifying the effects of noise on speech recognition. *J Speech Hear Disord* 1982;47:114-123.

Downs, M. Contributions of mild hearing loss to auditory language learning problems. In Roeser, R., and Downs, M., Eds. Auditory Disorders in School Children. New York: Thieme-Stratton, 1988.

Finitzo-Hieber, T. Classroom acoustics. In Roeser, R., Ed. Auditory Disorders in School Children, 2nd ed. New York: Thieme-Stratton, 1988:221-233.

Finitzo-Hieber, T., and Tillman, T. Room acoustics effects on monosyllabic word discrimination ability for normal and hearing-impaired children. *J Speech Hear Res* 1978;21:440-458.

Flexer, C. Turn on sound: An odyssey of sound field amplification. *Educ Audiol Assoc Newslett* 1989; 5:6-7.

Flexer, C., Millin, J., and Brown, L. Children with developmental disabilities: The effects of sound field amplification in word identification. *Lang Speech Hear Serv Schools* 1990;21:177-182.

Gearheart, B.R., and Weishahn, M.W. The Handicapped Child in the Regular Classroom. St. Louis: C.V. Mosby, 1982.

Goetzinger, D., Harrison, C., and Baer, C. Auditory discrimination and visual perception in good and poor readers. *Ann Otol Rhinol Laryngol* 1960;69: 121-136.

Kalikow, D.N., Stevens, K.N., and Elliott, L.L. Development of a test of speech intelligibility in noise using sentence materials with controlled word predictability. *J Acoust Soc Am* 1977;61:1337-1351.

Keith, R., and Talis, H. The effects of white noise on PB scores of normal-hearing and hearing-impaired listeners. *Audiology* 1972;11:177-186.

Kenworthy, O.T., Klee, T., and Tharpe, A. Speech recognition ability of children with unilateral sensorineural hearing loss as a function of amplification, speech stimuli and listening condition. *Ear Hear* 1990;11(4):264-270.

Kodaras, M. Reverberation times of typical elementary school settings. *Noise Control* 1960;6:17-19.

Kurtovic, H. The influence of reflected sound upon speech intelligibility. *Acoustica* 1975;33:32-39.

Lochner, J., and Burger, J. The influence of reflections in auditorium acoustics. *J Sound Vibration* 1964;4:426-454.

Markides, A. Speech levels and speech-to-noise ratios. *Br J Audiol* 1986;20:115-120.

McCroskey, F.L., and Devens, J.S. Acoustic characteristics of public school classrooms constructed between 1890 and 1960. *Noisexpo Proceedings* 1975:101-103.

Nabelek, A., and Nabelek, I. Room acoustics and speech perception. In Katz, J., Ed. *Handbook of Clinical Audiology*, 3rd ed. Baltimore: Williams & Wilkins, 1985.

Nabelek, A., and Pickett, J. Reception of consonants in a classroom as affected by monaural and binaural listening, noise, reverberation, and hearing aids. *J Acoust Soc Am* 1974;56:628-639.

Niemoeller, A.F. Acoustical design of classrooms for the deaf. *Am Ann Deaf* 1968;113:1040-1045.

Northern, J., and Downs, M. *Hearing in Children*, 3rd Ed. Baltimore, MD: Williams & Wilkins, 1991.

Olsen, W.O. Acoustics and amplification in classrooms for the hearing impaired. In Bess, F.H, Ed. *Childhood Deafness: Causation, Assessment and Management.* New York: Grune & Stratton, 1977.

Olsen, W.O. The effects of noise and reverberation on speech intelligibility. In Bess, F.H., Freeman, B.A., and Sinclair, J.S., Eds. *Amplification in Education.* Washington, D.C.: Alexander Graham Bell Association for the Deaf, 1981.

Olsen, W.O. Classroom acoustics for hearing-impaired children. In Bess, F.H., Eds. *Hearing Impairment in Children.* Parkton, MD: York Press, 1988.

Paul, R.L. An investigation of the effectiveness of hearing aid amplification in regular and special classrooms under instructional conditions. Unpublished doctoral dissertation, Wayne State University, 1967.

Pearsons, K., Bennett, R., and Fidell, S. Speech levels in various noise environments. EPA 600/1-77-025. Washington, D.C.: Office of Health & Ecological Effects, 1977.

Peutz, V.M. Articulation loss of consonants as a criterion for speech transmission in a room. *J Audiol Eng Soc* 1971;19:915-919.

Plomp, R. A signal-to-noise ratio model for the speech reception threshold for the hearing impaired. *J Speech Hear Res* 1986;29:146-154.

Quigley, S., and Thomure, F. Some effects of hearing impairment on school performance. Springfield, IL: Illinois Office of Education, 1968.

Ray, H., Sarff, L.S., and Glassford, F.E. Sound field amplification: An innovative educational intervention for mainstreamed learning disabled students. In *The Directive Teacher*. 1984:18-20.

Ross, M. Classroom acoustics and speech intelligibility. In Katz, J., Ed. *Handbook of Clinical Audiology*, 2nd ed. Baltimore: Williams & Wilkins, 1978.

Ross, M., Brackett, D., and Maxon, A. *Hard of Hearing Children in Regular School.* Englewood Cliffs, NJ: Prentice-Hall, 1982.

Ross, M., and Giolas, T.G. Effects of three classroom listening conditions on speech intelligibility. *Am Ann Deaf* 1971;December:580- 584.

Sanders, D. Noise conditions in normal school classrooms. *Exceptional Child* 1965;31:344-353.

Sarff, L.S. An innovative use of free field amplification in regular classrooms. In Roeser, R., and Downs, M., Eds. *Auditory Disorders in School Children*. New York: Thieme-Stratton, 1981.

Sarff, L.S., Ray, H.R., and Bagwell, C.L. Why not amplification in every classroom? *Hear Aid J* 1981;11:44-52.

Shepard, N.T., Davis, J.M., Gorga, M.P., and Stelmachowicz, P.G. Characteristics of hearing-impaired children in the public schools: Part I-demographic data. *J Speech Hear Disord* 1981; 46:123-129.

Suter, A. Speech recognition in noise by individuals with mild hearing impairments. *J Acoust Soc Am* 1985;78:887-900.

Waldman, J.S., Wade, F.A., and Aretz, C.W. *Hearing in the School Child.* Philadelphia: Temple University, 1930.

Acknowledgments

The Author would like to thank Alyssa Needleman and Susan Karasik-Rush for their assistance in contacting and evaluating subjects for this investigation.

Address reprint requests to Carl C. Crandell, Ph.D., Callier Center for Communication Disorders, University of Texas at Dallas, 1966 Inwood Road, Dallas, TX 75235.

Received May 20, 1992; accepted November 2, 1992.

Portions of this research were presented at the American Speech-Language-Hearing Association Annual Convention, Seattle, WA, November, 1991. This research was supported by a Texas Advanced Research Project (TARP) grant (#009741-031).

Children with Minimal Sensorineural Hearing Loss: Prevalence, Educational Performance, and Functional Status

1998

Fred H. Bess

Department of Hearing and Speech Sciences, Vanderbilt Bill Wilkerson Center for Otolaryngology and Communication Sciences, Vanderbilt University Medical Center, Nashville, Tennessee

Jeanne Dodd-Murphy

Department of Language, Reading and Exceptionalities, Appalachian State University, Boone, North Carolina

Robert A. Parker

Biometrics Center, Beth Israel Deaconess Medical Center, Boston, Massachusetts

Objective: *This study was designed to determine the prevalence of minimal sensorineural hearing loss (MSHL) in school-age children and to assess the relationship of MSHL to educational performance and functional status.*

Design: *To determine prevalence, a single-staged sampling frame of all schools in the district was created for 3rd, 6th, and 9th grades. Schools were selected with probability proportional to size in each grade group. The final study sample was 1218 children. To assess the association of MSHL with educational performance, children identified with MSHL were assigned as cases into a subsequent case-control study. Scores of the Comprehensive Test of Basic Skills (4th Edition) (CTBS/4) then were compared between children with MSHL and children with normal hearing. School teachers completed the Screening Instrument for Targeting Education Risk (SIFTER) and the Revised Behavior Problem Checklist for a subsample of children with MSHL and their normally hearing counterparts. Finally, data on grade retention for a sample of children with MSHL were obtained from school records and compared with school district norm data. To assess the relationship between MSHL and functional status, test scores of all children with MSHL and all children with normal hearing in grades 6 and 9 were compared on the COOP Adolescent Chart Method (COOP), a screening tool for functional status.*

Results: *MSHL was exhibited by 5.4% of the study sample. The prevalence of all types of hearing impairment was 11.3%. Third grade children with MSHL exhibited significantly lowere scores than normally hearing controls on a series of subtests of the CTBS/4; however, no differences were noted at the 6th and 9th grade levels. The SIFTER results revealed that children with MSHL scored poorer on the communication subtest than normal-hearing controls. Thirty-seven percent of the children with MSHL failed at least one grade. Finally, children with MSHL exhibited significantly greater dysfunction than children with normal hearing on several subtests of the COOP including behavior, energy, stress, social support, and self-esteem.*

Conclusions: *The prevalence of hearing loss in the schools almost doubles when children with MSHL are included. This large, education-based study shows clinically important associations between MSHL and school behavior and performance. Children with MSHL experienced more difficulty than normally hearing children on a series of educational and functional test measures. Although additional research is necessary, results suggest the need for audiologists, speech-language pathologists, and educators to evaluate carefully our identification and managament approaches with this population. Better efforts to manage these children could result in meaningful improvement in their educational progress and psychosocial well-being.*

Moderate to profound (41 to 100 dB HL; American National Standards Institute, 1996) early childhood hearing impairment is known to impose burdens on the affected child, the child's family, and society. Early onset of sensorineural hearing impairment (>41 dB HL) compromises communication skills, academic performance, psychosocial behavior, and emotional development (Bess & McConnell, 1981; Davis, 1990; Davis, Shepherd, Stelmachowicz, & Gorga,

1981; de Villiers, 1992; Holt, 1993; Karchmer, 1991). Even children with significant unilateral sensorineural hearing impairment (>40 dB HL) may experience problems with speech recognition in noise, educational difficulties, and psychosocial development (Bess & Tharpe, 1984, 1986; Bess, Tharpe, & Gibler, 1986; Jensen, Borre, 1989; Martini et al., 1988; Oyler &Matkin, 1988; Oyler, Oyler, & Matkin, 1987; Stein, 1983). Significant bilateral hearing impairment also causes economic adversities--the estimated lifetime costs of congenital deafness exceeds $1,000,000 for each affected individual (Northern & Downs, 1991). Other indirect costs affecting the child and family may include family tension, family disruption, breakdowns in family communication, and social isolation (Bess & Paradise, 1994; Davis, 1988, Maliszewski, 1988, Maliszewski, Reference Note 1).

Far less is known about children with milder degrees of sensorineural hearing impairment--prevalence data are almost nonexistent and information pertaining to the psychosocial and educational impact of mild losses is limited. Minimally hearing-impaired children (15-40 dB HL) do experience difficulty understanding speech under adverse listening conditions (Blair, 1977; Boney & Bess, Reference Note 2; Crandell, 1993; Goetzinger, 1962; Goetzinger, Harrison, & Baer, 1960; Ross & Giolas, 1971). It has not been determined, however, whether such speech recognition problems produce wider ripple effects by compromising psychoeducational achievement and other basic areas of human performance such as social and emotional function. Indeed, anecdotal reports, intuitive beliefs, and clinical experience suggest that some children with minimal sensorineural hearing impairment can experience a variety of communicative and learning problems. Numerous clinical reports and essays refer to the potential psychosocial and educational problems of children with minimal sensorineural hearing loss (MSHL) and encourage a more proactive approach to the identification and management of this population (Bess, 1985; Downs, 1995; Edwards, 1996; Flexer, 1995, 1996; Matkin, 1988; Sarff, 1981; Stein, 1983; Tharpe & Bess, 1991).

Despite increasing interest in the consequences of mild hearing loss, limited information exists with regard to MSHL and its relationship to social and emotional health. Data on self-ratings of social-emotional health status are limited even for children with moderate to profound sensorineural hearing. loss. Blake and Bess (Reference Note 3) found several indicators of functional health problems in children with mild to severe losses but tested relatively few subjects. In another study, Pudlas (1996) indicates a comparatively negative self-concept in a small sample of school children who were deaf or heard of hearing. Much of the research tat exists in this area has focused on teacher or parent perception of the child's social-emotional status. Stein (1983) notes that a small number of children (*N*=19) with unilateral hearing loss were rated by parents to exhibit a high frequency of behavior problems. Culbertson and Gilbert (1986) report negative teacher ratings of social compe-

tence in children with significant unilateral losses; however, the rating measure was relatively informal, pilot tested only in a local school system.

Several studies have attempted to assess systematically the educational impact of milder forms of hearing loss. Quigley and Thomure (Reference Note 4) examined the educational performance of 116 school-age children, grades 2 through 10, who exhibited hearing loss but did not receive special educational services. The children received a comprehensive audiologic and educational evaluation using selected subtests of the Stanford Achievement Test (Form W). Most of the children (83%) exhibited average hearing levels of less than 26 dB HL in the better ear. The educational performance of the children with hearing levels of less than 26 dB HL was poorer than would be expected from their intellectual potential. Even children with hearing levels less than 15 dB HL lagged behind expected educational performance.

Blair, Peterson, and Viehweg (1985) studied the educational performance of 24 children, grades 1 through 4, with mild (20 to 45 dB HL) sensorineural hearing impairment. Achievement test scores (Iowa Test of Basic Skills) were compared with a control group matched for age, sex, socioeconomic status, and school experience. Third and fourth grade children with hearing impairment performed poorer than their normal-hearing peers on several subtests of the Iowa Test of Basic Skills.

Finally, Davis, Elfenbein, Schum, and Bentler (1986) conducted a prospective study on 40 children with mild to moderately severe hearing impairments and demonstrated that degree of hearing loss was not a good predictor of a child's language or educational performance. That is, a child with minimal hearing loss could exhibit as much or more difficulty on verbal, educationa, and psychosocial tasks as a child with a mild to moderate hearing loss. Davis and colleagues conclude that "....children with any degree of hearing loss appear to be at risk for delayed development of verbal skills and reduced academic achievement." Similar findings have been reported by others (Bess & McConnell, 1981; Boyd Reference Note 5; Kodman, 1963; Sarff, 1981; Young & McConnell, 1957).

Inherent in all of the above studies are design limitations that preclude definitive interpretation and generalizability of the data. Some of the limitations are small sample size, selection bias, inadequate sampling procedures, incomplete description of the study population, ambiguous definition of minimal hearing loss, questionable matching of cases and controls or failure to employ a control group, and failure to report compliance data.

Clearly, a need exists to develop a better understanding of children with MSHL. If it is true that MSHL imposes a handicapping condition for some children, it would present important implications for the identificaiton, placement, and intervention strategies used with this population. We report here the results of a clinical, education-based study designed to determine the prevalence of MSHL in school-age children and to determine whether an association exists between MSHL and school performance and function.

METHODS

SAMPLE

The study sample comprised 1228 children in grades 3, 6, and 9 from the Nashville Metropolitan School District. A single-stage sampling frame of all schools in the district was created, listing separately schools with 3rd, 6th, and 9th grades. Schools were selected with probability proportional to size in each grade group. All children in grades 3 and 6 enrolled in the selected schools were asked to participate as subjects. For the other subjects, a complete roster of the 9th graders was prepared and individuals assigned a number in sequential order. A random number table of the students to be surveyed then was generated by computer. Consent forms were distributed to the subset of students based on the computer-assigned numbers, and those students who returned a signed parental consent form participated in the study.

INSTRUMENTATION AND PROCEDURES

All testing of children was conducted at the school site in a mobile unit that housed several examination stations and two sound-treated rooms suitable for the measurement of hearing (American National Standards Institute, 1991). Each child proceeded through the test stations to allow for data collection on: 1) background information (e.g., name, grade, school, sex, race) and ear-related history; 2) functional status; and 3) hearing status. Otoscopic examinations and pure-tone and middle-ear screenings also were performed on each child (findings from these tests are bing prepared for a separate report). For educational status, data were taken from school records. Children's behavior and potential for educational risk were assessed by using standardized questionnaires completed by the classroom teachers. The period of data collection spanned two years (November 1991 to June 1993).

Audiologic Evaluation - Hearing sensitivity was assessed using a standard pure-tone audiometer (MAICO, MA-40) equipped with TDH-39 earphones and Amplivox earcups. Hearing threshold levels were obtained using a standard protocol (Carhart & Jerger, 1959). Air-conduction pure-tone thresholds were obtained at octave intervals ranging from 0.5 to 8 kHz with 3 and 6 kHz also tested. Bone-conduction thresholds were obtained if the subject fit the criteria for minimal hearing loss. Bone-conduction thresholds were not obtained at 0.5 kHz, however, because of concerns regarding the possible influence of ambient noise.

Middle-ear function was determined using a GSI-33 Middle Ear Analyzer (Grason-Stadler, Inc.). Quantitative immittance values such as ear canal volume and peak admittance and pressure were collected on each subject. In addition, the supervising audiologist categorized each tympanogram as general type A, B, or C (Jerger, 1970). Type A tympanograms were those with peak admittance occuring between +100 and -150 and -400 daPa. Type B tympanograms had no peaks observed between +100 and -400 daPa. Tympanogram type was used as supplemental evidence for identifying a hearing loss as conductive or sensorineural.

Electronic calibration of audiometric equipment was carried out at least onece every 3 mo. A biologic calibration check of all measurement instruments was conducted twice each day of testing, before data collection began and after testing was completed.

Educational Performance - To establish educational performance for children identified with minimal hearing loss, test scores from the Comprehensive Test of Basic Skills (4th Edition) (CTBS/4) (Macmillan/McGraw-Hill, 1991) were obtained from school files for all children. The CTBS/4 is a series of comprehensive achievement tests designed to measure the outcome of learning at different levels in the educational sequence. It is a valid and reliable tool that has served as one of the nation's most popular test batteries for more than a decade (Macmillan/McGraw-Hill, 1991). The test assesses the objectives of general eduation from kidergarten through high school. The tests have been used widely as norm-referenced, objectively scored measures of educational achievement in reading, language, spelling, mathematics, reference skills, science, and social studies. Performance scores (percentile ranks) were compared between the children with MSHL and normal-hearing controls.

The Screening Instrument for Targeting Education Risk (SIFTER) (Anderson, 1989) was administered to the teachers of the children with MSHL in grades 3, 6, and 9. For each child with MSHL, at least three control subjects were selected randomly from the normal-hearing children. Teachers of the control subjects also completed the SIFTER. Teachers who completed the

SIFTER were not informed of the children's status (control versus MSHL group). The SIFTER is a test designed to provide a valid method by which children with hearing problems can be screened educationally. The SIFTER is a short, 15-item teacher rating test that explores several areas of school performance including academics, attention, communication, class participation, and school behavior. The SIFTER has been field tested and has been shown to have good content and score reliability (Anderson, 1989).

The Revised Behavior Problem Checklist (RBPC) (Quay, 1983; Quay & Peterson, 1987) also was administered to the teachers of children with MSHL in grades 3, 6, and 9 and to teachers of a randomly selected subsample of children with normal hearing. The teachers wo completed the RBPC were blind to student groups (control/MSHL). The RBPC assesses behavior in children and adolescents. This teacher rating scale is considered one of the most valid of all currently available teacher rating scales in terms of factor structure and related measures of validity. Based on a three-point scale, the test is composed of several subtests including conduct disorder, socialized aggression, attention problems-immaturity, anxiety-withdrawal, psychotic behavior, and motor access.

Finally, data on grade retention for children with MSHL were tallied from the school records. These data then were compared with school district norms.

Functional Status - The COOP Adolescent Chart Method (COOP) (Nelson, Wasson, Johnson, & Hays, 1996; Nelson et al., 1987; Wasson Kairys, Nelson, Kalishman, Baribeau, & Wasson, 1994, 1995; Wasson Landgraf, Berger, Kairys, Bracken, & Wasson, Reference Note 6) was used to measure functional status for all children in grades 6 and 9. The original COOP charts are office-based functional health measures that have been shown to produce reliable and falid data on a core set of functional dimensions: physical, emotional, and social (Nelson et al., 1981a, 1981b, 1983, 1987); the children's version of these charts was developed in 1987. The screening charts are based on a five-point scale with five representing the greatest dysfunction. The charts take 1 to 3 minutes to administer, are easy to use, and produce important clinical data. The limited available data suggest that the charts are acceptable, reliable, and valid for children in grades 6 through 12 (Nelson, et al., 1987; Wasson, et al., Reference Note 6). The patterns of correlations between the charts and validity indicator variables provide evidence for both convergent and discriminant validity. The children were assessed using 10 different dimensions of function: emotional feelings, schoolwork, social support, stress, family, self-esteem, behavior, energy, getting along with other, and overall health. Sample charts appear in the Appendix. The examiners instructed each child to select a category (1 through 5) that best represented the child's perception of his or her function in that dimension. Children responded either verbally or by pointing to the category on the chart. Examiners then recorded the responses on data forms.

EXAMINERS

The background information, ear-related history, and functional status data were collected by graduate students in speech-language pathology or audiology; the tests of middle ear function and pure-tone audiometry were conducted by more experienced graduate students in audiology (second year Master's or Ph.D. students). All graduate students who participated in the project underwent an extensive training period before data collection; additional periodic instruction was provided throughout the data-collection phase of the project. Graduate student examiners were supervised on site by a certified audiologist.

DESCRIPTION OF HEARING LOSS CATEGORIES

We defined MSHL for three distinct groups of children--unilateral sensorineural hearing loss (USHL), bilateral sensorineural hearing loss (BSHL), and high-frequency sensorineural hearing loss (HFSHL).

USHL was defined as average air-conduction thresholds (0.5, 1, 2 kHz) ≥20 dB HL (American National Standards Institute, 1996) in the impaired ear, with an average air-bone gap no greater than 10 dB at 1, 2, and 4 kHz. Average air-conduction thresholds in the good ear needed to be ≤15 dB HL.

BSHL was defined as average pure-tone thresholds between 20 and 40 dB HL bilaterally with average air-bone gaps no greater than 10 dB at frequencies 1, 2, and 4 kHz.

HFSHL was defined as air-conduction thresholds greater than 25 dB HL at two or more frequencies above 2 kHz (i.e., 3, 4, 6, 8 kHz) in one or both ears with air-bone gaps at 3 and 4 kHz no greater than 10 dB.

Tympanometry was used to rule out obvious middle-ear pathology in ears that were judged to have sensorineural loss based on the pure-tone criteria. Ears with hearing loss designated as sensorineural had Type A tympanograms with a peak admittance of 0.3 ml or greater.

Several other hearing loss categories were used. Conductive hearing loss (CHL) was defined as an average air-conduction threshold of 20 dB HL or greater in

TABLE 1. Selected demographic characteristics of a sample of 1218 school-age children.*

Grade	Number	Age (yr)	Sex		Race		
			Male	Female	Black	White	Other
3	565	8.6	264	299	194	360	11
6	350	11.4	166	183	155	183	11
9	303	14.7	135	168	188	111	4

Missing data for two children in grade 3 (sex) and one child in grade 6 (sex, race)

one or both ears with average bone-conduction thresholds (1, 2, 4 kHz) for the hearing-impaired ears more than 10 dB better than their air-conduction pure-tone average at the same frequencies or an average air-bone gap of 10 dB with a Type B tympanogram in the affected ear. Normal hearing was defined as no more than one pure-tone air-conduction threshold per ear greater than 25 dB HL and average pure-tone air-conduction thresholds of $\leq$15 dB in both ears. An "other" category was used to denote any child who did not fit into the above five categories (e.g., mixed hearing loss, previously identified children with hearing loss beyond the boundaries of MSHL).

DATA ANALYSIS

For prevalence of hearing loss, a weighted analysis using weights appropriate for the single-stage sampling design gave similar overall prevalence estimates to those using an unweighted analysis. Hence, prevalence is presented as the number and percentage of children from the study sample who met the criteria for MSHL and other hearing loss categories.

To assess the association of MSHL with educational performance, children with MSHL were assigned as cases into a subsequent case-control study. To increase statistical power, we matched at least three children with normal hearing to each child with MSHL. Controls were matched for school, school grade, gender, and race. To assess the relationship between MSHL and functional status, all children in grades 6 and 9 with MSHL and with normal hearing were included in the study.

For comparing the effects of hearing loss on measures of educational performance and functional status (available on all children with normal hearing), standard two-group methods of comparison were used, e.g., Fisher's exact test for contigency tables and the Mantel-Haenszel test for trend for ordered categorical data. For the results in the case-control study, continuous variables were averaged across the controls for each case, and a paired t-test (or equivalent nonparametric test, the Wilcoxon Signed Rank test) was used to assess differences between means. For binary variables, conditional logistic regression was used. Statistical significance was defined by p <0.05 (two-sided). Finally, exact 99% confidence intervals were calculated for the retention rate observed among cases. Conditional logistic regressions were done using EGRET V1.02.10 (Statistics and Epidemiology Research Corporation, Seattle, WA). All other analyses were done using SAS V6.22 (SAS Institute, Cary, NC). Missing values account for slight differences in totals in the tables.

We did not use formal methods to adjust p values because, in general, statistically significant results are reported only when there appeared to be a consistent response among several related variables. Formal methods of adjusting p values are most appropriate when multiple statistical tests are performed and the number of statistically significant findings are scattered throughout the variables examined. In our analysis, in contrast, we have focused on consistent patterns across variables rather than on the precise level of statistical significance for each comparison.

RESULTS

RESPONSE RATES

A total of 2816 children were recruited from grades 3, 6, and 9. Of these, 1228 children returned parental consent forms to participate in the study for an overall response rate of 44%. The following response rates were obtained for each grade level: 3rd grade - 65%; 6th grade - 48%; 9th grade - 30%. A review of the characteristics of responders and nonresponders in grades 3, 6, and 9 revealed that the two groups were similar with regard to race, sex, and school performance. Ten children were excluded from the study sample because of missing data or poor reliability. Our final study base consisted of 1218 children. Selected group characteristics for this sample as a function of grade level are summarized in Table 1.

Table 2. Number and prevalence of minimal sensorineural hearing loss, conductive hearing loss, and other types of hearing loss (e.g., mixed) in a sample of 1218 school-age children.

Hearing Loss Category	Number	Percentage
Bilateral sensorineural hearing loss	12	1.0
High-frequency sensorineural hearing loss	17	1.4
Unilateral sensorineural hearing loss	37	3.0
Subtotal	**66**	**5.4**
Conductive hearing loss	41	3.4
Other	30	2.5
Subtotal	**71**	**5.9**
Total	**137**	**11.3**

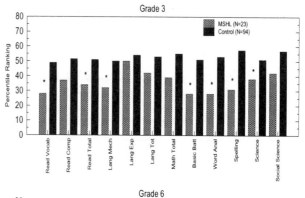

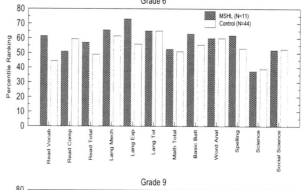

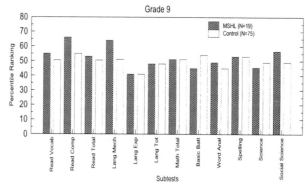

Figure 1. Median percentile test scores on the Comprehensive Test of Basic Skills (4th Edition) for children with minimal sensorineural hearing loss (MSHL) and for a group of normal-hearing counterparts presented as a function of subtests for grades 3, 6, and 9. Asterisks denote subtests in which significance ($p < 0.05$) was achieved between groups (paired t-test).

PREVALENCE

Table 2 summarizes the number and percentage of school-age children who exhibited MSHL or other categories of hearing loss (conductive, other). It is noted that 5.4% of the study sample exhibited one of the three types of MSHL. USHL was the most prevalent category (3.0%), more than BSHLs (1.0%) and HFSHLs (1.4%) combined. For HFSHL, 8 of the 17 cases (47%) were bilateral hearing losses. Interestingly, when the three types of MSHL were combined, more children exhibited MSHL (5.4%) than CHL (3.4%). Finally, when all categories of hearing loss were included, the prevalence of hearing impairment in this sample of school-age children was 11.3%.

The number and prevalence of school age children exhibiting MSHL as a function of grade, race, and sex are shown in Table 3. In general, the prevalence (%) of MSHL remained fairly constant over grades 3, 6, and 9. HRSHL and BSHL increased slightly with increasing grade. As noted above USHL was the most common hearing loss category. It is also observed that HFSHLs were more common among whites than blacks, FSHLs were more frequent among boys than girls, and USHLs were more common among girls than boys. CHLs were most frequent in the 3rd grade and were more common among white children.

Table 3. Number and prevalence (%) of school-age children (N = 1218) exhibiting minimal sensorineural hearing loss, conductive hearing loss, and other hearing loss (e.g., mixed) as a function of grade, race, and sex.

Hearing Loss Category	Grade 3 (%)	6 (%)	9 (%)	Race Black (%)	White (%)	Other (%)	Sex Male (%)	Female (%)
Bilateral sensorineural hearing loss	5 (0.88)	3 (0.86)	4 (1.32)	5 (0.93)	7 (1.07)	0 (0)	3 (0.53)	9 (1.38)
High-frequency hearing loss	6 (1.06)	5 (1.43)	6 (1.98)	5 (0.93)	12 (1.83)	0 (0)	11 (1.95)	6 (0.92)
Unilateral sensorineural hearing loss	23 (4.07)	5 (1.43)	9 (2.97)	20 (3.72)	16 (2.45)	1 (3.85)	12 (2.12)	25 (3.85)
Conductive hearing loss	28 (4.96)	9 (2.57)	4 (1.32)	9 (1.68)	31 (4.74)	1 (3.85)	21 (3.72)	20 (3.08)
Other	18 (3.19)	10 (2.86)	2 (0.66)	13 (2.42)	17 (2.60)	0 (0)	10 (1.77)	20 (3.08)

EDUCATIONAL PERFORMANCE

The primary analysis for educational performance was a comparison of CTBS/4 test scores for children with MSHL and a matched group of normal-hearing counterparts using a paired t-test. Figure 1 presents the median percentile test scores for the two groups of children as a function of subtests for grade levels 3, 6, and 9. In the 3rd grade, children with MSHL exhibited significantly lower scores than the control group for subtests reading vocabulary ($p < 0.002$), reading total ($p < 0.02$), language mechanics ($p < 0.03$), basic battery ($p < 0.05$), word analysis ($p < 0.0002$), spelling ($p < 0.02$), and science ($p < 0.05$). For grade levels 6 and 9, no significant differences were found between groups on any of the subtests.

The SIFTER was distributed to teachers of all children with MSHL and a matched group of children with normal hearing. Figure 2 summarizes the SIFTER data for the children whose teachers returned the questionnaire (response rate for children with MSHL was 44%; 29/66). This figure depicts the percentage of children with MSHL ($N = 29$) and their normal-hearing counterparts, collapsed across grades 3, 6, and 9, who displayed either marginal or failure scores for the various subtests. Many children from both groups exhibited failure or marginal ratings on each of the subtests. However, children with MSHL consistently performed more poorly than their normal-hearing peers. When one considers both failure rates and marginal passes, more than one-half of the children with MSHL experienced difficulty in academics (66%), attention (48%), and communication (79%). More than one-third of the children with MSHL were placed in the failure category for academics, attention, and communication.

Odds ratios and associated p values were calculated for each SIFTER subtest using a matched-pairs analysis of the case-control data. Odds ratios express the increase in likelihood of experiencing a problem (marginal or failure) for a child with MSHL compared with a normally hearing child. For example, a child with MSHL is 4.30 times more likely to experience trouble in the area of communication ($p < 0.01$) than a matched control child with normal hearing. Moreover, a child with MSHL is 3.42 times more likely than a normally hearing child to experience trouble if any one of three subtests (academics, attention, and communication) exhibited a problem (marginal or failure) ($p = 0.06$) and 2.59 times more likely than a normally hearing child to have difficulty with academics alone ($p = 0.06$). For other SIFTER subtests (attention, class participation, school behavior) the difference between groups were negligible.

The teacher response rate for children with MSHL on the RBPC was similar to the response rate obtained for the SIFTER (46%; 30/66). The RBPC data for a sample of children with MSHL in grades 3, 6, and 9 ($N = 30$) were compared with RBPC data of the normal-hearing controls ($N = 105$). No significant differences were found between groups for any subtests at any grade level.

Finally, in an attempt to obtain insight into the classroom performance of children with MSHL, we tallied the retention rates (i.e., repeating one or more grades) for children with MSHL. The average retention rate for all children with MSHL in grades 3, 6, and 9 was 37%. Figure 3 summarizes the retention rates for children with MSHL at each grade level. School district norm retention rates are included for comparison. The retention rate increased with increasing grade, from 29.2% (7/24), 99% confidence interval: 9.3 to 57.3%) in grade 3 to 36.4% (4/11, 99% confidence interval: 6.9 to 76.7%) in grade 6 and 47.4% (9/19, 99% confidence interval: 19.2 to 76.8%) in grade 9. All these rates are significantly higher than the district norm rates ($p < 0.01$). Retention rates were proportionally similar across the three categories of MSHL.

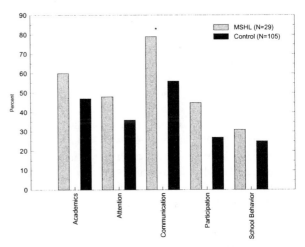

Figure 2. Percentage of children with minimal sensorineural hearing loss (MSHL) ($N = 29$) and with normal-hearing ($N = 105$) collapsed across grades 3, 6, and 9 who displayed either marginal or failure scores for subtests on the Screening Instrument for Targeting Education Risk. Asterisk denotes subtest in which significance ($p < 0.05$) was achieved between groups.

Functional Status

Functional statpus first was assessed by comparing mean COOP subtest scores for all children in grades 6 and 9 with MSHL and all children with normal hearing. A Mantel-Haenszel Chi-square test was used to determine whether the COOP scores for the different functional dimensions differed significantly between groups. For 6th graders, COOP scores were higher for the MSHL group (more dysfunctional) in 9 of the 10 domains. A significant difference between groups was achieved on the energy domain ($p < 0.03$); however, differences between groups on other subtests failed to reach significance. For the 9th graders, COOP scores wer also higher on 9 of 10 domains for the MSHL group. Children with MSHL

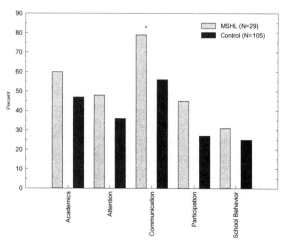

Figure 3. School retention rates for children with minimal sensorineural hearing loss (MSHL) at each grade level (3, 6, 9). School district norm retention rates are included for comparison. Asterisks denote the grades in which significance (*p* < 0.05) was achieved between groups.

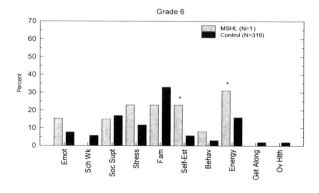

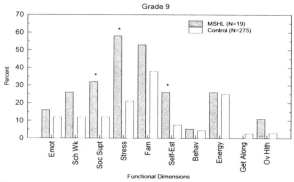

Figure 4. Percentage of children with minimal sensorineural hearing loss (MSHL) and normal-hearing counterparts in grades 6 and 9 who exhibited scores of 4 or 5 (greater dysfunction) on the various subtests of the COOP adolescent chart method. Asterisks denote domains in which significance (*p* < 0.05) was achieved between groups. (Fishers Exact test-2 tail).

exhibited significantly higher scores on the functional dimensions of stress (*p* < 0.001) and behavior (*p* < 0.05).

A second analysis of the COOP data contrasted all children (grades 6 and 9) with MSHL and all children with normal hearing who exhibited scores of 4 or 5 (more dysfunction) on the various subtests. Figure 4 illustrates the percentage of children from both groups who demonstrated the greatest amount of dysfunction along the various social/emotional domains. It is seen that children with MSHL tended to perform more poorly than their normal-hearing counterparts on some of the subtests, especially at the 9th grade level. A Fishers Exact test was used to determine whether the observed differences between groups achieved significance. For grade 6, significant differences were found between the two groups for self-esteem (*p* < 0.05) and energy (*p* <0.04). In grade 9, children with MSHL exhibited significantly higher dysfunction for three subtests: social support (*p* < 0.03), stress (*p* < 0.05), and self-esteem (*p* < 0.01).

DISCUSSION

The purpose of this study was to determine the prevalence of MSHL in school-age children and to determine whether an association exists between MSHL and educational performance and functional status. In a sample of 1218 children, prevalence of MSHL was 5.4%. Stated otherwise, 1 in 20 school-age children exhibited MSHL. USHL was the most prevalent form of MSHL in children followed by HFSHL and BSHL, respectively. When all forms of hearing loss were considered, the prevalence was 11.3%--approximately two times the 5 to 6% prevalence rate typically reported in the schools

using as the criterion an average of 25 dB or more through the speech frequency range (Bess & Humes, 1995; Bess & McConnell, 1981; Eagles, Wishik, & Doerfler, 1967).

Several possible factors may be contributing to the MSHL. First, it is well documented that noise-related hearing impairment poses a serious health problem to our youth (Mills, 1975). Montgomery and Fujikawa (1992), Axelsson, Jersen, Lindberg, and Lindgren (1981), and Axelsson, Aniansson, and Costa (1987) all attributed an increasing prevalence of sensorineural hearing loss to noise exposure from leisure activities. In the present study, the percentage of students reporting noise exposure was high throughout the sample. A higher percentage of 9th graders (89%) reported noise exposure compared with either the 3rd or 6th graders (approximately 77% in each grade). There was no significant difference in the percentage of boys and of girls who reported exposure to high-level noise. Reported exposure to intense noise levels was higher in children with MSHL (89%) than in children with normal hearing (79%).

Another possible explanation for the increased prevalence of sensorineural hearing loss can be found in the research by Hunter, Margolis, Rykken, Le, Daly, and Giebink (1996). They demonstrated that children with repeated episodes of middle ear disease can experience high-frequency hearing impairment, especially if the management history includes multiple intubations. It is theorized that basal cochlear damage occurs from the transmission of bacterial products through the round window. The authors questioned whether the high-frequency hearing loss related to recurrent otitis media might progress to the lower frequencies as age increases. The older children (7 to 11 yr) with histories of repeated episodes of otitis media showed slightly poorer thresholds from 250 to 4000 Hz when compared with the control group. Age was correlated positively with number of intubations. For the current study, data related to history of middle ear disease has increased markedly in the past several years (Schappert, 1992); many of the acute episodes of the disease will be unilateral (50 to 90%) (Hoberman, Paradise, Block, Burch, Jacobs, & Balanescu, 1996; Paradise, et al., 1990). A past history of repeated otitis media conceivably could contribute to a minimal to mild USHL or BSHL.

Finally, we have witnessed a marked increase in the survival rate of premature at-risk infants treated in neonatal intensive care units. Many at-risk conditions are associated with sensorineural hearing impairment--5 to 12% of these children exhibit mild sensorineural hearing impairments (Kenworthy, Bess, Stahlman & Lindstrom, 1987; Nield, Schrier, Ramos, Platzker, & Warbarton, 1986; Salamy, Eldredge, & Tooley, 1989; Walton & Hendricks-Munoz, 1991). In the present study, we did not have access to the prenatal and perinatal records of the children with MSHL.

The obtained prevalence rate of HFSHL (1.4%) is significantly lower than prevalence rates previously reported by other investigators. Montgomery and Fujikawa (1992) report the prevalence of HFSHL among school-age children as 6% for 2nd graders, 11% for 8th graders, and 12% for 12th graders. Similarly, Axelsson and coworkers (1981, 1987) report that prevalence rates of HFSHL in children at ages 7, 10, and 13 are 6%, 13.9%, and 12.3%, respectively. The probable difference in prevalence between the present investigation and the above studies is the difference in criteria for HFSHL. The aforementioned studies defined hearing loss as $\geq$ 25 dB HL at any test frequency. Montgomery and Fujikawa (1992) included three test frequencies (2, 4, 8 kHz) in their definition, whereas Axelsson and colleagues (1981, 1987) used six frequencies (0.5, 1, 2, 4, 6, 8 kHz). When the Montgomery and Fujikawa criteria were applied to these data, the prevalence of HFSHL for the older children became comparable in the two studies (14% for 9th graders in the present study versus 11% for 8th graders in the Montgomery and Fujikawa study). Based on the Mongomery and Fujikawa definition of loss, there would have been a 21% prevalence of

HFSHL for the 3rd graders in this study. A higher incidence of conductive loss in the 3rd graders would explain the higher prevalence in the current study. Importantly, Montgomery and Fujikawa did not obtain bone-conduction thresholds or conduct tympanometric assessments. The prevalence of HFSHL in the present study is actually higher than the rates reported by Axelsson and coworkers when using their definition of hearing loss. Regional differences also may account for some of the discrepancies between studies.

A somewhat surprising finding was that MSHL was more prevalent than CHL. Such a finding may be due to the time at which the testing was conducted--it is well recognized that otitis media is seasonal and occurs more frequently in spring and winter. Testing in the present study was performed throughout the entire school year.

It appears that children with MSHL experienced far greater difficulty in the educational system than one might predict from the audiometric data alone. Third grade children with MSHL exhibited significantly lower scores on many subtests of the CTBS/r. Interestingly, however, no such differences were found in the older children (grades 6 and 9). It is possible that MSHL imposes subtle problems that contribute to the test performance of younger children, who have less test-taking experience. Another possibility is that the effects of MSHL may not be long lasting, at least in terms of performance on standard aptitude tests. That is, children with MSHL may catch up in the later grades after a slow start. Finally, the CTBS/4 may not be sensitive enough at the higher grades to reflect the insidious problems of children with MSHL.

The CTBS/4 data are in agreement with Blair and coworkers (1985), who showed that a small sample of 3rd (N = 4) and 4th (N = 8) grade children with mild sensorineural hearing impairment (20 to 45 dB HL in better ear) performed significantly more poorly than a normally hearing matched control group on several subtests of the Iowa Test of Basic Skills. The largest between-group differences were apparent on the vocabulary and reading comprehension subtests. Even hearing-impaired children in the lower grades exhibited lower mean scores than those of their normal-hearing counterparts. Interestingly, Blair and coworkers speculated that the negative effects of mild hearing impairment may worsen as children reach the higher grades. Data from the CTBS/4 did not support this supposition; however, the educational performance (retention rate) of children with MSHL was poorer in the older children.

Although older children with MSHL performed within a normal range on the CTBS/4 and did not differ from their normally hearing counterparts, many were judged to be at risk for academic failure or at least marginally at risk as determined by the SIFTER. The largest discrepancy between children with MSHL and normally hearing children occurred on the subtest of communication. This subtest focuses on students' understanding ability, vocabulary, word usage skills, and story telling abilities--all fundamental skills essential for learning in the classroom. In support of the SIFTER data, 37% of all children with MSHL failed at least one grade in the educational system. Hence, similar to findings in previous studies on USHL (Bess, 1982; Bess & Tharpe, 1984, 1986), children can demonstrate normal aptitude for educationl performance yet continue to experience difficulty in school. The data on educational performance extend our understanding of this population to milder hearing impairments ($\leq$ 20 dB HL).

The high retention rate for children with MSHL imposes an economic burden on the education system. Of the approximately 46 million school-age children in the United States (United States Department of Education, 1998), 2,484,000 (5.4%) will exhibit MSHL. Of these, 919,080 (37%) will be projected to fail at least one grade. Assuming an average cost of $6000 to educate a child for 1 yr (United States Department of Education, 1998), the total expenditure for grade repetition exceeds 5 and one-half billion dollars (919,080 x $6000 = $5,514,480,000).

The RBPC, a teacher questionnaire focusing on problem behaviors in the classroom, showed no significant differences between the MSHL group and the control group. This resul.ts corresponds to the SIFTER data--these two groups differed the least in the SIFTER behavior category. Research by Furstenberg and Doyal (1994) supports the current study, reporting that students with hearing impairment were within the normal ranges and consistent across grades for teacher ratings on a behavior checklist similar to the RBPC. In the Furstenberg and Doyal study, the degree of hearing loss did not affect the teacher ratings of child behavior.

In earlier studies of social and emotional development, children with moderate to profound hearing losses have been shown to exhibit a number of problems in these areas (Bess & McConnell, 1981; Goetzinger & Proud, 1975; Higginbotham & Baker, 1981; Raymond & Matson, 1989; Schein & Delk, 1974). Even children with significant unilateral hearing losses experience social, emotional, and behavior problems in school (Bess & Tharpe, 1984; Culbertson & Gilbert, 1986; Stein, 1983). The present study extends our knowledge of psychosocial effects on hearing impairment to children with MSHL, providing information about the children's own perceptions of their functional status in a number of domains. Even the mildest forms of permanent hearing impairment can be associated with poorer functional health status.

The findings obtained on functional status using the COOP suggested that children with MSHL exhibited greater dysfunction than their normally hearing counterparts on such social/emotional domains as stress, self-esteem, behavior, energy, and social support. It is interesting to note that the 6th grade children with MSHL reported less energy or were tired more frequently than their normally hearing controls. Such a finding may be due to the difficulties these children experience listening under adverse noise/reverberant conditions.

Individuals with hearing loss are known to expend considerable effort and processing time trying to understand speech under adverse listening conditions (Downs, 1982; Ross, 1992a). In fact, poor acoustical conditions increase learning effort and, at the same time, compromise the energy available for performing other cognitive tasks (Downs & Crum, 1978; Rabbitt, 1966; Ross, 1992a).

Social skills are known to play an important role in an individual's receipt of social, academic, and emotional rewards (Raymond & Matson, 1989). Emotional-behavior functioning of children with hearing impairment as rated by teachers has been shown to be a significant predictor of student competency on outcome measures (Furstenberg & Doyal, 1994). Moreover, problems in social and emotional behavior are linked to peer status, school maladjustment, dropping out of school, and juvenile delinquency. Such functional difficulties in early childhood even can lead to other more significant social problems in later life (Raymond & Matson, 1989). Because social competence is critical to later emotional health and development, it is important for us to develop a better understanding of the functional status of any child with MSHL. To this end, the COOP appears to have potential as a screening tool for functional status in children (grades 6 and 9) with mild forms of hearing impairment. The test is safe, quick, simple, cost-effective, acceptable, and reliable. Additional research is needed, however, on the validity and predictive values of the tool. The COOP also may prove valuable for determining the success of amplification and other intervention strategies used with these children.

The COOP findings in this study raise research questions pertaining to the underlying psychosocial factors that contribute to poor social development. Does a perceived lack of social support in children with MSHL reflect an active rejection by their peers or does it reflect ignoring or neglect by peers? What factors might underlie the poor peer relationships of children with MSHL? Children with MSHL are most likely unaware of their hearing loss, yet they report poorer functional status in the area of self-esteem. If the difficulties with self-esteem are not related to an awareness of a hearing problem or to being labeled as different by other people, what is the source of these difficulties? Does an MSHL have subtle effects on language use, social interaction, or school work that might contribute to lower self-esteem for some children? The current study measured functional status for one period of time. Do children with MSHL experience transient periods of poor function or are the social/emotional problems present over the long ter? Answers to these questions and others will provide audiologists, speech-language pathologists, and professional educators with valuable insight for developing appropriate prevention, identification, and intervention programs for children with MSHL.

Not all children with mild hearing losses experience functional difficulties; some children, on the other hand, are clearly at risk for these problems. Thus, it seems important to consider screening all children with hearing impairment for functional problems to ensure they receive proper intervention when necessary. For example, if a screening highlights the presence of peer relationship difficulties, it is important to assess the specific nature of these deficits to tailor the appropriate intervention. Children who are socially neglected are often very different from those who are socially rejected, and each requires different intervention strategies (La Greca & Stone, 1990; Stone & La Greca, 1990, 1994). It is also important to study children with MSHL who do not experience functional difficulties to learn more about protective mechanisms that may be at work.

The results of this study spotlight the need for audiologists, speech-language pathologists, and educators to reassess our identification and management approaches for children with MSHL and to take a more proactive stance with these children. It is important to recognize that very few children from our target group had been identified with hearing impairment before this study. Two-thirds of the children with MSHL exhibited thresholds no greater than 25 dB HL at 1, 2 , and/or 4 kHz--it is likely that many of these children passed previous hearing screenings. Other reasons for a failure to identify these children may be that they had not been screened or they had late-onset hearing losses. Unfortunately, however, screening records for these children were not available for review. Clearly, we must do better. Early identification is a critical first step in the appropriate management of these children and poses some practical challenges to the audiologist. Preliminary data from the present study suggest that the performance characteristics of pure-tone audiometry (hand-held audioscope) under routine screening conditions in the schools are at best fair. If we lower the cutoff criteria to identify children with MSHL, more screening errors can be expected. That is, when the cutoff for hearing loss is lowered, the sensitivity of the tool will improve but specificity will be compromised. Such an uncomfortable spector highlights the need for audiologists to develop more effective screening procedures for identifying children with MSHL under field-testing conditions. To this end, greater emphasis on infant and school-age screening research seems warranted.

Because the hearing loss of many children with MSHL had not been identified, it is unlikely that any of them were receiving some form of management. To our knowledge, none of the children with MSHL wore hearing aids. Furthermore, none of the children with MSHL whose parents chose to seek further testing had veen receiving any hearing-related educational services. As noted earlier, identification of MSHL is only the first step for children with MSHL. It is also necessary to determine whether a child with MSHL is in need of special services to reduce risk for educational difficulties. Children at risk then should be provided with strategies that work for them. Further research is needed to find out how to

discern which children with MSHL are at risk for problems and which treatments are the most successful.

Many professionals advocate the use of FM amplification as a preference over personal hearing aids for children with MSHL who experience toruble in the schools. The primary difficulty experienced by these children is understanding speech in a background of noise/reverberation. The goal then is to improve the speech to noise ratio reaching the child's ear via an FM system or a sound field amplification device. The appropriate selection and evaluation of FM amplification for a child with MSHL poses unique challenges to the audiologist. Detailed discussions on this topic appear elsewhere (Bess, Gravel, & Tharpe, 1996; The Pediatric Working Group, 1996; Ross, 1992b). It is emphasized here that the potential for overamplification with such mild impairments is ever present. Moreover, the prospect of FM amplification should be considered on a case-by-case basis, and such factors as speech-language development, handicapping conditions, academic progress, communication needs, functional status, and parental support all should be factored into the decision about amplification. A possible alternative to a personal FM system is the use of sound-field amplification (Crandell, Smaldino, & Flexer, 1995; The Pediatric Working Group, 1996; Sarff, 1981). One important advantage of soundfield amplfication is that it benefits all students in the classroom, including any who may have transient conductive losses or any not yet identified as having minimal loss. Because this type of interention does not label the child with MSHL as different, the use of sound-field amplification may avoid self-esteem issues sometimes associated with the use of personal hearing aids or an FM system.

Although amplification appears to be a reasonable management strategy for children with MSHL, additional research on the efficacy of amplification for children with various forms of minimal hearing loss is critical (The Pediatric Working Group, 1996). Other management strategies such as enhancement of listening skills, especially for suprasegmental and segmental information, auditory programming, and modifications of the listening environment have been detailed by others (Edward, 1991, 1996).

Interpretation of the data should be made with caution in view of the study limitations. We were concerned about the small number of children whose parents consented to their participation in the study (44%)--response rates declined in the higher grade levels even when tangible incentives were offered to the children and teachers. The parental consent letter described the information to be collected and the testing to be performed. It is possible that our sample may have been somewhat biased toward higher prevalence of hearing loss if the response rate was higher for parents who had concerns about their child's hearing than for parents who had no such concerns. We did not have access to information regarding parental suspicion of hearing loss. Nevertheless, we were unable to discern any differences in baseline characteristics (age, race, sex, school performance) between the responders and the nonresponders for grades 3, 6, and 9. Although we sampled a large number of school-age children, the actual number of children with MSHL ($N = 66$) was relatively small, especially when the target group was analyzed as a function of grade. In several analyses, missing data precluded us from using all of the children with MSHL. Educational records such as the CTBS/4 scores were unavailable in some cases, and the response rates on the teacher questionnaires were somewhat low (44 to 46%). In addition, the limitations inherent within a between-subjects design along with a paired-matching technique long have been recognized. Prospective research with a larger sample of children with MSHL might serve to confirm and expand on the present findings and to delineate the contribution of MSHL, relative to other factors, to the educational and functional difficulties reported. It is also important to recognize that the data from the present study imply an association between MSHL and educational and functional difficulties--one cannot infer from these data a cause and effect relationship.

Finally, it would have been preferable to compare our retention rate data with a matched group of normal-hearing children in the same classroom rather than to use district norm data. Unfortunately, we were unable to use a normal-hearing control group for this part of the study. Even when one considers the shortcomings of this investigation, it seems evident that some children with MSHL experience difficulty in educational performance and functional status.

In summary, we conducted a clinical, education-based study to determine the prevalence of MSHL in children and to assess whether a relationship exists between MSHL and educational performance and functional status. The prevalence of MSHL was 5.4%. The prevalence for all forms of hearing loss was 11.3%. Some children with MSHL experienced more difficulty on educational measures than children with normal hearing. A somewhat surprising finding of this study was that children with MSHL exhibited greater dysfunction than their normal-hearing counterparts on several subtests of the COOP. Thus, even very mild losses can be associated with increased social and emotional dysfunction among school-age children. Efforts to manage these children more aggressively could result in a significant and meaningful improvement in educational performance and functional status. Further research is needed to determine whether prevention, early identification, and management strategies will lead to better educational and functional outcomes of school-age children with MSHL.

ACKNOWLEDGMENTS:

This investigation was supported, in part, by the Robert Wood Johnson Foundation. We express our gratitude to former doctoral students Jane Baer and Patricia Chase, who assisted in the data collection, as well as to numerous graduate students from the Department of Hearing and Speech Sciences, Vanderbilt Bill Wilkerson Center. Eileen Lawrence, Roberta Bradley, and Mitchell Schwaber all aassisted in otoscopic examinations. Don Riggs provided technical support for numerous components of the study. We are grateful to Tennessee Lion's Club Districts 12I and 12S for the use of their soundproof testing van as well as to their volunteer drivers including Bob Sewell, Chuck Schreiber, and George Syner. We thank the Nashville Metropolitan School District for allowing us to conduct this study. Principals, teachers, and students from the Metropolitan School District made this study possible. Finally, we express our gratitude to Dan Ashmead, Larry Humes, Michael Lichtenstein, Walter Murphy, Eugene Nelson, Anne Marie Tharpe, and Terry Wertz for their thoughtful comments and suggestions.

Address for correspondence: Fred H. Bess, Ph.D., 1114 19th Avenue South, Nashville, TN 37212.

Received October 28, 1997; accepted April 22, 1998

REFERENCES

American National Standards Institute (1991). *Maximum permissible ambient noise levels for audiometric test rooms. (ANSI S3.1-1991)*. New York: ANSI.

American National Standards Institute (1996). *Specification for audiometers. (ANSI S3.6)*. New York: ANSI.

Anderson, K.L. (1989). *SIFTER Screening Instrument for Targeting Educational Risk in Children Identified by Hearing Screening or Who Have Minimal Hearing Loss. Users Manual*. Danville, IL: The Interstate Printers and Publishers, Inc.

Axelsson, , A., Aniansson, G., & Costs, O. (1987). Hearing loss in school children. *Scandinavian Audiology, 16,* 137-143.

Axelsson, T., Jersen, U., Lindberg , & Lindgren, F. (1981). Early noise-induced hearing loss in teenage boys. *Scandinavian Audiology, 10,* 91-96.

Bess, F.H. (1982). Children with unilateral hearing loss. *Journal of the Academy of Rehabilitative Audiology, 15,* 131-144.

Bess, F.H. (1985). The minimally hearing-impaired child. *Ear and Hearing, 6,* 43-47.

Bess, F.H., Gravel, J.S. & Tharpe, A.M. (Eds.) (1996). *Amplification for children with auditory deficits.* Nashville, TN: Bill Wilkerson Center Press.

Bess, F.H., & Humes, L.E. (1995). *Audiology: The Fundamentals.* Baltimore, MD: Williams and Wilkins.

Bess, F.H., & McConnell, F.E. (1981). *Audiology, Education and the Hearing Impaired Child.* St. Louis, MO: The C.V. Mosby Company.

Bess, F.H., & Paradise, J.L. (1994). Universal screening for infant hearing impairment: Not simple, not risk-free, not necessarily beneficial, and not presently justified. *Pediatrics, 93(2),* 330-334.

Bess, F.H., & Tharpe, A.M. (1984). Unilateral hearing impairment in children. *Pediatrics, 74,* 206-216.

Bess, F.H., & Tharpe, A.M. (1986). Case history data on unilaterally hearing impaired children. *Ear and Hearing, 7,* 14-19.

Bess, F.H., Tharpe, A.M., & Gibler, A. (1986). Auditory performance of children with unilateral sensorineural hearing impairment. *Ear and Hearing, 7,* 20-26.

Blair, J.C. (1977). Effects of amplification, speech reading and classroom environments on reception of speech. *The Volta Review, 79,* 443-449.

Blair, J.C., Peterson, M.E. & Viehweg, S.H. (1985). The effects of mild sensorineural hearing loss on academic performance of young school-age children. *The Volta Review, 87,* 87-93.

Carhart, R., & Jerger, J.F. (1959). Preferred method for clinical determination of pure-tone threshold. *Journal of Speech and Hearing Disorders, 24,* 330-345.

Crandell, C.C. (1993). Speech recognition in noise by children with minimal degrees of sensorineural hearing loss. *Ear and Hearing, 14,* 210-216.

Crandell, C.C., Smaldino, J.J., & Flexer, C. (1995). *Sound-field FM amplification - theory and practical applications.* San Diego, CA: Singular Publishing Group, Inc.

Culbertson, J.L., & Gilbert, L.E. (1986). Children with unilateral sensorineural hearing loss: Cognitive, academic, and social development. *Ear and Hearing, 7,* 38-42.

Davis, J.M., Shepherd, N.T., Stelmachowicz, P.G., & Gorga, M.D. (1981). Characteristics of hearing-impaired children in the public schools: Part II-Psychoeducational data. *Journal of Speech and Hearing Disorders, 46,* 130-137.

Davis, J.M. (1988). Management of the school age child: a psychosocial perspective. In Bess, F.H. (Ed.), *Hearing Impairment in Children.* Parkton, MD: York Press.

Davis, J.M. (Ed.) (1990). *Our forgotten children: hard of hearing pupils in the schools.* Washington, D.C.: U.S. Department of Education pp. 1-2.

Davis, J.M., Elfenbein, J., Schum, D., & Bentler, R.A. (1986). Effects of mild and moderate hearing impairment on language, educational, and psychosocial behavior of children. *Journal of Speech and Hearing Disorders, 51,* 53-62.

de Villiers, P.A. (1992). Educational implications of deafness: language and literacy. In Eavey, R.D. and Klein, J.O. (Eds.), *Hearing Loss in Childhood: A Primer, pp. 127-135.* Report of the 102nd Ross Conference on Pediatric Research, Columbus, OH: Ross Laboratories.

Downs, D.W. (1982). Effect of hearing aid use on speech discrimination and listening effort. *Journal of Speech and Hearing Disorders. 47,* 189-193.

Downs, D.W., & Crum, M.A. (1978). Processing demands during auditory learning under degraded listening conditions. *Journal of Speech and Hearing Research. 21,* 702-714.

Downs, M.P. (1995). Contribution of mild hearing loss to auditory language learning problems. In Roeser, R.J. and Downs, M.P. (Eds.), *Auditory Disorders in School Children.* New York, NY: Thieme Medical Publishers, Inc.

Eagles, E.L., Wishik, S.M. & Doerfler, L.G. (1967). Hearing sensitivity and ear disease in children: A prospective study. *Laryngoscope suppl.*

Edwards, C. (1991). Assessment and management of listening skills in school-aged children. *Seminars in Hearing, 12,* 389-401.

Edwards, C. (1996). Auditory intervention for children with mild auditory deficits. In Bess, F.H., Gravel, J.S., and Tharpe, A.M. (Eds.), *Amplification for Children with Auditory Deficits, pp. 383-398.* Nashville, TN :Bill Wilkerson Center Press.

Flexer, C.L. (1995). Rationale for the use of sound-field FM amplification systems in classrooms. In Crandell, C., Smaldeno, J.J., & Flexer, C.L., *Sound-Field FM Amplification-Theory and Practical Applications, pp. 3-16.* San Diego, CA: Singular Publishing Group.

Flexer, C.L. (1996). Amplification for children with minimal hearing loss. In Bess, F.H., Gravel, J.S., & Tharpe, A.M. (Eds.), *Amplification for Children with Auditory Deficits, pp. 321-337.* Nashville, TN: Bill Wilkerson Center Press.

Furstenberg, K., & Doyal, G. (1994). The relationship between emotional-behavioral functioning and personal characteristics on performance outcomes of hearing impaired students. *American Annals of the Deaf, 139,* 410-414.

Goetzinger, C. (1962). Effect of small perceptive losses on language and on speech discrimination. *Volta Review, 64,* 408-414.

Goetzinger, C. P., & Proud, G.O. (1975). The impact of hearing impairment upon the psychological development of children. *Journal of Auditory Research, 15,* 1-60.

Goetzinger, D.P., Harrison, P., & Baer, C.J. (1960). Auditory discrimination and visual perception in good and poor readers. *Annals of Otology, Rhinology, and Laryngology, 69,* 121-136.

Higgenbothan, D.J., & Baker, B.M. (1981). Social participation and cognitive play differences in hearing-impaired and normally hearing pre-schoolers. *Volta Review, 83,* 135-149.

Hoberman, A., Paradise, J.L., Block, S., Burch, D.J., Jacobs, M.R., & Balanescu, M.I. (1996). Efficacy of amoxicillin/clavulante for acute otitis media: relation to Streptococcus pneumoniae susceptibility. *Pediatric Infectious Disease Journal, 15(10),* 955-962.

Holt, J.A. (1993). Stanford Achievement Test - 8th Edition [Reading Comprehension Subgroup Results]. *American Annals of the Deaf, 128,* 172-175.

Hunter, L.L., Margolis, R.H., Rykken, J.R., Le, C.T., Daly, K.A. & Grebunk, G.S. (1996). High frequency hearing loss associated with otitis media. *Ear and Hearing, 17,* 1-11.

Jensen, J.H., Børre, S., & Johansen, A. (1989). Unilateral sensorineural hearing loss in children: cognitive abilities with respect to right/left ear differences. *British Journal of Audiology, 23,* 215-220.

Jensen, J.H., Johansen, P.A., & Børre, S. (1989). Unilateral sensorineural hearing loss in children and auditory performance with respect to right/left ear differences. *British Journal of Audiology, 23,* 207-213.

Jerger, J. (1970). Clinical experience with impedence audiometry. *Archives of Otolaryngology, 93,* 311-324.

Karchmer, M.A. (1991). *Stanford Achievement test norms for hearing impaired students.* Washington, D.C.: Gallaudet University, Office of Demographic Studies.

Kenworthy, O.T., Bess, F.H., Stahlman, M.T., & Lindstrom, D.P. (1987). Hearing, speech and language outcome of infants with extreme immaturity. *American Journal of Otology,* 419-425.

Kodman, F. (1963). Educational status of the hard of hearing children in the classroom. *Journal of Speech and Hearing Research, 28,* 297-299.

La Greca, A.M., & Stone, W.L. (1990). Children with learning disabilities: The role of achievement in their social, personal, and behavioral functioning. In H.L. Swanson and B. Keogh (Eds.) *Learning disabilities: Theoretical and research issues (pp. 333-352).* Hilldale, NJ: Lawrence Erlbaum.

Macmillan/McGraw-Hill (19931). *Comprehensive Test of Basic Skills,--Technical Report,* Fourth Edition (C.T.B.S./4).

Maliszewski, S.J. (1988). The impact of a child's hearing impairment on the family: a parent's perspective. In Bess, F.H. *Hearing Impairment in Children.* Parkton, MD: York Press.

Martini, A., Bovo, R., Milani, M., DeVitis, M., Liddeo, M., Zangagla, A.M., & Carengnoto, D. (1988). Unilateral sensorineural deafness in children: Results of a questionnaire on 115 children suffereing from unilateral deafness. *Quaderni di Audiologia, 4,* 318-323.

Matkin, N.D. (1988). Re-evaluating our approach to evaluation: demographics are changing--are we? In Bess, F.H. (Ed.), *Hearing Impairment in Children,* Parkton, MD: York Press.

Mills, J.H. (1975). Noise and children: A review of literature. *Journal of the Acoustical Society of America, 58,* 768-779.

Montgomery, J., & Fujikawa, S. (1992). Hearing thresholds of students in the second, eighth, and twelfth grades. *Language, Speech, and Hearing Services in Schools, 23,* 61-63.

Nelson, E.C., Carger, B., Douglas, R., Gephart, D., Kirk, J., Page, R., Clark, A., Johnson, K., Stone, K., Wasson, J., & Zubkoff, M. (1983). Functional health status levels of primary care patients. *Journal of the American Medical Association, 249,* 3331-3338.

Nelson, E.C., Kirk, J.W., Bise, B.W., Chapman, R.C., Hale, F.A., Stamps, P.L., & Wasson, J.H. (1981a). The Cooperative Information Project Part 1: A sentinel practice network for service and research in primary care. *Journal of Family Practice, 13,* 641-649.

Nelson, E.C., Kirk, J.W., Bise, B.W., Chapman, R.C., Hale, F.A., Stamps, P.L., & Wasson, J.H. (1981b). The Cooperative Information Project Part 2: Some neutral clinical, quality assurance, and practice management studies. *Journal of Family Practice, 13,* 867-876.

Nelson, E.C., Wasson, J., Kirk, J., Keller, A., Clark, D., Dietrich, A., Stewart, A., & Zubkoff, M. (1987). Assessment of function in routine clinical practice: Description of the COOP Chart Method and preliminary findings. *Journal of Chronic Diseases, 40, Suppl. 1,* 555-635.

Nelson, E.C., Wasson, J.H., Johnson, D., & Hays, R. (1996). Dartmouth COOP Functional Health Assessment Charts: Brief Measures for Clinical Practice. In B. Spilker (Ed.) *Quality of Life and Pharmacoeconomics in Clinical Trials, (2nd Ed.),* Lippencott-Raven Publishers: Philadelphia.

Nield, T.A., Schrier, S., Ramos, A.D., Platzker, A.C.G., & Warburton, D., (1986). Unexpected hearing loss in high-risk infants. *Pediatrics, 78,* 417-422.

Northern, J.D., & Downs, M.P. (1991). *Hearing in Children, 4th ed.* Baltimore, MD: Williams and Wilkins.

Oyler, R.F., & Matkin, N.D. (1988). Unilateral hearing loss: Demographics and educational impact. *Language, Speech, and Hearing Services in Schools, 19,* 201-209.

Oyler, R.F., Oyler, A.L., & Matkin, N.D. (1987). Warning: A unilateral hearing loss may be detrimental to a child's academic career. *The Hearing Journal, September,* 18-22.

Paradise, J.L., Bluestone, C.D., Rogers, K.D., Taylor, F.H., Colborn, K., Bachman, R.Z., Bernard, B.S., & Schwarzbach, R.H. (1990). Efficacy of adenoidectomy for recurrent otitis media in children previously treated with tympanostomy-tube placement: Results of parallel randomized and nonrandomized trials. *The Journal of the American Medical Association, 263(15),* 2066-2073.

Pudlas, K.A. (1996). Self-esteem and self-concept: Special education as experienced by deaf, hard of hearing and hearing students. *British Columbia Journal of Special Education, 20(1),* 23-39.

Quay, H.C. (1983). A dimensional approach to children's behavior disorder: The revised behavior problem checklist. School *Psychology Review, 12,* 244-249.

Quay, H.C., & Peterson, D.R. (1987). *Manual for the revised behavior problem checklist.* Coral Gables, FL: University of Miami.

Rabbitt, P.M. (1966). Recognition: Memory for whole words correctly heard in noise. *Psychonomic Science, 6,* 383-384.

Raymond, K.L., & Matson, J.L. (1989). Social skills in the hearing impaired. *Journal of Clinical Child Psychology, 18,* 247-258.

Ross, M (1992a) Room acoustics and speech perception. In Ross, M. (Ed) FM *Auditory Training Systems-Characteristics, Selection and Use pp 21-43.* Timonium, MD: York Press.

Ross, M. (Ed.) (1992b). *FM Auditory Training Systems - Characteristics, Selection, and Use.* Timonium, MD: York Press.

Ross, M., & Giolas, T.G. (1971). Effect of three classroom listening conditions on speech intelligibility. *American Annals of the Deaf, 116,* 580-584.

Salamy, A., Eldredge, L., & Tooley, W.H. (1989). Neonatal status and hearing loss in high risk infants. *Journal of Pediatrics, 114,* 847-852.

Sarff, C.S. (1981). An innovative use of free-field amplification in regular classrooms. In Roeser, R.J. & Downs, M.P. (Eds.), *Auditory Disorders in School Children pp. 263-272.* New York, NY: Thieme Medical Publishers, Inc.

Schappert, S.M. (1992). Office visits for otitis media: U.S., 1975-1990. *Advance Data from Vital and Healthy Statistics. No. 214.* Hyattsville, MD: National Center for Health Statistics.

Schein, J.D., & Delk, M.T. (1974). *The deaf population of the United States.* Silver Spring, MD: National Association of the Deaf.

Stein, D. (1983). Psychosocial characteristics of school-age children with unilateral hearing loss. *Journal of the Academy of Rehabilitative Audiology, 16,* 12-22.

Stone, W.L., & La Greca, A.M. (1990). The social status of children with learning disabilities: A re-examination. *Journal of Learning Disabilities, 23,* 32-37.

Stone, W.L., & La Greca, A.M. (1994). Social deficits in children with learning disabilities. In A.J. Capute, P.J. Accardo, & B.K. Shapiro (Eds.) *Learning disabilities spectrum: ADD, ADHD, & LD (pp 155-175).* Baltimore: York Press.

Tharpe, A.M., & Bess, F.H. (1991). Identification and management of children with minimal hearing loss. *Journal of Pediatric Otorhinolaryngology, 21,* 41-50.

The Pediatric Working Group of the Conference on Amplification for Children with Auditory Deficits. (1996). Amplification for infants and children with hearing loss. *American Journal of Audiology, 5,* 53-68.

United States Department of Education National Center for Education Statistics. (1998). *Public elementary and sec-ondary education statistics: School year 1997-98, NCES 98-202,* by Lena M. McDowell. Washington, D.C.

Walton, J.P., & Hendricks-Munoz, K. (1991). Profile and stability of sensorineural hearing loss in persistent pulmonary hypertension of the newborn. *Journal of Speech and Hearing Research, 34,* 1362-1370.

Wasson, J. H., Kairys, S.W., Nelson, E.C., Kalishman, N., Baribeau, P., & Wasson, E. (1994). A short survey for assessing health and social problems of adolescents. *Journal of Family Practice, 38,* 489-494.

Wasson, J.H., Kairys, S.W., Nelson, E.C., Kalishman, N., Baribeau, P., & Wasson, E. (1995). Adolescent health and social problems - a method for detection and early management. *Archives of Family Medicine, 4,* 51-56.

Young, C., & McConnell, F.E. (1957). Retardation of vocabulary development in hard-of-hearing children. *Exceptional Children, 23,* 368-370.

REFERENCE NOTES

1. Maliszewski, S.J. (In press). Reflections of family support: One parent's perspective. In Bess, F.H. (Ed.), *Children with Hearing Impairment: Contemporary Trends,* Nashville, TN: Vanderbilt Bill Wilkerson Center Press.

2. Boney, S., & Bess, F.H. (1984). *Noise and reverberation effects on speech recognition in children with minimal hearing loss.* Paper presented at the American Speech-Language-Hearing Association, November, San Francisco.

3. Blake, P.E. and Bess, F.H. (1992). *The use of functional health assessments with hearing impaired adolescents.* Poster presented at the annual convention of the Florida Language Speech and Hearing Association. Tarpon Springs, FL.

4. Quigley, S.P., & Thomure, F.E. (1968). *Some effects of hearing impairment upon school performance.* Springfield, IL: Illinois Office of Education.

5. Boyd, S.F. (1974). *Hearing loss: Its educationally measurable effects on achievement.* Master's degree research requirement, Department of Education, Southern Illinois University.

6. Wasson, L., Landgraf, J., Berger, D., Kairys, S., Bracken, A., & Wasson, J. (1988). *The COOP Adolescent Chart Pilot Project: Final Report.* Dartmouth COOP Project, Department of Community and Family Medicine, Dartmouth Medical School, Hanover, NH, 03755.

Requests for reprints should be sent to Fred H. Bess, Ph.D., Vanderbilt Bill Wilkerson Center for Otolaryngology and Communication Sciences, Department of Hearing and Speech Sciences, 1114 19th Avenue South, Nashville, TN 37212.